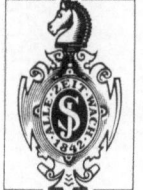

W. Wallace Park

# The Histology
# of Borderline Cancer

With Notes on Prognosis

With the collaboration of James W. Corkhill

314 illustrations

Springer-Verlag
Berlin  Heidelberg  New York

W. Wallace Park, MD (Edin.), FRCPath.
University Department of Pathology
Ninewells Hospital
Dundee, Scotland
United Kingdom


James W. Corkhill, FIMLT
Senior Technician (ret.)
Department of Pathology
The University
Dundee, Scotland
United Kingdom

ISBN-13: 978-1-4471-1297-6     e-ISBN-13: 978-1-4471-1295-2
DOI: 10.1007/978-1-4471-1295-2


**Library of Congress Cataloging in Publication Data**

Park, W      W
   The histology of borderline cancer, with notes on
prognosis.

   Includes index.
   1.  Cancer—Diagnosis.   2.   Histology, Pathological.
I.   Corkhill, James W., joint author.   II.   Title.
RC269.P37        616.9′94′07583        79-26151

This book
Is for fellow-pathologists
But is dedicated
To surgeons, of all sorts,
Who withstand,
With such patience
And friendly forbearance,
Our forever peering over their shoulder

It is dedicated also to
Dorothy, Jill and Daphne

# Preface

Often enough, in diagnosing cancer the last word rests with the pathologist and his or her microscope. Often enough, too, the pathologist is thought to dispense absolute truth: he does his best, but the truth he dispenses is not absolute. Rather, with a greater or lesser degree of confidence, he is making a prediction or expressing a probability of a certain kind of biological behaviour, and the degree of confidence with which he operates is based on experience. This experience is, in turn, based on the recollection of earlier events, counsel from his mentors, from his studies, and from discussions with colleagues. It would be going too far to agree with those clinicians said to prefer their pathologist, as they prefer their cheese, slightly mouldy, but there is no substitute for lengthy practice, consultation and debate. Every such effort is designed the better to define the correlation between the pattern of a tissue and its likely future behaviour.

For many years, with exactly this object in mind, it has been the custom within the University Department of Pathology, Dundee, to hold regular slide sessions at which sections of interest have been examined by some six to twelve pathologists of varied experience. Throughout, all sections have been examined initially in the absence of any information, not even the sex or age of the patient or the anatomical site being revealed. This practice, of which more is said in Chapter 1, is not one that commends itself immediately to all, but few who have come as critics have failed to leave as converts, and none has failed to find it educative and revealing.

This book is based largely on the experience gained from these meetings. Few lesions, even tropical lesions, are not represented in the collection of slides that accrued, some neoplastic or possibly neoplastic, some not. In essence, the book is concerned with interpretation of the borderline or histologically equivocal case and the clinical implications thereof. It is based on some 390 examples of which most are individually described in brief. No useful purpose is served by giving in detail the clinical and pathological circumstances of every patient with, say, a dubious lesion of endometrium or larynx, or with a similarly borderline papilloma in bladder or rectum, for each of these lesions exemplifies a familiar and 'standard' problem. Problems of this kind will be examined as such but not the details of every patient who posed them. Circumstances have been described individually, in most instances simply because each seemed to have something useful to teach. At the same time, they can hardly avoid giving much of the text a strongly parochial, even anecdotal, ring. We offer in explanation that very many of the diagnostic and prognostic difficulties can or could be matched exactly in countless laboratories everywhere: none is peculiar to this area or even to the United Kingdom or Western Europe; their relevance is universal.

A further possible shortcoming is that not all the cases individually described are accompanied by illustrations as perhaps, in the context of morphology, they should be. Rightly or wrongly, considerations of space were allowed to prevail in the belief that the more important cases have been illustrated and in the hope that, for the rest, the text will suffice. We refer in places to lesions or circumstances not represented in the local series. Their inclusion has been prompted by a wish to include supplementary information wherever it seemed likely to be useful as a guide to prognosis.

So essential to the quality of prediction, which

is the giving of a prognosis, is knowledge of the later events in the life of a lesion and its owner that it seems surprising that departments of histopathology did not long antedate departments of radiotherapy in instituting a system of regular follow-up enquiry for borderline cases.

The explanation may simply be that the necessary ingredients rarely coincided; a relatively stable population, a geographically stable pathologist, and cooperative clinical colleagues. All these have coincided here and allowed the analysis that follows.

# Acknowledgements

We owe our most appreciative thanks to many for help in compiling this book. First, we warmly thank all our past and present colleagues and associates in the Department of Pathology, initially of the University of St Andrews, then of the University of Dundee. Over a period of some 25 years, all have contributed in some measure by discussion, debate and friendly collaboration. We are equally indebted to our clinical colleagues, mostly surgeons of all disciplines, whether general, gynaecological, orthopaedic or others, but also on occasion physicians and dermatologists, and indeed virtually all those, including haematologists, microbiologists and biochemists, who have clinical responsibilities: all have given all the cooperation we could have wished. For help with the tracing of patients we owe much to our Department of Radiotherapy and the local Cancer Registry, and also to many of our General Practitioner colleagues in and around Dundee. In the early stages of the project, generous support was given for the same purpose by the former Board of Management for the Dundee General Hospitals.

The essential prerequisite for an acceptable photomicrograph is the proper fixation, processing, cutting and staining of the tissue, and this has been the responsibility of our many technical associates. Without their skills, the production of our volume would have been virtually impossible: we pay tribute to this skill, and extend to them our deep appreciation. As fellow-patholo-gists in the UK know, much of the credit for the technical standards attained and maintained within the Department goes to our former colleagues Professor A. C. Lendrum and Mr D. S. Fraser, FIMLT.

Our special thanks go to Mr R. S. Fawkes who, with the help of Mrs Sheila Gibbs, prepared many of the more recent illustrations after one of us (JWC) had retired; to Mrs Isla Bloomer who typed most of the script and also to Mrs Elizabeth Cargill who started it; and to the various other members of the secretarial staff who have without exception been ever willing to help on many occasions.

We could not have enjoyed greater help and cooperation from a publishing firm than we have had from Messrs Springer-Verlag. At all times our contacts with Mr Michael Jackson, Medical Editor (UK), and his associate, Mr S. Whittingham Boothe, and with Mr Chester Van Wert, Production Editor (NY), have been of the friendliest and carried out on their part (though rather less so, we regret, on ours!) with an impressive efficiency.

We finally mention with deep gratitude the understanding, tolerance and help of our families. All have been generous in their help, patience and, so much appreciated, keen interest in the production of the 'borderline' book.

W. Wallace Park
James W. Corkhill

# Contents

1   A Philosophy of Cancer Diagnosis by Microscopy        1

    Series of Cases Analysed        1
    Rationale of Histopathological Diagnosis        3
    Validity of Histological Criteria of Malignancy        6
    Use of Clinical Data        8
    The Histopathological Audit        10


2   Lesions of the Breast        13

Local Series        14
    Summarised Totals        15
    Case Data        15
    Commentary on Local Series        27
General Commentary        28
    Dysplasia        28
    Lobular Carcinoma In Situ        28
    Intraduct Carcinoma        30
    Paget's Disease of the Nipple        32
    Cystosarcoma Phyllodes        33
    Prognosis        33
Conclusions        38


3   Lesions of the Thyroid Gland        41

Local Series        42
    Summarised Totals        42
    Case Data        42
    Commentary on Local Series        57
General Commentary        57
    Microfollicular Adenoma        57
    Papillary Carcinoma        59
    Multifocal Carcinoma        60
    Medullary Carcinoma        60
    Lymphoreticular Neoplasms        61
    Hyperthyroidism        62
    Cryptic Carcinoma        62
Conclusions        63

4    Lesions of Lymph Nodes        67

Local Series        71
    Case Data I: ? Hodgkin's Disease        73
    Case Data II: ? Malignant Lymphoma Other than Hodgkin's Disease        104
    Commentary on Local Series        123
General Commentary        124
    Hodgkin's Disease        124
    Non-Hodgkin's Lymphomas        128
    Lesions that may Simulate ML        130
Conclusions        138


5    Lesions of the Soft Tissues        143

Local Series        144
    Summarised Totals        144
    Case Data        146
    Commentary on Local Series        193
General Commentary        194
    Pseudo-sarcomatous Lesions        194
    Myxoma        195
    Mesenchymoma, Benign and Malignant        196
    Neoplasms of Fat        198
    Fasciitis (Pseudo-sarcomatous, Nodular)        200
    Histiocytoma        201
    Juvenile Fibromatoses        206
    Desmoid Tumour        207
    Fibrosarcoma        207
    Granulation Tissue Sarcoma: Haematoma-sarcoma        208
    Granular Cell Myoblastoma        209
    Proliferative Myositis        210
    Myositis Ossificans        210
    Bony Neoplasms of Soft Tissue        211
    Synovial Overgrowths        213
    Epithelioid Sarcoma        214
    'Staging' of Soft Tissue Sarcomas        214
Conclusions        215


6    Lesions of Bone and Cartilage        221

Local Series        221
    Summarised Totals        221
    Case Data        222
    Commentary on Local Series        240
General Commentary        240
    Clinical Evidence vs Histological Evidence        242
    Inflammatory Patterns vs Neoplastic Patterns        242
    Chondroma vs Chondrosarcoma        245
    Callus vs Osteosarcoma vs Chondrosarcoma        247
    Predominantly Fibroblastic Lesions Containing Giant Cells        250
Conclusions        255

# 7    Lesions of the Skin        259

*Part A: Epithelial Lesions Other than Melanocarcinoma      260*
Overgrowths of Stratified Squamous Epithelium        260
    Local Series      260
    General Commentary      261
Basal Cell Carcinoma      265
Extramammary Paget's Disease (EMPD)        266
Conclusions      266

*Part B: The Problem of Mycosis Fungoides and Comparable Conditions      267*
Local Series      267
General Commentary      269
Lymphocytic Infiltrations of the Skin        271
Other Pseudo-malignant Lesions        271
Conclusions      273

*Part C: Melanocarcinoma      274*
Local Series      275
    Summarised Totals      275
    Case Data      276
    Commentary on Local Series        308
General Commentary      311
    Classification      311
    Constituent Cells      313
    Lentigo Maligna      314
    Spitz Naevus      316
    Diagnosis by Frozen Section        316
    Trauma      317
    Lymphadenectomy      317
    Pregnancy      319
    Influence of Age      320
    Delay in Metastasis      320
Conclusions      320

# 8    Lesions of the Digestive Tract        325

Local Series      325
    Summarised Totals      325
    Case Data      326
    Commentary on Local Series        356
General Commentary      356
    Oral Cavity      356
    Salivary Tissue      357
    Palate      358
    Pharynx      358
    Oesophagus      359
    Stomach      360
    Small Intestine      361
    Large Intestine      362
    Carcinoid Tumour      363
    Malignant Lymphoma and Pseudo-lymphoma        365

Plasma Cell Lesions     366
Pancreatic Biopsy     366
Serosal Metaplasia     367
Endometriosis     367
Conclusions     368


9     Lesions of the Respiratory Tract     371

Local Series     371
Case Data     371
General Commentary     382
Nose and Nasopharynx     382
Larynx     383
Bronchus and Lung     384
Conclusions     388


10     Lesions of the Female Genital Tract     391

Local Series     391
Case Data     391
Commentary on Local Series     399
General Commentary     402
Vulva     402
Cervix Uteri     403
Endometrium, the Glandular Component     405
Endometrium, the Stromal Component, and Myometrium     409
Ovary     412
Trophoblast     415
Endometriosis     416
Conclusions     416


11     Some Miscellaneous Lesions     421

Case Data     421
General Commentary     436
Nervous System     436
The Eye and Orbit     439
Urinary Tract     440
Bladder     443
Vasculature     444
Conclusions     446


12     General Assessment     451
Comment in Summary     455


Index     459

# 1 A Philosophy of Cancer Diagnosis by Microscopy

Cancer is suspected by clinicians; it is diagnosed by pathologists. Clinical acumen plus some or all of direct observation or endoscopy or radiology or endocrinology may be compellingly suggestive and, indeed, be more than adequate to justify active treatment; nevertheless, even then, were it to become available, the tissue concerned could provide evidence of a higher order. Few doctors would elect for themselves or their patients to have this or that viscus or limb removed without histopathological confirmation of malignancy. That, at any rate, is the general position but there are exceptions. Thus, the pathologist may find a never-suspected cancer quite by chance, as, for example, in the cervix of the uterus removed at a pelvic floor repair or in the seemingly simple ovarian cyst, but such instances are few and, *because so early*, often clinically unimportant. Or again, there are circumstances where histopathological examination is unnecessary to establish the simple diagnosis of cancer as, for example, in the patient found at necropsy to be 'riddled' with metastases; gross examination will not reveal the type and thus probably not the origin of the growth but a diagnosis simply of 'cancer' is nevertheless self-evident. Histological diagnosis at this stage may well have an academic or scientific significance in the study of cancer as a biological phenomenon; its clinical significance will be slight except to the extent that study of the case-history in retrospect may enable the clinician to diagnose any similar case in the future at an earlier and therefore potentially treatable stage. However, consideration of accidentally discovered cancer or advanced cancer is not the purpose of this study. We are concerned rather with those exceptions to the general rule that are neither few nor clinically unimportant, namely, those situations where the

pathologist has been in doubt: that is, with the interpretation of abnormal tissue patterns that may or may not indicate cancer.

## SERIES OF CASES ANALYSED

This book has been written in an attempt to gain some idea of the accuracy of histopathological diagnosis in the borderline case, and also to convey some information on the likely behaviour of most of the neoplasms under discussion. Certainly, some information of this kind is often included in textbooks or monographs on neoplastic disease but it tends to be limited. With some exceptions shortly to be mentioned, the analysis is based essentially on the after-history of 390 patients whose original biopsies had raised significant doubt whether the histology indicated malignant disease or not. The histological reports of these patients' lesions were found by searching the approximately 90 000 reports issued from the University Department of Pathology in Dundee during the years 1948–1972. How comparable this 'index of doubt' of 390/90 000 or 0.4% is to similar indices that could be calculated in other departments of pathology is unknown and of little consequence: so subjective in this context is the term *significant* that valid comparison between departments could be achieved only if the histological reports were assessed by the same observer. Comparability is not the primary aim of this study and, so, to the strictly departmental cases have been added a few others received from elsewhere which seem to be instructive. The exceptions to the inclusion of all equivocal lesions are, first, papillomas of bladder and large intestine, and salivary adenomas, all of which are almost by definition equivocal, and, second, carcinoma in situ of the cervix uteri. None of these has been considered in a formal way, for the zone of debate that surrounds them is well known to all.

Attempts to trace the 390 patients were made along the usual routes: general practitioners, local authorities and, ultimately, Registrars General. Positive information in the sense of being alive or dead was obtained in the case of 378 patients. Information that the patient was alive is, of course, informative in a way that knowledge of the patient's death is not: the possibly malignant neoplastic lesion may have contributed nothing at all to the patient's dying, and this was judged to be so in 30 of the 88 patients who had died. In many cases a further biopsy either from another site or at a later time revealed appearances no longer equivocal but sufficient to establish the diagnosis. The distribution of cases is shown in Table 1.1.

As with the 'index of doubt', the pattern of distribution in Table 1.1 has no particular significance: it does no more than illustrate the histological population under analysis. Some factors, however, did have a bearing on the distribution of cases. For local reasons, over the 25 years, relatively few examples were seen of lesions of lung and brain: also, more than one half of the 22 specimens from respiratory tract were equivocal biopsies of larynx and have not been individually described in detail. Further, unlike the practice in some hospitals, all gynaecological specimens were reported upon in this Department. The lesions from the female genital tract included in Table 1.1 concern mainly overgrowths of the endometrium and ovary: here in particular the 'significance' of any doubt expressed in a report is difficult to assess. The figure of 80 (including 20 from the uterus and 40 from the ovary) is therefore only approximate and is included primarily for comparison with a figure of some 700 cases each of cancers of uterus and ovary diagnosed in the hospital concerned during the years under survey.

As will be seen from Table 1.1, most of the problems have been met in skin, female genital tract and lymph nodes, and of individual organs, in the breast and thyroid gland.

Each of the cases, grouped by organs or anatomical system, has been briefly described and analysed either individually or with others of its like, with a final assessment whether, in retrospect, the diagnosis at the relevant time

**Table 1.1.** Numbers of borderline lesions, by systems or organs, comprising the series under analysis.

| | |
|---|---|
| Breast | 21 |
| Thyroid gland | 26 |
| Lymph nodes | 40 |
| Connective tissue and muscle | 36 |
| Bone and cartilage | 15 |
| Skin | 114 |
| Digestive tract | 26 |
| Respiratory tract | 22 |
| Female genital tract | 80 |
| Miscellaneous | 10 |
| Total | 390 |

appears to have been an over-diagnosis, an under-diagnosis or an appropriate or inappropriate diagnosis. As mentioned in the Preface, virtually all of the sections comprising the series were at some time the subject of retrospective panel discussion: furthermore, few if any can have been reported at the time on the basis of a single opinion. Nevertheless, the final allocation throughout to one of the four categories, even if based on these corporate views, has been essentially my own. There then follows, where appropriate, a commentary on the local series, a short general commentary and conclusions. Some of the 'conclusions' may not have been derived directly from the cases individually described but from various experiences over the years.

In a survey such as this, seeking as it does to prove or assess the validity of histopathological assessment of abnormal tissue, the response of the patient's disease to whatever treatment seemed optimum in the circumstances is obviously important. As emphasised earlier, the essence of cancer histodiagnosis is correlation between tissue pattern and clinical outcome. The well-acknowledged biological variability of neoplasms, even of the same histogenetic type, introduces an unavoidable element of uncertainty into this correlation: treatment introduces another. To some extent analysis here is necessarily speculative but it may be educative nevertheless. If a histologically equivocal lesion is not really cancer but is nevertheless for pragmatic reasons treated as such, a successful outcome will be gratifying to patient, relatives and therapist but adds a false-positive diagnosis to statistics and leaves the honest histologist with a lingering doubt: and it is only further experience of the same kind, and a growing number of unexpectedly gratifying 'cures', that will tilt his diagnostic balance towards the benign. If, on the other hand, a totally excised lesion is diagnosed as benign but really is malignant, even though no one can know, the therapist has been cheated of a cure and statistics impaired by a false-negative diagnosis.

However, to one type of observer at any rate, the therapeutic nihilist, the response to treatment may be disregarded as a factor complicating the assessment of equivocal or borderline histology. If, after the excision or ablation of a histologically disturbing lesion, the patient is trouble-free $x$ years later, then, says the nihilist, such appearances were innocuous and may be safely regarded as such in the future; had the lesion been capable of metastasis it would have metastasised long before it was diagnosed. Quite similar reasoning will apply to appearances thought to indicate a strong likelihood of local recurrence despite seemingly adequate excision. If, $x$ years later, there has been no recurrence, again, says the nihilist, such appearances may be accepted in future as innocuous; non-excised remnants, if any, will have regressed for that will have been the intrinsic nature of the neoplasm; therapy would have done nothing to prevent metastasis in the first instance, and done no more in the second instance than comprise a universally reputable practice, the removal of irremediably diseased tissue.

There is, of course, a good deal of substance in this attitude, since it is based on the obvious fact that time and again lesions metastasise widely or recur at the site or do both despite radical treatment within days of diagnosis; this is why the histological diagnosis of cancer is essentially an expression of probability. In the lesion diagnosed as unequivocal carcinoma of stomach, for example, the diagnosis is implying a virtually 100% probability of lethal spread if not treated, and a not much lesser probability even if it is treated. The granulosa cell neoplasm of ovary is a lesion with a well-known intermediate probability of spread, possibly some 50%, and this 50:50 position is reflected in the equally well-known uncertainty, should the designation be granulosa cell carcinoma or the escapist granulosa cell tumour? At the opposite end of the probability scale from carcinoma of

the stomach and pancreas is the aberrant polypoid adenoma of rectum with an estimated associated risk of later carcinoma of, say, 1%.

These three examples of different histological problems posed by malignant disease have their counterpart clinical problems in the solution of which the histologist has a considerable part to play. In relation to the matter immediately in hand, the influence of treatment on the clinical outcome, and thus on the interpretation of borderline histology, the situation is simply stated: all patients in the present series had what was judged at the time to be optimum treatment even if on occasion this meant continued observation or supervision only.

RATIONALE OF HISTOPATHOLOGICAL DIAGNOSIS

As analysed before (Park, 1956), along with some of its attendant difficulties, the histological diagnosis of cancer is based on the establishment of a predictive correlation based upon the experience, however gained, of the pathologist, namely, the correlation between a certain tissue pattern and the subsequent likely behaviour of that tissue. Histological 'proof' is not proof in the mathematical or legal sense. Properly, the word should be understood in its original and now almost archaic sense of tried, tested or assessed. In practice it means, and should be taken to mean, no more than that in the opinion of the pathologist(s) the tissue pattern in question has a probability of being followed, if untreated, by metastasis and death of some 95%–99% (with even the most flagrant tissue patterns, few pathologists would care to put the figure at 100%). Sometimes, and often enough to be a source of worry, there is difficulty in giving a diagnosis of malignancy with a confidence figure as high even as, say, 75%, and the difficulty may take one or three main forms.

*First*, the change from the histological norm may be so relatively small that adequately accurate prediction of future behaviour is not possible. The earlier the lesion is histologically, that is, the less it departs from the structural norm, the greater the margin of uncertainty and the likelihood of variation in individual prediction. To be sure, wide experience of a particular type or group of neoplasm will reduce this margin but it will not abolish it; the general principle still holds. Examples of this kind of difficulty are familiar, as in the case, for instance, of uterine cervical dysplasia/carcinoma in situ/carcinoma-microinvasive/carcinoma-frankly invasive. Even the most expert have their zones of uncertainty in subdividing this particular histopathological spectrum or continuum and others like it.

*Second*, the correlation between even blatantly diagnostic histological abnormality and subsequent clinical or biological behaviour is sometimes proved by events to be inexplicably low. I refer here to the kind of tissue pattern that could be used in a teaching set of sections for a class of medical students; the flagrant carcinoma of pancreas or textbook picture of Hodgkin's disease, the type of histological pattern that even the most enthusiastic team of pathologists/surgeons/radiotherapists would hesitate to forecast cure in more than, say, 5% of patients. These still-baffling circumstances exemplify and emphasise the variability of the patient/cancer battle. By all current knowledge we say that the cancer will win; nature confounds us somehow or other by letting the patient win. No doubt there will emerge a means of identifying these lesions, and thus allowing more accurate prognosis, but the techniques are not yet available. Certainly we already know well from many observations that cancers may be dormant for 15 years or more, and we should perhaps not be as surprised as we are when a patient who had a mastectomy, hysterectomy or amputation of a limb at age 60 for undoubted cancer, dies at age 75 with no signs of a recurrence. The patient might have died at age 110 with multiple metastasis, and so proved the accuracy of histological prediction; that might be of some comfort to the academic and scientific histopathologist, but it hardly lessens the limitations of current techniques.

*Third*, there have emerged over the years certain groups of lesions of relatively well-defined histological character which were once thought to indicate cancer but now no longer are; or, at any rate, are followed by the clinical expression of cancer much less frequently than was thought probable at the time of diagnosis. Examples of this are some of the melanotic lesions, some spindle-cell growths of connective tissue, and the keratoacanthoma. All have emerged as a result of continued observation of

patients and a gradual realisation that, for a 'sarcoma' or a 'carcinoma' the behaviour was quite unexpectedly benign. These comprise the pseudocancers: not all such groups are yet sharply defined but as knowledge of their existence spreads increasing accuracy in diagnosis will follow, and, with it, a more accurate framing of prognosis. Cancer diagnosis, in fact, *is* prognosis.

It seems proper to note, in parenthesis, the term 'pseudotumour' which still appears in many texts though, certainly, mostly clinical rather than pathological. Its use is unfortunate for it causes confusion and sometimes needless alarm. The oddly paradoxical element in pseudotumour is that the lesions so termed are always, in the literal sense, proper tumours: they are abnormal masses or swellings of tissue (even the simple nasal polyp has been designated a pseudotumour, as, for example, in the AFIP series of fascicles (Ash et al., 1964). Only the implication of neoplasia is 'pseudo-': and for this we ourselves, as pathologists, are largely to blame for condoning or insufficiently condemning use of the term 'tumour' as a synonym for 'neoplasm' (I recently heard the comment, "The lesion is a mass but it is not a tumour"; this seems to me nonsensical). The term 'pseudotumour' is doubtless here to stay but that is no reason for not condemning its use.

The problems posed by the three main obstacles to accurate prognosis are not of the same order. In the third group, that of the pseudocancers, uncertainty concerns the nature of the lesions: are they truly cancer or not? As just mentioned, answers will gradually be provided by continuous clinicopathological observation of the patients. In the other two groups, it is not the nature of the lesion that is in question, in the sense that such tissue patterns are indeed known to be followed sufficiently often by metastatic spread and shortening of life to warrant the term 'cancer'. The problem we face is the long-familiar, How malignant?, in other words the quality of the lesions, and the answer to this, in turn, operates at two levels, what may be called 'group' level and 'individual' level. That is, a patient diagnosed as having malignant disease, and assessed on signs and symptoms as being in, say, a clinical Stage II, has been allocated to a group known on past actuarial evidence to have a calculable rate of morbidity/mortality/survival.

The next assessment, at individual level, lies with the pathologist rather than the statistician yet the technique is still basically statistical. The position was well stated by Blanco and his colleagues (1977) with reference particularly to neoplasms of the ovary but of general relevance nevertheless, thus, "Although such studies indicate, in statistical terms, which tumours are to be regarded as more malignant and which less, they are not very accurate in prognosticating the course of an individual tumour". The pathologist will search within the individual neoplasm for features either known or suspected from past experience to be associated with a particular form of behaviour, essentially recurrence or metastasis, and on these he will base his estimate or degree of probability. An interesting parallel, incidentally, has emerged in relation to the interpretation of ECGs by computer-based pattern-recognition. The situation was described thus (Editorial, 1974):

> Presentation of results in statistical terms, as a set of probabilities, may be difficult for clinicians to assimilate at first. In fact, despite the conceptual difficulties and the need for careful interpretation, presentation as a set of probabilities is a more realistic expression of the interpretation of an E.C.G. than a bald single diagnosis which increases the risk of confusion from conflict with the clinical findings.

If, in this passage, we substitute a histological pattern for an ECG, the parallel is exact. Fortunately for histopathologists, analysis of an ECG tracing is one thing, analysis of a histological pattern very much another.

To some extent, indeed, expression of risk as a percentage probability is already practised. For example, in the days when it seemed possible that degree of trophoblastic hyperplasia in a hydatidiform mole was usefully correlated with subsequent liability to choriocarcinoma, it was the practice of some pathologists to express the risk as 1%, 5% or 10% depending on the degree of trophoblastic hyperplasia, and thus the clinician could make his decision on further treatment. This is now well out of date, overtaken by the accuracy of HCG assay, but the general principle still holds. In a multiparous woman of 40, a 1% risk of subsequent choriocarcinoma could have been enough to warrant, at one time, hysterectomy. In a nulliparous woman aged 20, even an expressed risk of 10%

might not have been enough to warrant this. *Every* borderline tissue pattern can be given a mathematical expression of risk: the odds are just more easily calculated in some than in others. Paradoxically, as the amount of information about a patient and his neoplasm grows, the calculation of the probabilities becomes more complex.

Ultramicroscopy has introduced a whole new generation of facts, so has the continuing discovery of various cancer-associated metabolites and their accurate assay, further sophistication in isotopic scanning, and very possibly CAT-scanning. The time has come now when the computer has been enlisted to help with the making of diagnostic and therapeutic decisions in Hodgkin's disease (Safran et al., 1977). As Safran and his colleagues clearly explain, "Decision theory consists of a set of mathematical rules for simplifying complex decisions into several equivalent decisions which are less complex and easier to solve". Decision theory itself has been analysed by Henschke and Flehinger (1967): pathologists who may not have realised how their mind worked when framing their diagnoses and prognoses will find an explanation here.

Many attempts have been made in the past to devise 'scoring systems' for various neoplasms, for example, carcinoma of the breast and melanocarcinoma, in the hope of defining the lesion more accurately for prognostic and therapeutic purposes. The use of the computer is but the logical extension of this, necessitated by the almost daily accession of new data. Its impact on histopathology is clear: it makes precision in morphological interpretation all the more imperative, not less.

In submitting a biopsy, the clinician is asking not only whether the lesion is cancerous or not, he is also and on all occasions asking, if only by implication, whither, how far and how fast is it likely to spread: and this is the information the pathologist must try to convey, in mathematical terms it may be, for on the answers to these questions obviously depends the therapeutic strategy of the clinician. The histopathologist has thus a frequently overlooked but nevertheless crucial and direct clinical responsibility: the better informed he is about the behaviour of a neoplasm, the more useful will his clinical contribution be. A point made by Scully (1970), again in relation particularly to cancers of the ovary but of universal relevance, is that the pathologist is ". . . expected not only to make a correct microscopic diagnosis using modern terminology but also to supply accurate information about the natural history of a given tumor, thereby guaranteeing the possibility of optimal treatment". For this reason, in the various chapters that follow, some information on the natural history and implied prognosis of lesions has been included where it seemed to be relevant. For the same reason, the list of 'conclusions' at the end of each section may concern topics not represented by cases in the local series.

In the flagrant case, with which we are not primarily concerned in this study, a diagnosis of carcinoma of bronchus, stomach or pancreas, just of itself, tells all. Rather, we are primarily concerned with the histologically early or dubious case in these and all other tissues: and it is here that even a detailed and analytical report may be no substitute for a personal discussion with the clinician at the time and perhaps later also at the operating table. It is here also that the reconciliation will be achieved between the shades-of-grey concept so familiar, from what he sees down his microscope, to the pathologist, and the black-or-white decision that of necessity so often confronts the surgeon. Sometimes, some intermediate procedure such as segmental or strictly local resection is possible but all too often either the larynx or limb, stomach or rectum has to be removed in toto or not at all. The biological niceties of shades of grey have to yield to hard practicality, and this the pathologist will acknowledge with understanding.

This all-or-none situation is an expression of the fact that much of the treatment of cancer, surgery and radiotherapy, is based on the simple mechanical concept that if all cancer cells are removed or destroyed, cure will result, but that if any cells remain beyond the line of excision or field of irradiation, recurrence and/or metastasis is inevitable. This obviously over-simplifies the matter. Cancer is much more of a systemic disorder, albeit usually with a dominant local expression, and the growing use of chemotherapy and interest in immunotherapy are an acknowledgment of this, but the mechanical concept has hitherto been, and in large part remains, a reasonably sound working principle.

## VALIDITY OF HISTOLOGICAL CRITERIA OF MALIGNANCY

The standard histological criteria of malignancy are, of course, cellular and nuclear aberrancy, mitotic activity abnormal in amount and/or type, and transgression of normal tissue boundaries, yet none of these has a definable value beyond which the diagnosis of cancer is absolute.

So-called breaching of the basement membrane is a simple and tidy concept, and one suspects this is the main reason for its popularity, but it is quite misleading and of little or no value in practice. Its role has been described thus by Hamperl (1967), a histopathologist of immense experience: "The presence or absence of a basement membrane around developing or established cancer cells is therefore to be considered as a purely secondary feature without significance in any theoretical or diagnostic respect", and also, in later discussion, "The presence or absence of the basement membrane does not influence diagnosis or prognosis". To cite but one example in support of this view, examination of sections of the chronically inflamed cervix uteri, however stained, will frequently show stretches of epithelium wholly devoid of a subjacent basement membrane, while similarly stained examples of an invasive carcinoma of the cervix will commonly show an apparent basement membrane around the invading clusters of cells. In the context of the cervix in particular, the comment was earlier made by Song (1950) that, 'Use of the term 'basement membrane' in light microscopy for the purpose of differentiating carcinoma *in situ* from early invasive cancer appears to be improper. Furthermore, emphasis on the status of the combined structure called a basement membrane as a criterion in determining invasiveness of cervical carcinoma seems to be invalid". It is true that, in early squamous carcinoma, changes may be seen at the dermo-epidermal junction by ultramicroscopy (Kobayasi, 1969) but the relevance of this to everyday biopsy practice is meantime remote.

A more clearly dependable criterion of malignant growth is mitotic aberrancy but even this may be found in circumstances such as actively reparative tissue and proliferating bone marrow where the tissue is shown by subsequent events to have been certainly non-neoplastic. Such actively growing tissue may mimic cancerous overgrowth virtually completely, and not just in isolated high-power fields. Wide areas of tissue may show hypercellularity, aberrant mitotic figures and apparent infiltration of surrounding tissue in high degree. Granulation tissue provides most of the examples of this, essentially because soft tissues are damaged more often than others, but callus may be equally misleading in its capacity to mimic osteosarcoma, while the difficulty in distinguishing between gliosis and the well-differentiated glioma is well known. We have recently seen a needle-biopsy specimen of liver from a patient with infectious mononucleosis, initially jaundice of uncertain origin, in which triaster forms of mitosis were conspicuous. No other features suggested malignant neoplasia, and the phenomenon was doubtless purely regenerative in character. This was the eighth local example, in a period of some 10 years, of one or more aberrant mitotic figures being seen in tissue judged by its other features to be not neoplastic. Whether this indicates a basic tendency towards malignant neoplasia is a matter of speculation; all we can say is that none of the earlier-seen patients has been seen again, at least at Ninewells Hospital, with a cancerous lesion.

There is still uncertainty about the time of arrest or rate of decay of mitotic figures in tissue removed from the body, and also problems of sampling, but the pathologist still leans heavily on the presence of even apparently normal mitotic figures in his assessment of a possibly malignant biopsy; and he is largely justified in doing so. Apart from the allowance to be made for what experience teaches is the normal mitotic frequency for a given tissue, care is required not to be misled by the mitotic mimicry of squashed or pyknotic cells of other kinds, often polymorphonuclears. A good working rule is that, when in doubt, no structure should be accepted as a mitotic figure unless it could be photographed and used in a text for students.

All neoplastic tissue patterns are obviously enough departures from the normal but there are many departures from the normal that are not even semineoplastic. The pathologist comes to acquire a wide knowledge of what may be called paranormal histology; the epithelial surface distorted by past or present injury, inflammatory or mechanical; the possible hamartoma or other structural variant; the bizarre character of the degenerate and dying nucleus and others besides. There is a wide no-man's land between the strictly physiological norm on the one side and the certainly neoplastic on the other; and always in their earliest stages, and for a generally unknown length of time, neoplastic cells will lie here. Every cancer must have a beginning, 'Hodgkin's disease must start somehow,' and the problem for the pathologist is to distinguish between the paranormal pattern and that of the early cancer whether the abnormality be aberrancy of cell type or of cell site. The foregoing is, of course, platitudinous and no doubt a lengthy way of stating the obvious. Nevertheless, it sets out the essence of a situation that is frequently ignored or overlooked to the extent at any rate that only rarely, if at all, do published figures or series of the incidence or prevalence or curability of this or that cancer make mention of it. In some cases the pathologist will have diagnosed cancer only with reluctance. For scientific purposes he will retain some doubt; for practical purposes, to minimise the risk and in the best interests of the patient, he cannot do otherwise.

This is a delicate and debatable area, and the following short examination of it is made against the background of two assumptions. First, that in all borderline situations, pathologist and surgeon are agreed on the best course of action to be followed. Second, the treatment used is the optimum. The dangers to the patient will therefore be either the possibly *false-positive* diagnosis and the not negligible effects of treatment for a lesion that really was not a cancer; and the possibly *false-negative* diagnosis and irremediable spread of a lesion that really was cancer. Very likely, when confronted on some occasion with this problem, most pathologists will have asked themselves, Would I have my arm off for this, or my stomach out for that, or would I advise it in the case of one of my family?; and often enough this will be his final court of appeal. Few would quarrel with this, and yet we may wonder. For a pathologist, who probably understands the situation as thoroughly and accurately as anyone can, to run the risk himself is one thing; to ask, in effect to require, someone else to run the same risk is another, and perhaps not ethically legitimate. The ultimate decision is, of course, that of the clinician, for it is on the other side of *his* table, not the pathologist's, that the patient sits, and only the clinician knows all the facts. Only he knows, for example, how his patient is going to react to the suggestion of many months' or years' surveillance for mammary masses, on the one hand, or of mastectomy, on the other. Nevertheless, often enough, and most clinicians would concede the point, the procedure adopted is based wholly on what the pathologist says. So, in that sense it is the pathologist in making his report of 'malignancy' who is requiring the patient to undergo this or that form of treatment, which may be severe, or, in making his report of 'borderline but not malignant' requiring the patient to run a risk of which (unless an oncological pathologist himself) he has little or no technical understanding at all.

It is an old story, and surely apocryphal, that the pathologist most praised by surgeons in some part of the country was one whose biopsy reports came from one or other of two rubber stamps on his desk, 'Malignant' and 'Not malignant'. The picture has changed since then. Therapeutic techniques of whatever kind are more specialised, and much more information is required of the lesion if they are to be used to the full. This is why a main part of the obligation of a histopathologist is to convey to the clinician all the facts about the lesion which the pathologist believes are or may be relevant to its understanding and its treatment; and this means that the pathologist must try as best he can to keep abreast of current knowledge about the biology and general behaviour of neoplasms. The following passage is quoted almost verbatim from a current surgical text on the pathology of a certain type of neoplasm (I shall not identify it any more closely); "Pathologists, impressed by the frequency with which true infiltrating carcinoma develops subsequent to the demonstration of this type of lesion, have generally advocated radical removal of the organ. Surgeons, most of whom are unaware of other basic facts concerning the natural history of this disease entity, have blindly followed the recommendations of their pathologists". This is a sadly revealing passage. It betrays a situation that simply should not be. For the construction of their prognoses pathologists and surgeons alike use the same raw material, their accumulated experience however acquired. It is difficult to understand what the basis of such an attitude really is, for, unless a surgeon is his own pathologist, his patients have been diagnosed as having cancer by a pathologist.

## Use of Clinical Data

> In the first step the evidence displayed by the biopsy must be observed and analyzed as objectively as possible. During the first step . . . our chief interest should be to study the appearance of the tissues without reference to the other information that may be available regarding the patient's illness. (Wartman, 1959)

Beyond any doubt, maximum use should be made of clinical data supplied, and further information sought if necessary, for none would deny that the more information the clinician gives the pathologist, the more information the pathologist can give him in return; but at what stage should the clinical data be used? As emphasised on an earlier occasion (Park, 1956), I remain in no doubt that the proper time to evaluate the clinical information and its significance is after the histology has been assessed, not before. By this practice the pathologist will in effect say: in circumstances *a* this histological pattern suggests this diagnosis, in circumstances *b* it means that diagnosis, in circumstances *c* it means another diagnosis. Then, learning from the clinical data that the circumstances are *a, b* or *c* his report to the clinician will suggest this, that, or the other diagnosis. For the sake of scientific precision, so far as it can be attained in diagnostic histopathology, and entirely in the interests of the patient, the pathologist should be wholly prepared to construct his opinion as outlined above, put his microscope aside, then consult the clinical data and make his correlation. There is no risk to the patient in this. Some may have read the remark of a pathologist when asked to pronounce on a section 'blind': 'Would you have me play games with you or do you wish my considered opinion?' This misjudges the situation completely. In working initially blind the pathologist is gaining a keener appreciation of tissue patterns that he otherwise could; indeed, diagnostic possibilities that might otherwise be quite overlooked will offer themselves. In these circumstances, the pathologist may find that he has diagnosed glioblastoma multiforme in a uterine mass or chordoma in a tibial neoplasm (for both these 'mistakes' are entirely possible) but no matter; the pathologist has widened his familiarity with abnormal tissue patterns and the patient may indeed be more thoroughly investigated than would otherwise be the case. After all, this is no more than an extension of the analytical process by which the pathologist tries to diagnose the nature of, say, a lump in the neck or skin of a vaguely ill or even apparently fit patient. He is then operating in effect in the absence of clinical data, and has to summon up his recollections of, for example, metastatic carcinoma of different kinds, the malignant lymphomas, brucellosis, infectious mononucleosis, drug responses in nodes, tissue ectopias and many others besides.

Now it clearly matters not to the patient that her uterine sarcoma may exactly mimic a malignant glioma or her synoviosarcoma a carcinosarcoma. The essential diagnosis, that a malignant neoplasm is present, has been made. What the pathologist should on only the rarest occasions find himself doing is making a diagnosis of malignancy *before* he knows the clinical circumstances, then changing his diagnosis to nonmalignant *after* he knows the clinical circumstances: for equally clearly this does matter to the patient, and crucially. If the pathologist does this he is saying that a particular tissue pattern can mean *cancer* in one set of circumstances but *not cancer* in another; and this is at the least a debatable proposition. For the sake of clarity and at the cost of some repetition it should be noted that we are not considering here the tissue pattern that one pathologist says is cancerous and another says is not, for this is a problem well known to all. We are considering rather the interpretation in two different ways of the one tissue pattern by the same pathologist. Certainly the situation can be approached very closely and sometimes, I believe, attained completely, but just how often this happens is virtually impossible to appreciate unless the blind approach is practised. The matter will arise for consideration again from time to time in later chapters but it may be helpful to give some examples now.

One of the clearest examples is provided by the keratoacanthoma (molluscum sebaceum). If a pathologist knows in advance that the biopsy comes from a crateriform lesion on the cheek that has reached a diameter of 15 mm in 3 months he cannot be other than strongly biased towards diagnosing the exuberant and perhaps even mitotically aberrant epidermal tissue as keratoacanthoma. If he examines the tissue not knowing the clinical circumstances he may well diagnose squamous cell carcinoma. With experience, and having recognised the situation blind, he will admit his helplessness and base his diagnosis on the clinical data: if present for only a few months, keratoacanthoma; if present for longer, squamous cell carcinoma. With more experience still he will add to this a note of caution for he will recall that sometimes, though admittedly rarely, an apparently typical keratoacanthoma has not only recurred more than once but has metastasised.

The interpretation of aberrant melanonaevi in children provides another example of the pitfall into which foreknowledge of the clinical circumstances, in this case the age of the patient, may precipitate the pathologist. Aware of the fact that the patient is aged, say 10 years, the pathologist is strongly conditioned to interpret even a highly aberrant pattern as not malignant melanoma but juvenile melanoma; and yet, even if on the rarest occasions only, malignant melanoma does occur in children. There is an argument in this context which holds that, since malignant melanoma in children is so extremely rare, the probability of a borderline pattern's indicating malignancy is so small that all doubt may be dismissed. This reasoning is quite illogical; if it were valid there would be no point in using the microscope at all except for the peripheral purpose of showing, perhaps, that the lesion was not of melanotic character in the first place, but, say, a haemangioma. The real position is that if the pattern is by general consent that of a malignant melanoma, then *either* that is the diagnosis *or* we are admitting that the situation just outlined does exist, namely, that a histological pattern can have two opposite meanings: cancer in the adult; not cancer in the child; and not every pathologist is convinced that this is so.

In parenthesis we may note the difficult question that confronts those who support the dominating role of age: at what age does the change-over occur; at what age is the abnormal tissue pattern to be regarded as no longer benign but malignant? These diagnostic and prognostic problems arise, not only with the melanotic growths of children; they are not infrequent in the adult also and apply with particular relevance to lesions of the breast. For this reason they are considered again later in that important context.

Age of the patient is not the only feature of a neoplasm sometimes allowed weight in a borderline diagnostic balance. On one occasion I recall, the approach to the diagnosis of a lesion submitted (with a preferred diagnosis) for further opinion included, in essence, the following statements:

1) The patient is very old for this tumour.

2) The history is much too short.

3) The tumour is much too big and much too cystic.

This line of reasoning is open to question. If the histology, of itself, indicates Tumour *A*, then, either:

a) That is the proper diagnosis, or

b) If the lesion is proved independently (i.e. by some means other than histology) to be not Tumour *A* but, say, Tumour *B*, then the histological pattern is common to two lesions: Tumour *A*, in youth, with a long history, small and minimally cystic; and Tumour *B*, at older ages, with a short history, large and maximally cystic.

That is, either this is the first (or an exceptional) example of Tumour *A* at older ages, with a short history, large and maximally cystic, *or* the histology is literally equivocal and common to two different tumours which cannot be separated by histological techniques but only by those that are biochemical, immunological, virological, or of some other kind.

It therefore seems evident that if beliefs 1, 2 and 3 are held inflexibly, Tumour *A* will 'never' be found at older ages and/or with a short history and/or be large or markedly cystic. Again, however, as with the melanocytic lesions, what of the lesions in middle age, of intermediate duration, intermediately sized and cystic? There was a time when neuroblastoma 'never' occurred in the adult but later events have proved otherwise.

The day has already come when the microscope has been superseded in some areas by other techniques as the best predictor of neoplastic behaviour. The patient with a known or even only suspected choriocarcinoma can be supervised by hormonal assay in a way far more effective than any microscopy could achieve. The controllability and curability of choriocarcinoma are still almost unique but already some other cancers can at least be monitored by assays of various metabolites, and here one thinks of, for example, CEA and catecholamines. Few doubt that such assays will increasingly acquire an initially diagnostic significance. Few doubt also, with Ravitch (1969), that discovery of the ultimate diagnostic 'cancer test', detection of the first cell whose descendants will produce a clinically diagnosable cancer in 5 or 10 years' time, would, in the absence of perfect chemotherapy, be, as he says, an 'unmitigated catastrophe'.

## THE HISTOPATHOLOGICAL AUDIT

There is a growing and legitimate interest in the rightness or wrongness, accuracy or inaccuracy, of diagnosis in medicine whether at the bedside or in the laboratory, and the greater the problem at the bedside, the nearer it comes to the laboratory for solution. Even then, of all the laboratory services, it is within the histopathological that the difficulties of final solution are in one sense the greatest. The biochemist can use known standards and measure constituents with precision. The bacteriologist and virologist can identify micro-organisms with a high degree of accuracy: even if a usually virulent organism is found as an unexpected commensal, or vice versa, its correct identification is almost always possible. In consequence, techniques of audit in these disciplines are not difficult to apply. The histopathologist is not in this position. There is little he can identify, like a micro-organism, that can establish the diagnosis absolutely (he may be able to identify acid-fast bacilli but only the bacteriologist, from further material, can say *Mycobacterium tuberculosis*), and little he can measure. The basic difficulty for the histopathologist is that already mentioned, that of assessing the closeness and, thus, correctness of the correlation between abnormal tissue pattern and clinical result: even when the newer techniques of histometry allow the more accurate measurement of such features as nuclear size, nucleo-cytoplasmic ratio and the like, they can only at best, as it were, increase the correlation coefficient.

### Assessing Validity of Diagnosis in Prospect

Many tissue patterns are distinctive enough to allow a virtually absolute diagnosis, and thus prognosis. The correlation cannot be 100%, and the diagnosis thus absolute, if only because a seemingly 'obvious' cancer does rarely regress: nevertheless, for practical purposes, these may be regarded as diagnoses of a yes/no order. Here, for purposes of assessment, we have to assume a theoretical panel of, say, ten pathologists all of omniscient experience: if all ten agree independently that the diagnosis is entity $X$, then that is the diagnosis. Failure by another pathologist to make the diagnosis will be due either to inexperience or a poor memory. In practice, matters are different for we have to remember that an entity seen weekly by one specialist pathologist may be seen only once in a lifetime, if at all, by another specialist pathologist or a general pathologist. The hope here is that the pathologist will know that he doesn't know, and seek help: the danger is the pathologist who doesn't know that he doesn't know. In this context, at any rate, a diagnosis can be recognised as a wrong diagnosis. For practical purposes, if a scoring system were to be used, only two possibilities exist, 100% or 0%.

Let us now assume a tissue pattern that is less distinctive, one that is unanimously agreed by the panel to be equivocal but where, for pragmatic purposes, the opinion given has to be either malignant or not malignant. It would appear that we can do one of two things here: (a) accept a majority verdict as right, a score of 100%, and the minority wrong, a score of 0%, or (b), more logically, work in terms of probability according to the distribution of the panel's opinion; that is, if $8/10$ or $2/10$ of the panel say malignant, the pathologist under test who has also said malignant should be regarded as having an 80% or 20% chance of being correct. In practice, of course, with a panel of such experienced pathologists, matters would not work in this way, and here the complexity of framing a histopathological audit begins to emerge. Each of the ten panel members would have couched his own opinion in terms of probability, and necessarily so. The borderline situation considered above is one where the point at issue is *whether* it is malignant. Yet further complexity appears when we add to this the problem of *how* malignant, and here again opinions may differ. A panel may agree that the lesion is entity $X$, say, a carcinoma of ovary, but not agree on how aggressive it may be. Here at least, however, the pathologist under audit is at little more of a disadvantage than the panel; all are relatively helpless in the face of intrinsic biological variability (as with the earlier-cited example of choriocarcinoma and HCG, it may yet be found that, with many a cancer, knowledge of the serum level of some metabolite will be a much better predictor than the histology).

### Assessing Validity of Diagnosis in Retrospect

At first sight this may seem the more valuable way of establishing diagnostic histopathological criteria. A patient dies from the dissemination of a neoplasm initially represented on biopsy $x$ years ago by a tissue pattern that had then caused doubt. Therefore, it would seem, the same tissue pattern on a future occasion would allow a confident diagnosis; for this is the means whereby histopathological knowledge has grown. But again there are problems, one major and real, the other minor and in part artificial.

The major difficulty is that, even if the changes in pattern were by some hypothetical technique shown certainly to be a manifestation of the ultimately fatal disease, they may be at too early a stage to be diagnostic. To be sure, a study and growing experience of such subtle changes in pattern will push further back in its life the time when a lesion becomes certainly diagnosable, but even the most experienced pathologist will reach a stage where the clues become too faint. This at present is an insoluble difficulty and it seems likely to remain so (who, if cancer of the breast were shown incontestably to be caused by a particular virus, would recommend mastectomy or cytotoxic therapy on the discovery at biopsy of a single virus particle? Our immune defences are destroying pathogens all the time). This is not to say that a retrospective study of such lesions is valueless. On the contrary, it is highly valuable, for therein lies the best hope of sharpening our diagnostic criteria. There is the further complication that not all malignant neoplasms, even of the same histogenetic type, show a progressive structural change, and also that, among those that do, the rate or speed of change varies greatly.

The minor difficulty is simply that imposed by sampling. This applies in particular in systemic disorders such as the malignant lymphomas where, as is well known, one lymph node of a group may show equivocal appearances, and another be diagnostic. If, in these circumstances, only a single node were available or taken for biopsy, it might be at the equivocal stage. A further biopsy may prove diagnostic or it may not: if it does, not only is the matter resolved, it offers a perfect opportunity to study the earlier equivocal pattern of the now firmly diagnosed disease. In this way, an equivocal section may be correctly diagnosed with virtual certainty, but no such retrospectively diagnosed section could in fairness be used for purposes of an audit.

It would appear, therefore, that degree of diagnostic accuracy in histopathology can be measured only in terms of degree of concordance with an accepted majority opinion given predictively or prospectively. The 'correct' opinion and the 'attempted' opinion are equally no more than expressions of probability. Also, the majority opinion given in prospect has of necessity been based *au fond* on accumulated knowledge gained in retrospect. Such complexities as these, and the others mentioned above, make the difficulties of devising a histological audit not surprisingly great. Ingenious and valuable schemes for the assessment and comparison of levels of diagnostic histological accuracy have been described by Owen and Tighe (1975) and, with reference also to cytology, by Langley (1978).

# References

Ash JE, Beck MR, Wilkes JD (1964) Atlas of tumor pathology, sect IV, fasc 12. Tumors of the upper respiratory tract and ear. Armed Forces Institute of Pathology, Washington, D.C.

Blanco AA, Gibbs ACC, Langley FA (1977) Histological discrimination of malignancy in mucinous ovarian tumours. Histopathol 1: 431–443

Editorial (1974) E.C.G. interpretation by computer. Br Med J 3: 702

Hamperl H (1967) Early invasive growth as seen in uterine cancer and the role of the basal membrane. In: Denoix P (ed) Mechanisms of invasion in cancer, UICC Monograph Ser, vol 6. Springer, Berlin Heidelberg New York, pp 17–27

Henschke UK, Flehinger BJ (1967) Decision theory in cancer therapy. Cancer 20: 1819–1826

Kobayasi T (1969) Dermo-epidermal junction in invasive squamous cell carcinoma. An electron microscopic study. Acta Derm Venereol (Stockh) 49: 445–457

Langley FA (1978) Quality control in histopathology and diagnostic cytology. Histopathol 2: 3–18

Owen DA, Tighe JR (1975) Quality evaluation in histopathology. Br Med J 1: 149–150

Park WW (1956) On diagnosing cancer histologically. Lancet 1: 701–704

Ravitch MM (1967) Early cancer detection—blessing or bombshell? Resident Physician: Oct., 59–61

Safran C, Tsichlis PN, Bluming AZ, Desforges JF (1977) Diagnostic planning using computer assisted decision-making for patients with Hodgkin's disease. Cancer 39: 2426–2434

Scully RE (1970) Recent progress in ovarian cancer. Hum Pathol 1: 73–98

Song J (1950) The epithelial-stromal junction of human cervix uteri. Am J Clin Pathol 50: 102–103

Wartman WB (1959) Evaluation of biopsy diagnosis. Am J Clin Pathol 32: 468–471

# 2 Lesions of the Breast

Carcinoma of the breast is in many ways *a* crucial cancer. It has fair claim to be held to be *the* crucial cancer; for in it, as the exemplar of a killing cancer, the value of surgical extirpation finds its greatest test. The terms are relative but, compared with other regularly lethal cancers such as those of bronchus, pancreas and stomach, it is superficial, easily and early diagnosable, and potentially removable in toto. If local extirpative measures have limited success here, they can hardly be expected to do better with the deeper-seated cancers. To be sure, when each form of cancer is shown to have its own therapeutically exploitable difference from the others in biological behaviour, this view will require revision but, despite hints, that day is not yet.

Clearly enough, many cancers kill by their essentially mechanical and local effects such as pressure or obstruction, perhaps in the urinary, digestive or respiratory tracts, and their removal may then be curative. It is then difficult to know whether, by its removal, the patient has been cured of the cancer or, as with a non-neoplastic lesion, of the obstruction it was causing; for few can doubt that some cancers of whatever viscus metastasise early, some late, and some, on necropsy evidence, not at all. None of these considerations applies to carcinoma of the breast; it cannot cause death in a purely mechanical way, hence its almost unique status as a therapeutic challenge; hence, also, the massive attention it receives. Only four other types of cancer are comparable as localised lesions excisable in toto, namely, melanocarcinoma of the eye, seminoma/teratoma testis, and melanocarcinoma and osteosarcoma of a limb, but each of these has its differences. For ocular melanocarcinoma, possible forms of treatment are few in comparison with mammary carcinoma. With the testicular lesions, nodes cannot be comparably assessed and their excision is out of the question. For melanocarcinoma of a limb, rarely if ever nowadays is amputation performed as part of the primary treatment, yet logically it should be. The justification for its not being done can only be based on past experience when amputation, logically founded on the mechanistic concept of the spread of cancer, so frequently failed; so, gradually and thankfully was the surgeon able to stop amputating and yet feel fully justified in his decision. The distal osteosarcoma thus remains as probably the closest analogue to mammary carcinoma, yet even here circumstances are not totally comparable.

The practice of 'irradiation, wait for 6 months, then, if apparently no metastasis, amputation', is not applied to the cancerous breast. Mammary carcinoma therefore stands alone as the great therapeutic challenge, and the carefully planned attempts at treatment by chemotherapy which are increasingly being practised (Editorial, 1976a; Editorial, 1976b; Conference, 1977) are fully justified. Their triumph will come when, with the ending of mutilation, tylectomy ('lumpectomy') plus chemotherapy is shown to achieve results no worse than those achieved by regimes requiring mastectomy. What total triumph would be is obvious but even this partial version would be an immense therapeutic advance. The assessment of tylectomy by Atkins and his colleagues (1972) has been valuable. This procedure, with adjuvant radiotherapy, was practised on 370 patients all aged over 50 years. In patients with clinically involved axillary nodes there was a significantly higher incidence of local and distant recurrence in association with local excision, and survival was less than in those who had had a radical mastectomy. In those with clinically uninvolved nodes, although there was a significantly higher incidence of local recurrence, there was no increased incidence of distant recurrence, and survival rates were similar to those having a radical mastectomy. Some encouragement at least may be derived from these findings and from others of comparable character reported more recently by Calle and his colleagues (1978). The outcome after tylectomy was not so catastrophic as to rule it out for all time as an acceptable procedure. Further improvements in chemotherapy may yet make it the preferred procedure. Meantime, the practice of partial mastectomy with prosthetic reconstruction appears to be growing, and, as an operation more akin to tylectomy than radical mastectomy, its accumulating results are awaited with interest. A noteworthy report has been published by Crile (1975) whose experience so far has led him to state that '. . . from the standpoint of contracting a new cancer the hazard of leaving part of the original breast is no higher than that of leaving the contralateral breast'. The importance of this observation needs no emphasis: nor does its significance for the contralateral breast.

Increasingly, cytologists and pathologists will have to accustom themselves to receiving material obtained by needle biopsy; with such material, simply in terms of amount of tissue or cells sampled, borderline problems are likely to increase whether the specimen be a 'core' of tissue or an aspirate for cytology. A representative core from an undoubted carcinoma can, as would be expected, be totally diagnostic: the specimen, after all, differs only in size from that obtained by open biopsy. A more important matter is how helpful the techniques are in the investigation of lumps in the breast in general.

The outcome in a series of 368 patients on whom 'Tru-Cut' needle biopsy was used, and of whom 278 were later shown certainly to have a carcinoma, was reported by Elston and his colleagues (1978). In a population already quite highly selected, the carcinoma was diagnosed in only 73.5% of the 278 patients; it was not diagnosed in 19.5% and was 'suspicious' in the remaining 7% (these figures stand in substantial contrast to the generally agreed 95%–99% accuracy for cryostat sectioning of an open biopsy). The population of 368 patients was selected in that those with lesions of certain kinds were excluded at the outset, namely, those with diffuse nodular areas in the breast; those under age 30 '. . . in whom the lesion was thought to be a fibroadenoma'; and those with lesions shown by aspiration to be cystic. Therefore, the effectiveness of the technique as a diagnostic procedure overall was, to the extent of this degree of selection, further diluted.

These same authors, who usefully review the experiences and results of earlier users of needling procedures, investigated also the value of fine needle aspirates for cytology in 163 of the same original population of patients; of the 163, 119 were subsequently shown to have carcinoma. The carcinoma was detected in only 52%: not only that, 5 of 44 patients subsequently shown to have benign breast disease were diagnosed as having carcinoma: that is, a rate of false positive diagnosis of 11%. As the authors themselves say, '. . . the occurrence of a single false positive from aspiration cytology renders the method unacceptable as a means of eliminating frozen section and proceeding directly to mastectomy'. A rather similar criticism of the technique had been made earlier (Park, 1977). In general, from results such as those just cited and others, published and unpublished, it seems possible, even probable, that investigation of mammary masses by aspiration cytology will be abandoned. The procuring of 'cores' may spread, but is perhaps best regarded meantime as a practice still sub judice. To most histopathologists, all single lumps are ipso facto suspicious and should be excised. For the surgeon, practicalities may make this policy difficult, while the multinodular breast remains a problem for all.

## Local Series

The local series of borderline cases comprises 19 in which prognostic concern had been caused, one in which infiltrating carcinoma was discovered fortuitously, and one in which an infiltrating carcinoma was initially 'missed'. During the same period of time, the number of cases firmly diagnosed within the same Department of Pathology (Dundee Royal Infirmary) as primary malignant disease of the breast in women, including Paget's disease and cystosarcoma phyllodes, was 1149. The large subjective element involved in the decision whether or not an intraductal proliferation of epithelium represents carcinoma means that a degree of over-diagnosis may be concealed within the diagnoses made firmly as intraduct carcinoma. This possibility has not been investigated since the purpose here is to assess the significance of cases in which the diagnosis had been made not firmly but with reservations. However, as the figures emerged for the diagnosis of mammary cancer from year to year, their consistency suggested that the amount of over-diagnosis concealed in this was, if any, small.

SUMMARISED TOTALS

*Intraduct carcinoma* or epitheliosis (seven cases):
In six cases (2.1–2.6 inclusive), mastectomy
In one case (2.7), no mastectomy
All alive 7–20 years later

*Intraduct carcinoma* or papilloma (five cases; 2.8–2.12 inclusive):
Mastectomy in all
All alive 7–18 years later

*Intraduct papilloma* or carcinoma (one case; 2.13):
Supervision rather than mastectomy
Alive 5 years later

*Extreme hyperplasia* or early carcinoma (three cases):
Mastectomy in two cases (2.14, 2.15)
Both alive 17 and 14 years later respectively
Pregnancy reaction suspected and confirmed in one case (2.16)
No further treatment
Well 12 years later

*Fibroadenoma* with ? carcinomatous transformation (one case; 2.17):
No further treatment
Well 8 years later

*Adenomatosis of nipple* with recurrence (one case; 2.18):
Undue alarm because lesion not identified as one intrinsically benign

No further trouble for at least 12 years

*Sclerosing adenosis* or carcinoma (one case; 2.19):
No mastectomy
Well 18 years later

*Infiltrating carcinoma* discovered fortuitously (one case; 2.20):
Intraduct carcinoma diagnosed on biopsy; mastectomy, no further lesions; extra blocks from biopsy showed more intraduct carcinoma, also two foci of infiltrating carcinoma
Well 12 years later

*Infiltrating carcinoma* 'missed' (one case; 2.21):
Biopsy diagnosis sclerosing adenosis of apocrine type; recurrence at 8 months, lesion now diagnosed carcinoma; mastectomy
Alive 8 years later

> *Review has yielded:*
> Appropriate diagnoses, 15
> Over-diagnoses, 5
> Under-diagnoses, 1

The 21 cases thus regrouped comprise Table 2.1

CASE DATA

*Case 2.1*

Age, 46 years; lump just beneath nipple present for 1 year. A 3-cm diameter mass was excised.

Mildly hyperplastic fibrocystic disease was present throughout but one section included a cluster of some 12 ductules, all 1 mm across, half of which showed a well-marked cribriform pattern. The cells were uniform and only rarely in mitosis, but the finding was held sufficient to warrant a diagnosis of 'early intraduct carcinoma'.

Mastectomy was performed, sections showing one other similarly minute focus of intraduct epithelial overgrowth though, on this occasion, solidly cellular and not cribriform.

Radiotherapy followed mastectomy, and the patient was well 18 years later. Evidence of malignancy here seems, on review, less than convincing, and it is difficult to regard this as other than a marginal *over-diagnosis*. Epitheliosis now seems a more appropriate designation.

**Table 2.1.** Twenty-one cases of equivocal lesions of breast.

| Case No. | Diagnosis on review | Treatment | Outcome |
|---|---|---|---|
| *1 case under-diagnosed* | | | |
| 21 | Carc. > 'apocrine' scl. adenosis | Excision | Recurrence: mastectomy + R/th alive @ 7 yr |
| *5 cases over-diagnosed* | | | |
| 1 | Epitheliosis > I-duct carc. | Mastect. + R/th | Alive @ 18 yr |
| 3 | Epitheliosis > I-duct carc. | Mastect. + R/th | Alive @ 20 yr |
| 9 | Pap/osis > I-duct carc. | Mastect. only | Alive @ 16 yr |
| 14 | Prognosis over-serious | Mastect. + R/th | Alive @ 17 yr |
| 18 | Nipple duct adenomatosis > I-duct papillomatosis | Excision | Recurrence @ 4 yr: re-excision: well for next 8 yr to date |
| *15 cases appropriately diagnosed* | | | |
| 2 | Intraduct carcinoma | Mastect. + R/th | Alive @ 18 yr |
| 4 | Intraduct carcinoma | Mastect. + R/th | Alive @ 18 yr |
| 5 | Intraduct carcinoma | Mastect. only | Alive @ 9 yr |
| 6 | Intraduct carcinoma | Mastect. + R/th | Alive @ 11 yr |
| 7 | Intraduct carcinoma | Local excision | Alive @ 10 yr |
| 8 | I-duct carc. + sc. carc. | Mastect. + R/th | Alive @ 18 yr |
| 10 | Papillomatosis ++ | Mastect. + R/th | Alive @ 8 yr |
| 11 | Intraduct carcinoma | Mastect. + R/th | Alive @ 9 yr |
| 12 | Intraduct carcinoma | Mastect. only | Alive @ 7 yr |
| 13 | Intraduct papilloma | Local excision | Alive @ 5 yr |
| 15 | Intraduct carcinoma | Mastect. only | Alive @ 14 yr |
| 16 | Lactational hyperplasia | Local excision | Alive @ 12 yr |
| 17 | Fibroadenoma + ? carc. | Local excision | Alive @ 8 yr |
| 19 | Sclerosing adenosis | Local excision | Alive @ 18 yr |
| 20 | I-duct + infiltr. carc. | Mastect. + R/th | Alive @ 12 yr |

*Case 2.2*

Age, 39 years; slight discharge from nipple for 2 months. A 3 × 3 × 2 cm mass of 'sub-areolar' tissue was removed.

In general, there was mildly hyperplastic fibrocystic disease throughout but also a single focus of ductal epithelial overgrowth sufficiently pronounced to have led to its being diagnosed as 'intraduct carcinoma'.

In section, the area was 2 × 1 mm and included some six ducts or ductules of which the largest, 0.25 mm across, was filled by cells; the others showed a varying amount of papillary overgrowth. The cells were uniform throughout and showed, on average, two (normal) mitotic figures per section. There was no indication of extension into the stroma.

Mastectomy was performed.

Radiotherapy followed the mastectomy, and the patient was well 18 years later. Some might regard this as having been an over-diagnosis but on balance it still seems *appropriate*.

*Case 2.3*

Age, 45 years; discharge from nipple for 2 years. The clinical evidence of itself was held sufficient to warrant mastectomy.

No papilloma was found on dissection, nor any notably localised nodule. The parenchyma was generally nodular with scattered 1–5 mm cysts. Blocks were cut from three areas rather firmer than the rest, sections showing lobular hyperplasia with, in one 3-mm area, a focus of intraductal epithelial overgrowth that was diagnosed as 'intraduct carcinoma' with 'no evidence of invasion'.

Radiotherapy followed, and the patient was well 20 years later. On review, this appears as a diagnosis of carcinoma made on less than wholly convincing evidence; to a degree, at any rate, an *over-diagnosis*.

### Case 2.4

Age, 45 years; lump in breast noticed 5 weeks earlier. A 3 × 3 × 2 cm mass was excised.

Scattered amongst a mildly hyperplastic fibrocystic background were occasional foci of what were regarded as 'intraduct carcinoma', small ducts totally occupied by epithelium that showed no cribriform interruption of the cellular sheets.

Mastectomy was performed, further representative sections showing no areas diagnosable as carcinoma.

Radiotherapy followed the mastectomy. During the year after the mastectomy a lump was noticed in the other breast accompanied by 'one gland in the axilla'. Simple mastectomy was carried out but yielded only a tense 3-cm cyst and a 5-mm fibroadenoma in a generally fibrocystic parenchyma; the axillary 'gland' was not removed.

There was no further trouble and the patient was well 18 years later. The original diagnosis was *appropriate*.

### Case 2.5

Age, 31 years; lump in breast, duration unknown (patient an imbecile). Excision produced a mass, 25 × 15 × 15 mm, with a 'prominently and unusually speckled cut surface'.

Throughout virtually the whole of the nodule the appearances were those shown in Fig. 2.1; that is, ducts in varying degree distended and wholly or partly filled by epithelium in papillary, cribriform or solid patterns. At cellular level there was no undue polymorphism and only scanty normal mitotic figures. The sheer amount of the epithelial overgrowth, however, throughout all of the three blocks that were taken, was regarded as enough to warrant diagnosis as 'intraduct carcinoma'.

Mastectomy was performed, to reveal the pattern of a generalised fibrocystic mastopathia with frequent overgrowth of ductal epithelium but, on the whole, less pronounced than in the originally removed nodule.

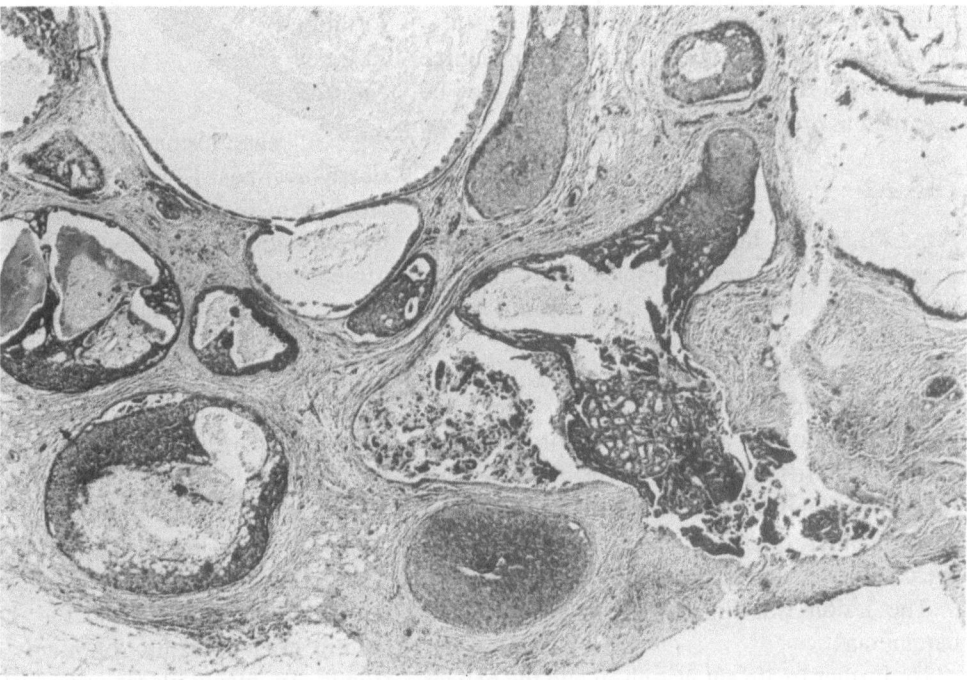

**Fig. 2.1.** Ducts filled partially or wholly by hyperplastic epithelium. In some places, in detail, it was cribriform but not significantly polymorphic; mitoses were few. Even so, in toto, the amount of epithelial overgrowth was great. H & E, × 26

Radiotherapy was *not* used, and the patient was well 9 years later. The diagnosis may reasonably be considered as *appropriate*.

### Case 2.6

Age, 45 years; noticed painless lump in breast a week earlier. The excised mass, 6 × 4 × 3 cm, contained a solitary 4-cm cyst, sections showing a background of fibrocystic disease. Two years later a lump was again palpable, the two excised masses together measuring 5 × 3 × 2 cm. Again the pattern was that of fibrocystic disease.

After 13 months a further mass, 6 × 6 × 3 cm, was excised.

Eight representative blocks were taken. All again showed fibrocystic disease but in one there was a focus of eight ductules wherein the epithelium showed a degree of polymorphism and mitotic activity meriting diagnosis 'for practical purposes' as 'early intraduct carcinoma'. Mastectomy followed within 1 month to reveal a single similar focus in 1 of 12 representative blocks. The diagnosis could be taken no further.

The patient remains well 11 years later. As in all such cases, there is no way of knowing how the patient would have fared had mastectomy not been performed. However, after the two earlier operations, mastectomy did at least remove what must have been an increasing source of anxiety. For this reason the diagnosis may be regarded as *appropriate*.

### Case 2.7

Age, 40 years; lump in breast for about 3 months. The excised mass, 5 × 3 × 3 cm, was notably firm and contained two obvious cysts, 15 mm and 4 mm.

In scattered areas, ducts were wholly or partly occupied by hyperplastic epithelium, sometimes with production of a partly cribriform pattern. The cells were generally uniform and rarely in mitosis. A comment was made that none of the cells, in many sections, had been seen beyond the confines of any of the ducts.

The lesion was finally designated 'intraduct carcinoma'.

No further treatment was given and the patient was known to be well 10 years later. Contact was lost thereafter but at least no enquiry has been received to suggest further trouble. Even if the subsequent history, no further trouble

despite no mastectomy, suggests that this had been an over-diagnosis, review of the sections still makes it seem *appropriate*.

### Case 2.8

Age, 68 years; history of discharge from nipple for 2 weeks. Wedge resection was performed.

Sections from the 3 × 2 × 2 cm mass revealed a 1-mm papillary structure within one of the ducts. It was essentially a duct papilloma but of such high cellularity that, despite a generally uniform pattern and rarity of mitotic figures, the diagnosis of 'early intraduct carcinoma' was given.

Simple mastectomy was performed and no macroscopically identifiable mass was seen. One of several representative sections, however, showed a single 1-mm focus of what, in view of its cellular aberrancy and seeming invasiveness, was reasonably diagnosed as 'scirrhous carcinoma'; it was an anatomically independent lesion.

Radiotherapy followed the mastectomy, and the patient was well 18 years later. The original diagnosis was *appropriate*. The fact that the consequent mastectomy revealed an independent and probably more dangerous lesion was purely fortuitous.

### Case 2.9

Age, 50 years; history of lump in breast growing slowly over past 18 months. The clinical features alone were regarded as sufficiently suggestive to warrant simple mastectomy. Dissection revealed a moderately well circumscribed mass, firm but not typically scirrhous, 2 cm in diameter.

As shown in Fig. 2.2 the mass consisted of a multitude of ductular structures uniformly distributed throughout an almost purely fibrous stroma but with, in addition, scattered larger ducts largely filled and distended by hyperplastic epithelium in a generally papillary arrangement. None of these larger ducts was solidly filled; rather, the papillary pattern was generally maintained although, as seen in Fig. 2.3, a laciform pattern was a feature of many of the larger fronds. In many places, as in that illustrated here, a delicate fibrovascular stroma supported the pattern; elsewhere, such a stroma was lacking, the arrangement then being more truly cribriform.

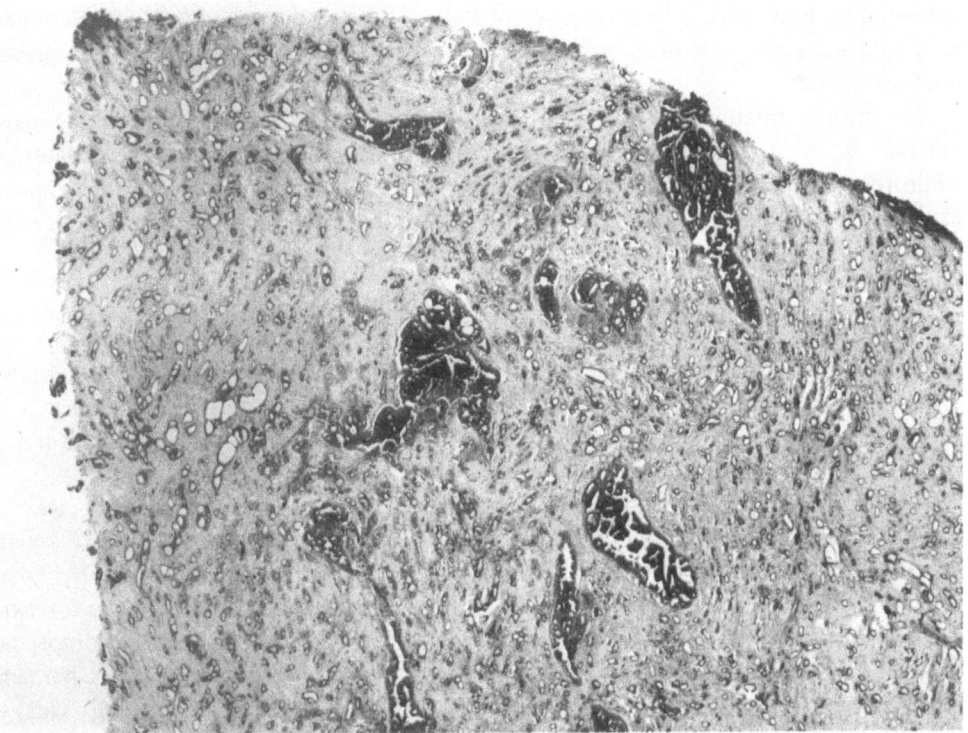

**Fig. 2.2.** Scattered ducts are largely occupied by hyperplastic epithelium of papillary pattern. H & E, × 13

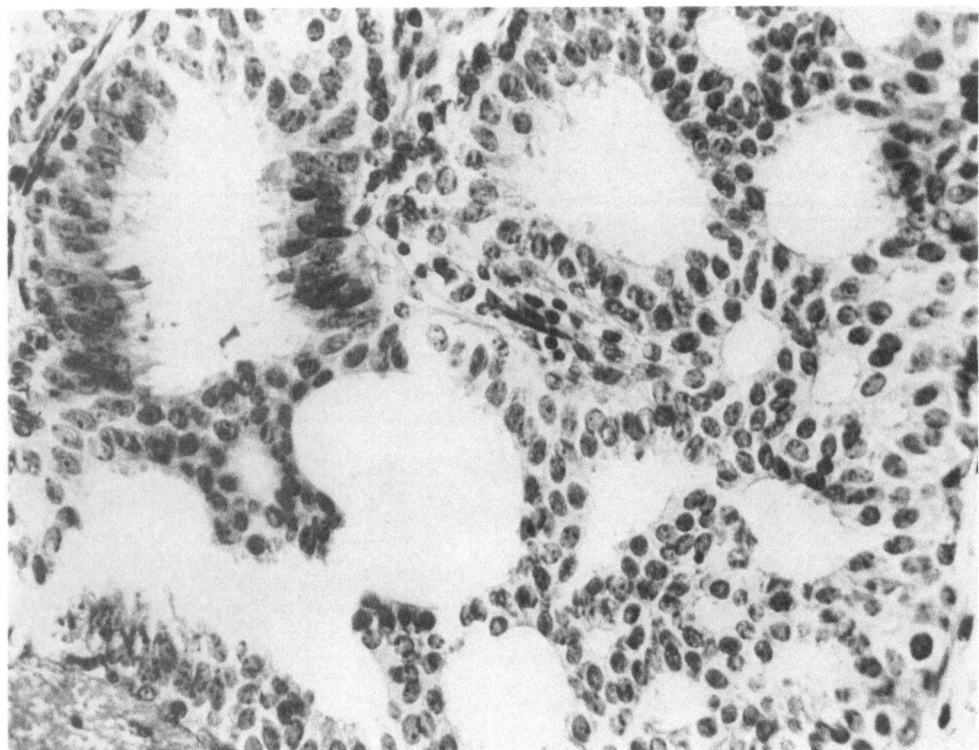

**Fig. 2.3.** Many of the papillary fronds had this laciform pattern. The cells are generally uniform and rarely in mitosis. H & E, × 476

The cells were uniform but in some places the appearances were held to be 'suggestive of invasion' and the lesion was diagnosed as an 'intraduct carcinoma'.

No further treatment was given, and the patient was well 16 years later. In retrospect, while recognising the intraductal overgrowth as exuberant, a likelier diagnosis would be pericanalicular fibroadenoma with interspersed ductal papillomatosis. Microcalcification was widespread throughout the mass, no more prominent around the papillomatous ducts than elsewhere. This must be accounted an *over-diagnosis*.

### Case 2.10

Age, 52 years; subareolar nodule and discharge from nipple, occasionally bloodstained, for 7 months. Mastectomy was performed without preliminary biopsy.

Dissection revealed a 14-mm firm nodule including dilated ducts containing gritty particles. The general appearances were as shown in Figs. 2.4, 2.5 and 2.6; that is, at the least, the pattern of a segmental duct papillomatosis. The cells were generally uniform and only infrequently in (normal) mitosis but the degree of cellularity

was in places so high and associated with scattered areas of overgrowth apparently outwith ducts that the diagnosis was given for practical purposes as 'carcinoma'.

Radiotherapy followed the mastectomy, and the patient was well 8 years later. An element of doubt remains but, like the original report itself, the diagnosis seems 'for practical purposes' *appropriate*.

### Case 2.11

Age, 33 years; lump in the breast noticed for 3 weeks. Excision produced a 3 × 3 × 2 cm mass of tissue with a firm 10-mm nodule in the centre.

The nodule was mostly well circumscribed and unaccompanied by any scirrhous reaction though accompanied by outlying satellite foci at places around the edge as, for example, in Fig. 2.7. The cells formed an almost confluent sheet and were generally uniform but sufficiently often in mitosis to be disquieting. This, plus the sheer amount of the abnormal tissue, despite a still broadly intraductal pattern, was held to make the diagnosis of 'carcinoma' inescapable; the overgrowth seemed more florid than could be

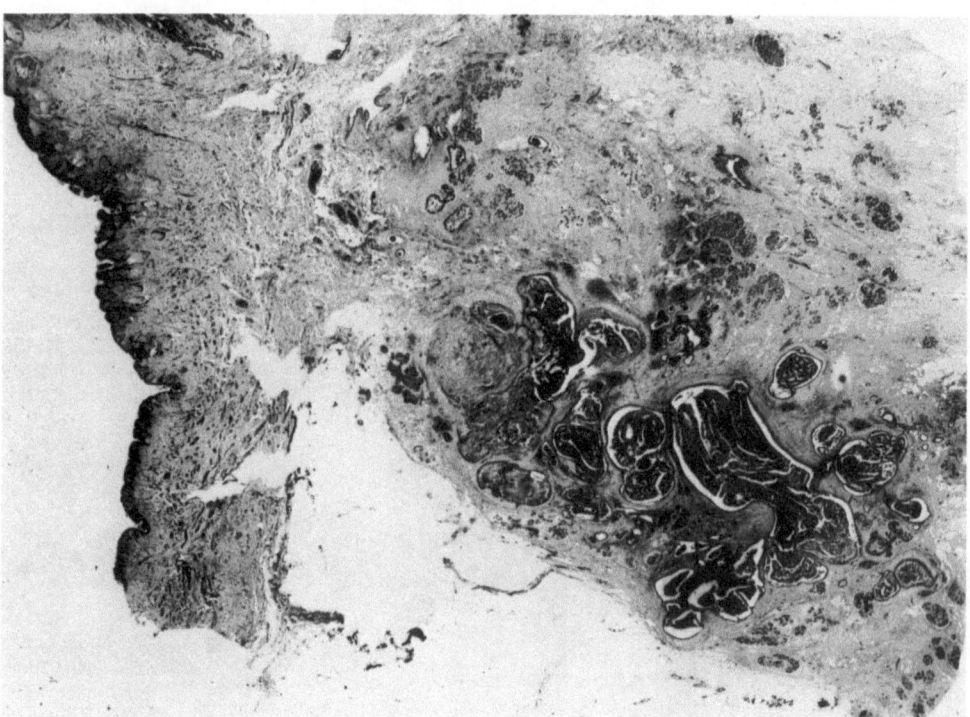

**Fig. 2.4.** Shows the only area of abnormality found within the breast. It was relatively superficial and close to the nipple. H & E, × 5

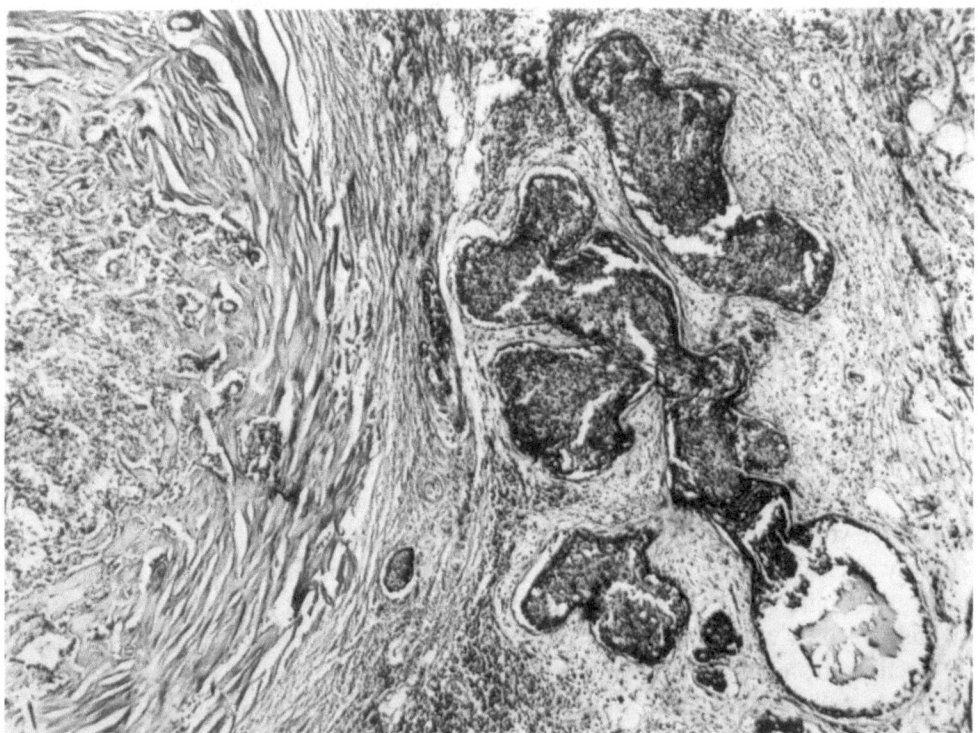

**Fig. 2.5.** One of the groups of smaller ducts, all of which were largely occupied by solid masses of epithelium. Associated epithelial overgrowth is seen on the left. H & E, × 60

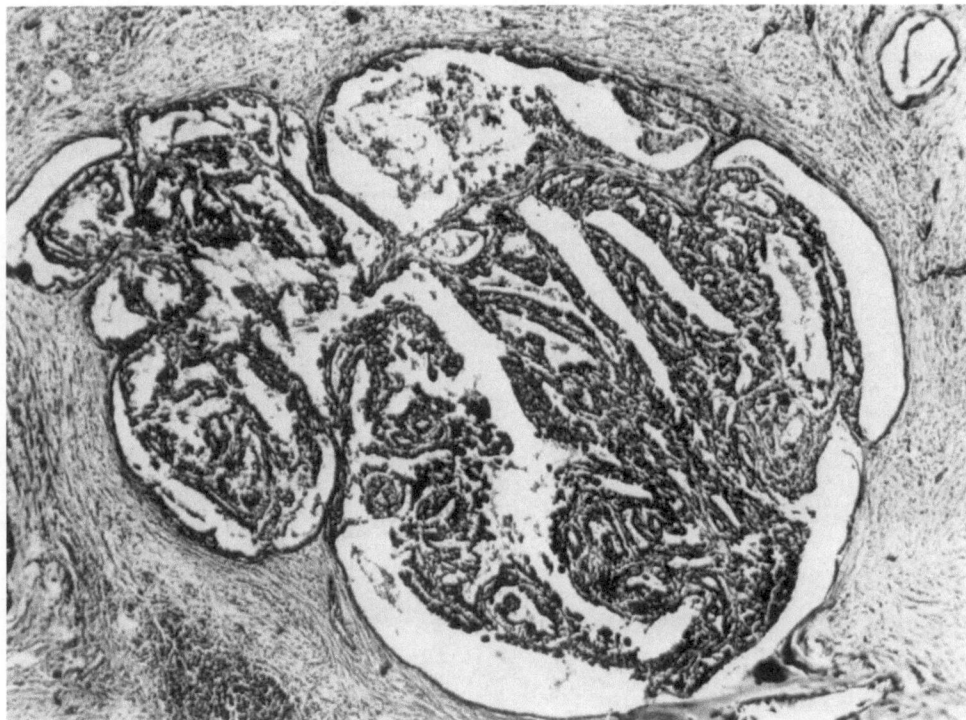

**Fig. 2.6.** A more papillary or open-work mass of tissue. It lacks a truly cribriform pattern and amounts to a state of papillomatosis rather than the diagnosis that was suggested, intraduct carcinoma. H & E, × 60

admitted for even a confluent ductal papillomatosis. In a few places, as in Fig. 2.8, the possibility of lymphatic permeation could not be excluded with certainty. In the space shown here the lining cells were so uniformly flat that an endothelial nature seemed much likelier than one of compressed epithelium.

Mastectomy was performed, many further sections showing no other areas of carcinoma.

Radiotherapy followed the mastectomy and the patient was well 9 years later. An element of uncertainty remains but the diagnosis still, in retrospect, seems reasonable and *appropriate*.

### Case 2.12

Age, 32 years; lump in breast for 2 months. Biopsy produced a fibrofatty mass, 5 × 3 × 3 cm, containing a thick-walled 20-mm cyst largely filled by a soft papillary growth.

Sections from across the whole mass showed a highly cellular papilloma within a cystically dilated duct which itself had a lining of hyperplastic epithelium, and several adjacent groups of ducts all distended and filled wholly or partly by epithelium in cribriform or solid arrangement. The epithelium in all areas showed an appreciable though not extreme degree of nuclear polymorphism and mitotic activity; occasional high power fields (hpf) contained as many as five mitotic figures.

The appearances were held to warrant a diagnosis of 'early carcinoma'; though not expressly designated as such, the implication was that the carcinoma was still of intraduct type, and simple mastectomy was advised. This was performed and revealed throughout the rest of the parenchyma a pronounced degree of lobular hyperplasia and also multiple small fibroadenomata or fibroadenomatoid nodules. Close search produced no other lesion with the exuberance of the original.

Radiotherapy was not used, and the patient was well seven years later. She had had a normal pregnancy one year after the mastectomy. There must be some suspicion that this was an over-diagnosis, yet review of the sections by a group of pathologists found none prepared to say 'not malignant', so on this basis the diagnosis was *appropriate*.

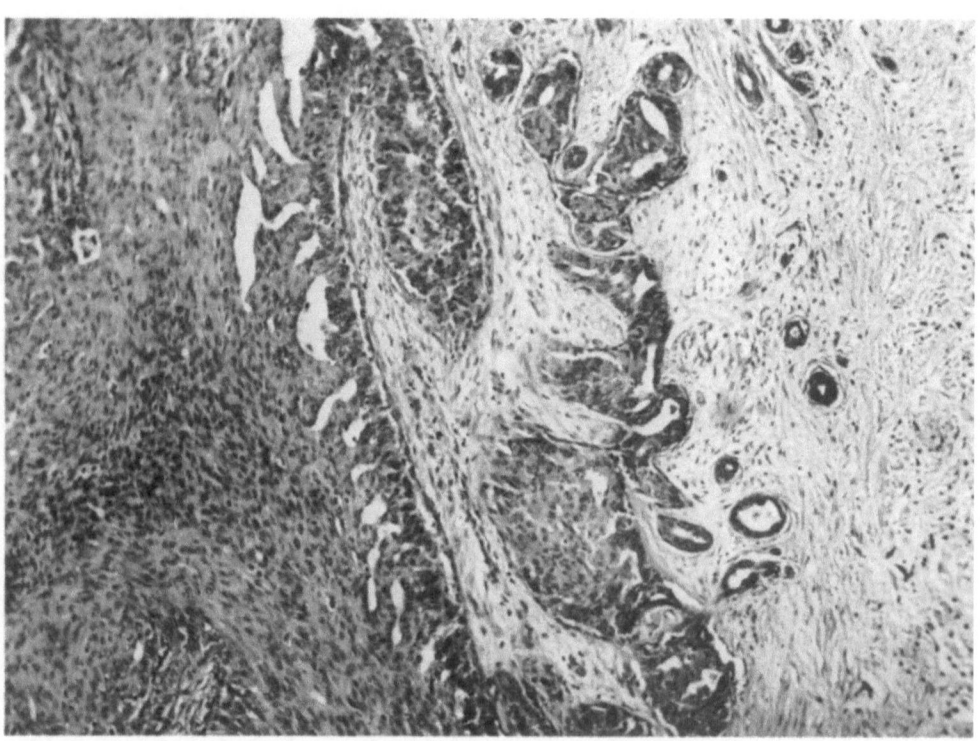

**Fig. 2.7.** The left half of the field shows the high and almost confluent cellularity of the central 10-mm nodule noted macroscopically. The outlying foci seen on the right strongly suggest a truly invasive stromal permeation. H & E, × 119

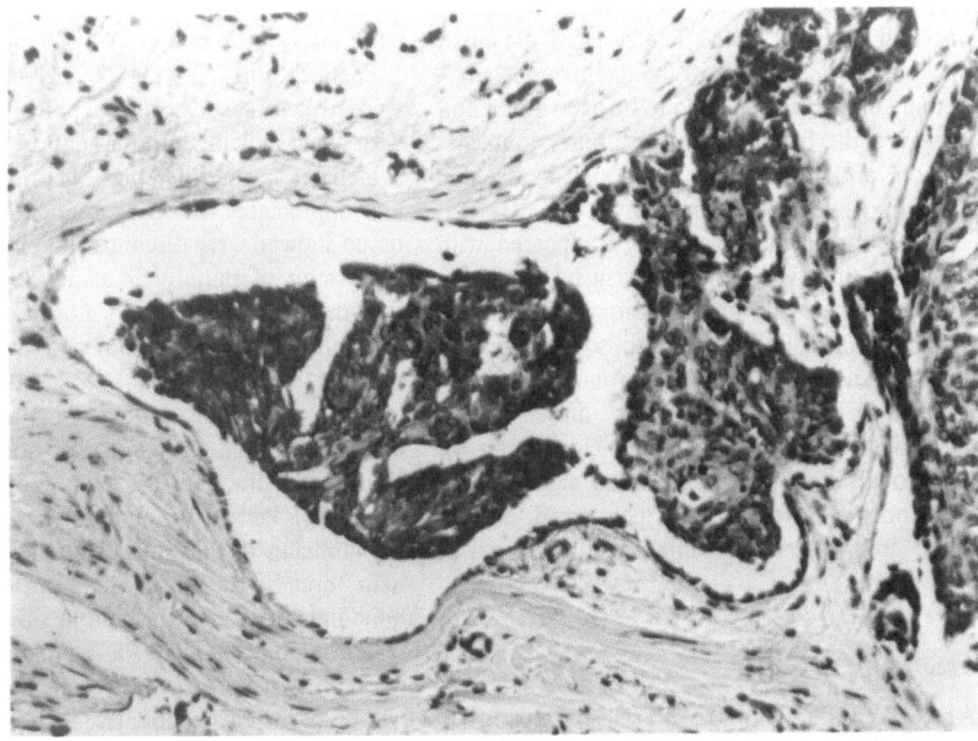

**Fig. 2.8.** Possibly simulated, possibly truly, lymphatic permeation. In the absence of an indicative valve within the vessel, certain distinction between a lymphatic and a dilated duct is not possible. H & E, × 238

*Case 2.13*

Age, 39 years; discharge from nipple for 3 months. A 15 × 10 mm nodule was removed and found to be a simple fibroadenoma. The discharge continued. Further exploration produced an irregular mass of tissue, 20 × 6 × 5 mm.

The mass of tissue contained a fragmented, quite highly cellular 'intraduct papilloma'. The degree of cellularity combined with uncertainty whether the whole of the lesion had been removed led to the recommendation of regular supervision.

The discharge ceased, and the patient was well and trouble-free 4 years later. The diagnosis and course recommended were *appropriate*.

*Case 2.14*

Age, 40 years; lump in breast noticed for 4 weeks. Fibrofatty mass, 4 × 2 × 2 cm excised.

Sections showed generally hyperplastic changes with widespread intraduct epitheliosis, sclerosing adenosis and cyst formation. The appearances were regarded as 'not malignant' but so prominent that "it might be unsafe to leave any such tissue behind". Accordingly, mastectomy was performed, representative sections showing similar though less markedly hyperplastic changes in many areas.

Radiotherapy followed the mastectomy, and the patient was well 17 years later. In some degree, therefore, this was an *over-diagnosis*.

*Case 2.15*

Age, 42 years; lump in breast for 9 years since breast-feeding last baby; it had been painful for the past 6 months. Excision produced a firm fibrofatty mass, 4 × 3 × 2 cm.

Microscopy showed an extremely florid lobular hyperplasia with papillary overgrowth of ductal epithelium and widespread adenosis as yet minimally 'sclerosing'. Despite much mitotic activity, the appearances were considered as *not* malignant but held nevertheless to represent a high risk of the development of carcinoma eventually.

Mastectomy was performed. Sections from various areas showed a generally hyperplastic picture but nowhere as striking as in the original biopsy.

Radiotherapy was *not* given, and the patient was well 14 years later. The original diagnosis was *appropriate* even if the subsequent mastectomy may have appeared to be over-treatment. However, the decision was taken after joint discussion, and justification for it may be seen in the happenings in the other breast.

Two years later the patient reappeared with a lump in the other breast, present for 6 months and syn-menstrually painful. Biopsy showed appearances closely similar to those seen on the earlier occasion, essentially a prominent lobular hyperplasia with many areas of sclerosing adenosis, but now with a single 2-mm area of overgrowth within ducts regarded as 'intraduct carcinoma'. Mastectomy was performed, and no other areas of similar intraductal overgrowth were found.

## Case 2.16

Age, 22 years; lump in breast present for 1 month. Excision produced an irregularly shaped mass 5 cm across composed of many firm pale nodules amongst fibrofatty tissue; some of the nodules had been transected by the line of excision.

Sections showed (Fig. 2.9) that the nodules were hyperplastic and hypercellular lobules with ducts showing intraluminal proliferation and sometimes cystic dilatation. The high cellularity and appreciable mitotic activity that the acinar tissue showed were disconcerting, but the general uniformity of pattern at acinar level suggested that this was an unusually florid 'adenosis' and 'epitheliosis', not malignant neoplasia, and so it was reported.

Some of the dilated ducts contained colostrum or colostrum-like corpuscles, so the report concluded with the question, Was the patient pregnant? This led to the finding that, unknown to the clinician at that time, she was indeed pregnant though so early in its course that only a quite unusually vigorous and localised end-organ response could explain the mammary histology: in some parts of the mass there were still some wholly unresponsive lobules.

Nothing further was done and a successful delivery of twins was achieved 26 weeks later. After another 2 years the patient had a second

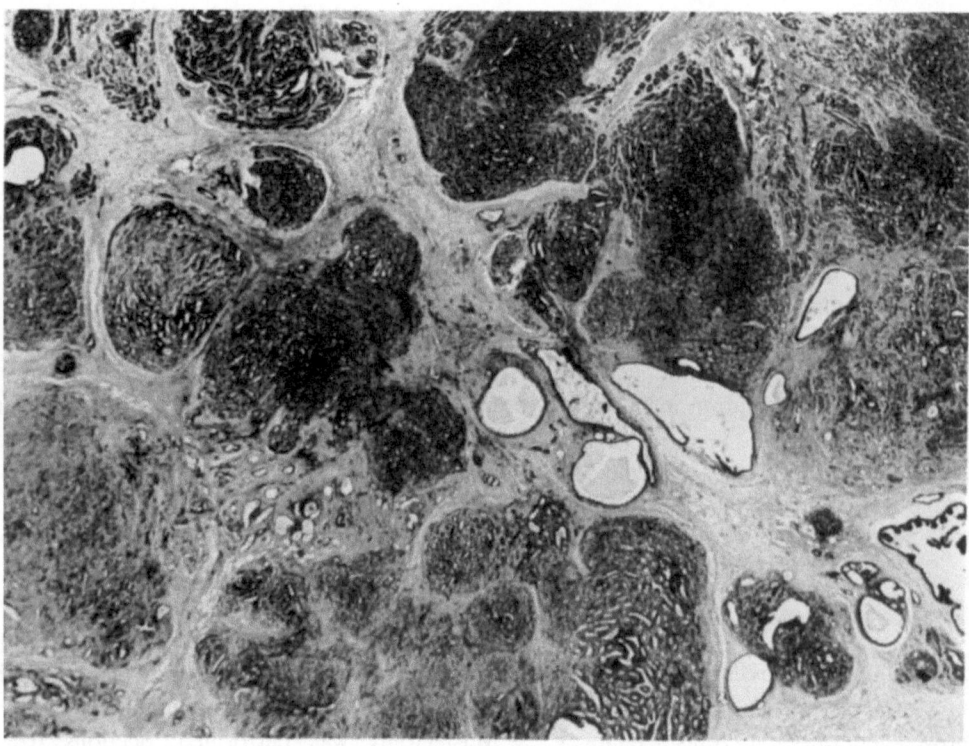

**Fig. 2.9.** These hypercellular (and mitotically active) lobules were disconcerting but proved to be a product of the early pregnancy suspected and suggested by the pathologist but not at that time entertained by patient or surgeon. H & E, × 13

and trouble-free pregnancy; she remains well 12 years later. An *appropriate* diagnosis.

### Case 2.17

Age, 36 years; lump in breast present for 11 months. Excision produced a moderately well-circumscribed mass, 6 × 4 × 4 cm, surrounded by fibrofatty tissue. It was firm and rubbery, and had a mucoid cut surface.

In general, as shown in Figs. 2.10 and 2.11, there was a mixture of appearances with foci of lobular hyperplasia, sclerosing adenosis, ductal epitheliosis and some nodules of fibroadenomatoid pattern. The stroma was mildly mucicarmine-positive. In some places the degree of cellularity and impression of early 'infiltration' was disquieting but the mass was concluded to be 'a type of fibroadenoma' and thus not malignant.

No further treatment was given, and the patient was well 8 years later. The diagnosis appears to have been *appropriate*.

### Case 2.18

Age, 16 years; discharge from nipple during past few weeks. A 10-mm nodule, pressure on which produced discharge, was present beneath the areola. Excision yielded a partly firm, partly spongy, 5 × 3 × 1 cm mass with cut surface showing an occasional 1–2-mm cyst and one 4-mm polypoid structure.

The general pattern was that of a fine spongework of ductular spaces, none wider than 0.5 mm, with most of the larger lumina wholly or partly occupied by plexiform papillary ingrowth. The lumina were lined, and the papillary processes covered, by a simple cubical or columnar epithelium frequently bearing so-called apocrine 'snouts'. In a few places the epithelium showed a double-layered arrangement, and in a similarly scattered fashion there were foci of 'pink epithelium'.

The lesion was diagnosed as widespread 'intraduct papillomatosis' with the advice that, since the abnormal tissue appeared to have been transected at many places by the line of excision, recurrence was very possible.

No further treatment was given until the patient reappeared 4 years later with a lump at the site of the earlier operation. The excised mass, 3 × 2 × 2 cm, was occupied to half its extent by a relatively well-circumscribed mass of what was described as microcystic mucoid tissue.

Histology showed essentially the same appearances as before, and on this occasion it seemed much more likely that excision had been complete. However, the advice was proffered, almost certainly misguided as mentioned below, that there remained at least the possibility a similar lesion would develop elsewhere within the ductal system of the breast.

In fact, this seems with little doubt to be a typical example of the papillary adenoma or 'adenomatosis of the ducts of the nipple' as described by Perzin and Lattes (1972) and some earlier workers. It appears to be a lesion exclusively of the nipple, has no premalignant significance and is associated with other lesions in the breast no more frequently than could occur by chance. It was thus that the advice given with the second biopsy was in error, an *over-diagnosis* in effect, and possibly a source of needless anxiety.

The patient was trouble-free at least for a further 10 years.

### Case 2.19

Age, 36 years; lump in breast present for 8 months. Excision produced a disc of firm white tissue, 4 × 1 cm.

The pattern was that of 'sclerosing adenosis', rather more exuberant than most but, after examination of many sections, finally diagnosed as that.

No further treatment was given, and the patient was known to be trouble-free for at least 18 years. The diagnosis was *appropriate*.

### Case 2.20

Age, 50 years; lump in breast noticed for 1 month. Two masses of tissue were received, each 5 × 4 × 3 cm.

The macroscopic appearances were those of fibrocystic disease with no area visibly or palpably more suggestive of neoplasia than any other. However, one of the five blocks originally sectioned showed a 1-mm focus of undoubted 'intraduct carcinoma' and also what seemed with little doubt to be occupation of two neighbouring lymphatics by malignant cells.

Mastectomy was performed, and many sections from around the biopsy-cavity and elsewhere showed no residual carcinoma. For no certainly recollected reason but possibly because of this negative finding in the amputated breast, and also the minute size of the original lesion, the pathologist cut a further eight blocks from the original biopsy, essentially at random and still without macroscopic suspicion of any particular area. These yielded further areas of intraduct carcinoma and two 3-mm foci of typically 'scirrhous carcinoma'.

The patient was treated by radiotherapy and was well 12 years later. But for the examination of the further tissue, the patient would have been regarded as having been cured of an intraduct carcinoma rather than the typically, albeit extremely small, scirrhous carcinoma that she undoubtedly had. The original diagnosis, inadequately representative though it was, was within its limits *appropriate*.

### Case 2.21

Age, 44 years; lump in breast present for 3 months. A mass, 6 × 5 × 3 cm, was excised. It was generally fibrofatty, contained occasional cysts up to 8 mm in diameter and one 10-mm area rather firmer than the rest of the tissue.

There was widespread epithelial overgrowth in many forms—lobular hyperplasia, ductal epitheliosis and early papilloma formation, all in association with chronic inflammatory cell reaction, and also several small areas of apparently infiltrative, notably uniform pale cells. These cells, all present within the rather firmer 10-mm focus, were identified as certainly epithelial and as representing 'almost certainly sclerosing adenosis of apocrine type, not carcinoma'.

In all, the diagnosis was given as 'fibrocystic mastopathia'.

Within 8 months a nodule was again palpable; its anatomical relation to the one removed earlier was not specified. Sections from the two pieces of tissue (the larger 3 × 2 × 2 cm) now showed an even more marked degree of lobular hyperplasia and areas of what had to be diagnosed as lobular carcinoma. Further sections from a 10-mm nodule still within the amputated breast showed a uniformly spheroidal-cell 'carcinoma' predominantly within ducts but also undoubtedly infiltrative in some places.

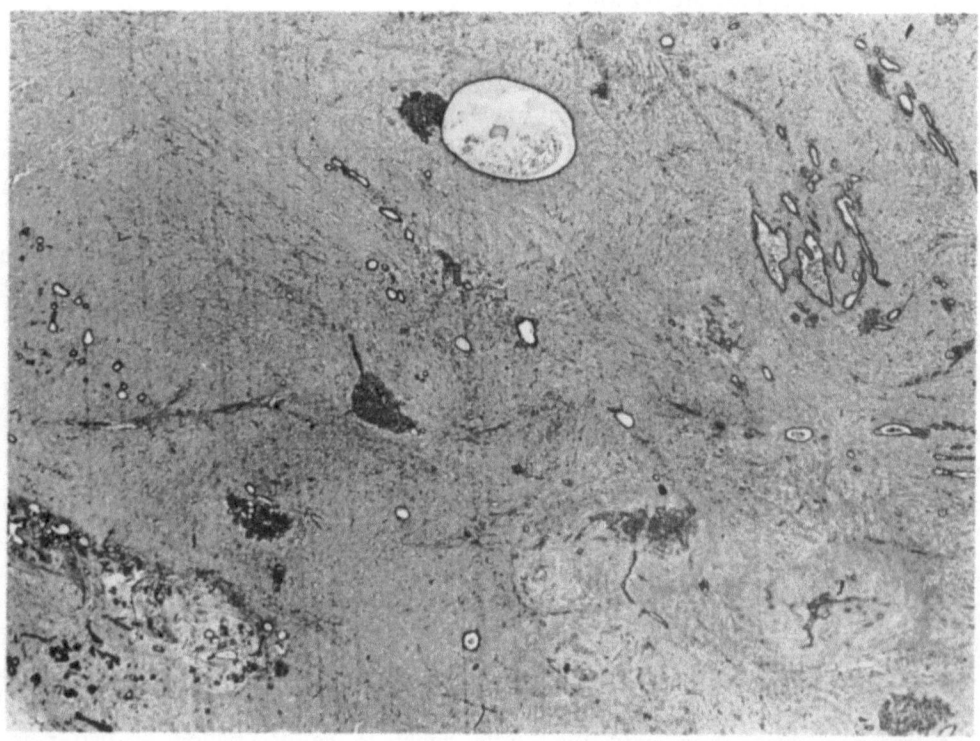

**Fig. 2.10.** In a generally hypercellular fibroblastic stroma there are foci of ductal and fibroadenomatoid overgrowth and, on the left, at least an approach towards sclerosing adenosis. H & E, × 7

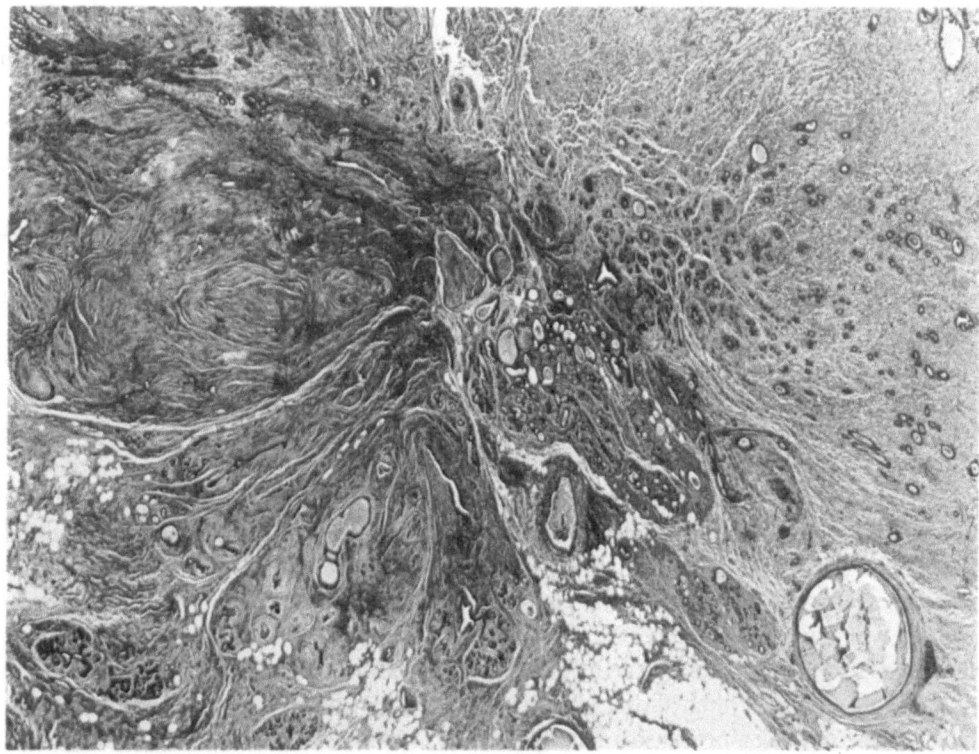

**Fig. 2.11.** Some of the complexities of tissue pattern are shown here. The general distortion and apparently scirrhous pattern were interpreted as due to sclerosing adenosis and fibro-adenomatoid stromal overgrowth. H & E, × 13

The question naturally arises, Had the carcinoma been 'missed' on the first occasion? In retrospect, when the cells of the undoubted carcinoma became available for comparison, the answer must be 'Yes'. Even so, however, few experienced colleagues to whom the first sections have been shown 'blind' over the years have not expressed a degree of uncertainty; most have said they were glad not to have been confronted with the lesion in a frozen section. It was, in fact, with a frozen section that the whole sequence of events began.

The error-based deferral of mastectomy may or may not have prejudiced the course of the disease. We cannot know but at any rate the patient remains alive and well 7 years later. Even so, this must be accounted as an *under-diagnosis*.

### COMMENTARY ON LOCAL SERIES

There has been a tendency towards the over-diagnosis as carcinoma of epithelial overgrowths still apparently confined to ducts. In view of the persisting uncertainties of diagnostic criteria for the confirmation of intraduct carcinoma, shortly to be discussed, this is not surprising. What is surprising, as with enlarged prostates, multiple myomas in the uterus, and large ovarian tumours, is that no patient has reappeared with an obvious carcinoma months or years after the diagnosing as innocuous of a mass removed at biopsy. The explanation may be that the identification and selection of areas as 'suspicious' by the pathologist has been skilful, or that areas which certainly are malignant are always obviously so (this is hardly likely and certainly is not applicable in the case of myomas in the uterus) but at any rate the state of affairs is reassuring. Much the same applies to the selection of areas from a biopsy for frozen-section examination. However, of recent years we have experienced two instances where the larger number of paraffin sections showed carcinoma in a biopsy specimen that was reported, on frozen-section, to be benign. If a first section shows no evidence of malignancy, further blocks must be cut: the surgeon should be asked to continue to wait.

## General Commentary

Not every neoplastic or possibly preneoplastic lesion that may occur in the breast will be considered here. Attention will be given rather to those lesions in the local series that have posed particular problems and to prognostic difficulties in general.

### Dysplasia

For manifest reasons, probably more has been written about the dysplasias of the breast than about any other precancerous or possibly precancerous lesion. The extent to which the various types of lesion are precancerous has been endlessly debated, but however the data are collected and assessed, few authorities now doubt that women who have had a lesion of some dysplastic type removed from a breast are at greater risk of subsequent cancer than those who have not. One of the most comprehensive surveys, based on reports world-wide, was provided by Davis and his colleagues (1964) who concluded that the risk to a patient with 'cystic disease' of developing carcinoma was double that to a patient without it. In continuation of his long interest in the matter Dr Shields Warren in company with co-authors (Monson et al., 1976) concluded from the history of 733 women with 'chronic mastitis' over 30 years that the risk of their developing carcinoma was 2½ times that of normal women. A slightly different attitude is held by Haagensen and his colleagues (1972) who consider it wrong to include all the forms of dysplastic lesion as simple 'fibrocystic disease'. They believe that some forms are innocuous but, even so, are of the opinion that at least grossly cystic change and multiple intraduct papillomatosis must be regarded as precancerous. A main and universal difficulty in the way of study of the significance of fibrocystic disease (FCD), whether prospective, retrospective, or current, is variation in the quality and/or consistency of diagnostic criteria. This has long been acknowledged and is still short of solution. Thus, Silverberg and his associates (1972), who studied the tissues from 398 mastectomy specimens and found no increased incidence of FCD in carcinomatous breasts, still were obliged to remark that ". . . the variation in criteria of different authors for accepting this diagnosis (i.e. FCD) makes any detailed quantitative comparison meaningless". The complexities of the matter were well described in a recent account (Editorial, 1972) that suggested the desirability of a ". . . well-designed interdisciplinary study of benign and malignant breasts . . ." in an attempt to lessen the still-prevailing uncertainty. Until this comes about there is much to be said for applying to the dysplastic lesions in general the phrase that Gallager and Martin (1969) apply to the hyperplastic variety, namely, ". . . a non-obligate preneoplastic lesion". The slightly paradoxical element in the phrase expresses well the uncertainty inherent in the diagnosing of any cancer at an early stage by microscopy (and thus the parallel uncertainty how best to treat the lesion). If a lesion could be regarded beyond question as no longer non-obligate but obligate, we should find ourselves in the position well described by Hutter (1971): ". . . if we can consistently identify an obligate precursor to metastasizing cancer we can establish a cure rate of 100%. However, once we become that successful we may be told that the reason our cure rate is so high is that we are not really treating an obligate precursor to metastasizing cancer". In cold logic, the implication of a lesion in the breast, regarded by a pathologist as a cause for concern, is clear. Maximum safety still lies only in bilateral mastectomy. Anything less than this involves a risk of some degree and it is the responsibility of the pathologist to help his clinical colleague to calculate the risk. The limitations in this are severe, and the pathologist can usually do little more than say, from his histological evidence and accumulated experience, that the risk is high or low, and this, in turn, will generally mean a risk of at least 50% at one extreme and 1% or less at the other. Thereafter the decision lies with the surgeon, for only he knows fully the clinical circumstances including technical possibilities and the psyche of his patient.

### Lobular Carcinoma In Situ

Lobular carcinoma in situ (LCIS), possibly described first by Sheild (1898) though by no specific name, and recognised and designated by Muir (1941) as 'intra-acinous carcinoma', was given prominence and its present name by Foote and Stewart (1941). Since then, its histological features have been well described by many observers, for example, McDivitt et al., 1968; Hutter and Foote, 1969; and Warner, 1969, as has its infiltrating form (Ashikari et al., 1973) and variants thereof (Fechner, 1975). The histology will not be further described here. Rather, it is appropriate to consider the prognostic and therapeutic implications, an aspect that has for years understandably concerned surgeons and pathologists.

Like carcinoma in situ elsewhere, LCIS is an early cancer at least in the sense that it is diagnosable only by microscopy. It is referred to by Farrow (1970) as one of the two "earliest of early breast cancers" (his other is intraduct carcinoma, referred to presently). Time had to pass after 1941 before its prognostic significance emerged, and this is now available. The history of 40 patients was given by Lewison and Finney (1968). All but one were living and well 2–11 years later: local excision had been used in three, and some form of mastectomy[1] in the others. A similar study was made by Hutter and Foote (1969) on 46 patients followed for 4–27 years. Only 6 had mastectomy, the other 40 had no treatment after the biopsy. None of the 6 subsequently developed cancer; of the 40, 15 subsequently developed cancer, mostly ipsilateral but in some cases contralateral or bilateral. Of the cancers (in 15 of 46 or 33% of the patients), 75% were regarded as 'infiltrating'; 2 patients died with metastases, and 2 were alive with metastases. Understandably, the authors recommended mastectomy as the treatment of choice for LCIS. The series of 270 patients reported by Farrow (1970) had been under observation for a much shorter time but this author also recommends mastectomy, as does Schiodt (1971). LCIS was included with several other lesions of the breast such as non-infiltrating duct carcinoma and Paget's disease with non-infiltrating carcinoma, by Wanebo, Huvos and Urban (1974) in a category of 'minimal breast cancer' which these workers also believe should be treated by mastectomy. In contrast to this attitude is that of Ackerman and Katzenstein (1977) who state that ". . . lobular carcinoma in situ should not be considered 'minimal' cancer. It may be only a marker for cystic disease and it is even possible that it could spontaneously regress". Similarly, Haagensen and colleagues (1972) and Wheeler and colleagues (1974) believe that prolonged and careful supervision of patients with LCIS is an adequate safeguard. In line with this approach, Haagensen, both here and elsewhere (1971), campaigns strongly for abolition of the term LCIS and for its replacement by 'lobular neoplasia'. He believes essentially that for a lesion so seldom followed by metastasising cancer, designation as a form of carcinoma is unjustifiable and, since perhaps needlessly alarming, also unwarranted. The same group of workers (Haagensen et al., 1978) have further underlined their attitude, thus: "We all agree and wish to emphasize that our data regarding the predisposition to subsequent carcinoma in patients with lobular neoplasia do not justify prophylactic subcutaneous mastectomy and plastic reconstruction of the breasts".

The debatable nature of this line of reasoning may be emphasised by quoting the prognostic assessment of the lesion as given by Haagensen and his colleagues in their 1972 paper, "The chance of developing carcinoma during a subsequent 4 to 25 year period is approximately 25 per cent for the breast in which lobular neoplasia was found, and 10 per cent for the contralateral breast".

The even higher figure of 30% for involvement of the opposite breast in association with LCIS was found by Urban (1969), and almost exactly the same proportion, 14 of 49 patients (and in 3 of these 14 invasive carcinoma was discovered at the subsequent mastectomy) by Carter and Smith (1977). This would seem to many to be an ample reason for ringing an alarm bell of some kind: how muffled or modified the tone for the patient is ultimately the surgeon's decision.

---

[1] No consideration is given in this chapter to the type of mastectomy performed: simple, radical, modified radical or ultraradical. Those with a mainly surgical interest know well the pros and cons of the various procedures. So far as the patient is concerned, either the breast(s) is removed or it is not. For these two situations, I shall use the terms 'mastectomy' and 'local excision' (or biopsy) respectively. The procedure of partial mastectomy, briefly mentioned on p. 14, is not yet used widely enough to be relevant in this general assessment but its impact on the whole question of the treatment of carcinoma of the breast is likely to be great.

In practice, for various reasons, certainty in the diagnosing of LCIS is difficult to attain. Not only are there qualitative differences, there are quantitative differences as well. Thus, according to Ashikari et al. (1974) ". . . no diagnosis of in situ lobular carcinoma should be made if only a single microscopic lobule was involved by cells otherwise meeting the criteria of lobular carcinoma", a concept introduced earlier by Hutter (1971) when he asked, "How many lobules must be involved before we can make a diagnosis of lobular in situ carcinoma?" This is a novel concept, wide in its implications, dubious in its logic. The pathologist frequently makes a diagnosis of cancer, perhaps in bronchus or oesophagus, on much less tissue than there is in a mammary lobule, and does so with confidence. The hesitation to make a diagnosis of LCIS on the changes in just a single lobule is understandable but is no more than an index of the uncertainty and fallibility unavoidably inherent in the assessment. Either the tissue pattern is regarded as truly neoplastic or it is not. If tissue of identical appearance in many lobules (should it be 2 or 3 or $x$?) is regarded as neoplastic, then it must in logic be regarded equally as neoplastic if present in only one lobule. LCIS may clinically be a low-grade carcinoma but histologically, like other cancers, its diagnosis should properly rest on qualitative rather than quantitative evidence.

Current texts make scarcely a mention of the changes that precede the stage most would accept as warranting diagnosis as LCIS; LCIS would seem almost an all-or-none condition, yet there are such changes. They were recognised by the original observers (thus Muir [1941], "It is impossible to state when malignancy actually occurs"; and Foote and Stewart, "there is . . . a graded progressive increase in cell size so gradual that demarcation is impossible"), and they comprise a classical borderline situation with all its attendant difficulties. The circumstances are closely analogous to those surrounding carcinoma in situ of the cervix. There is uncertainty amongst pathologists, and, as we have been, even when the pathologist has made a positive diagnosis, uncertainty also amongst surgeons on how best to treat the lesion. Unless great care is taken, and the lesion always classified separately, the widening recognition of LCIS and its being increasingly diagnosed correctly or incorrectly, represents a significant threat to the reliability of statistics relating to what is still widely accepted as a single uniform entity, namely, 'carcinoma of the breast'.

Opinions vary on the value of frozen section examination. Whatever the effort, the risk will still remain that tissue obtained for frozen sections will be 'negative' and the later paraffin sections 'positive', and the prudent surgeon will no doubt anticipate this by appropriate advice in advance to his patient. Sampling error apart, it is assessment of the recognisably abnormal tissue itself that is debatable. Thus, to quote McDivitt and his colleagues (1968), "If in situ lobular carcinoma is contained in the frozen section, it is, in most instances, sufficiently distinctive to be diagnostic. The use of the cryostat for frozen sections has helped tremendously in this respect". In contrast is the opinion of Warner (1969) that ". . . diagnosis of lobular carcinoma in situ by frozen section is hazardous and unreliable", an opinion confirmed by his further experience in company with other workers (Benefield et al., 1972) and also that of Farrow (1970) with his 270 cases of LCIS; in 176 cases (65%) the tissue was reported on frozen section as benign, i.e. false-negative diagnosis, in the remaining 94 as "suspicious or malignant with quick paraffin sections recommended". As Farrow virtually acknowledged, unreliability of this order is unacceptable.

INTRADUCT CARCINOMA

Besides fibrocystic disease or 'chronic mastitis', of which LCIS may be a feature, and LCIS per se, the intraductal proliferations pose an equal problem. The question essentially is, To what extent may epithelial cells occupy a duct and still be regarded as benign? The epithelium may be arranged around or be supported by few or many cores of fibrovascular tissue. Then, at least, the overgrowth is a papillary lesion: the problem is that of papilloma vs papillary carcinoma, one frequently difficult to solve and substantially the same as that commonly met with in the urinary bladder or nasal cavity. Its relevance to lesions in the breast has been described by Kraus and Neubecker (1962). At other times, the exuberant epithelium does not have this papillary arrangement but is 'solid', whether sheet-like or cribriform, and whether occupying the whole or only part of a duct or ducts. The cytology of the hyperplastic epithelium may be such that it would in any context be diagnosed as indicating carcinoma in situ; the diagnosis then is intraduct carcinoma. With a minor exception, the infrequency of mitoses, this was in essence the criterion used by Ashikari and his associates (1971), thus, "The loss of cell polarity and variation in size and shape of duct-lining cells are the most significant histologic alterations in intraductal carcinoma. Nuclear hyperchromasia and increased numbers of mitotic cells were rarely seen". The same stand is taken by Fechner (1971) where cellular pleomorphism is taken as the distinguishing feature between, on the one hand, intraduct carcinoma involving lobules and, on the other, LCIS. The importance of this distinction lies in the implications for the other breast. LCIS is relatively frequently bilateral, thus raising the question of bilateral mastectomy; intraduct carcinoma seems much less likely to be bilateral. As Fechner says, "Carcinoma in a lobule is not necessarily lobular carcinoma". Guidance on the significance of cellular polymorphism by Mc-Divitt and co-workers (1968) is equivocal. Their textual description emphasises the atypia, hyperchromatism and anaplasia of the cells; yet many of the examples they illustrate have notably uniform cytology.

The problem therefore reduces itself to the significance of overgrowing cells that are uniform, whether solid or cribriform in pattern, occupying the duct(s) in whole or in part. This pattern was well described many years ago by Dawson (1933) and designated 'epitheliosis', that is, a benign overgrowth. It was used in the same sense by McGillivray (1969) who examined the implications of the lesion and concluded very reasonably that almost certainly much of the wide variation in figures of incidence of mammary carcinoma in association with 'chronic mastitis' is owed to variation in interpretation of the significance of intraductal epitheliosis; the incidence of carcinoma will vary directly with the diagnostic threshold of the pathologist. Undoubtedly, the lesion is commonly innocuous or, at least, sufficiently slow in development to allow its removal at an innocuous

stage. Thus, in McGillivray's 30 cases of 'chronic mastitis with epitheliosis', the incidence of invasive carcinoma after excision 2–12 years earlier was nil.

The so-called cribriform pattern in intraductal growths, whether with polymorphic or monomorphic cells, merits examination. Its general appearance is well known. Sometimes the spaces are lined by radially arranged columnar cells to produce well-formed glandular differentiation; at others, the spaces appear to be simply holes in a flat sheet of cells with no such radial margination. The two patterns are clearly expressions of different degrees of differentiation, yet there are few if any accounts of the possible prognostic significance of the difference; there may be no difference but it is surprising that information on the matter is so scanty if not nonexistent. The pattern per se is widely regarded as virtually diagnostic of intraduct carcinoma; thus, Haagensen (1971) states dogmatically that it is an "unmistakable sign" and an "absolute indication" of carcinoma. The implication of this is that a cribriform pattern can never be formed by benign cells, or, vice versa, that all cells that form such a pattern are ipso facto carcinomatous.

In examining this further, let us recall that we have disposed of the cases where the cells are sufficiently aberrant to justify a diagnosis of, in effect, carcinoma in situ. We are considering cells that are essentially uniform, sometimes showing glandular differentiation and sometimes not. We must then ask: (a) whether a duct can ever be totally occupied by cells that are benign and simply hyperplastic; that is, is epitheliosis in its original sense an acceptable entity?; (b) whether, if so, the appearance per se of round holes in a sheet of such cells transforms the cells from benign to malignant? If the answer to the second question is 'Yes' we are saying that a mammary duct or ductule can never be wholly occupied by cells that are benign; that is, that a benign hyperplasia never occurs and that epitheliosis is not an acceptable entity. This seems to me either untenable or forcing us to acknowledge that the epithelium of mammary ducts is unique amongst epithelia in being able to exist in two forms only, normal or malignantly neoplastic, never hyperplastic. It is surely more reasonable to believe that the epithelium of the mammary duct can, like any other epithelium, indulge in a benign hyperplasia and, again like other epithelia, suffer a gradual change with growing aberrancy to become acceptable at some stage as carcinoma in situ. This was the original concept as held by Muir (1941) who went even further in saying that "The forms and arrangement of epithelial cells in precancerous hyperplasia are of endless variety". On general pathological principles this appears a sounder assessment of the histology than the just-mentioned all-or-none principle that current attitudes seem to demand. Direct evidence on which to judge is harder to provide but I can say at any rate that in some laboratories it has been the practice over many years to make a diagnosis of intraduct epitheliosis when ducts have been occupied by seemingly benign epithelium, even in the presence of a cribriform pattern of some degree, without the patients appearing later with manifest carcinoma.

Much obviously depends on the significance accorded to cytological detail. As mentioned earlier, somewhere along the line of increasing aberrancy the pathologist will decide that the epithelium, whether intraduct or intra-acinous, is so aberrant as to merit diagnosis as 'malignant'. At the other end of the scale, paradoxically, the very uniformity of the epithelium may raise suspicion. If, for example, the epithelium were as regular as that of, say, an argentaffin carcinoma, would it have the same neoplastic significance? Thus, McDivitt and his colleagues (1968) remarked of the ductal lesion with a cribriform pattern that it may infiltrate and metastasise even though, as they frequently comment, there is little cellular pleomorphism and a generally uniform and monotonous pattern. Perhaps, sometimes, utter uniformity can be a sinister uniformity. The possibility has not to my knowledge been closely examined; it seems ripe for histometric analysis.

The cribriform pattern should not be confused with the rather similar pattern that may be produced by the relatively uncommon *adenoid cystic carcinoma* of the breast. An important prognostic point is that carcinoma of this type does not have in the breast the gloomy prognosis that it has at other sites. The explanation may be its usually smaller size at the time of diagnosis, and the greater likelihood of total removal when in the breast than elsewhere (Cavanzo and Taylor, 1969).

## PAGET'S DISEASE OF THE NIPPLE

No one likely to read this text will be unfamiliar with debate on the origin and evolution of Paget's disease. It is still not wholly resolved. There is no intention to add to that debate here but only to cite some data concerning its prognostic significance. Even this would have seemed unnecessary but for a realisation, from random casual questioning, that surgeons and pathologists are generally less familiar with the outlook for a patient with Paget's disease than with straightforward mammary carcinoma; and also a statement recently received from a surgeon of some experience that many still believe thelectomy alone to be adequate treatment. In fact, few surely now doubt that, even for Paget's disease with no associated palpable mass in the breast, simple mastectomy is the least that is required.

A series of 140 patients with the disease was described by Maier and his colleagues (1969). Of these patients 88 had been under observation long enough to reveal a 5-year survival rate of 52.3%. The extremes of the range were, at one end, a rate of the order of 90% for those with no palpable mass in the breast and no involvement of axillary nodes, and, at the other, inoperability. Further points worth citing from this report are that Paget's disease in the premenopausal woman is more dangerous than in the postmenopausal, and that absence of a palpable mass in the breast is no guarantee against metastasis. This last finding was the experience also of Ashikari and his associates (1970) who found amongst patients with no palpable mass an incidence of axillary involvement of 6% and 17% respectively in those diagnosed early (6 months or less from first recognition) and late. In all, in their series of 214 cases, 96 had no preoperatively palpable mass, and of these 13% had axillary nodal metastasis. All of the 209 operable cases were treated by some form of mastectomy with an overall survival rate of 60% at 10 years. As would be expected, and as was found also by Gregl and co-workers (1968), the overriding prognostic factor is the involvement or noninvolvement of axillary nodes.

## CYSTOSARCOMA PHYLLODES

In the case of Paget's disease, histological diagnosis is usually straightforward and the prognostic implications relatively clear: mastectomy is virtually mandatory. In the case of cystosarcoma phyllodes, matters are otherwise. Histological diagnosis is again usually straightforward but the prognostic implications are uncertain and the place of mastectomy debatable. All too often a satisfyingly sharp distinction between 'benign' and 'malignant' cannot be made: the level of histoclinical correlation is too low. However, useful guidance has been given by Norris and Taylor (1967) who found a broad correlation between cellular atypia and survival. No example proved fatal that was less than 4 cm in diameter or had fewer than three mitotic figures per 10 hpf in any area, while of 30 showing 'minimal cytologic atypism' of stromal cells, only two proved fatal. Their recommendation is wide local excision for the 'smaller' neoplasm (presumably less than 4 cm in diameter) and simple mastectomy for the larger, with low axillary nodal dissection in addition for patients with palpable nodes and/or neoplasms greater than 4 cm in diameter and/or showing more than two mitotic figures per 10 hpf. Radical mastectomy produced no better survival rates than simple mastectomy. In the smaller series (32 cases) of Maier and co-workers (1968), ten patients were regarded histologically as having a 'malignant' lesion, and of these seven died within five years.

A series of 42 patients with the lesion was divided by Pietruszka and Barnes (1978), on the basis of the Norris/Taylor criteria, into 18 benign, 19 malignant and 5 borderline examples. Local recurrence occurred in all three groups but metastasis was seen only among those in the 'malignant' group (it occurred in four patients, three of whom died). The essential morphological distinction between the three groups was incidence of mitotic figures per area of tissue, namely, 0–4, 5–9 and 10 or more respectively per 10 hpf ($\times$ 400 magnification).

According to Hoover and his associates (1975), some 34 examples have been reported in patients aged less than 20 years, all but four of them benign (the four regarded as malignant were treated surgically and all were well at the time of reporting). These authors were themselves reporting an example that recurred locally then fatally metastasised in a girl of 14 years. The neoplasm may occasionally show squamous metaplasia, and one such case was included in the series of squamous-celled carcinoma of the breast reported by Cornog and his colleagues (1971). Here, however, as with its occurrence in other mammary neoplasms, squamous-celled differentiation carries no prognostic message of value. Cystosarcoma phyllodes should be accorded more than the 'rarely malignant' reputation it widely enjoys.

## PROGNOSIS

### Influence of Age

Apart from the generally acknowledged worsening of prognosis with pregnancy and the puerperium, opinions have varied whether younger age per se is similarly significant: even Haagensen (1971) states no more than a 'clinical impression' that his younger patients had a rather poorer prognosis than the older. Three representative series have figures pointing in the same direction. In the almost 9,000 patients analysed by Mausner and his associates (1969), where carcinoma was confined to the breast, survival rates for those aged 39 or less were marginally poorer than those of the others but survival rates were convincingly poorer in patients with axillary node involvement (rather surprisingly, of those with axillary involvement, the group with the best survival figures were those aged 40–49). A group of 101 patients all aged less than 35 years was studied by Brightmore and his colleagues (1970). These authors used for comparison the overall figures 'in most series' of 50% survival at 5 years, 30% at 10 years; in their own series of younger patients, the corresponding figures were 36% and 18%. From their study of 135 patients aged less than 30 years, Norris and Taylor (1970) consider the prognosis 'slightly poorer' than in older women but that this is due to some extent in most series to the inclusion of patients pregnant or in the puerperium. In contrast to this, however, are the results of an analysis by Wallgren and colleagues (1977) of the outcome in 75 patients also aged less than 30 years. These authors found not only that the survival rate for this group was not significantly worse than for patients of all ages but also that the survival rate of their 15 patients either pregnant or diagnosed as having mammary carcinoma within 1 year of delivery was no worse than that of their other patients whose carcinoma was not thus complicated.

It is difficult to know how truly comparable a group of such series is, especially internationally, and in this context the study by Norris and Taylor is particularly valuable in showing the need for careful analysis of the many factors involved before generalisations can be made about the relationship between age and prognosis. However, it is probably true, on the basis of evidence like the above, that the prognosis is rather worse for the younger woman. It is also probably true that this has little bearing on the elements of treatment that are technical. It is certainly true that it has a very large bearing on the elements of treatment that are psychological. If we ask, may it also have an influence on the diagnosing of the lesion by the pathologist, the answer must be almost always 'Yes'. This merits a closer look, for attitudes are oddly ambivalent.

In the case of borderline mammary lesions, foreknowledge of the age of the patient, here as elsewhere, inescapably and ineradicably conditions the pathologist; objective assessment is virtually impossible. A lesion of this kind is with little doubt more likely to be diagnosed as malignant than nonmalignant in the peri- or postmenopausal patient but nonmalignant rather than malignant in the younger patient (and the younger the patient, the greater the leaning towards the nonmalignant diagnosis). There is, therefore, a tendency at least towards overdiagnosis in all but the youngest patient; its degree will never be known for its existence is not even suspected. That this is so becomes clear when so often the first question from a pathologist examining such a section is "How old is the patient?" The comment, if the pathologist is told 'aged 55' may well be "At this age, very suspicious, almost certainly malignant, mastectomy is the only safe course"; on the other hand, if the information is 'aged 25', the comment may equally be, "At this age, with malignancy so rare, almost certainly no more than extreme hyperplasia, mastectomy should not be performed". By acting like this, so reluctant are we to counsel mastectomy in the young woman, we stretch histology to its limits and in so doing, perhaps without fully realising

it, take so much the greater a gamble. This approach is saying in effect that the one histological pattern may mean two different things depending on the age of the patient; if aged 55, 'cancer', if aged 25, 'not cancer'. Quite apart from the difficulties of decision with the same lesion at ages 45 and 35, this is a most dubious proposition with little evidence to support it. The paradox is that the younger the patient, the greater the number of years of life that would be saved by removing a presumably early cancer: logically, attempts to remove all possible risk should be all the more energetic. This, of course, is not done: minimal mutilation or no mutilation is the wish of all, and many would defend the view that to incur some extra risk is justified in trying to achieve it. This attitude is understandable and reasonable but, when we adopt it, as histopathologists we should be clear what we are doing. We are 'bending' the histology, fixed and factual though it be, to fit the desired therapeutic end. Defensible as this may be, it blunts pathological precision. The hope must be that the spreading practice of partial mastectomy with reconstruction will provide a way round the problem or, in the current phrase, let everyone 'off the hook'. In the case of malignant disease of the breast this will be a practical solution but it does not make the problem go away. Quite the same problem remains elsewhere, as, for example, in rectum and uterus, and there is no comparable way round there.

The dangers of age-induced diagnostic bias were fully appreciated by Elston and his colleagues (1978) in their just-cited report. They stated that the assessment of both 'Tru-Cut' and cytological specimens was reported ". . . without knowledge of patients' ages or other clinical details".

## Clinical 'Staging'

The cancer literature is replete with data on the survival rates of patients with carcinoma of the breast grouped according to generally agreed schemes of clinical 'staging'. At some sites, for example the cervix uteri, the staging of the lesion has a great bearing on the type of treatment used. In the case of the breast this matters less, to the extent, at any rate, that a diagnosis of carcinoma, however classified, will mean some form of mastectomy. By this time the patient will be assignable to one of the recognised clinical stages, and to that further extent will have a predictable prognosis. Can the pathologist now, considering the individual patient, define the prognosis any more narrowly: and, if so, will it help?

### Size of Neoplasm

The main factor determining the prognosis for an individual patient is with little doubt the intrinsic biological aggressiveness of the neoplasm. Nevertheless, the broad belief remains that smaller neoplasms are prognostically less gloomy than larger neoplasms, and confirmation of this has been provided by Fisher and his colleagues (1969). Even so, according to the careful observations and calculations of these authors (data from more than 2000 patients), the advantages accruing to a patient from smallness of tumour per se are relatively restricted: if all tumours of 20 mm had been removed when 10 mm, recurrence rates might have decreased, and five-year survival rates increased, by some 10%–20%.

Fisher and his colleagues also usefully analyse an immediately relevant topic, one more widely familiar now than a few decades ago, namely, the implications—and potentially misleading implications—of the terms 'early' and 'late' when applied to the growth of cancers.

### Structural Differentiation

Many schemes have subdivided mammary carcinoma in accordance with many variables such as degree of glandular (tubular) differentiation, cellular polymorphism, and nuclear character as, for example, those of Bloom (1950, 1974), Tough and co-workers (1969) and Black along with others (1975). As would be expected, there is a degree of correlation between increasing anaplasia and decreasing survival but generally it is low; neoplasms of any histological grade may be found at any clinical stage. The medullary and predominantly syncytial form of carcinoma, however, has been reported by Ridolfi and his associates (1977) as having appreciably better survival rates than the commoner infiltrating duct carcinoma. In the hope of achieving greater precision, individual characteristics have been assessed such as the nuclear grade (Bell et al., 1969), the general character of individual neoplastic cells (Hartveit, 1971), and the size of the neoplasm as a whole (Fisher et al., 1969), and all have some, although again limited, predictive value. The discovery of wild anaplasia and massive lymphatic invasion might help to determine a more aggressive policy for the radiotherapist but this is debatable; much would depend on local practice and procedure. It is doubtful if even the most detailed pathological grading can do much more for the individual patient. Indeed, the general position at present has been well summarised by Hutter (1974) when he says that ". . . the most and the least favorable breast cancers are usually clinically evident and pathologic parameters add little prognostic information". However, this is not to say that the definition of histological minutiae is of academic interest only. With the spreading use of chemotherapy, and immunotherapy always in the background, all information is important and may at any time turn out to be prognostically and therapeutically vital.

### Involvement of Lymph Nodes

The predictive value of extent of nodal involvement is limited. Some hold that it increases in direct proportion to the number of nodes examined and found to be, or not to be, invaded. In the light of the detailed analysis by Fisher and Slack (1970) of specimens from more than 2000 patients, this may be doubted. These observers found that patients with 5 to 10 nodes negative had essentially the same prognosis as those with 25 to 30 negative. Similarly, in patients with positive nodes, little difference existed between those with one to five involved and those with more than 30 involved: also, patients with two nodes positive out of five examined were at no greater risk than those with two nodes positive out of 30 examined. These observations bring into question the often expressed opinion that the outlook for patients with fewer than four nodes involved is markedly better than for those with four nodes or more involved. There is a difference, it is true, but in some series at any rate hardly enough to weigh heavily in prognosis. A series of 826 patients (from 25 centres) observed over 10 years was analysed by Fisher and his colleagues (1975). These observers found that 76% of all patients with positive nodes 'demonstrated a treatment failure' during the 10 years: the figure of 76% was derived from 65% of the patients with one to three, and 86% of those with four or more nodes involved. Overall, the survival rate of patients with one to three nodes involved was 37.5%, and of those with four or more involved only 13.4%. Further, ". . . even one of every four patients with negative nodes had a treatment failure". The more realistic dividing line would appear to be, not four nodes involved or less, but one node or none.

A related investigation was carried out by Fisher and his colleagues (1978) into the significance of 'occult' metastases: that is, nodal metastases discovered only on the semiserial sectioning of nodes originally, on a single section, reported as negative. In a series of 78 patients, metastasis of this type hitherto unsuspected was discovered in 24%: yet its presence bore no relation to the 5-year survival rate. The summarising conclusion of these investigators was that, ". . . attempts to detect occult metastases by extending histopathological methods may be more academic than practical or therapeutically significant".

There is even so a belief in some quarters that anything less than the detailed examination by the pathologist of every node and nodule, if necessary as small as 1 mm, in an excised axillary mass is a shortcoming. On the other hand, the observations just cited suggest otherwise. Be that as it may: either detailed information on every node is demonstrably essential or it is not. If it is essential, the pathologist will try to ascertain it so far as is possible (the serial sectioning of nodes, if not impracticable, is not realistically practical, yet simple bisection is inadequate: a feasible compromise suggested by Wilkinson and Hause (1974) is division of a 5-mm node into 1-mm slices, and division of a larger node into four equally spaced blocks). If such detailed information is not demonstrably essential, the pathologist will want to know how many nodes the surgeon would wish him to examine.

The whole topic is meantime surrounded by some uncertainty and stands in need of rigorous review, not least because quite the same considerations apply elsewhere, as, for example, with cervical nodes in relation to carcinoma of the tongue or larynx, or with pelvic nodes in the case of carcinoma of the uterus, or in similar

circumstances anywhere. Since international comparisons are understandably being increasingly made, particularly in search of better chemotherapy, it is desirable that international agreement be reached at least on the technique of examination of lymph nodes: unless some such technique as that suggested by Wilkinson and Hause is adopted, there can be no guarantee that a 'negative' node really is a negative node.

A sombre comment on the significance of axillary nodal metastasis made by Fisher and many colleagues (1977), from their observations on 1665 patients, is that "These observations provide substance to the conviction that positive axillary lymph nodes are not the predecessor of distant tumor spread but represent one manifestation of disseminated disease".

Of associated phenomena, the significance of sinus histiocytosis in lymph nodes (Black and Asire, 1969; Silverberg et al., 1970) has yet to be assessed as has that of elastosis (Azzopardi and Laurini, 1974), now recognised as the true nature of the yellow streaks seen in a scirrhous carcinoma rather than the formerly believed necrosis. Its presence may indicate early infiltration from an intraduct carcinoma and should be regarded with suspicion when seen in the apparent absence of carcinoma (further blocks should be taken) but, as Azzopardi and Laurini say, its importance and predictive value have yet to be fully evaluated. A potentially misleading appearance may be seen sometimes in benign lesions of the breast, namely, the invasion of nerves or nerve sheaths (Taylor and Norris, 1967; Davies, 1973) or the walls of blood vessels (Eusebi and Azzopardi, 1976) in sclerosing adenosis or other benign dysplasias. In the experience of Taylor and Norris this had led on three occasions to mastectomy but the above authorities are all agreed that the 'invasion' is harmless and benign. Attention should be paid to the character of the infiltrating cells: they were described by Taylor and Norris as ". . . uniform cells with bland nuclei and no appreciable cytologic atypism".

An axillary node may on occasion contain glandular or glanduliform structures superficially resembling carcinoma. The phenomenon is rare but, as described by Garret and Ada (1957), when found in association with sclerosing adenosis or intraduct hyperplasia in the breast, its potential significance in relation to diagnosis and treatment is obviously great. Similar structures may be found in nodes elsewhere, most commonly in those related to salivary glands. They are believed by Garret and Ada to be of maldevelopmental origin comparable to that of the dermoid cyst of skin.

A further potentially prognostic, and directly measurable, feature yet to be fully assessed is the incidence of mast cells in axillary nodes. A retrospective survey of the nodes of 43 patients by Bowers and his colleagues (1979) yielded a five-year survival rate of 23/27 with 11 cells or more, but one of only 3/16 with 10 cells or less, per sq mm ($p < 0.001$).

### Apparent Stromal Invasion

The frailty of 'breaching of the basement membrane' as a criterion of malignancy has already been noted. Its status in lesions of the breast and particularly its correlation with ultramicroscopic observations have been studied by Busch (1969) and also by Ozzello and Sanpitak (1970) who concluded, inter alia, that "no correlation can be demonstrated between the PAS-positive 'basement membranes' seen with the light microscope and the 'basal laminae' visualised with the electron microscope. In corresponding sections, the latter may be clearly visible while the former are not, and vice versa", and also that "no clear-cut causal relationship between invasive process and absence of basal laminae was demonstrated". Their investigations confirm the earlier observations of Ozzello (1970) that the epithelial-stromal junction in the breast, and by inference elsewhere, is a zone of great biological activity and far from a band or lamina that may or may not be simply 'breached'. For these reasons, and since many examples are on record of carcinoma's metastasising while still apparently intraductal (in 4 of 38 examples reported by Carter and Smith, 1977 for example), any operative procedure less than mastectomy for intraduct carcinoma is hazardous.

The mimicry of stromal invasion by sclerosing adenosis is now widely familiar. Advice on another diagnostically potential pitfall, pseudo-invasive but benign sclerotic papillary overgrowth around mammary ducts, has been given by Fenoglio and Lattes (1974). The pattern as shown in their illustrations has some similarity to that of sclerosing adenosis but, in their words,

"The 'pseudoinvasion' is limited to the immediate periductal zone. Involvement of the interlobular fat should suggest a true carcinoma".

### The Contralateral Breast

The possibility of carcinoma's developing later, or perhaps being already present, in the contralateral breast is an obvious prognostic problem. Several workers, from the time of the comprehensive analysis of Robbins and Berg (1964) onwards, have agreed that the risk of such a 'second' carcinoma is much greater than for a 'first' carcinoma. Thus, Schröder and Hüttner (1968) calculated from their 400 postmastectomy cases that such patients were at 20 times greater risk of contralateral carcinoma than the rest of the population. In the series of Urban (1969) already cited, the incidence of such 'second' carcinomas amongst 422 patients with carcinoma of all types was 15%: in the subgroup of LCIS, it will be recalled, the incidence was 30%. In Farrow's series (1970) bilateral involvement by some form of carcinoma, past, present or later, was experienced by as many as 44% of his patients. A similar difficulty is presented by patients who have had a biopsy revealing a benign lesion, whether neoplastic or dysplastic. According to Potter and his coworkers (1968) they are at risk of subsequent carcinoma of nearly fivefold compared with women who have never had a biopsy.

How best to obviate or reduce these risks varies from clinic to clinic. In some, continued close supervision is practised: in others, biopsy of the other breast at the time of mastectomy, with, if indicated, the second mastectomy: in a few, especially when the first breast contains LCIS, 'prophylactic' mastectomy of the other is performed. Mostly, however, it appears that a conservative approach is the more usual practice, and for understandable reasons. As Donegan and Perez-Mesa (1972) have said, "pressures for preservation of a culturally valued organ are allied with the general impression that routine harvest of breasts even among high risk patients is a task out of proportion to the expected benefits". These and other matters of current concern, including population-screening, are comprehensively described in the recently published proceeding of a Conference on Breast Cancer (Conference 1977).

It seems doubtful whether technical advances, be they mammographic, ultramicroscopic, immunological or other, will do much to reduce the amount of diagnostic uncertainty inherent in the microscopically borderline lesions of breast: rather, they may increase it, as did merely the designation of a particular pattern as LCIS. It may be that measurement of degree of nodal sinus histiocytosis, or of numbers of perilesional lymphocytes, will sharpen prognostic assessment but even then we shall still be drawing an arbitrary line across a range of values for both criteria, with 'mastectomy' in some form on the one side, and 'no further treatment' on the other. The same might apply if a causative virus were found: how many particles would warrant mastectomy?

## Conclusions

1) Lesions that may be overdiagnosed as carcinoma are intraduct epitheliosis and, less likely, sclerosing adenosis.

2) The lesion most likely to be underdiagnosed as carcinoma is a finely infiltrative carcinoma that mimics sclerosing adenosis.

3) The intraductal papillary growths remain diagnostically and prognostically a debatable group.

4) Diagnostic thresholds for LCIS vary widely.

5) Invasion of nerves, nerve sheaths and the walls of vessels may be seen in benign lesions: the morphology of the invading cells is important as a criterion for identification as benign.

6) Elastosis in seemingly non-neoplastic breasts is suspicious.

7) Papillary adenoma of the nipple may be mistaken for glandular carcinoma, especially on frozen section.

8) The explanation for a florid lobular overgrowth may be an unsuspected pregnancy.

9) An 'unusual' malignant tumour should prompt thoughts of metastasis from elsewhere including, in particular, malignant lymphoma and a leukaemic deposit (see Gralnick and Dittmar, 1969; Mambo et al., 1977). However, the rare, histologically misleading pseudolymphoma (Fisher et al., 1979) should not be forgotten.

10) The larger a mass submitted by a surgeon for frozen section, the longer he should be prepared to wait.

11) The practice of needle-biopsy as a preliminary procedure seems likely to grow.

## References

Ackerman LV, Katzenstein AL (1977) The concept of minimal breast cancer and the pathologist's role in the diagnosis of "early carcinoma". Cancer 39: 2755–2763

Ashikari R, Park K, Huvos AG, Urban JA (1970) Paget's disease of the breast. Cancer 26: 680–685

Ashikari R, Hajdu SI, Robbins GF (1971) Intraductal carcinoma of the breast (1960–1969). Cancer 28: 1182–1187

Ashikari R, Huvos AG, Urban JA, Robbins GF (1973) Infiltrating lobular carcinoma of the breast. Cancer 31: 110–116

Ashikari R, Huvos AG, Snyder RE, Lucas JC, Hutter RVP, McDivitt RW, Schottenfeld D (1974) A clinicopathologic study of atypical lesions of the breast. Cancer 33: 310–317

Atkins H, Hayward JL, Klugman DJ, Wayte AB (1972) Treatment of early breast cancer: A report after ten years of a clinical trial. Br Med J 2: 423–429

Azzopardi JG, Laurini RN (1974) Elastosis in breast cancer. Cancer 33: 174–183

Bell JR, Friedell GH, Goldenberg LS (1969) Prognostic significance of pathologic findings in human breast carcinoma. Surg Gynecol Obstet 129: 258–262

Benefield JR, Fingerhut AG, Warner NE (1972) A multidiscipline view of lobular breast carcinoma. Am Surg 38: 115–116

Black MM, Asire AJ (1969) Palpable axillary lymph nodes in cancer of the breast. Structural and biologic considerations. Cancer 23: 251–259

Black MM, Barclay THC, Hankey BF (1975) Prognosis in breast cancer utilizing histologic characteristics of the primary tumor. Cancer 36: 2048–2055

Bloom HJG (1950) Prognosis in carcinoma of the breast. Br J Cancer 4: 259–288

Bloom HJG (1974) Value of histology in prognosis and treatment policy in breast cancer. Frontiers of radiation therapy and oncology. 9th edn. The relationship of histology to cancer treatment. Karger, Basel, pp 112–136

Bowers HM, Mahapatro RC, Kennedy JW (1979) Numbers of mast cells in the axillary lymph nodes of breast cancer patients. Cancer 43: 568–573

Brightmore TGJ, Greening WP, Hamlin I (1970) An analysis of clinical and histopathological features in 101 cases of carcinoma of breast in women under 35 years of age. Br J Cancer 24: 644–669

Busch W (1969) Elektronenmikroskopische Untersuchungen an der Tumor Bindegewebsgrenze beim Mammacarcinom der Frau. Virchows Arch [Pathol Anat] 346: 15–28

Calle R, Pilleron JP, Schlienger P, Vilcoq JR (1978) Conservative management of operable breast cancer. Ten years experience at the Foundation Curie. Cancer 42: 2045–2053

Carter D, Smith RRL (1977) Carcinoma in situ of the breast. Cancer 40: 1189–1193

Cavanzo FJ, Taylor HB (1969) Adenoid cystic carcinoma of the breast. An analysis of 21 cases. Cancer 24: 740–745

Conference on Breast Cancer (1977). Cancer 39: 2697–2964

Cornog JL, Mobini J, Steiger E, Enterline HT (1971) Squamous carcinoma of the breast. Am J Clin Pathol 55: 410–417

Crile G (1975) Multicentric breast cancer. The incidence of new cancers in the homolateral breast after partial mastectomy. Cancer 35: 475–477

Davies JD (1973) Neural invasion in benign mammary dysplasia. J Pathol 109: 225–231

Davis HH, Simons M, Davis JB (1964) Cystic disease of the breast: Relationship to carcinoma. Cancer 17: 957–978

Dawson EK (1933) Carcinoma in the mammary lobule and its origin. Edinb Med J 40: 57–82

Donegan WL, Perez-Mesa CM (1972) Lobular carcinoma—an indication for elective biopsy of the second breast. Ann Surg 176: 178–187

Editorial (1972) Benign and malignant breasts. Lancet II: 218–219

Editorial (1976a) Early cancer of the breast: The way ahead. Lancet I: 1116

Editorial (1976b) Treating breast cancer—true light or false dawn? Br Med J 2: 263–264

Elston CW, Cotton RE, Davies CJ, Blamey RW (1978) A comparison of the use of the 'Tru-Cut' needle and fine needle aspiration cytology in the pre-operative diagnosis of carcinoma of the breast. Histopathol 2: 239–254

Eusebi V, Azzopardi JG (1976) Vascular infiltration in benign breast disease. J Pathol 118: 9–16

Farrow JH (1970) Current concepts in the detection and treatment of the earliest of the early breast cancers. Cancer 25: 468–477

Fechner RE (1971) Ductal carcinoma involving the lobule of the breast. Cancer 28: 274–281

Fechner RE (1975) Histologic variants of infiltrating lobular carcinoma of the breast. Hum Pathol 6: 373–378

Fenoglio C, Lattes R (1974) Sclerosing papillary proliferations in the female breast. A benign lesion often mistaken for carcinoma. Cancer 33: 691–700

Fisher B, Slack NH (1970) Number of lymph nodes examined and the prognosis of breast carcinoma. Surg Gynecol Obstet 131: 79–88

Fisher B, Slack NH, Bross IDJ (1969) Cancer of the breast: Size of neoplasm and prognosis. Cancer 24: 1071–1080

Fisher B, Slack N, Katrych D, Wolmark N (1975) Ten year follow-up results of patients with carcinoma of the breast in a co-operative clinical trial evaluating surgical adjuvant chemotherapy. Surg Gynecol Obstet 140: 528–534

Fisher B, Montague E, Redmond C, Barton B, 16 others (1977) Comparison of radical mastectomy with alternative treatments for primary breast cancer. A first report of results from a prospective randomized clinical trial. Cancer 39: 2827–2839

Fisher ER, Swamidoss S, Lee CH, Rockette H, Redmond C, Fisher B (1978) Detection and significance of occult axillary node metastases in patients with invasive breast cancer. Cancer 42: 2025–2031

Fisher ER, Palekar AS, Paulson JD, Golinger R (1979) Pseudolymphoma of breast. Cancer 44: 258–263

Foote FW, Stewart FW (1941) Lobular carcinoma in situ: A rare form of mammary cancer. Am J Pathol 17: 491–496

Gallager HS, Martin JE (1969) Early phases in the development of breast cancer. Cancer 24: 1170–1178

Garret R, Ada AEW (1957) Epithelial inclusion cysts in an axillary lymph node. Report of a case simulating metastatic adenocarcinoma. Cancer 10: 173–178

Gralnick HR, Dittmar K (1969) Development of myeloblastoma with massive breast and ovarian involvement during remission in acute leukemia. Cancer 24: 746–749

Gregl A, Stankovic P, Eydt M, Yu D (1968) Paget-Karzinom der Brustdrüse (Morphologie, Klinik, Therapie). Strahlentherapie 136: 650–656

Haagensen CD (1971) Diseases of the breast, 2nd edn. Saunders, Philadelphia

Haagensen CD, Lane N, Lattes R (1972) Neoplastic proliferation of the epithelium of the mammary lobules: Adenosis, lobular neoplasia, and small cell carcinoma. Surg Clin North Am 52: 497–524

Haagensen CD, Lane N, Lattes R, Bodian C (1978) Lobular neoplasia (so-called lobular carcinoma in situ) of the breast. Cancer 42: 737–769

Hartveit F (1971) Prognostic typing in breast cancer. Br Med J 4: 253–257

Hoover HC, Trestioreanu A, Ketcham AS (1975) Metastatic cystosarcoma phylloides in an adolescent girl: An unusually malignant tumor. Ann Surg 181: 279–282

Hutter RVP (1971) The pathologist's role in minimal breast cancer. Cancer 28: 1527–1536

Hutter RVP (1974) Pathology and progress in breast cancer. In: Vaeth JM (ed) Frontiers of radiation therapy and oncology, vol 9. The relationship of histology to cancer treatment. Karger, Basel, pp 96–111

Hutter RVP, Foote FW (1969) Lobular carcinoma

in situ: Long term follow-up. Cancer 24: 1081–1085

Kraus FT, Neubecker RD (1962) The differential diagnosis of papillary tumors of the breast. Cancer 15: 444–455

Lewison EF, Finney GG (1968) Lobular carcinoma in situ of the breast. Surg Gynecol Obstet 126: 1280–1286

MacGillivray JB (1969) The problem of 'chronic mastitis' with epitheliosis. J Clin Pathol 22: 340–347

McDivitt RW, Stewart FW, Berg JW (1968) Atlas of tumor pathology, 2nd ser, fasc 2. Tumors of the breast. Armed Forces Institute of Pathology, Washington, D.C.

Maier WP, Rosemond GP, Wittenberg P, Tassoni EM (1968) Cystosarcoma phyllodes mammae. Oncology 22: 145–158

Maier WP, Rosemond GP, Harasym EL, Al-Saleem TI, Tassoni EM, Schor SS (1969) Paget's disease in the female breast. Surg Gynecol Obstet 128: 1253–1263

Mambo NC, Burke JS, Butler JJ (1977) Primary malignant lymphomas of the breast. Cancer 39: 2033–2040

Mausner JS, Shimkin MB, Moss NH, Rosemond GP (1969) Cancer of the breast in Philadelphia hospitals, 1951–1964. Cancer 23: 260–274

Monson RR, Yen S, MacMahon B, Warren S (1976) Chronic mastitis and carcinoma of the breast. Lancet II: 224–226

Muir R (1941) The evolution of carcinoma of the mamma. J Pathol Bacteriol 52: 155–172

Norris HJ, Taylor HB (1967) Relationship of histologic features to behavior of cystosarcoma phyllodes: Analysis of ninety-four cases. Cancer 20: 2090–2099

Norris HJ, Taylor HB (1970) Carcinoma of the breast in women less than thirty years old. Cancer 26: 953–959

Ozzello L (1970) Epithelial-stromal junction of normal and dysplastic mammary glands. Cancer 25: 586–600

Ozzello L, Sanpitak P (1970) Epithelial-stromal junction of intraductal carcinoma of the breast. Cancer 26: 1186–1198

Park WW (1977) Pinning down the diagnosis in breast cancer. Br Med J 2: 519

Perzin KH, Lattes R (1972) Papillary adenoma of the nipple (florid papillomatosis, adenoma, adenomatosis). A clinicopathologic study. Cancer 29: 996–1009

Pietruszka M, Barnes L (1978) Cystosarcoma phyllodes. A clinicopathologic analysis of 42 cases. Cancer 41: 1974–1983

Potter JF, Slimbaugh WP, Woodward SC (1968) Can breast carcinoma be anticipated? A follow-up of benign breast biopsies. Ann Surg 167: 829–838

Ridolfi RL, Rosen PP, Port A, Kinne D, Miké V (1977) Medullary carcinoma of the breast. A clinicopathologic study with 10 year follow-up. Cancer 40: 1365–1385

Robbins GF, Berg JW (1964) Bilateral primary breast cancers. A prospective clinicopathological study. Cancer 17: 1501–1527

Schiodt T (1971) Lobulaert carcinoma in situ mammae. En oversigt. Nord Med 85: 45–49

Schröder H, Hüttner J (1968) Über Zweitkarzinome in der gesunden Brust bei Zustand nach Mammaradikal-operation. Fortschr Rontgenstr 109: 770–775

Sheild AM (1898) A clinical treatise on diseases of the breast. Macmillan, London

Silverberg SG, Chitale AR, Hind AD, Frazier AB, Levitt SH (1970) Sinus histiocytosis and mammary carcinoma. Study of 366 radical mastectomies and an historical review. Cancer 26: 1177–1185

Silverberg SG, Chitale AR, Levitt SH (1972) Prognostic implications of fibrocystic dysplasia in breasts removed for mammary carcinoma. Cancer 29: 574–580

Taylor HB, Norris HJ (1967) Epithelial invasion of nerves in benign diseases of the breast. Cancer 20: 2245–2249

Tough ICK, Carter DC, Fraser J, Bruce J (1969) Histological grading in breast cancer. Br J Cancer 23: 294–301

Urban JA (1969) Biopsy of the "normal" breast in treating breast cancer. Surg Clin North Am 49: 291–301

Wallgren A, Silfverswärd C, Hultborn A (1977) Carcinoma of the breast in women under 30 years of age. A clinical and histopathological study of all cases reported as carcinoma to the Swedish Cancer Registry 1958–1968. Cancer 40: 916–923

Wanebo HJ, Huvos AG, Urban JA (1974) Treatment of minimal breast cancer. Cancer 33: 349–357

Warner NE (1969) Lobular carcinoma of the breast. Cancer 23: 840–846

Wheeler JE, Enterline HT, Roseman JM, Tomasulo JP, McIlvaine CH, Fitts WT, Kirshenbaum J (1974) Lobular carcinoma in situ of the breast. Long-term followup. Cancer 34: 554–563

Wilkinson EJ, Hause L (1974) Probability in lymph node sectioning. Cancer 33: 1269–1274

# 3　Lesions of the Thyroid Gland

The thyroid is unusual in having more, and histologically more sharply divisible, forms of cancer than most other monoepithelial organs or tissues such as, for example, breast or prostate. Classification into papillary, follicular, medullary and anaplastic types is now generally accepted, and many large series of cases thus subdivided have been published with analyses of clinical features, treatment and outcome. Two such, each particularly illustrative with their survival tables for the various forms of carcinoma, are those of Halnan (1966) and Woolner and his colleagues (1968). However, neither here nor in most other series is much consideration given to diagnostic borderline difficulties, whether the tissue in question is carcinomatous or not, and, if it is cancerous, of which type; for the subdivision is not always as easy to make as most texts would have us suppose. One communication that does illustrate the difficulty is that by Saxén and his colleagues (1969) who re-examined and retyped all 392 cases of "thyroid cancer" notified to the Finnish Cancer Registry during 1958–1962. Their Table 1 shows, inter alia, that of 67 cases originally diagnosed as *anaplastic carcinoma*, 47 were rediagnosed as such, 3 as benign lesions; of 53 *follicular carcinomas*, 15 were confirmed, 17 considered benign; of 64 *papillary carcinomas*, 53 were confirmed, 4 considered benign; of 38 diagnosed *malignant adenoma*, 4 were rediagnosed as that, 23 as benign. In all, of the 345 histologically assessable cases of 'carcinoma', 82, or almost one quarter, were on re-examination considered to be benign.

Thyroid cancer varies so much in its clinical behaviour, from virtually innocuous to rapidly fatal, that generalisation is hazardous but one such, published many years ago by Ward (1944) and widely recorded, remains broadly valid. This author, in analysing a series of "malignant goiter" concluded, of 5-year survivals, that for cancers first discovered by the pathologist, the rate was 80%; for those discovered at operation, the rate was 40%; for those discovered or suspected preoperatively, the rate was 20%. This again emphasises at the least that the pathologist has a considerable influence in establishing the rate of incidence and curability or, at any rate, apparent curability.

A pathologist confronted by a borderline lesion of thyroid, and reluctant scientifically to issue a firm diagnosis of cancer or not cancer, may nevertheless be quite properly asked, for practical purposes, to do so. If he decides 'cancer' the logical demands of the matter seem clear. A cancer of any type may evidently be multifocal and bilateral and may also already have metastasised [the magnitude of this possibility may be measured by the statement of Taylor (1969) that, of follicular carcinomas, 50%–60% first appear, not as local lesions, but as metastases especially to bones and lungs]. The demand, therefore, is for extirpation of the gland, regional nodes and possibly distant metastases by whatever technique(s) offer the best hope of total ablation. However, depending on many other circumstances such as the patient's age, general condition and personality, techniques available and technical feasibility, including risks of operation, that is, circumstances that are the concern of the surgeon rather than the pathologist (though joint discussion will usually be the rule), some middle course may be chosen but the choice will rarely be easy. What, for example, should best be done for the young patient with a carcinoma in the light of such evidence as that reported by Tawes and Delorimier (1968) who, in patients aged 21 or less, encountered local recurrence in 3 of 17 patients treated by lobectomy, in none of 25 treated by subtotal thyroidectomy, and none of 23 who had total thyroidectomy? The papillary lesions are often minimally aggressive, the undifferentiated lesions maximally aggressive, and age does have some influence (Halnan, 1966; Exelby and Frazell, 1969; Russell et al., 1975; Byar et al., 1979) but it remains generally sound, as Cline and Shingleton (1968) have said, that ". . . the variation in host response of these tumors should promote caution when one attempts to offer prognosis, even in the presence of widespread tumor".

## Local Series

The local series of equivocal cases numbered 26; of these, 7 were diagnosed as 'for practical purposes' malignant. During the same years, the total number of cases diagnosed as malignant was 33, and that figure includes these 7. Therefore, by coincidence, the number of cases diagnosed 'firmly' was the same as the number presenting a borderline problem.

### SUMMARISED TOTALS

*'Lateral aberrant thyroid' syndrome* (four cases):
Case 3.1: two cervical node dissections; no thyroidectomy; well 18 years later.
Case 3.2: node dissection; subtotal thyroidectomy; well 1 year later and probably cured.
Case 3.3: node dissection; lobectomy after 1 year; further node dissection 1 year later; well 7 years after that.
Case 3.4: cervical node histologically highly mimetic of the 'LAT' syndrome; in fact, metastasis from a true carcinoma of thyroid rapidly fatal thereafter.

*Papillary adenoma vs papillary carcinoma* (six cases; 3.5–3.10 inclusive):
All alive at 6–18 years.
Two had been diagnosed as carcinoma, the others as doubtfully carcinoma.

*Microfollicular adenoma vs carcinoma* (ten cases):
Cases 3.11–3.15 inclusive, diagnosed as carcinoma; all alive at 4–15 years.

Cases 3.16–3.20 inclusive, diagnosed as adenoma or suspicious adenoma: one patient died after 20 years; one was certainly alive at 4 years, the others probably alive for up to 20 years.

*Hyperplasia vs 'early malignancy'* (five cases; 3.21–3.25 inclusive):
All examples of markedly hyperplastic tissue in a thyrotoxic patient. None, though regarded with suspicion, was followed by malignancy.

*Chronic thyroiditis vs '? lymphoma'* (one case; 3.26):
Lymphoid hyperplasia not only within but also without the thyroid parenchyma; no lymphoma emerged; well 10 years later.

*Review has yielded:*
Under-diagnoses, 1
Over-diagnoses, 6
Appropriate diagnoses, 19
Details of the 26 cases are shown in summarised form in Table 3.1.

### CASE DATA

*Case 3.1*

F (28 years). Complained of swelling in right side of neck for 1 year, thought to have started after episode of tonsillitis. Exploration showed two nodes in the anterior, one in the posterior, triangle, the largest 20 × 15 × 10 mm and the others only slightly smaller.

The two larger nodes were 90% occupied by mostly highly papillary but sometimes more solidly cellular neoplastic thyroid-type tissue. Adjacent areas of the two types of tissue are shown in Fig. 3.1; the dark wedge at the top is remnant lymphatic tissue and fairly represents the degree of replacement of normal structure by the neoplasm.

The lesion was diagnosed as 'metastatic papillary thyroid carcinoma' presumably derived from a primary source in the ipsilateral lobe of thyroid. For whatever reason, thyroidectomy was not performed.

The patient reappeared 15 months later, again with swelling in the neck. Operation yielded a further four nodes, 20, 20, 15 and 8 mm in maximum dimension respectively. The two

**Table 3.1.** Twenty-six cases of equivocal lesions of thyroid.

| Case No. | Diagnosis on review | Treatment | Outcome |
|----------|---------------------|-----------|---------|
| *1 case under-diagnosed* | | | |
| 3.20 | Follicular carc. > 'cellular adenoma' (M, 16 yr) | Prob. subtotal thyroidectomy | Recurrence 18 yr later: death 2 yr after that |
| *6 cases over-diagnosed* | | | |
| 3.10 | Microfollic. adenoma > papillary carcinoma | Subtotal thyroidectomy | Alive @ 8 yr |
| 3.11 | Microfollic. adenoma > 'adenocarcinoma' | Subtotal thyroidectomy | Alive @ 15 yr |
| 3.12 | Microfollic. adenoma > 'well-differentiated carc.' | Subtotal thyroidectomy | Alive @ 8 yr |
| 3.13 | Microfollic. adenoma > 'carcinoma' | Subtotal thyroidectomy | Alive @ 5 yr |
| 3.14 | Prob. follic./papillary adenoma > carcinoma | Lobectomy | Alive @ 13 yr (abn. tissue transected) |
| 3.15 | Prob. microfollic. adenoma > carcinoma | Partial lobectomy | Alive @ 14 yr |
| *19 cases appropriately diagnosed* | | | |
| 3.1 | Pap. carc. metastatic in cervical nodes | Lymphadenectomy only | Alive @ 18 yr |
| 3.2 | Papillary/follic. carcinoma | Subtotal thyroidectomy | Alive @ 1 yr: untraced |
| 3.3 | Pap. carc. originally in cervical nodes | Lobectomy | Alive @ 7 yr |
| 3.4 | Follic. carc. originally in cervical nodes | (see text) | |
| 3.5 | Papillary adenoma | Nodule excised | Alive @ 8 yr |
| 3.6 | Partially pap. adenoma | Part. lobectomy | Alive @ 16 yr |
| 3.7 | Pap. adenomas, multiple | Part. lobectomy | Alive @ 17 yr |
| 3.8 | Partially pap. adenoma | Subtotal lobectomy | Alive @ 18 yr |
| 3.9 | Papillary carcinoma | Subtotal lobectomy | Alive @ 8 yr |
| 3.16 | Microfollic. adenoma, ? premalignant | Partial lobectomy | Alive @ 18 yr |
| 3.17 | Follicular adenoma | Nodule excised | Alive @ 4 yr |
| 3.18 | Adenoma, probably benign | Nodule excised | Not traced |
| 3.19 | Adenoma, probably benign | Nodule excised | Not traced |
| 3.21 | Hyperplasia, ? invasive | Subtotal thyroidectomy | Alive @ 12 yr |
| 3.22 | Hyperplasia + intramuscular invasion | Subtotal thyroidectomy | Alive @ 5 yr |
| 3.23 | Suspicious hyperplasia in regrown remnant | Subtotal thyroid-ectomy + re-excision | Alive @ 11 yr |
| 3.24 | Unduly hyperplastic | Subtotal thyroidectomy | Not traced |
| 3.25 | Unduly hyperplastic | Subtotal thyroidectomy | Not traced |
| 3.26 | Struma lymphomatosa > lymphosarcoma | Subtotal thyroidectomy | Alive @ 10 yr |

smaller were normal. The two larger were, as before, almost totally replaced by carcinoma, still largely papillary but now solidly cellular over much wider areas.

Again, for whatever reason, nothing was done to the thyroid itself, and the patient was well and trouble-free 18 years later. She had had no treatment beyond the lymph node dissections.

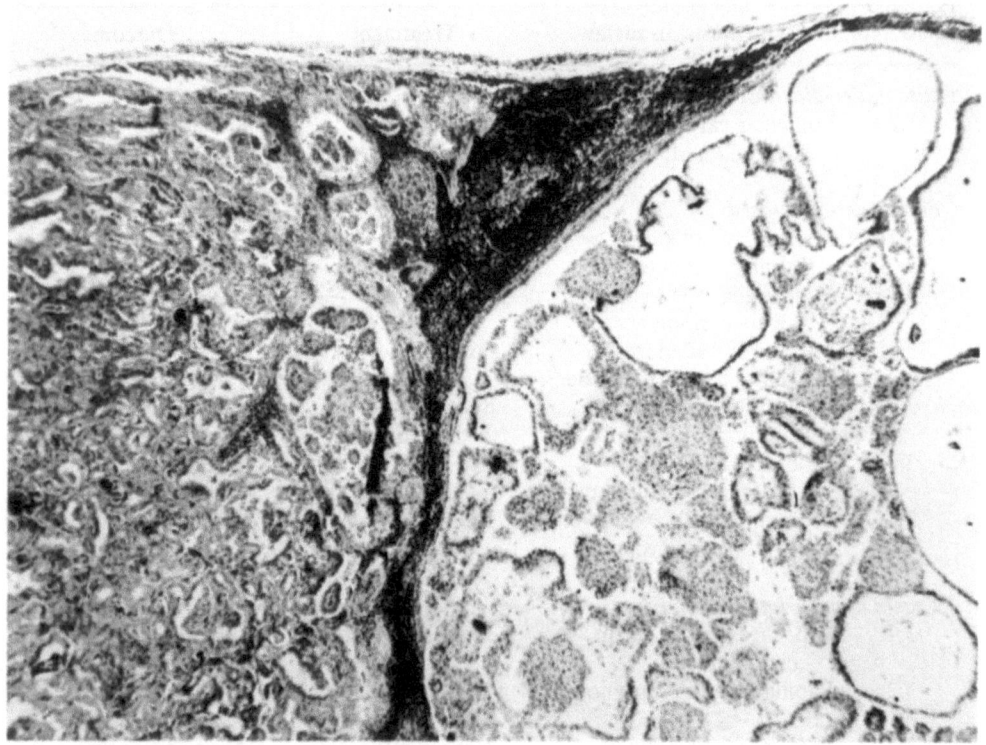

**Fig. 3.1.** Part of one of the nodes showing the degree of replacement of normal architecture by partly papillary (*right*), partly more solidly cellular (*left*) tissue with only a wedge and narrow band of remnant lymphatic tissue. H & E, × 62

Even 18 years may not be long enough to induce total confidence that further trouble may not yet develop but, even if it does, the patient will have been fortunate in having so dormant a neoplasm.

Despite the unusual clinical circumstances and the after-history this must still be counted an *appropriate* diagnosis.

*Case 3.2*

F (35 years) with mass in the side of the neck present for 3 months. Excision produced a nodule, 25 × 10 × 10 mm.

Sections showed the (partly cystic) mass to be a lymph node almost wholly replaced by a largely papillary but quite frequently follicular *carcinoma* of thyroid type. Ipsilateral thyroid lobectomy and nodal dissection was advised.

Subtotal thyroidectomy was performed: it revealed two firm white nodules, each 5 mm in diameter, within the suspected lobe. Each con-

sisted of partly papillary, partly follicular 'carcinoma'. Many 1-mm pale nodules in both the isthmus and the other lobe were of lymphoid tissue. Simultaneous exploration of the neck yielded only one node, from the affected side, 25 × 10 × 7 mm and as completely and identically invaded as the original node.

The patient was known to be trouble-free 12 months later but then emigrated and could no longer be traced. At least, however, no further enquiry has been received on her behalf but the matter can be taken no further than that. The diagnosis had been *appropriate*.

*Case 3.3*

F (23 years) while under supervision and treatment for an unrelated condition, was noticed to have a swelling in the neck. This was excised, 40 × 20 × 15 mm and thus a relatively large mass.

Sections showed a lymph node 95% replaced

by an obvious 'carcinoma' of mixed papillary (predominant) and follicular thyroid character. The virtual certainty of its being metastatic from an ipsilateral primary lesion in thyroid was reported.

For some obscure reason no further treatment was given at that time.

The patient reappeared exactly 1 year later with a submandibular nodule, 4 × 2 × 2 cm, found on section also to be a node similarly replaced by tissue identical with that seen originally.

Thyroid lobectomy with removal of two other nodes from beside the carotid bifurcation showed within the lobe an 8-mm focus of 'papillary carcinoma'; similar tissue filled the lymph nodes.

The patient recovered fully and was well 7 years later.

As in Case 3.1, this was a borderline lesion only in the sense that all papillary overgrowths in the thyroid always are, but its behaviour was illustrative of their usually indolent character: despite the year's delay before removal of the primary focus, cure may have been achieved. The diagnosis was *appropriate*.

### Case 3.4

F (74 years) with a swelling in the neck present for 2 years. There were several palpable cervical nodes of which one was excised.

The node was almost completely replaced by obviously recognisable thyroid tissue, well differentiated but with a greater-than-normal tendency to form small areas of sheet-like, follicle-free tissue. In the thyroid itself the lesion could have been diagnosed as a 'true' adenoma. In its present site, a cervical node, it apparently exemplified the 'lateral aberrant thyroid' complex. It was reported as such and, as such, a 'carcinoma' doubtless metastatic from a primary ipsilateral lesion within the thyroid.

By the time of delivery of the biopsy report, strong radiological evidence was available of skeletal metastases; now also, on further clinical examination, there seemed little doubt that the thyroid itself was largely replaced by a malignant neoplasm, presumably carcinoma. The patient died within 3 weeks of the biopsy, ultimately of bronchopneumonia; there was no necropsy.

This case is included primarily as a contrast

to Case 3.1 where, also, the circumstances were those of the 'lateral aberrant thyroid' complex yet the outcome was so different. In fact, this present case was not truly comparable. The more detailed clinical information that became available only after the biopsy was performed made it clear that the cervical node was only the first-discovered of many already extant metastatic sites. Even so, the high grade of differentiation and virtually complete absence of cytological and mitotic aberrancy made the lesion a good example of, if not " 'benign' metastasising goitre", then " 'insidiously' metastasising goitre". The diagnosis was *appropriate* despite the marked discrepancy between the histology of the tissue and its behaviour.

### Case 3.5

F (19 years) with a non-toxic goitre which had grown gradually since the menarché at age 13. Sections from the subtotally removed gland showed no significant abnormality. The mass recurred and was removed 4 years later; it was generally uniform but contained a quite well-demarcated 20 × 10 × 10 mm pale nodule.

The nodule was of distinctly papillary pattern and accordingly diagnosed as a 'papillary adenoma' with a suggestion that the patient be kept under review against the possibility that metastasis to cervical nodes might already have happened.

No further treatment was given; there were no sequelae; the patient was trouble-free for at least 8 years thereafter. The diagnosis and advice given were *appropriate*.

### Case 3.6

F (27 years) with one-sided swelling in the neck present for 3½ years, then, for past three months a feeling of "something sticking on swallowing". There was no indication of thyrotoxicosis. Partial thyroidectomy performed.

The specimen was a lobulate fleshy mass 6 cm in diameter. Most consisted of relatively uniform well-filled follicles as seen at the centre lower edge of Fig. 3.2. In one 10-mm localised area, however, there was a distinctly papillary pattern as shown throughout the rest of that illustration. Furthermore, as seen in Figs. 3.3 and 3.4, not only do many of the follicles in this

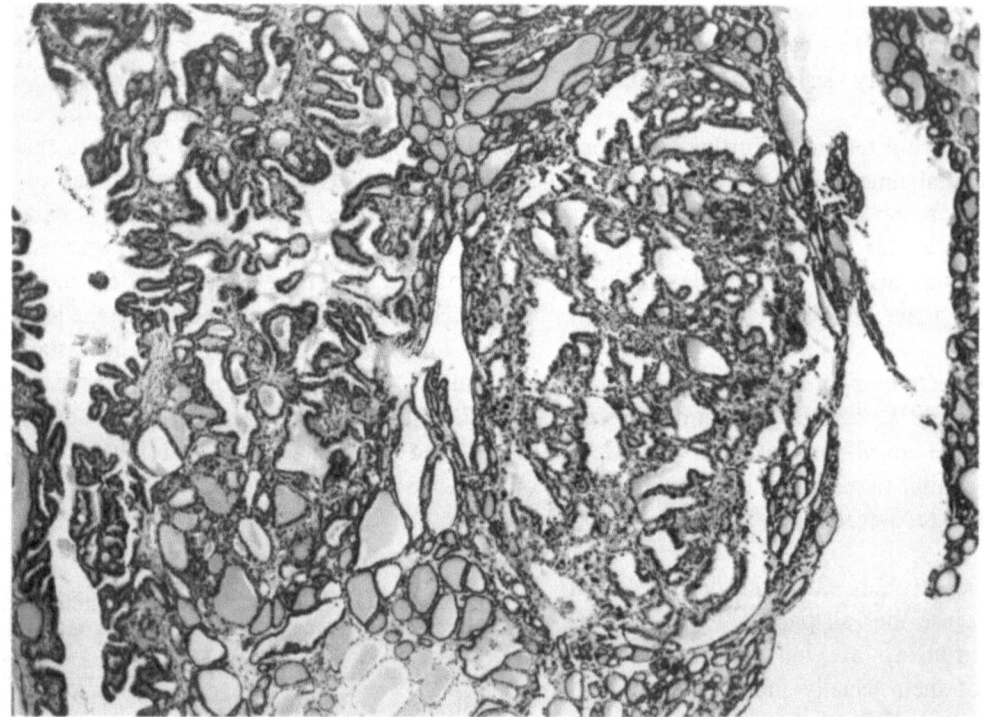

**Fig. 3.2.** A small area of normally follicular architecture remains at the bottom of the field. Elsewhere the pattern is highly papillary and/or irregularly follicular. H & E, × 60

area have a notably hyperplastic type of epithelium, their cells quite frequently show marked nuclear enlargement and polymorphism. Despite this, mitotic figures, though present, were extremely few and not aberrant.

The mass was reported as a colloid 'adenoma' with a single focus of papillary hyperplasia considered to represent at any rate some possibility of metastasis.

There was no further trouble and the patient was well 16 years later. Two points merit comment. First, though nuclear abnormality of this kind is sometimes regarded as 'regressive', it was occurring here only in an area where the epithelium was otherwise notably hyperplastic. Second, nuclear change such as this is, as an alternative explanation, sometimes attributed to antithyroid medication whether by drugs or radio-iodine. There was no mention that this patient had been receiving either.

In this instance, at least, both the papillary pattern and the nuclear changes were innocuous, and the diagnosis, from the after-history, still remains *appropriate*.

*Case 3.7*

F (33 years) with a swelling over one side of the thyroid for some 6 months. There was no dysphagia but the patient was thought to have mild toxicosis; she had not, however, received any antithyroid medication. A relatively well circumscribed mass was removed.

The mass was 3 × 3 × 2 cm, lobulate, micronodular and, as seen in Fig. 3.5, sometimes microcystic. Part of the tissue within the uppermost cyst in this illustration is shown in Fig. 3.6; it is finely papillary as was the tissue in the two nodules at the lower margin of Fig. 3.5 and in others of similar size scattered with about this frequency throughout the mass.

The many foci of papillary differentiation were recorded as possibly representing some risk of metastasis.

There was no recurrence and no metastasis, and the patient was well 17 years later. In the absence of antithyroid medication as a possible explanation, this remains an example of multifocal papillary hyperplasia that was innocuous.

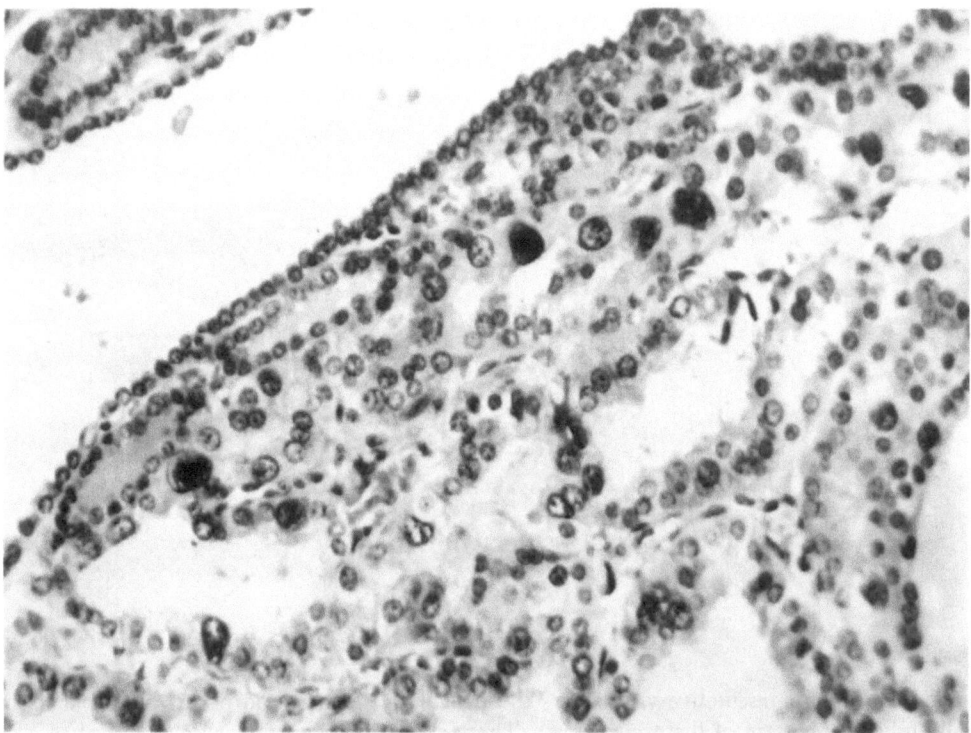

**Fig. 3.3.** Marked nuclear polymorphism is evident in the lining of follicles and in other areas showing no follicular differentiation. H & E, × 476

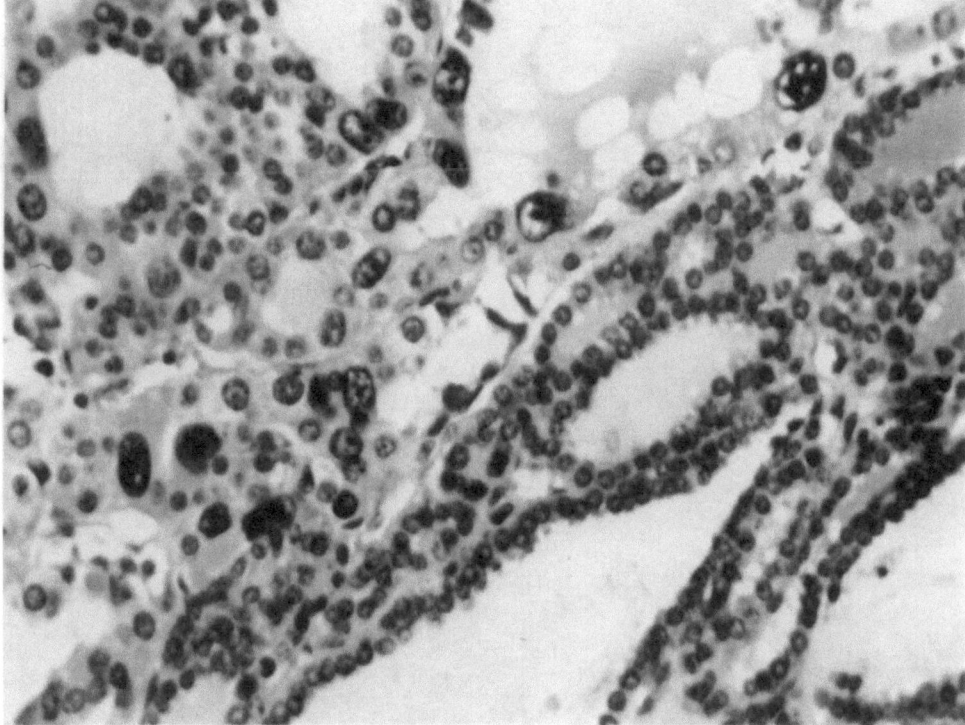

**Fig. 3.4.** Conspicuous enlargement of nuclei and a general polymorphism throughout the upper left half of the field stands in marked contrast to the normal cellular pattern of the follicular epithelium in the lower right half. H & E, × 540

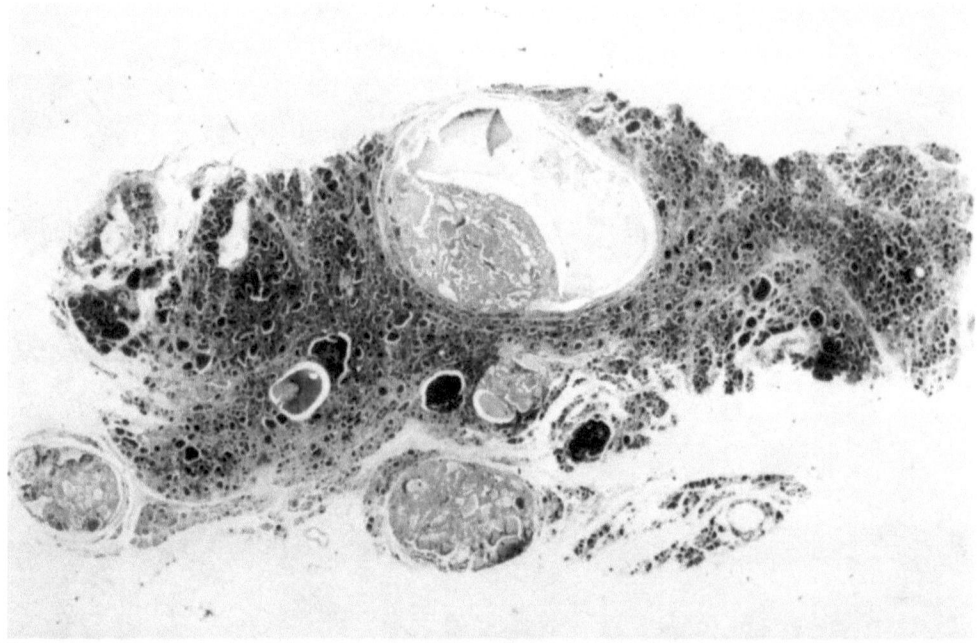

**Fig. 3.5.** This representative view shows the irregularly nodular and partly cystic but basically follicular pattern of the excised mass. There are three relatively well-circumscribed nodules. H & E, × 11

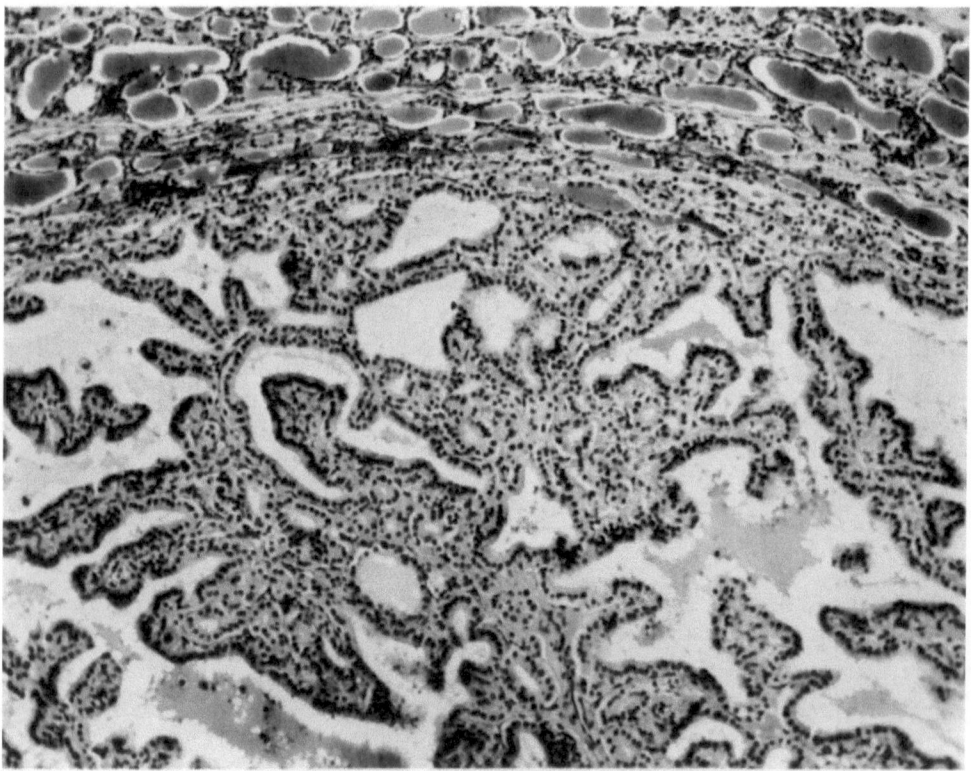

**Fig. 3.6.** Papillary differentiation of this degree was common but, as shown at the tissue-interface, such areas were almost always confined within the nodule. H & E, × 123

Circumstances were closely similar to those in the preceding case, and the diagnosis similarly *appropriate*.

## Case 3.8

F (65 years) with an asymptomatic swelling in the neck present for 4 months. The greater part of the affected lobe was excised.

The excised tissue consisted largely of a 20-mm microfollicular adenoma but adjacent to it was a 5-mm nodule of highly papillary, non-follicular tissue. In Fig. 3.7, the right two-thirds shows the obviously follicular component: the left third is devoid of any follicular pattern and has the papillary architecture shown in Fig. 3.8. It is fairly well demarcated by a fibrous wall in this area but was much less sharply circumscribed in many other areas.

As in Cases 3.6 and 3.7, the possibility of metastasis was recorded.

No further treatment was required and the patient was well 18 years later: an *appropriate* diagnosis.

## Case 3.9

M (66 years) with complaint of a swelling in the neck for 2 months associated with dyspnoea and hoarseness. Subtotal lobectomy was performed. The lobe contained a 30-mm haemorrhagic cyst and a 10-mm white nodule.

Interest centred on the white nodule. Though its cells were generally uniform it had the structure of a 'papillary carcinoma' albeit relatively closely packed.

Adequate removal appeared to have been achieved and no further treatment was given. A warning was given of the possibility, even likelihood, of nodal metastasis, but none occurred. The patient was still trouble-free 8 years later.

There seems no way of knowing whether this was a papillary adenoma that never would have metastasised or truly a carcinoma for whose timely removal the patient could thank the haemorrhage into the pre-existing cyst; for that was almost certainly the reason for the relatively short duration of the swelling and dyspnoea. The diagnosing of carcinoma rather than papillary adenoma made no difference to the treat-

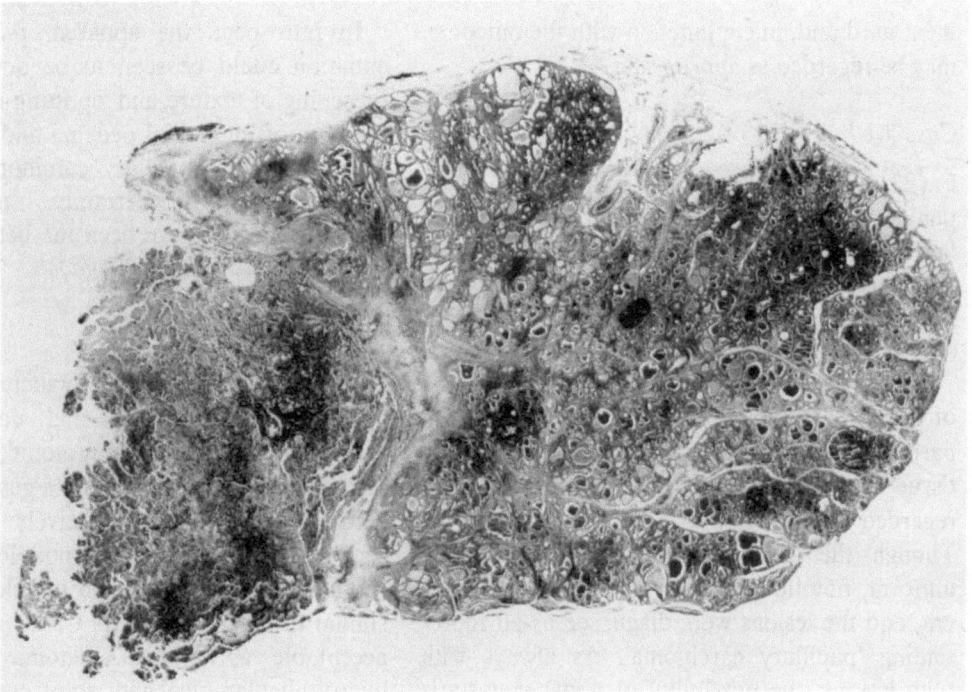

**Fig. 3.7.** The right two-thirds of the field shows an essentially normal follicular pattern; the rest of the field has no follicular pattern but is of a varyingly close papillary pattern. H & E, × 11

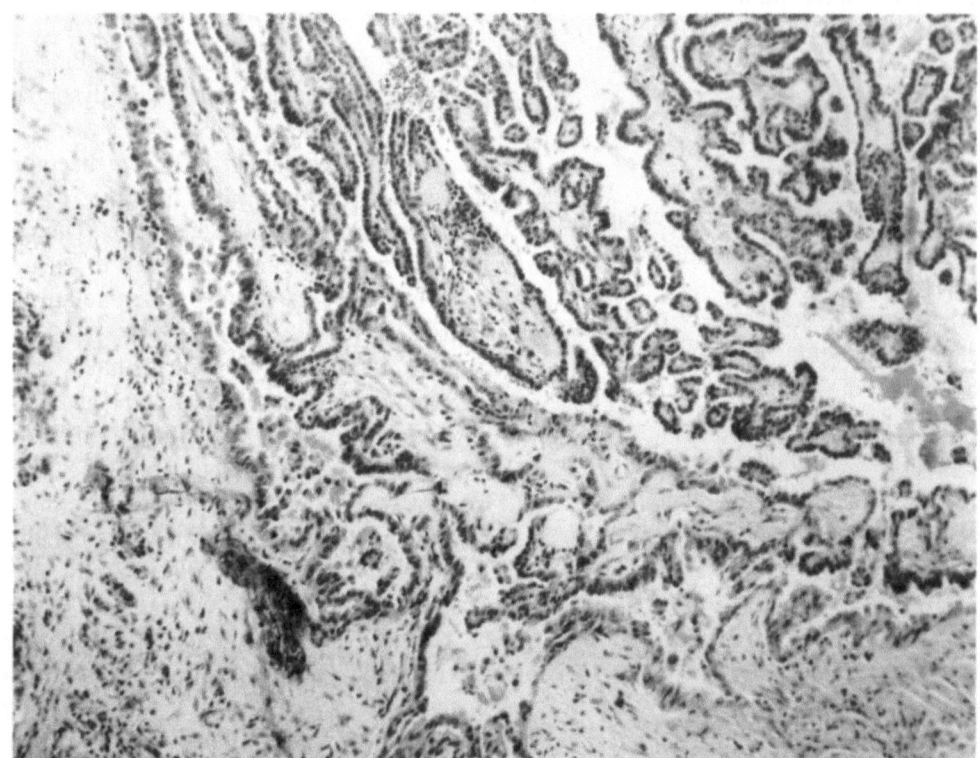

**Fig. 3.8.** In this area the papillary tissue is fairly well circumscribed but less so than in the rather similar overgrowth in Case 3.7. H & E, × 123

ment used and, in conjunction with the outcome, may be regarded as *appropriate*.

### Case 3.10

F (23 years) with swelling in the neck accompanied by dysphagia and dyspnoea for 5 weeks. Subtotal thyroidectomy yielded four pieces of tissue containing, between them, one 20 mm and two 10 mm quite well circumscribed nodules of soft grey-white tissue.

All three nodules consisted of the same type of tissue, partly microfollicular but for the most part large sheet-like areas of solidly cellular tissue occasionally loosening to form what were regarded as foci of papillary differentiation. Though the cells were almost monotonously uniform, mitotic figures were occasionally present, and the lesions were diagnosed as all representing 'papillary carcinoma'. As always with such lesions, the possibility of nodal metastasis was mentioned.

There were no sequelae and the patient was well 8 years later.

In retrospect, the apparent papillary differentiation could be seen to be due rather to a loosening of texture and 'splitting-up' by a combination of interstitial oedema and haemorrhage than to a truly papillary carcinomatous differentiation. Almost certainly, 'microfollicular adenoma' would have been the better term: this may be judged an *over-diagnosis*.

### Case 3.11

F (62 years) with a gradually increasing swelling in the neck for 35 years and, during the past year, signs of mild thyrotoxicosis. Subtotal thyroidectomy revealed, amid a generally normal fleshy parenchyma, a relatively well circumscribed 30-mm paler firmer nodule.

The tissue pattern of the nodule was notably similar to that seen in both Cases 3.12 and 3.15, acceptable as a true adenoma of generally microfollicular type with solid areas sometimes and a mild degree of epithelial nuclear variability. The lesion was diagnosed as 'adenocarcinoma'.

No further treatment was given and the patient was known to be well 15 years later. The good result might be attributed to the fortuitous removal of a carcinoma at an early stage. The evidence suggests rather that this was an *over-diagnosis*.

### Case 3.12

F (68 years) with complaint of tightness of the throat for many years but increasingly so for the past 2 years.

Subtotal thyroidectomy revealed, in one lobe (7 × 6 × 3 cm) a centrally calcified mass of uniform, white, opaque tissue. The other lobe appeared normal.

The pattern throughout the opaque white tissue was uniformly microfollicular and was diagnosed as a well-differentiated "carcinoma . . . that does not have a highly aggressive appearance . . .", an opinion based essentially on uniformity of cell type and scarcity of mitotic figures.

No further treatment was given and the patient was well 8 years later.

This was probably an instance of *over-diagnosis*. Classification as 'microfollicular adenoma' would probably have been the more accurate.

### Case 3.13

F (28 years) with nodule over thyroid, increasing over past 2 years. Excision produced an oval mass, 3 × 2 × 2 cm.

The tissue was, on average, 20% microfollicular, 80% solid or, when traversed by vessels, trabeculate. The cells were generally large with abundant eosinophilic cytoplasm; their nuclei varied greatly in size with a range of diameter from 10 to 70 $\mu$m: Mitotic figures were present but relatively scarce at 1 per 50 hpf. This scarcity of mitoses favoured a diagnosis of adenoma rather than carcinoma but undoubted excursion of the abnormal tissue through its most sharply circumscribing capsule and into surrounding normal parenchyma determined the decision to diagnose the mass as 'carcinoma'.

All but a posterior flake of thyroid on both sides was excised and was found to contain three pale nodules, each 3 mm across. Each was

reasonably classifiable as microfollicular adenoma: all had a larger proportion of well-differentiated follicles, and none showed any comparable or even significant degree of nuclear aberrancy.

No further treatment was given and the patient was well 5 years later. This was possibly another instance of *over-diagnosis*. The discrepancy between the relative scarcity of cells in mitosis and the prominent degree of nuclear polymorphism rather suggests that the nuclear change, which contributed appreciably towards the decision 'malignant', was regressive.

### Case 3.14

F (30 years) with a swelling over one side of the thyroid present for 6 months; no toxicosis. Lobectomy yielded tissue containing three nodules.

Two of the nodules had the structure of straightforward microfollicular adenomas though one appeared to have been transected. The other had a varied pattern with areas of follicular, papillary and, relatively extensively, solid sheet-like disposition; it also appeared to have been transected. Though nuclear aberrancy was slight, and mitoses few, the lesion was regarded as a microfollicular 'carcinoma'.

The patient was well, without further treatment, 13 years later. This also was possibly an instance of *over-diagnosis*, especially in view of the absence even of regrowth despite the evident transection of two of the three hypercellular nodules.

### Case 3.15

M (33 years) with swelling on the left side of his neck for 1 year, nausea and loss of weight for 1 year, vomiting for 3 months. He was hypertensive and judged to be mildly thyrotoxic. Left partial thyroidectomy produced 30 g of friable yellowish-pink tissue.

The tissue had a universally microfollicular pattern. This can be seen in Fig. 3.9, where the abnormal tissue abuts on its capsule of compressed normal parenchyma. The tissue was at the least adenomatous: was it carcinomatous? The answer to this depended almost entirely on assessment of the cytology: degree of differentiation was of no help since the microfollicular

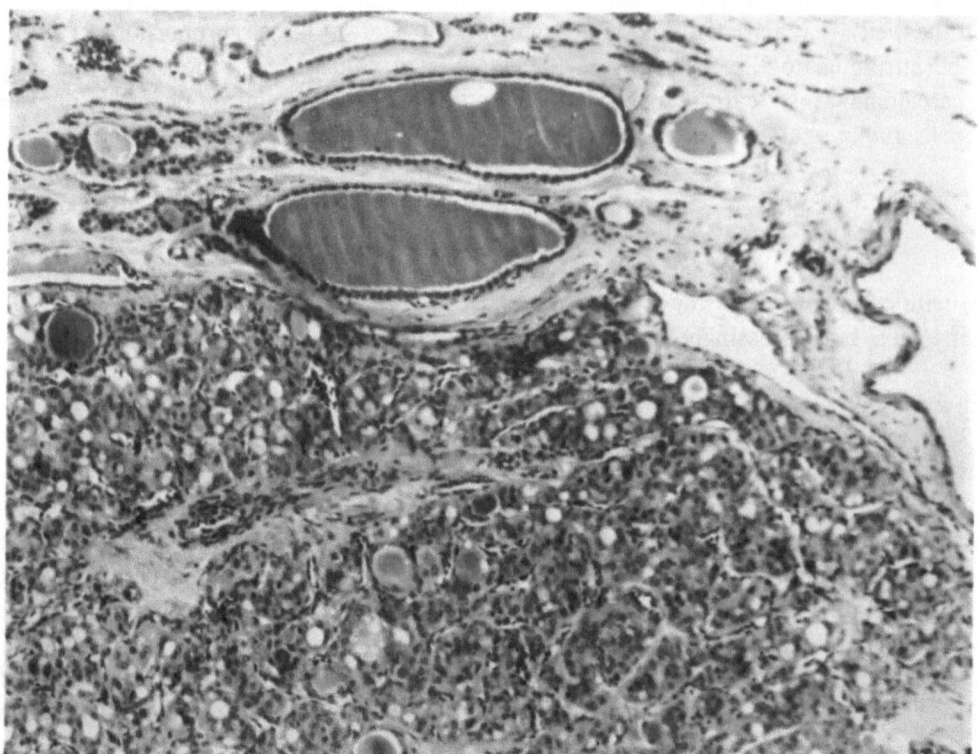

**Fig. 3.9.** The abnormal tissue, of microfollicular differentiation and relatively high cellularity, is seen here, as it was around most of its circumference, fairly well demarcated from the adjacent normal parenchyma. H & E, × 60

arrangement, with some variation in size of follicle and amount of contained colloid, was present virtually throughout. The disquieting features were the presence of occasional nuclei very much larger than the rest (Fig. 3.10) and, amongst the nuclei in general, a greater degree of polymorphism than is seen in the 'usual' adenoma of thyroid. Mitotic figures, however, were extremely few.

With acknowledgement that other opinions might differ, the lesion was diagnosed as a well-differentiated 'carcinoma'.

The excision alone was deemed adequate and no further treatment was given. The patient remains well 14 years later. This after-history, in a patient with a lesion of such size and histology, can only suggest strongly that the lesion was *not* a carcinoma: almost certainly, therefore, this was an *over-diagnosis*. However, in prospect, with its expressed reservations, the report that was given led to no over-treatment: the uncertainties had been adequately conveyed to the surgeon.

*Case 3.16*

F (22 years) with history of swelling in the neck for 5 years, thought to have become more prominent during past 6 months. Partial lobectomy was performed.

The tissue included four nodules differing from the parenchyma in general in being, by comparison, microfollicular and almost devoid of colloid content, with a minor degree of epithelial nuclear variability and an occasional cell in mitosis. The appearances were regarded as 'premalignant', and supervision recommended.

There was no further treatment and no further trouble in the neck for at least the next 18 years. The diagnosis was *appropriate* and the expectant policy fully justified.

*Case 3.17*

F (36 years) with swelling in the neck and dysphagia for 2 months. Exploration and excision produced a spherical mass, 35 mm in

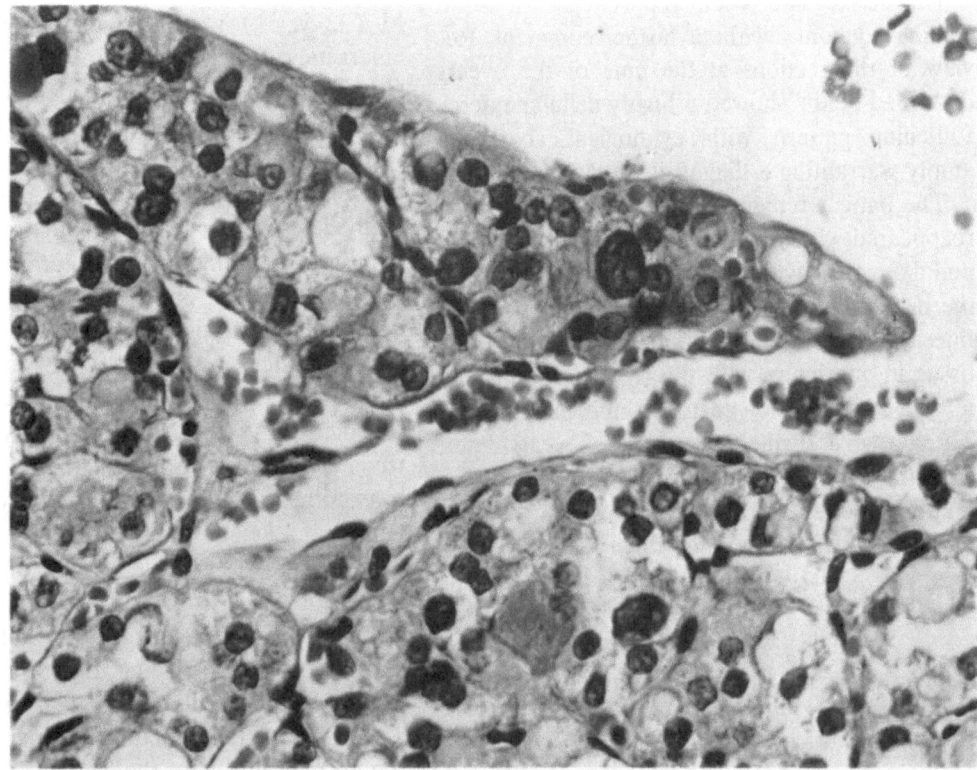

**Fig. 3.10.** This tissue forms part of the lining of a relatively large space partly filled with blood. In the lower part of the field the tissue is covered by a single-cell layer of flattened cells, possibly endothelium. In the upper part the layer does not exist. The appearance, therefore, could be interpreted as 'invasion of a vein'. However, since the space is not unequivocally a vein, this interpretation would not be justified. The cellular polymorphism present in many places throughout the tissue is also seen here. H & E, × 765

diameter, brown and glistening on the cut surface in contrast to the paler duller appearance of adjacent parenchyma.

The nodule was, in terms of structural demarcation and intrinsic histological difference from surrounding parenchyma, a true follicular 'adenoma'. Some prognostic uncertainty was induced by its high cellularity, mild but definite nuclear polymorphism and occasional mitotic figure. Continued supervision was advised, but no further treatment.

There were no sequelae and the patient was well 4 years later (the pallor of the adjacent parenchyma was owed to massive lymphoid tissue infiltration or overgrowth, of which there was a small amount also in the adenoma: its significance in relation to the patient's general well-being appeared to be nil: she was systemically fit before the operation and for at least the

4 years of follow-up thereafter). Circumstances were essentially similar to those in the preceding case, and the diagnosis similarly *appropriate*.

### Cases 3.18, 3.19

Cases 3.18 and 3.19 were of women aged 49 and 39 respectively, each with an adenoma regarded as 'borderline' but probably benign.

Later information is lacking but no enquiry has been received during the 20 years since their operations. To that rather restricted extent the diagnoses were *appropriate*.

### Case 3.20

M (16 years) with symptomless swelling in neck for 6 months, 'never very large, can wear soft collar of normal size'; no toxicosis. The dimensions of the excised mass are not on record.

The tissue had been reported as 'a solid cellular adenoma' without further comment. Review of the sections at the time of the events described below showed a highly cellular microfollicular pattern with cytological aberrancy amply warranting a diagnosis of carcinoma.

The patient remained well for 18 years, then reappeared with what was described as 'multiple nodular goitre with multiple enlarged nodes in the neck'. The operation for total removal produced a $15 \times 15 \times 6$ mm mass of solidly fleshy tissue in continuity with the right sternomastoid muscle and 8 nodes up to 30 mm in diameter. These was a further recurrence 2 years later, and the patient died shortly thereafter with multiple metastasis.

This clearly was an *under-diagnosis*.

### Case 3.21

F (37 years) subtotal thyroidectomy for toxicosis.

For the most part the appearances were typically those of a medicated 'toxic' gland. In some places, however, the relation between areas of parenchymatous hyperplasia and adjacent stroma were such as to satisfy completely any requirements for 'invasion of the stroma'. A comment to this effect was made in the report, 'prophylactically' some might say, but with the further comment that the appearance was almost certainly of no clinical significance.

No further treatment was given. The patient recovered fully and was well at least 12 years later.

Had the biopsy appeared two years later than it did, the report would probably have made no mention of 'invasion of the stroma'. At the time, an analysis was in process of some earlier-encountered neoplasms of thyroid (Park and Lees, 1955) and one of the conclusions eventually was, ". . . if infiltration is to be recognised by the presence of epithelial cells where epithelial cells have no right to be, it is almost impossible to recognise invasive properties as long as the suspected tissue remains within the capsular limits. 'Invasion of the stroma' is thus of little or no value as a criterion of malignancy in the thyroid".

Even so, the report had been essentially *appropriate*.

### Case 3.22

M (22 years) was admitted to hospital as an emergency case with thyrotoxicosis of considerable severity. Subtotal thyroidectomy produced 57 g of minimally colloid, notably fleshy tissue.

The tissue was highly hyperplastic, with relatively little content of colloid and prominent epithelial overgrowth in both follicular and papillary pattern. The epithelium was appreciably polymorphic and occasionally in mitosis, approximately 1 figure per 20 hpf of the close-packed follicles.

These features, it was considered, could be accepted as a consequence simply of the extreme hyperplasia. Concern was raised primarily by another feature, namely, the enclosure of bands of skeletal muscle by the hyperplastic tissue. This was present in one of the original blocks of tissue, and was present again in another of several extra blocks taken for the express purpose of trying to assess this feature, for it undoubtedly indicated 'invasiveness'. There was equally unequivocal permeation into the fibrous capsule of the gland.

Despite these features, it was decided that the lesion should *not* be diagnosed as carcinoma.

The patient was kept under observation but nothing untoward happened. He was fit five years later.

The undoubted 'invasiveness' here, even though achieved by highly hyperplastic tissue, clearly, in retrospect at any rate, did not indicate malignancy. Any permeating remnant presumably regressed either altogether or to normality, as did the portion of gland left after the subtotal removal.

This case stands in interesting, because rather paradoxical, contrast to the preceding Case 3.20. In the present example, 'invasion' was unequivocal yet the decision to say 'not malignant' was quite generally agreed. It is difficult to know, from the acknowledged infrequency of toxicosis in patients with thyroid carcinomas, to what extent foreknowledge of the clinical circumstances might have influenced the pathological report. However, the diagnosis was confirmed as *appropriate*.

### Case 3.23

F (25 years) whose initial complaint was 'eyes looking abnormal'. Thyroid swelling was found and subtotal thyroidectomy performed. Histology showed simply 'diffusely hyperplastic thyroid tissue'. Postoperative recovery was normal but, at review 2 months later, there was again a swelling in the neck. This was again explored and further tissue, $3 \times 2 \times 1$ cm, removed.

The tissue was again hyperplastic but now most irregularly so at both general architectural and cell level. As shown in Fig. 3.11, large misshapen follicles are separated by sheets of microfollicular tissue bearing thickened epithelial linings. The characters of this epithelium are shown in Figs. 3.12a and 3.12b. It is thick and asymmetrically arranged, and the nuclei, often abnormally large, vary greatly in size; some cells appear to be multinucleated, and, as seen in Fig. 3.12b, are sometimes in mitosis.

The varied pattern, follicular and cytological, was regarded as indicating 'irregular hyperplasia', not carcinoma, but was looked upon with considerable suspicion.

The second operation proved curative, and the patient was known to have remained well for at least the next 11 years. The 'suspicion' at least led to no further inconvenience for the patient; later events proved it groundless, and thus confirmed the diagnosis as *appropriate*.

### Cases 3.24, 3.25

Cases 3.24 and 3.25 concerned, respectively, a boy of 9 years and a woman aged 48 years, whose excised thyroid tissue had been sufficiently hyperplastic to raise suspicion.

Later information is lacking but no enquiry has been received during the 20 and 24 years since their respective operations. Again, the diagnoses appear to have been *appropriate*.

### Case 3.26

F (27 years) with an asymptomatic swelling of the neck existing for 2 years. Subtotal thyroidectomy was performed.

The tissue was pale, firm and finely nodular with many similarly pale 2–5 mm nodules among the fibrous capsule. Microscopically, the pallor was seen to be due to a relatively massive lymphoid tissue hyperplasia, without, however,

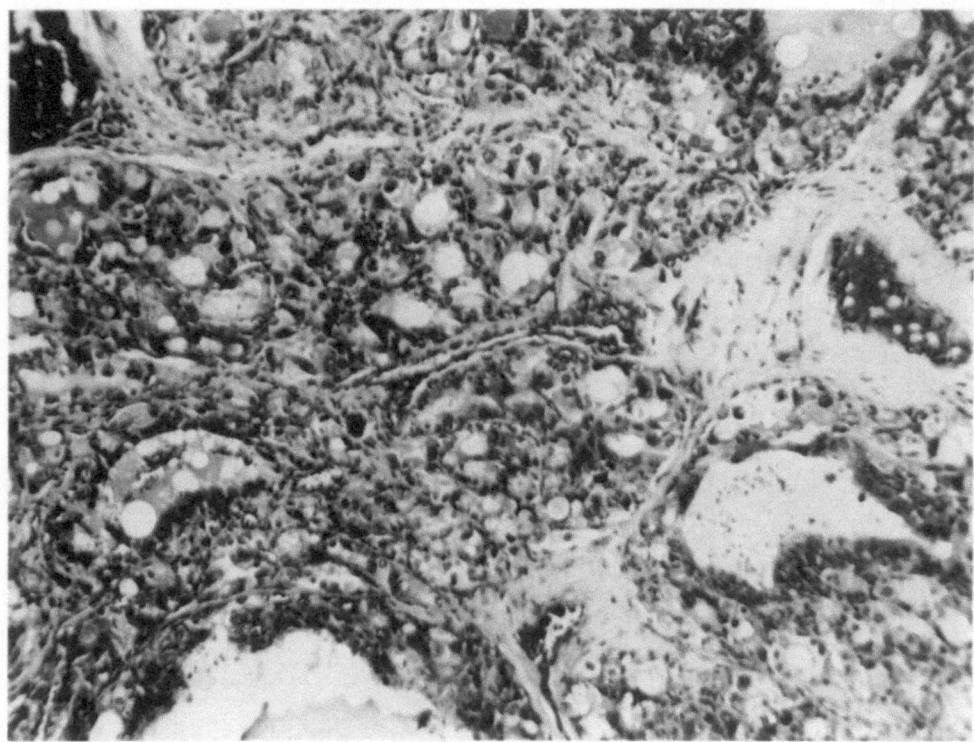

**Fig. 3.11.** The follicular pattern is markedly irregular, and the epithelium generally thick. H & E, $\times$ 126

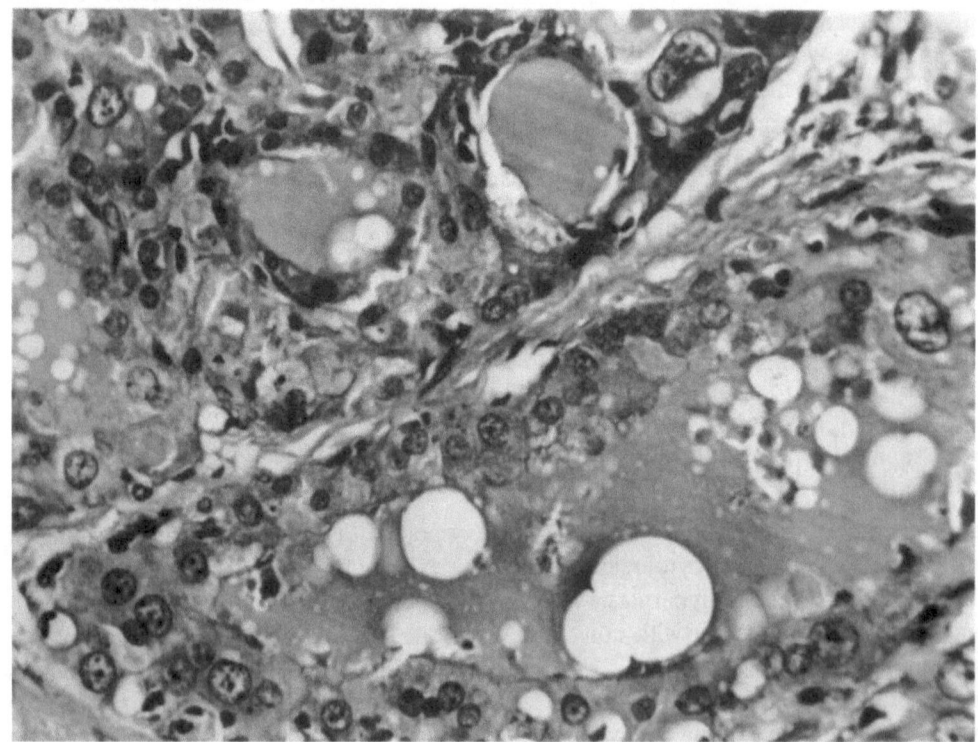

Fig. 3.12a

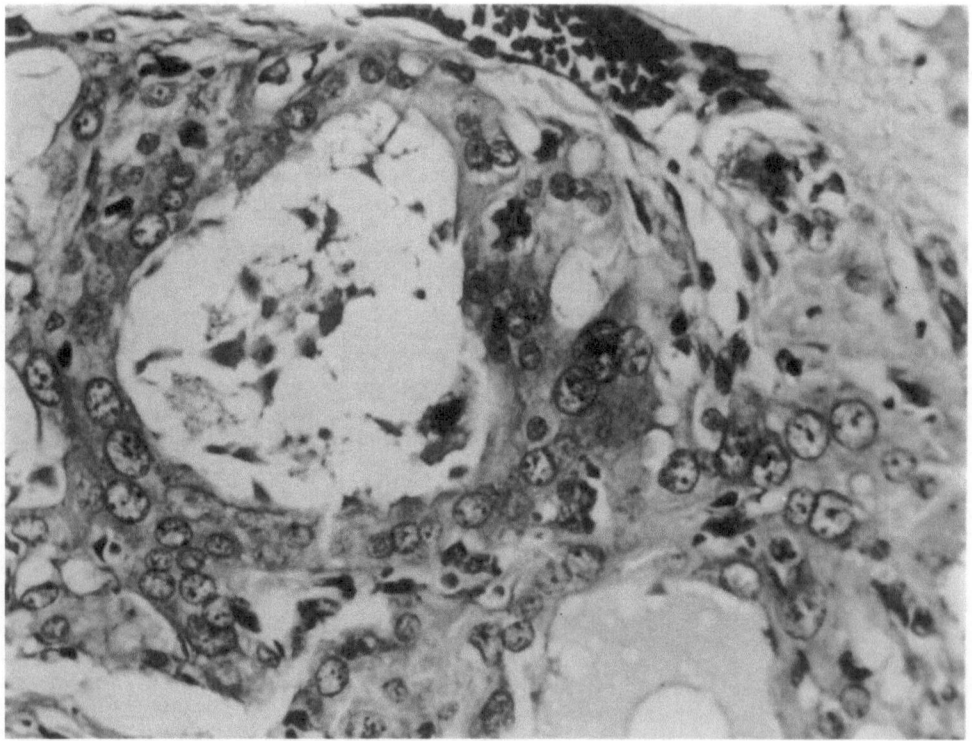

Fig. 3.12b

**Fig. 3.12 a and b.** The degree of epithelial hyperplasia and nuclear polymorphism is considerable. At 2 o'clock in the upper follicle at (b) is a cell in mitosis. The mitotic figure, if not frankly aberrant, is unusually large. H & E, × 476

any notable degree of alteration of the epithelial parenchyma or follicular pattern. For this reason, the lesion was diagnosed as a 'non-specific thyroiditis' rather than struma lymphomatosa (Hashimoto). Concern, however, was caused by the fact that all of the discrete capsular nodules were lymph nodes, and that all were as hyperplastic as the tissue throughout the thyroid, sometimes to the point of wide obliteration of normal architecture.

This was reported along with a recommendation that a search be made for splenic or nodal enlargement elsewhere, and for any abnormality in the blood.

No other abnormality was found, nothing further was done and the patient was still well 10 years later. The distinction between massive lymphoid hyperplasia and an early malignant lymphoma continues to be difficult sometimes. In this instance the cautious diagnosis of non-malignancy proved *appropriate*.

COMMENTARY ON LOCAL SERIES

In contrast to the status of the papillary and undifferentiated carcinomas, the unpredictability and general diagnostic difficulty surrounding the follicular carcinomas of the thyroid are confirmed again in this series: five of the six over-diagnoses concerned this group. This may indicate a general tendency amongst pathologists; it may be that, well aware of the insidious behaviour that gave rise to the term 'benign metastasising goitre', we give ourselves a low diagnostic threshold and thus an ample safety margin within which to work. If so, the six over-diagnoses could be regarded as the price paid in the hope of avoiding the one under-diagnosis that did occur. At least, however, the patients were not further inconvenienced by their being diagnosed, even if wrongly, as having cancer. The forms of treatment used for these six patients may be noted. Despite the diagnosis, none had a total thyroidectomy; four had a subtotal thyroidectomy; one had a lobectomy, the other a partial lobectomy only; and this conservatism was fully justified. However, in the light of the circumstances in Case 3.20, where the lesion that should have been diagnosed as carcinoma at age 16 recurred 18 years later, perhaps none of these five patients really has been cured. In them, as in Case 3.20, we cannot know whether

reappearance of the lesion, should it happen, would be regrowth of a long-dormant neoplastic remnant or, not a true recurrence like this, but a fresh development in the seemingly normal tissue left in situ.

# General Commentary

The problems surrounding the diagnosis of malignant neoplasms of the thyroid were analysed in some detail in an earlier article (Park and Lees, 1955). The possibility of bias is acknowledged but a re-reading of that analysis now finds the main points still reasonably valid and in little need of amendment. The analysis had been based on the reassessment of 66 cases originally diagnosed as some form of carcinoma or sarcoma, and their regrading in strictly practical terms had produced four groups: unequivocal cancer, 36; papillary neoplasm, 15; still doubtful, 7; not malignant, 8. There had thus been a minimum rate of over-diagnosis in the series of 8/66 or some 12%. The discussion that follows now is in the main supplementary to the comments made then on criteria of histological diagnosis.

MICROFOLLICULAR ADENOMA

The 'solitary nodule' of the thyroid, a notorious problem for the surgeon, is very often a microfollicular adenoma, an equally notorious problem for the pathologist; and, basically, the reason for the uncertainty of the surgeon is the uncertainty of the pathologist. The difficulties have been reviewed on many occasions (see, for example, Kendall and Condon, 1969; Taylor, 1969a; Editorials, 1971, 1973, 1976).

An apparently solitary nodule will almost always be excised. The first problem for the pathologist is then to decide (perhaps on frozen section, of which more later) whether the nodule is an adenoma or not, for the implications of the decision are important; 'adenoma' implies some threat of malignancy, 'adenomatoid nodule' does not. The decision is generally based on the well-known criteria of Meissner and Warren (1969), in essence, sharp demarcation and a distinct structural difference from, and compression of, the surrounding parenchyma; and by these criteria the distinction usually can be established. In addition to this, the further assumption is generally made that, to merit the diagnosis 'adenoma', the tissue comprising the nodule should be more highly cellular than that of the surrounding parenchyma; the adenoma is thus likely to be microfollicular. In the present series there were eight such cases: the adenoma was single in six, one of three nodules in one patient, and all of four nodules in the other[1].

The microfollicular adenoma is a lesion wherein the correlation between structure and behaviour is still frustratingly low; the 'benign metastasising goitre' has not yet disappeared. The pathologist can do little more than continue to rely on the standard criteria of structural and cytological aberrancy, and grade his assessment of clinical/biological probabilities accordingly. As the local series has shown, this is not completely worthless. Such assessment may lead to a degree of over-diagnosis but, *pace* the possible existence of potentially malignant adenomas in the opposite lobe, diagnosis of a nodule as 'only just' a carcinoma may spare the patient a total thyroidectomy; in these circumstances, the surgeon may consider that lobectomy, or even only local excision, will suffice, and often he will be right. Another criterion, 'invasion of blood vessels', has long been regarded as proof that a nodule is not an adenoma but a carcinoma. However, this morphological feature can no longer be given the high reputation it once had as a diagnostic and prognostic indicator. It is at any rate not a diagnostic sine qua non (Russell et al., 1963), and many a lesion kills in the seemingly certain absence of demonstrable venous invasion. Further, a review of the outcome in 301 patients with malignant disease of the thyroid led Greene (1969) to conclude that the significance of invasion of both capsule and vessels, and even of metastasis, had been unduly emphasised. An earlier report, by Branson and Houston (1949), speaks for itself. In describing the difficulties of identifying an adenoma as 'malignant', these authors wrote, ". . . it was

accepted that 60% of such cases could be diagnosed on morphological grounds, while, in the remainder, invasion of the blood-vessels, or the close relation of the neoplastic cells to vascular endothelium, was accepted as evidence of malignancy". Yet, of 50 patients with thus-diagnosed malignant adenoma, none was known to have died within 5 years, and only one within 10 years. It still seems sound to maintain the opinion given by Park and Lees (1955), and endorsed by Meissner and Warren (1969), that invasion of blood vessels may be of value ". . . but only if the 'epithelium' is unequivocally epithelium and the 'blood vessel' unequivocally a blood vessel".

Increasingly, the decision 'benign or malignant' will be requested on frozen-section. Examination of a frozen section can certainly allow a firm diagnosis in some cases of thyroid cancer but most reliably in those cases, the anaplastic cancers, where suspicion is already high on clinical evidence alone. Where clinical guidance is most needed, in the case of the solitary nodule, the uncertainties met with paraffin sections are accentuated since few would claim that diagnosis of thyroid lesions by frozen section is more accurate than by paraffin section. Since some help might be gained from frozen-section examination, it is worth doing, but the surgeon should not be disappointed if his pathologist colleague in the event has little to offer. Overall, the place for frozen sections in the assessment of lumps in the thyroid is, I believe, small. Either the tissue is diagnosable as unequivocally cancer or it is not, and if it is not, it is unreportable; paraffin sections must be awaited. Only then can an adenoma be fully assessed.

A point of both clinical and pathological significance is that an apparently solitary nodule is quite often not solitary; for example, in the series reported by Taylor (1969a), 207 nodules were believed on palpation to be solitary. Surgical exploration revealed further nodules and reduced the figure to 124; dissection by the pathologist of the removed tissue, usually one lobe, reduced it still further to 108. Perhaps, therefore, removal of an apparently solitary nodule should always be by lobectomy. Lobectomy is a middle course; it reduces the risk of later carcinoma represented by any further ipsilateral adenomas there may be but, necessarily, leaves as the price for avoidance of total thyroid-

---

[1] The Meissner/Warren criteria require also that the 'true adenoma' be solitary; yet, if all of four nodules have a structure that would, in a single nodule, be diagnosed as 'adenoma', it is hardly logical not to accept them as also adenomas unless multiplicity per se is to be given diagnostic precedence over histological structure.

ectomy the lesser risk of carcinoma from any contralateral adenomas there may be.

## PAPILLARY CARCINOMA

This lesion is intimately associated with the 'lateral aberrant thyroid' syndrome. Few now doubt that the presence within a cervical node of thyroid tissue, of either well-differentiated follicular or papillary pattern or a mixture of both, indicates metastasis from a focus within the thyroid itself, virtually always in the ipsilateral lobe. The association has been established abundantly often but the matter was reopened to some extent by Meyer and Steinberg (1969) who found in cervical nodes in 5 of 106 necropsies well-differentiated thyroid tissue not associated with carcinoma in the thyroid itself (a focus of carcinoma was present in one of the thyroids but in the contralateral lobe). However, these authors did believe that a reliable distinction could be made between such ectopic thyroid tissue and metastatic carcinoma, essentially by careful attention to histological detail; their Table 3 lists the characteristics of the benign tissue including uniformity of structure and cellular pattern, and absence of stromal proliferation and psammoma bodies. These observations have been evaluated by Sampson and his colleagues (1970) who do not dismiss altogether the possibility that such benign intrusions may exist. Also, the further support for the 'always-metastatic' interpretation of thyroid tissue in cervical nodes advanced by Butler and co-workers (1967) was critically assessed by Meyer and Steinberg and regarded as not invalidating their belief in its occasional benignity.

It may be that the presence of thyroid tissue of whatever architecture in cervical nodes has during the past 20 years been too uncritically accepted as metastatic from a focus of carcinoma in the thyroid, and thus led sometimes to an unnecessary thyroidectomy. More critical assessment of histological detail should minimise this risk. The possible value of psammoma bodies was emphasised by Klinck and Winship (1959) who found them in association with 48% of 473 primary thyroid carcinomas of various types but in only 1 of 2153 noncancerous thyroids. Their presence, therefore, in a gland apparently without an area of carcinoma is an indication for further search.

The questions raised by the presence of thyroid tissue within a cervical node or nodes are at any rate straightforward: (a) should the tissue be regarded as metastatic from the lesion in the thyroid?, and the answer, despite the occasional exception such as the local case (Case 3.1) must be virtually always 'yes', (b) should ipsilateral lobectomy or sub-total or total thyroidectomy be performed?, (c) should further prophylactic or putatively curative cervical lymphadenectomy be performed? The last two questions have for decades been and still are debatable and the subject of many contributions to the clinico-surgical literature as, for example, those by Noguchi and associates (1970, 1970a) and Otani (1972).

A problem more particularly for the pathologist is presented by the microscopic focus or even manifest nodule of papillary neoplastic tissue in the excised thyroid where there is no associated lymph nodal involvement. This is a borderline problem even harder to solve than that presented by the papillary neoplasms of rectum, bladder or ovary. At these sites there is a gradation of cytological aberrancy at some level of which the pathologist will draw his line, subjective and arbitrary though it be: in the papillary lesion of thyroid, on the other hand, one example may be innocuous, another of identical morphology may metastasise. As earlier shown in the 'summarised totals', this was met on six occasions. Two of the lesions were diagnosed as carcinoma and registered as such, the others as doubtfully carcinoma and so not registered, and none of these patients had any further trouble. These six cases exemplify well the threat to statistics that diagnostic frailty represents. With slight but wholly legitimate differences in the diagnostic thresholds of pathologists, these patients might have figured as six cases of thyroid cancer, or as none. The possibility that hyperplastic papillary infolding may be misinterpreted as carcinoma has been noted by Block and colleagues (1970) with particular reference to nodules in children and in cretins. In five cases in the present series, the presence of an extreme degree of papillary overgrowth in generally hyperplastic glands raised a deep suspicion of malignancy but in no case did this develop.

The notorious unpredictability of thyroid cancer is exemplified by the papillary forms no less than the others. Thus, Ibanez and his co-workers (1966) cite two patients, one dying 2 years after removal of a malignant nodule and the other 42 years after. In the local series, experience has ranged from a patient (Case 3.1) who is alive 18 years after the second of two 'positive' cervical node dissections, with thyroid gland still untouched, to one (Case 3.4) whose cervical node was diagnosed as containing not unduly aberrant papillary carcinoma yet was, as clinical details supplied later revealed, only one of many nodes accompanying a massive and widely invasive primary thyroid carcinoma from which the patient died within days: the histology in the two cases was nevertheless almost identical. A further factor adding to the difficulties of prognosis and classification is that the undifferentiated lesions may sometimes or perhaps always arise from a well-differentiated papillary or follicular carcinoma (Tollefsen et al., 1964; Silverberg et al., 1970; Nishiyama et al., 1972).

## MULTIFOCAL CARCINOMA

The possibility is considerable that a seemingly single focus of carcinoma in a gland is not so but, instead, one of several, a point that has been emphasised on many occasions and especially by those working at the M. D. Anderson Hospital. Thus, Russell and his associates (1963), using a whole-organ-sectioning technique reported intraglandular dissemination within, or spread to the contralateral nodes from, as many as 70 of 89 glands containing a primary carcinoma. That this is frequently 'real' cancer, and thus a real risk, and not 'histologist's' cancer is illustrated in another report from the same group (Rose et al., 1963) in a follow-up study of 116 patients whose thyroid carcinoma had been treated initially by unilateral lobectomy. In 34 of these patients the remaining tissue was removed immediately for, as the authors say, 'prophylactic' reasons: in 21 cases (61.7%) it contained carcinoma. In the remaining 82 followed for up to 19 years, 27 suffered recurrence including 8 who had nodal or more distant (some osseous) metastases. Similarly, intraglandular dissemination was found by Iida and his colleagues (1969) in 27.4% of 186 excised specimens.

These reports make it clear that, in contrast to circumstances mentioned earlier, there are other circumstances where nothing less than total thyroidectomy offers a hope of removing the carcinoma in toto. The difference lies in the nature, which means in effect the morphological character, of the carcinoma. For the borderline '? malignant' adenoma, lobectomy may suffice; for the histologically unequivocal carcinoma, only total thyroidectomy will suffice. The decision will largely lie with the pathologist.

## MEDULLARY CARCINOMA

This lesion, given its name by Hazard and his colleagues (1959), possibly first identified as an amyloid-containing neoplasm by Stoffel (1910) and now accepted as an entity with distinctive histological and endocrine associations, has been the subject of many reviews (see, for example, Melvin et al., 1972; Hill et al., 1973; Chong et al., 1975). It presents the familiar double problem for the pathologist, its histological identification and the relation of the histology to prognosis. Its histological variability, patchy distribution of amyloid and occasional patchy possession of a micro-follicular architecture represents some risk of a 'missed' diagnosis should only a single block of tissue be examined. This may happen with a frozen-section requested during operation, and I have had personal experience of this, but, even if no diagnostic amyloid substance is seen in these circumstances, the degree of structural variability shown even by most of the rather small blocks usually prepared for the cryostat should alert the pathologist to the possibility. Sometimes, however, even many H & E sections may leave the pathologist in doubt, and here it is that other techniques may help. The difficulties there may be have been described by Normann and his collaborators (1976) who note that both ultramicroscopy, with demonstration of secretory granules, and assay of serum calcitonin may establish the diagnosis beyond doubt in cases where the histology is equivocal.

The second problem, correlation of the histology with prognosis, finds the pathologist rather helpless, much as he may be, for example, with the bronchial 'adenoma' or granulosa cell tumour of the ovary. As yet, even reasonably accurate prediction of the risk of metastasis is not possible, and this is generally acknowledged. As with the granulosa cell tumour and some other cancers, there is probably a broad correlation between degree of polymorphism/mitotic activity and aggressiveness but little more can be said as yet than that. The series of 40 patients analysed by Gordon and his colleagues (1973) gives a general picture of the prognostic and therapeutic possibilities: the 10 year survival rate was nearly 70% for those who had had a radical dissection of the neck, nearly 43% for those who had not.

## Lymphoreticular Neoplasms

In one case in the local series (Case 3.25), unduly prominent lymphoid tissue overgrowth raised doubts whether it might represent a malignant lymphoma (ML); later events appeared to show that the overgrowth was either reactive or only coincidental, not neoplastic. This problem is not common but it is usually difficult and has three components.

*First*, can the thyroid be the site of a primary lymphoma? There is general agreement now that, as with most other organs, it can, and that the diagnosis of small-cell neoplasms as carcinoma has in the past been too uncritical and sometimes unjustified (Woolner et al., 1966). In the opinion of Heimann and his colleagues (1978), who analysed 12 cases in relation to the Kiel classification of ML (Lennert et al., 1975, 1975a), ". . . small cell carcinoma of the thyroid does not exist as a distinctive clinicopathological entity".

*Second*, with what confidence can the pathologist make this distinction, between the ML and the small-cell carcinoma? As Heitz and his colleagues (1976) have stressed, and in contrast to Heimann and colleagues just quoted, the greater the number of sections available, the greater the likelihood that a 'sarcoma', whether lymphoid or other, will somewhere show epithelial differentiation. If it does, the answer is evident. If it does not, the answer must be 'rarely, if ever', for even technically perfect special staining of reticulin or any other component is an uncertain guide. There are indeed those, such as Meissner and Warren (1969), who believe with some justification that response to radiotherapy is possibly the best discriminator. In the light of this, some reservations will remain about the true status of some cases of primary malignant lymphoma; for example the 46 reported by Woolner and his associates (1966) who, incidentally, make surprisingly little reference to the histopathological problem. All 46 patients received radiotherapy; of 30 patients with invasive or inoperable lesions, 21 died; of 16 patients with lesions confined to the thyroid alone, only one died.

For the same general reasons it remains an open question whether the versatility of thyroid carcinoma could perhaps explain the apparent coexistence, with Hashimoto's disease in each case, of fibrosarcoma and follicular carcinoma (Glass et al., 1956) and lymphosarcoma and follicular carcinoma (Ayala et al., 1968). In each instance, on reasonable grounds, the authors regarded the components as distinct.

*Third*, does the impressive lymphoid hyperplasia of Hashimoto's disease predispose to the development of a ML? Evidence that it does has been offered by Lindsay and Dailey (1955) who reported the co-existence of Hashimoto's disease in 7 of 8 patients with lymphosarcoma of the thyroid, by Cureton and associates (1956) who described two instances of reticulum cell sarcoma (RCS) in glands with Hashimoto's disease, and by Burke and his colleagues (1977) who have considered the matter against the more recent background of the classifications of ML proposed by Rappaport (1966) and Lukes and Collins (1975).

We may note in the general context of diagnostic accuracy and the borderline case that, of 60 cases originally diagnosed as ML of the thyroid, only 35 were finally accepted by Burke and his colleagues as unequivocal examples. Of these 35, 34 were reclassified as histiocytic lymphoma (formerly RCS), 29 diffuse and 5 'nodular becoming diffuse'; the histiocytes were considered to be 'immunoblasts', and 3 of the lesions contained large cells closely resembling R-S cells. In 27 of the cases there was remnant thyroid parenchyma; this showed 'chronic lymphocytic thyroiditis of the Hashimoto's type', and, like earlier workers, the authors emphasise how difficult the distinction of this from ML may be. The malignant lesions were characterised by transgression of the capsule of the thyroid and a generally monomorphous population of cells, the thyroiditis by non-transgression of the capsule and a generally polymorphous population of cells (mostly lymphocytes of varying size and plasma cells). Mitotic figures had been equally numerous in both the benign and malignant lesions and so were of no prognostic value. As would be expected, the probably immunoblastic nature of the 'histiocyte' suggested that the lesion was basically an immunoblastic sarcoma, and the authors believed that it had evolved from the lymphoid thyroiditis, perhaps from an aberrant clone provoked by chronic antigenic stimulation.

This possibly precancerous habit of lymphoid thyroiditis recalls an earlier-stated opinion of its significance in relation, not to ML, but to carcinoma, and this, in turn, has some bearing on prognosis and treatment. In a survey of over 9000 thyroidectomy specimens, Hirabayashi and Lindsay (1965) noted that, of glands showing chronic focal or diffuse thyroiditis, 22.5% contained carcinoma, whereas, of glands not showing such thyroiditis, only 2.4% contained carcinoma. This had led to a suspicion that chronic thyroiditis was a premalignant lesion sufficiently threatening to make total thyroidectomy the treatment of choice. However, from a further study of 436 cases of carcinoma, these authors concluded, as the most plausible explanation, that associated Hashimoto-type thyroiditis was more probably not the cause of the carcinoma (mostly papillary) but the consequence, due to the elaboration of antigens by the neoplasm. Hashimoto-type thyroiditis per se would therefore not be a precancerous state, and total thyroidectomy for it, therefore, not indicated. The observations of Burke and his colleagues (1977), recently endorsed by those of Heimann and associates (1978), would now seem to restore chronic thyroiditis to its role as a precancerous condition, in this case, however, as a prelymphoma, not a precarcinoma.

## HYPERTHYROIDISM

A matter of general relevance lies in the statement of Wade (1975) that 'As yet there is no accepted record of a thyroid carcinoma, without secondaries, producing hyperthyroidism'. The explanation for this stated fact may be either that nonmetastasising carcinomas can cause hyperthyroidism but that no case reports have been published, and this is possible, or that the malignant tissue can be metabolically active only when ectopic, not in situ, and this is not easy to explain. Be that as it may, the clinical reassurance that hyperthyroidism may give in the case of a patient with a thyroid under suspicion would have to be tempered by the thought that metastases might already be present but not as yet detectable. A recent local case at least throws doubt on the proposition, that of a man of 32 whose thyroid, after 3 years of treatment with radio-iodine, underwent 'fulminant' enlargement over 2 months. Thyroidectomy then revealed largely anaplastic but recognisably microfollicular carcinoma. No metastases were demonstrable at this time yet he was notably hyperthyroid. He died 5 months later but there was no necropsy. The true position vis-à-vis metastasis therefore remains uncertain.

## CRYPTIC CARCINOMA

The cryptic character of thyroid cancer is well illustrated by two reports. Of 94 patients shown at necropsy by Silliphant and his co-workers (1964) to have died directly of thyroid cancer, only 60 (64%) had been correctly diagnosed during life. These authors remark that this figure is almost the same as that reported sometimes for the level of correct antemortem diagnosis of bronchial carcinoma but it is still unexpectedly low. A diagnostic success rate as low as this is understandable in the case of carcinoma of the bronchus but is unexpected in the case of an organ as anatomically superficial as the thyroid. The other report was by Silverberg and Vidone (1966) who, in 300 consecutive unselected necropsies, found eight primary cancers of the thyroid: only two had been diagnosed clinically, three had been observed grossly at necropsy, three were found microscopically. In the light of findings like this, it is no surprise that published estimates of the incidence of the various types of cancer in the thyroid, whether in single nodules or smoothly enlarged glands or in the nodular goitre, are so varied and consequently of such relatively little help to the clinician or pathologist in the individual case. In commenting on the wide variation in figures of incidence of thyroid cancer, Winship (1967) remarked that "Some of the disparity is also due to the lack of uniform criteria for evaluating pathologic findings. Certainly the low incidence of malignant tumors in some areas reflects the failure of pathologists to recognize cancer of the thyroid". No doubt this is true, for not every thyroid is serially sliced at necropsy (as was done by

Silverberg and Vidone in their 300 cases). At the same time, the diagnostic certitude and at any rate the clinical significance of the microscopically discovered cancers, the 'histologists' cancers', is debatable.

The extent of diagnostic uncertainty with lesions of the thyroid that besets the pathologist is great: it has been further revealed in a recent report from the already mentioned Finnish Cancer Registry (Saxén et al., 1978). A total of 696 cases registered as cancer of the thyroid was reviewed by five pathologists independently. In 83% of the cases, three of the five observers were in agreement but in only 58% was unanimity achieved. Difference of opinion was least with the papillary carcinoma (disagreement in 7% of the cases) and most with the follicular carcinoma (disagreement in 27%). The commonest form of diagnostic divergence was between the follicular carcinoma and some form of benign overgrowth.

In one of the articles cited earlier (Editorial, 1976) the comment is made that "Many of the problems seen in the treatment of thyroid cancer stem from the clinician's failure to make an accurate diagnosis". If this be 'failure', it is failure of a fully excusable order, for, as has been stressed, even the much more strategically placed pathologist to whom the clinician gives the tissue itself cannot always be sure.

## Conclusions

1) For practical purposes, malignant neoplasms of the thyroid may still be divided into: (a) the unequivocally malignant, including malignant lymphoma; (b) the papillary carcinomas, from which papillary adenomas are sometimes not certainly distinguishable; and (c) others that present diagnostic difficulty of varying degree.

2) The reality of the 'benign metastasising goitre' remains. Over-diagnosis as carcinoma of lesions that probably are in truth follicular adenomas seems likely to persist. It is the price paid in the hope of 'catching' the occasional lesion of identical histological pattern that metastasises.

3) Prognosis in the unequivocal cancers is related much more closely to degree of local anatomical spread than to the histology.

4) Thyroid tissue within cervical nodes may not always be metastatic carcinoma.

5) The certain diagnosis of medullary carcinoma may sometimes be possible only by the use of ultramicroscopy and calcitonin assay.

6) Small-cell malignant neoplasms are much more likely to be ML than carcinoma.

7) The place of frozen-section techniques in the assessment of lumps in the thyroid is sharply restricted and small.

## References

Ayala A, Sloane J, Wolma FJ (1968) Coexistent lymphoma, adenocarcinoma and struma lymphomatosa. JAMA 204: 829–831

Block MA, Horn RC, Miller JM (1970) Hazards in the diagnosis and management of certain thyroid nodules in children. Am J Surg 120: 447–451

Branson KM, Houston W (1949) Malignant disease of the thyroid gland. Lancet 2: 979–982

Burke JS, Butler JJ, Fuller LM (1977) Malignant lymphomas of the thyroid. A clinical pathologic study of 35 patients including ultrastructural observations. Cancer 39: 1587–1602

Butler JJ, Tulinius H, Ibanez ML, Ballantyne AJ, Clark RL (1967) Significance of thyroid tissue in lymph nodes associated with carcinoma of the head, neck or lung. Cancer 20: 103–112

Byar DP, Green SB, Dor P, Williams ED, Colon J, van Gilse HA, Mayer M, Sylvester RJ, van Glabbeke M (1979) A prognostic index for thyroid carcinoma. A study of the E.O.R.T.C. thyroid cancer cooperative group. Europ J Cancer 15: 1033–1041

Chong GC, Beahrs OH, Sizemore GW, Woolner LH (1975) Medullary carcinoma of the thyroid gland. Cancer 35: 695–704

Cline RE, Shingleton WW (1968) Long-term results in the treatment of carcinoma of the thyroid. Am J Surg 115: 545–551

Cureton RJR, Harland DHC, Hosford J, Pike C (1956) Reticulosarcoma in Hashimoto's disease. Br J Surg 44: 561–566

Editorial (1971) The solitary thyroid nodule. Br Med J 2: 720–721

Editorial (1973) The solitary thyroid nodule. Br Med J 4: 310–311

Editorial (1976) Thyroid cancer. Br Med J 1: 113–114

Exelby PE, Frazell EL (1969) Carcinoma of the thyroid in children. Surg Clin North Am 49: 249–259

Glass HG, Waldron GW, Brown WG (1956) Coexistent sarcoma, adenocarcinoma, and Hashimoto's disease in a thyroid gland. Cancer 9: 310–316

Gordon PR, Huvos AG, Strong EW (1973) Medullary carcinoma of the thyroid gland: A clinicopathologic study of 40 cases. Cancer 31: 915–924

Greene R (1969) Treatment of thyroid cancer. Br Med J 4: 787–789

Halnan KE (1966) Influence of age and sex on incidence and prognosis of thyroid cancer. Three hundred forty-four cases followed for ten years. Cancer 19: 1534–1536

Hazard JB, Hawk WA, Crile G (1959) Medullary (solid) carcinoma of the thyroid—a clinicopathologic entity. J Clin Endocrinol Metab 19: 152–161

Heimann R, Vannineuse A, Sloover C de, Dor P (1978) Malignant lymphomas and undifferentiated small cell carcinoma of the thyroid: A clinicopathological review in the light of the Kiel classification for malignant lymphomas. Histopathol 2: 201–213

Heitz P, Moser H, Staub JJ (1976) A study of 573 thyroid tumors and 161 autopsy cases observed over a thirty-year period. Cancer 37: 2329–2337

Hill CS, Ibanez ML, Samaan NA, Ahearn MJ, Clark RL (1973) Medullary (solid) carcinoma of the thyroid gland: An analysis of the M. D. Anderson Hospital experience with patients and this tumor, its special features, and its histogenesis. Medicine (Baltimore) 52: 141–171

Hirabayashi RN, Lindsay S (1965) The relation of thyroid carcinoma and chronic thyroiditis. Surg Gynecol Obstet 121: 243–252

Ibanez ML, Russell WO, Albores-Saavedra J, Lampertico P, White EC, Clark RL (1966) Thyroid carcinoma—biologic behavior and mortality. Postmortem findings in 42 cases, including 27 in which the disease was fatal. Cancer 19: 1039–1052

Iida F, Yonekura M, Miyakawa M (1969) Study of intraglandular dissemination of thyroid cancer. Cancer 24: 764–771

Kendall LW, Condon RE (1969) Prediction of malignancy in solitary thyroid nodules. Lancet 1: 1071–1073

Klinck GH, Winship T (1959) Psammoma bodies and thyroid cancer. Cancer 12: 656–662

Lennert K, Mohri N, Stein H, Kaiserling E (1975) The histopathology of malignant lymphoma. Br J Haematol 31: suppl 193–203

Lennert K, Stein H, Kaiserling E (1975a) Cytological and functional criteria for the classification of malignant lymphomata. Br J Cancer 31: suppl II 29–43

Lindsay S, Dailey ME (1955) Malignant lymphoma of the thyroid gland and its relation to Hashimoto disease: A clinical and pathologic study of 8 patients. J Clin Endocrinol Metab 15: 1332–1353

Lukes RJ, Collins RD (1975) New approaches to the classification of the lymphomata. Br J Cancer 31: suppl II 1–28

Meissner WA, Warren S (1969) Tumors of the thyroid gland. Atlas of tumor pathology, 2nd ser, fasc 4. Armed Forces Institute of Pathology, Washington, D.C.

Melvin KEW, Tashjian AH, Miller HH (1972) Studies in familial (medullary) thyroid carcinoma. Recent Prog Horm Res 28: 399–460

Meyer JS, Steinberg LS (1969) Microscopically benign thyroid follicles in cervical lymph nodes. Serial section study of lymph node inclusions and entire thyroid gland in 5 cases. Cancer 24: 302–311

Nishiyama RH, Dunn EL, Thompson NW (1972) Anaplastic spindle-cell and giant-cell tumors of the thyroid gland. Cancer 30: 113–127

Noguchi S, Noguchi A, Murakami N (1970) Papillary carcinoma of the thyroid. I. Developing pattern of metastasis. Cancer 26: 1053–1060

Noguchi S, Noguchi A, Murakami N (1970a) Papillary carcinoma of the thyroid. II. Value of prophylactic lymph node excision. Cancer 26: 1061–1064

Normann T, Johannessen JV, Gautvik KM, Olsen BR, Brennhovd JO (1976) Medullary carcinoma of the thyroid: Diagnostic problems. Cancer 38: 366–377

Otani S (1972) Papillary adenomatous tumors of aberrant thyroid in cervical lymph nodes. Mt Sinai J Med NY 39: 70–75

Park WW, Lees JC (1955) The histology of cancer of the thyroid. Cancer 8: 320–335

Rappaport H (1966) Atlas of tumor pathology, sect III, fasc 8. Tumors of the hematopoietic system. Armed Forces Institute of Pathology, Washington, D.C.

Rose RG, Kelsey MP, Russell WO, Ibanez ML, White EC, Clark RL (1963) Follow-up study of thyroid cancer treated by unilateral lobectomy. Am J Surg 106: 494–500

Russell WO, Ibanez ML, Clark RL, White EC (1963) Thyroid carcinoma. Classification, intraglandular dissemination, and clinicopathological study based upon whole organ sections of 80 glands. Cancer 16: 1425–1460

Russell MA, Gilbert EF, Jaeschke WF (1975) Prognostic features of thyroid cancer. A long-term followup of 68 cases. Cancer 36: 553–559

Sampson RJ, Oka H, Key CR, Buncher CR, Iijima S (1970a) Metastases from occult thyroid carcinoma. An autopsy study from Hiroshima and Nagasaki, Japan. Cancer 25: 803–811

Saxén E, Franssila K, Bjarnason O, Norman T, Ringertz N (1978) Observer variation in histologic classification of thyroid cancer. Acta Pathol Microbiol Scand [A] 86: 483–486

Saxén EA, Franssila K, Hakama M (1969) Effect of histological typing of Registry material on the results of epidemiological comparisons in thyroid cancer. In: Hedinger E (ed) Thyroid cancer, UICC Monograph ser, vol 12. Springer, Berlin Heidelberg New York, pp 58–103

Silliphant WM, Klinck GH, Levitin MS (1964)

Thyroid carcinoma and death. A clinicopathological study of 193 autopsies. Cancer 17: 513–525

Silverberg SG, Vidone RA (1966) Adenoma and carcinoma of the thyroid. Cancer 19: 1053–1062

Silverberg SG, Hutter RVP, Foote FW (1970) Fatal carcinoma of the thyroid: Histology, metastases, and causes of death. Cancer 25: 792–802

Stoffel E (1910) Lokales amyloid der Schilddrüse. Virchows Arch [Pathol Anat] 201: 245–251

Tawes RL, Delorimier AA (1968) Thyroid carcinoma during youth. J Pediatr Surg 3: 210–218

Taylor S (1969) Carcinoma of the thyroid gland. J R Coll Surg Edinb 14: 183–192

Taylor S (1969a) The solitary thyroid nodule. J R Coll Surg Edinb 14: 267–271

Tollefsen HR, De Cosse JJ, Hutter RVP (1964) Papillary carcinoma of the thyroid. A clinical and pathological study of 70 fatal cases. Cancer 17: 1035–1044

Wade JSH (1975) The aetiology and diagnosis of malignant tumours of the thyroid gland. Br J Surg 62: 760–764

Ward R (1944) Malignant goiter. Surgery 16: 783–803

Winship T (1967) Management of patients with cancer of the thyroid. Cancer 20: 1815–1818

Woolner LB, McConahey WM, Beahrs OH, Black BM (1966) Primary malignant lymphoma of the thyroid. Review of forty-six cases. Am J Surg 111: 502–523

Woolner LB, Beahrs OH, Black BM, McConahey WM, Keating FR (1968) Thyroid carcinoma: General considerations and follow-up data on 1181 cases. In: Young S, Inman DR (eds) Symposium of thyroid neoplasia. Academic Press, London, pp 51–77

# 4 Lesions of Lymph Nodes

Many publications confirm the general belief that the ambiguous or equivocal lymph node presents one of the hardest and commonest problems in histopathological practice. Those cited below are retrospective analyses of abnormal lymph nodes in the course of which, we may note, almost all the observers emphasise that their reassessments were carried out 'blind'. This acknowledges the fact that the greater the histological difficulty, the greater the need to avoid the bias induced by foreknowledge of circumstances.

As the title of their paper shows, Coppleson and his colleagues (1970) set out avowedly to estimate the degree of 'observer disagreement' surrounding the histology of Hodgkin's disease. Their series was culled from 'all cases diagnosed as Hodgkin's disease' in their area during a 34-year period. From their series, some cases were excluded as being not Hodgkin's disease but their number, and thus the proportion of the original total they represented, was not stated. Three observers were unanimously agreed on classification in 76.0% and 54.2% of cases using the Jackson/Parker and Rye classifications respectively. There was, thus, a considerable variation in opinion, especially in terms of the Rye classification, and these authors went so far as to say in their summary that "individual observers, independently evaluating the histologic aspects of the classification of Hodgkin's disease, had a level of agreement too low to be scientifically useful". However, two out of three observers were in agreement in over 90% of cases in both classifications, a finding which led the authors to emphasise the value of consensus opinion: two opinions were better than one, and three better than two, with a likely result that even more than three would increase the degree of reproducibility of opinions still further. Pathological practice no doubt varies from area to area and country to country, but in the United Kingdom at any rate it would be surprising if the final decision on a borderline lymph node were *not* a consensus decision, however informally achieved. There is a great deal of passing or sending of difficult sections to colleagues for further opinion, and it is hard to believe that a singleton pathologist would, on such a section, expose a patient to the rigours of current investigation and treatment of a malignant lymphoma on the basis of his opinion alone.

Findings rather similar to those of Coppleson and his colleagues had been published earlier by Hall and Olson (1956) in analysing 119 slides from 96 patients with 'malignant lymphoma'. All were examined by three pathologists who found themselves in essential agreement in 72% of the cases. Even so, there were instances where all the examiners could not agree, not on the type of lymphoma but whether the lesion was a malignant lymphoma at all.

Figure 4.1 has been constructed from the data of Kreyberg and Iversen (1959) who reviewed 124 borderline nodes, 41 originally 'moderately' suspicious and 83 'gravely' suspicious. As the figure shows, on reassessment, 40 were judged to be certainly benign and 56 certainly malignant: that is, the review reduced the 124 borderline cases to 28 but simultaneously revealed the marginal over-diagnosis of 40 cases (33%) and the marginal under-diagnosis of 56 (45%).

A similar series of cases, 158 doubtful nodes from a total of 906 nodal biopsies, was reported by Dawson and co-workers (1964). Figure 4.2 represents their findings along the same lines as Fig. 4.1 but differs in that these observers included categories of 'reactive hyperplasia' and 'malignant lymphoma'. It is not possible, from

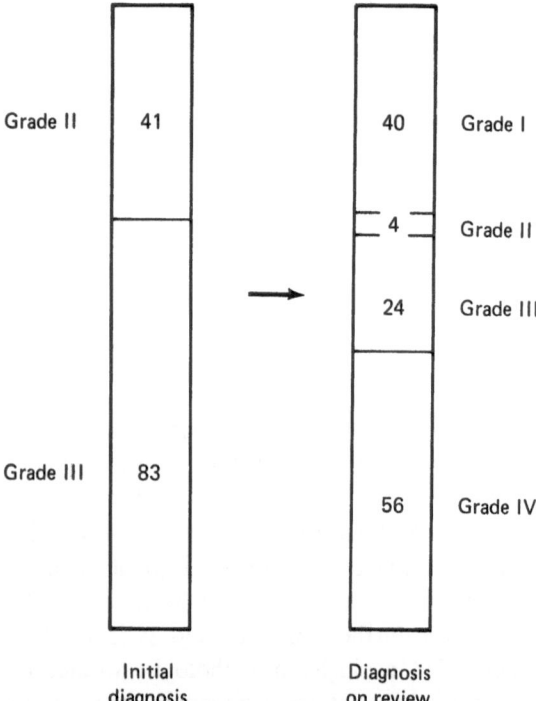

**Fig. 4.1.** Analysis of 124 cases of 'lymphoid hyperplasia—malignancy cannot be excluded'. Grade I: not malignant; grade II: moderately suspicious; grade III: gravely suspicious; grade IV: malignant (Kreyberg and Iversen, 1959).

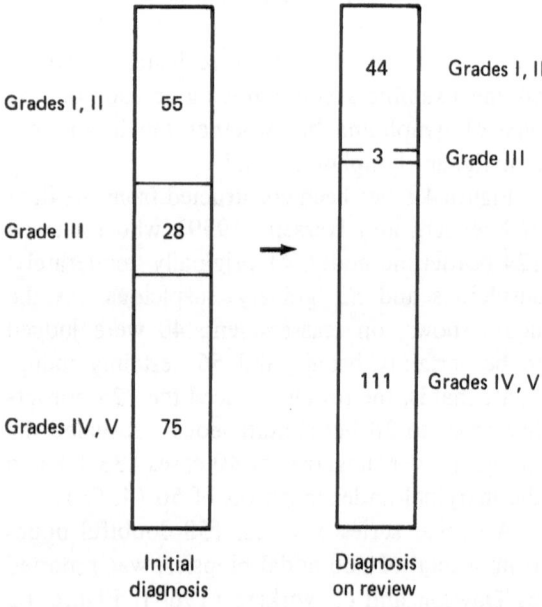

**Fig. 4.2.** Results on review of '158 difficult lymph node biopsies'. Grades I, II: reactive hyperplasia; grade III: equivocal; grades IV, V: malignant lymphoma (Dawson et al., 1964).

the mode of presentation of their figures, to calculate a percentage value for rates of apparent under/over-diagnosis as malignant but two points emerge: (*a*) as seen in Fig. 4.2, reconsideration of the nodes almost completely abolished the category of 'equivocal'; (*b*) the number of cases in the 'malignant' category became much larger, a more exact measure of this being given in their own statement that '. . . 35 examples of malignant lymphoma were recognized among 83 biopsy specimens originally reported as certainly reactive or equivocal'. That is, rather unusually, there had been originally a large degree of under-diagnosis.

Two remarkable papers have been published by Symmers (1968a, b), surveys and reassessments of 600 and 226 cases originally diagnosed as Hodgkin's disease and reticulum cell sarcoma respectively. The outcome of the analyses is shown in Fig. 4.3. The most striking feature is the relatively enormous degree of over-diagnosis as Hodgkin's disease of inflammatory/reactive nodal patterns: almost exactly one-third of the cases originally diagnosed as Hodgkin's disease were judged on review to be non-malignant. Admittedly, this review was not performed by panel consensus, and opinions might well vary on some of the cases, but even so the degree of discrepancy is revealing, disconcerting, and educative. The publication of these papers almost certainly aroused awareness of the size of the problem and so added something towards its solution. More recently, an analysis was made by Iversen and Sandnes (1971) of the opinions of eight pathologists on lymph nodes showing 'giant follicular hyperplasia or lymphoma' from 35 patients of known outcome (19 'benign clinical development', 16 'malignant clinical development'). In the final analysis, with decision by majority verdict, there emerged only four discrepant diagnoses, two false-positive, two false-negative. At the same time, complete unanimity was attained in only 8 of the 35 cases, while, amongst individual pathologists giving their initial opinion, the number of false-positive and false-negative diagnoses ranged from 1 to 12 and 1 to 10 respectively.

Another summary of lymph nodal pathology may be mentioned here, that of Moore and his associates (1957). It is not concerned primarily

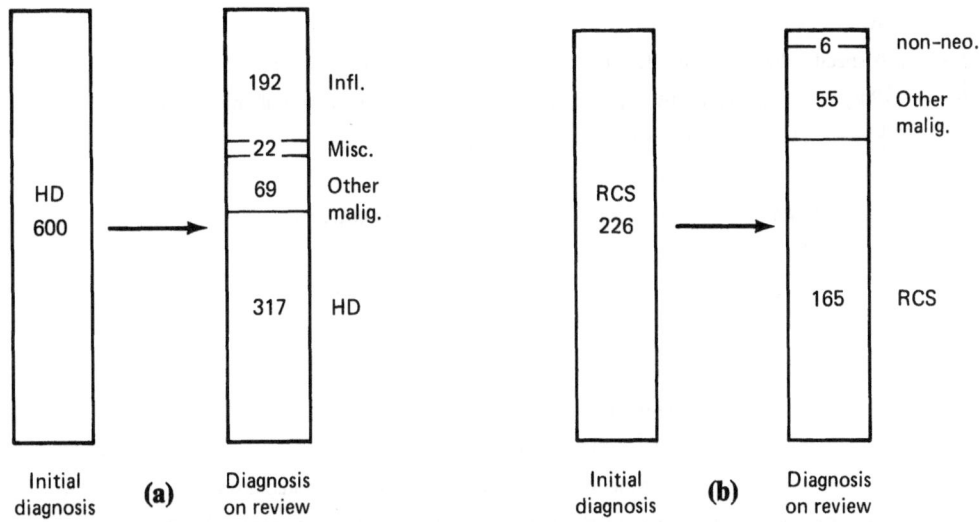

**Fig. 4.3.** Results on review of (a) 600 cases originally diagnosed as Hodgkin's disease, (b) 226 cases originally diagnosed as reticulum cell sarcoma (Symmers, 1968 a, b).

with the borderline lesion, though the need for diagnostic revisions did emerge, but rather with the prognostic implications simply of an enlarged node. These observers wished to find out what had happened to 'all patients who had had biopsies done on enlarged superficial lymph nodes' in their area during 1945–1955. Their findings in the case of 379 patients are shown, semidiagrammatically reproduced, in Fig. 4.4.

Points to note are that the review yielded six cases of malignant lymphoma previously undiagnosed, and that a further ten patients eventually developed either a malignant lymphoma or leukaemia. It is evident from the article that these ten cases were not all examples of outright under-diagnosis since seven had been included originally in a category of 'atypical hyperplasia' or 'hyperplasia with abnormal cells'. It is interesting, however, that within the same category were four patients with a 'collagen disease' and one who remains alive and well. Discussion on the nodal histology was concerned mainly with the changes in patients with lupus erythematosus, and as such it is particularly valuable.

Almost by definition, the best hope of reducing the relatively large amount of under- and over-diagnosis revealed by these various papers still lies in the sharper definition of entities, and this, in turn, still depends on the correct identification of morphological criteria of proven reliability. However, the recognition of morphological features may not always, or perhaps for

much longer, be the ultimate arbiter. The recent proposal by Lukes and Collins (1974, 1975) of a scheme of classification of the lymphomas along functional lines, in terms of the B- and T-cell systems and transformation of lymphocytes, is a portent. Our present preoccupation with cytological minutiae may in time be seen to be as irrelevant to certain diagnosis here as are the varied clinical expressions of syphilis, malaria, and brucellosis to certain diagnosis there. However, that day is not yet: still we must try to familiarise ourselves with emerging entities as they are proffered, and for the general pathologist the difficulties are considerable: new classifications abound and debate is endless. The difficulties have been well described by Symmers (1978) in his scholarly account of the pathology of the lymphoreticular system (with its 1643 references and many entertaining and educative footnotes). They also receive regular attention in a series of editorial annotations, mainly on Hodgkin's disease (Editorial 1969, 1973, 1974, 1975, 1975a, 1976c, 1979) which all surely hope will continue.

In the days when malignant lymphomas (ML) were classified as giant follicular lymphoma (or equivalent term), lymphosarcoma (LS), reticulum cell sarcoma (RCS) and Hodgkin's disease (HD), the position was relatively straightforward. We now know that, morphologically at least, this subdivision was too simple: new techniques and observations have revealed its

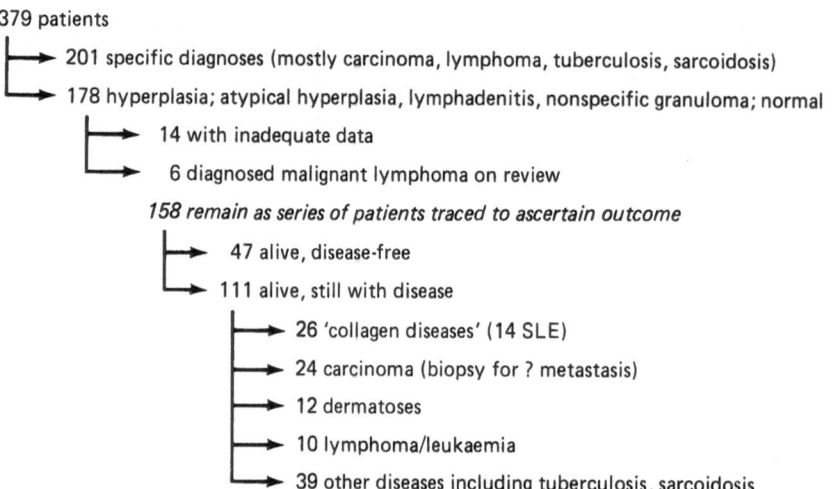

379 patients

▸ 201 specific diagnoses (mostly carcinoma, lymphoma, tuberculosis, sarcoidosis)

▸ 178 hyperplasia; atypical hyperplasia, lymphadenitis, nonspecific granuloma; normal

▸ 14 with inadequate data

▸ 6 diagnosed malignant lymphoma on review

*158 remain as series of patients traced to ascertain outcome*

▸ 47 alive, disease-free

▸ 111 alive, still with disease

▸ 26 'collagen diseases' (14 SLE)

▸ 24 carcinoma (biopsy for ? metastasis)

▸ 12 dermatoses

▸ 10 lymphoma/leukaemia

▸ 39 other diseases including tuberculosis, sarcoidosis

**Fig. 4.4.** An analysis of diagnosis in the case of 379 patients on whom a biopsy of lymph node(s) was performed (Moore et al., 1957).

shortcomings. In these circumstances, the general pathologist can do little but wait for the emergence from specialist centres of entities that seem likely to serve both clinician and pathologist as well in the future as did these others in the past. For they did serve well. It will be some time yet before such terms as, for example, 'diffuse centrocytic lymphoma (germinoblastoma) without sclerosis' or 'secondary centroblastic lymphoma (germinoblastic sarcoma)' convey the same immediate information as, say, 'lymphocytic lymphoma', which the patient might outlive, and 'reticulum cell sarcoma' with its implication of high and rapid mortality.

In the case of Hodgkin's disease the scheme that has emerged is the Rye classification (Lukes et al., 1966a), now widely accepted essentially because: (*a*) it can be used by pathologists with fair reproducibility (the 95% reproducibility of diagnoses attained on review after a 6 month interval by a single pathologist [Crum et al., 1974] might not be achieved by many individuals or most panels but is at any rate illustrative); and (*b*) it is prognostically helpful. At the same time it has its shortcomings. Even when proposed, the scheme was considered less than adequate, for the histopathologist at least (Lukes and Butler, 1966; Lukes, 1971), while recent histometric analysis of diffuse lesions has shown that '. . . lymphocytes are, in general, more numerous in the lymphocytic depletion than in the mixed cellularity subtypes' (Livesey et al., 1978). The implications of this surprising revelation are likely to be far-reaching. For the non-H

lymphomas, the terms proposed by Rappaport (1966) are widely used. In essence, they divide lymphosarcoma and reticulum cell sarcoma each into a well-differentiated and a poorly differentiated form, with appropriate name, and supplement these with a fifth intermediate or 'mixed-cell' form: any of these, it is held, may assume a follicular or nodular form; thus was follicular lymphoma, as a separate entity, abolished. The position of the Rappaport classification is at present closely similar to that of the Rye classification of HD: each has gained acceptance in practice by merit. Another scheme for the non-H lymphomas has been proposed more recently by Lennert and his colleagues (Gérard-Marchant et al., 1974; Lennert et al., 1975, 1975a), the so-called Kiel classification, and with this has come a further group of suggested names and proffered entities. This classification which, like that of Lukes and Collins (1975), takes note of the functional as well as the morphological character of cells, has yet to prove itself in practice; with its complex terminology, universal acceptance, even if this should become obviously desirable, will be neither quick nor easy.

A leading article on follicular lymphomas (Editorial, 1974), and the correspondence that followed, culminating in a communication by Dorfman (1974), together form a striking illustration of the detailed range of debate that classification of the lymphomas can generate or provoke. The effect on many a general pathologist, confused if not exasperated by his lymphadenologist colleagues, is counter-productive; in the confusion, with experts at odds, he tends to cling to entities long familiar. Years will probably pass before the older terms disappear altogether from the day-to-day reports of pathologists. However, increasingly the reports will be amplified by the explanatory addition of the more modern equivalent terms as these are shown to be more useful; and here there is some risk. The pathologist may, in his reporting, find himself using terms as yet unfamiliar to his clinical colleagues, and this should be avoided, perhaps by explanation at combined clinics. 'Blinding with science', whether intentional or unintentional, has no place in biopsy reporting, and the danger of doing so is nowhere greater than with the lesions of lymph nodes.

There is no intention here to analyse and evaluate the terminology of the lymphomas, for data on this are voluminous. Rather, as in the other chapters, it is to examine in retrospect the quality of histological diagnosis in routine practice with a comment on some of the main obstacles to accuracy. The original diagnosis as RCS of a malignant lesion now better understood and more appropriately given another name is not, in retrospect, a wrong diagnosis. It may be an outdated diagnosis but, as used at the time, it may have been wholly appropriate. A variant of this situation concerns the once much-used term 'atypical Hodgkin's disease'. No doubt, in this Department as elsewhere, some lesions that were not HD were placed in this category. At the same time, many such lesions, differing as they did from the pattern usually illustrated then as 'typical' HD, were indeed HD. For structural variants now comfortably accommodated within the Rye classification there was, until the advent of this classification, no other resting place but the category 'atypical'.

Local experience with lesions of lymph nodes is described in two parts, inevitably with some overlap: first, where the diagnosis of HD had been mainly at issue; second, where a lymphoma other than HD had been at issue. The short discussion at the end of the sections, as well as incorporating an analysis of the local borderline cases, now seen in retrospect, includes a note on circumstances, not met personally, where the pathologist is likely to be asked whether prognosis can be given any more accurately in the individual case, perhaps in childhood or during pregnancy, than is conveyed, it may be, by just the diagnosis 'HD' or 'LS'.

The practical difficulties in the way of achieving a comprehensive examination of lesions of lymph nodes seem not to be widely appreciated. Quite apart from clinical data collecting, preparations should be made from the node, either fresh or appropriately fixed, for at least imprints, immunohistological, serological, cytogenetic, ultramicroscopic and microbiological as well as 'ordinary' histological study. Ideally, to meet these needs, the pathologist, suitably equipped, should be in the operating theatre at the removal of any lymph node; best of all, with the node exposed, the final excision should be performed by the pathologist himself, for he, better than many, knows how tenderly the node should be treated. However, the time required would be great, for not every lymph node would be lymphomatous, nor every 'node' a lymph node. No doubt, in the matter of reporting, the standard descriptions of nodes, especially those of 'nonspecific reactive' type, are less informative than they might be. At the same time, it is not easy to decide what type of information should be sought and recorded. Guidance has been given here by Cottier and his colleagues (1973) who have offered a 'summary' protocol and an 'expanded' protocol by which various data could be recorded in a standard form with the immunological function of lymph nodes particularly in mind. As with the technical manipulation of a node, so with this scheme of reporting; it would take much time. Even the 'summary' protocol of Cottier and his colleagues requires consideration of 85 separate entries (the expanded has 330): the authors concede that the protocol '. . . may be considered too complex for the busy surgical pathologist . . .', and few would disagree with this. Nevertheless, the scheme is, as the authors intend, a guide to the kind of information that may be usefully recorded even if, at present, largely for posterity.

## Local Series

During the years in question, the diagnosis of Hodgkin's disease was made in the case of 58 patients and considered possible in a further 22; the diagnosis of a non-Hodgkin lymphoma was

**Table 4.1.** Analysis of 'quality of diagnosis' in 40 borderline lymph nodes.

| Nature of uncertainty | Under-diagnosis | Over-diagnosis | Appropriate diagnosis | Total |
|---|---|---|---|---|
| *I. Cases of ? Hodgkin's disease* | | | | |
| Reactive vs HD | 3 | 2 | 2 (1*) | 7 |
| Leukaemia vs HD | | | 1 | 1 |
| Early, atypical or suggestive of HD | 4 | 1 | 9 | 14 |
| Total | 7 | 3 | 12 | 22 |
| *II. Cases of ? (non-H) malignant lymphoma* | | | | |
| Reactive vs neoplastic | | 1 | 9 (6*) | 10 |
| Not reactive but ? lymphoma | | 1 | 4 | 5 |
| ? Lymphoma ? Carcinoma | | | 1 | 1 |
| ? Follicular lymphoma | 1 | 1 | | 2 |
| Total | 1 | 3 | 14 | 18 |

* Of the 26 cases 'appropriately diagnosed', the histology in 1 + 6 (7) instances was still, on review, judged ambiguous.

*Summarised total of 'quality of diagnosis' in the 40 borderline cases:*

| | |
|---|---|
| Under-diagnoses | 8 |
| Over-diagnoses | 6 |
| Appropriate diagnoses | 26 (7 still ambiguous) |

made in 75 and considered possible in a further 18. There are, thus, for analysis as the local series, a total of 40 borderline or ambiguous cases culled from a total of 173 instances during the relevant years where the diagnosis was considered to be possibly, probably, or certainly malignant lymphoma, as follows:

1)  80 Hodgkin's disease (HD) or ? HD

58 firmly diagnosed

22 borderline diagnoses

2)  93 (non-HD) malignant lymphoma or ? (non-HD) malignant lymphoma

75 firmly diagnosed

18 borderline diagnoses

That is, 40/173 or almost one-quarter of the cases had raised significant doubt. The results of a review of these 40 cases are shown in Table 4.1. A more detailed analysis of the two main groups, HD and non-HD, is shown later in Tables 4.2 and 4.3.

Consideration is given later, separately, to some of the main diagnostic problems surrounding the Hodgkin and non-Hodgkin lymphomas as they present themselves in practice; that is, with the interpretation of histological pattern rather than of fine details of nomenclature. Certainly, for obvious reasons, universal agreement on nomenclature is the ideal but that day is still some way away. To say that every new technique, whether instrumental or tinctorial, fathers a new classification would be an exaggeration but it cannot be far from the truth. No doubt it would be instructive to re-examine all of the 40 borderline cases by all possible techniques but, with only paraffin blocks to hand, this cannot be done. However, reclassification in retrospect is not the primary purpose of this analysis; assessment of diagnostic accuracy is, and accuracy can fairly be judged only in relation to terms and diagnoses generally accepted at the time. On this understanding, therefore, the present series may be assessed as follows:

## Under-diagnosis

There had been significant or marginal under-diagnosis in eight cases, seven of them cases of

? HD (all died, four of HD, two of RCS, one of lymphosarcoma; all but one had received radiotherapy); one of follicular lymphoma (died, without radiotherapy, of lymphosarcoma). In these patients, some time may have been lost in instituting therapy but it seems doubtful whether definitive diagnosis at the time of first biopsy would have significantly altered the outcome.

### Over-diagnosis

In the six cases significantly or marginally over-diagnosed, the only consequence of clinical significance was the unnecessary performance of a permanent colostomy. This was, of course, regrettable but would almost certainly not happen today. A lesion that led to a gastrectomy, plasmacytoma and not lymphosarcoma, would have required the gastrectomy in any event. In the four other cases, no specific local or systemic treatment was used, and all the patients were alive and well many years later.

### Appropriate Diagnosis

In 7 of the 26 cases the histology, seen 'blind' by several colleagues, remains ambiguous. Only one of the seven patients received specific treatment (radiotherapy) and was well 10 years later. Such doubt as the report contained had been so couched as to lead to an agreed clinical policy of 'expectancy'. The generally satisfactory outcome in most of these patients is possibly in some part a function of co-operation between pathologist, clinician and radiotherapist.

### CASE DATA I
### ? HODGKIN'S DISEASE (TABLE 4.2)

### Case 4.1

F (63 years) with what appeared to be a painless swelling of submaxillary salivary gland noticed for 4 months, ? ductal stenosis due to newly fitted denture. Dilatation of the duct produced no improvement, and the gland was excised. Of the specimen received, one half was salivary tissue, the other comprised two large lymph nodes (20 × 12 mm and 15 × 10 mm).

Only relatively scanty minute follicles remained (approximately 30, none larger than 1 mm, in a whole 20 × 12 mm section), all consisting purely of lymphocytes, none with germ-centres (Fig. 4.5). The rest of the parenchyma was composed of an equal and even mixture of lymphocytes and large pale cells with large vesicular nuclei, sometimes up to four nuclei per cell, usually with prominent nucleoli (Figs. 4.6, 4.7). Eosinophil polymorphonuclears were present though not abundant; even so, they averaged two per hpf. Mitoses in the large pale cells were relatively plentiful at, on average, one per hpf.

The diagnosis had been taken no further than 'suggestive of Hodgkin's disease'.

Receipt of the biopsy report led to further examination of the patient and discovery of further enlarged nodes, especially on both sides of the neck: biopsy of a cervical node, 1 month after the original operation, showed essentially identical appearances.

The disease progressed despite radiotherapy and the patient died 3 years later with marked enlargement of spleen and liver, and recurrent pyrexia (no necropsy).

It is difficult now to understand the reluctance to advance the original diagnosis beyond 'suggestive' of Hodgkin's disease: 'virtually diagnostic of' seems the more appropriate term. This was a significant *under-diagnosis*.

### Case 4.2

M (24 years) with a complaint of abdominal pain and nausea. A mass in the right inguinal region was found to consist of enlarged nodes (5 × 3 × 2 cm) around the iliac vessels.

The nodes showed almost total loss of normal architecture. A few places retained reasonably well-defined follicles with normal germ centres (Fig. 4.8) but most had disappeared. In addition, there was a thin diffuse infiltration by pale reticulum cells. Unduly large forms of these cells were scanty; they were no more frequent than 1 per 20 hpf. Figure 4.9 is uncharacteristic in being the only area of that size to contain more than one such cell but characteristic in its portrayal of the cells' morphology. Infiltration by eosinophil polymorphonuclears, and areas of early fibrosis, were relatively prominent but, as also shown in Fig. 4.8, wide areas showed no fibrosis at all.

These findings, though suggestive of Hodgkin's disease at an early stage, were regarded as in-

**Table 4.2.** Twenty-two cases of '? early' or 'atypical' Hodgkin's disease (HD).

| Case No. | Diagnosis on review | Treatment + or − | Outcome |
|---|---|---|---|
| *7 cases under-diagnosed* | | | |
| 4.1 | HD > suggestively HD | + | Death at 3 yr |
| 4.2 | HD > atypical HD | − | Death at 3½ yr |
| 4.5 | HD > suggestively HD | − | Death at 12 yr |
| 4.6 | HD > aberrantly reactive | + | Death at 7 yr |
| 4.13 | Lymphosarcoma > ? reactive | + | Death at 6 yr |
| 4.15 | Malig. lymphoma > ? reactive | + | Death at 1 wk |
| 4.16 | RCS > suggestively HD | + | Death at 1 yr |
| *3 cases over-diagnosed* | | | |
| 4.11 | Reactive > atypical HD | − | Probably unrelated death within 1 yr |
| 4.18 | 'Lymphocytoma' > probable HD | − | Alive at 15 yr |
| 4.21 | Sinus histiocytosis > ? HD | − | Alive at 15 yr |
| *12 cases appropriately diagnosed* | | | |
| 4.3 | HD | + | Unrelated death at 4½ yr |
| 4.4 | HD | − | Alive at 9 yr |
| 4.7 | HD | + | Alive at 12 yr |
| 4.8 | Atypical HD | + | Death at 4 yr |
| 4.9 | Atypical HD | + | Alive at 20 yr |
| 4.10 | Atypical HD | − | Death at 7 wk |
| 4.12 | Atypical HD | − | Unrelated death at 5 yr |
| 4.14 | Atypical HD | + | Death at 4 yr |
| 4.17 | ? Granulomatous, ? HD | + | Death at 2 yr |
| 4.19 | Malignant lymphoma | − | Death at 14 yr |
| 4.20 | Chronic lymphatic leukaemia | − | Death at 16 yr |
| 4.22 | Still ambiguous | − | Alive at 8 yr |

sufficiently typical to warrant firm diagnosis as such. It was suggested that bacteriological and serological testing be continued, and the situation reviewed when results were complete. All such tests were negative and the diagnosis remained at 'atypical Hodgkin's disease'.

It was decided no further treatment was indicated. The patient left the district but enquiry found that he had died 3½ years later. Clinical details for the intervening period are lacking but a necropsy had shown disseminated malignant disease with involvement of thoracic and abdominal nodes, spleen, liver and lungs. The tissue was highly polymorphic and undifferentiated but almost certainly basically lymphomatous; the reporting pathologist considered that 'Hodgkin's sarcoma' was a reasonable diagnosis.

Review suggests that this was at the least a marginal *under-diagnosis*. The appearances now seem to warrant a greater emphasis on possible malignancy than was given at the time. Whether this, and resulting therapy, would have influenced the outcome, we can only guess.

*Case 4.3*

M (67 years) with a swelling behind the ear, gradually growing larger for 1 year. During the year before that, swellings had appeared in groins and axillae, 'reached the size of marbles', then spontaneously subsided. Examination of the present swelling behind the ear revealed a similar swelling in the ipsilateral anterior triangle of neck.

The excised specimen was a soft fleshy nodule, 15 × 10 mm in outline. Microscopically it was an extensively necrotic lymph node. In the remaining surviving tissue, but especially in the subtotally necrotic areas, the cells were

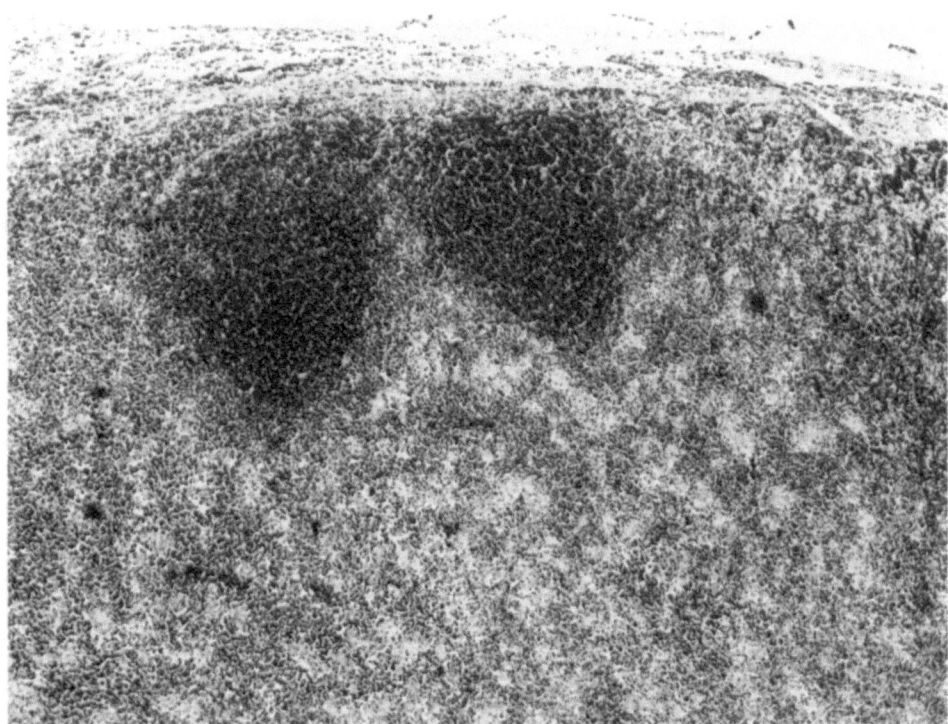

**Fig. 4.5.** This obliteration of architecture characterised the whole node. The dark clusters are not normal follicles but the scanty remains of the normal population of lymphocytes. H & E, × 62

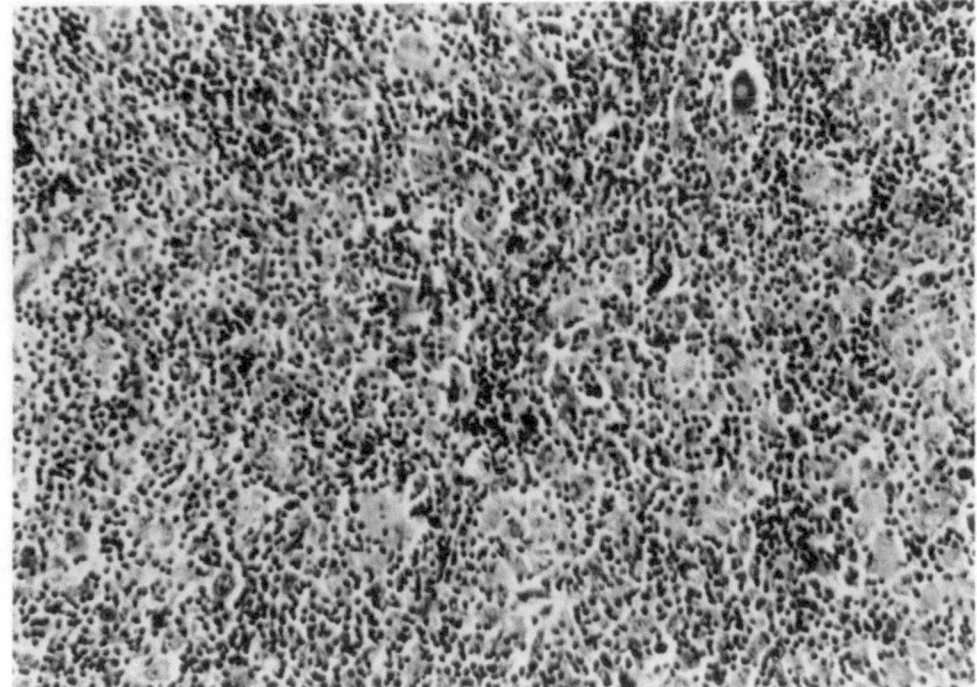

**Fig. 4.6.** An even mixture of lymphocytes and rather polymorphic large, pale cells. H & E, × 204

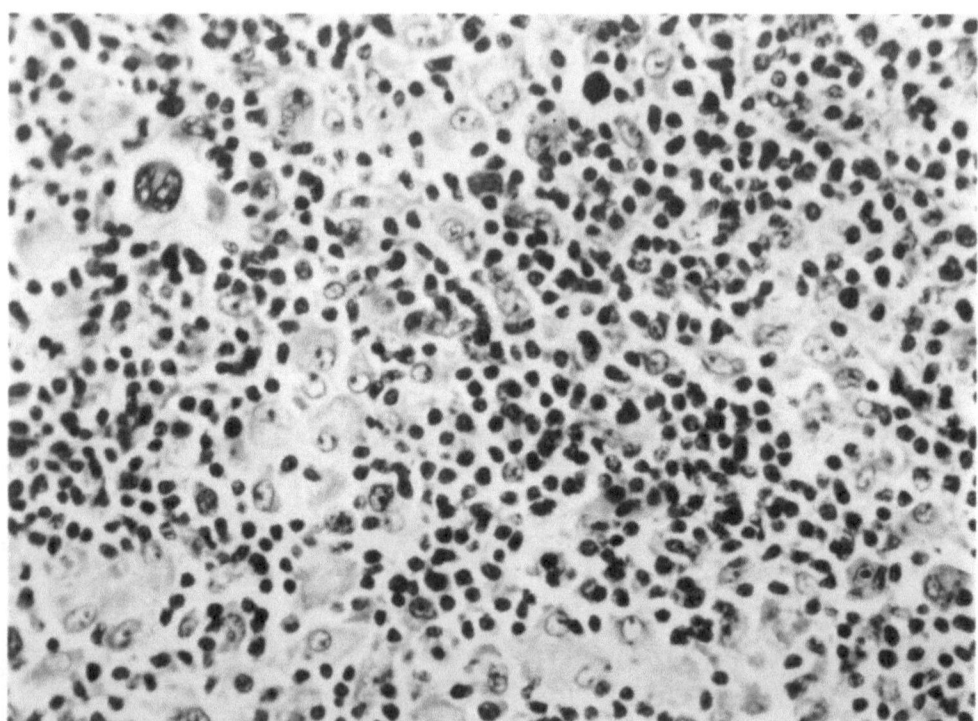

**Fig. 4.7.** Nuclear polymorphism of the large, pale cells is obvious. Most have a single nucleus with prominent nucleolus. Those with more than one nucleus, or, as at upper left and lower right, a multilobular nucleus, are acceptable as R-S cells. H & E, × 408

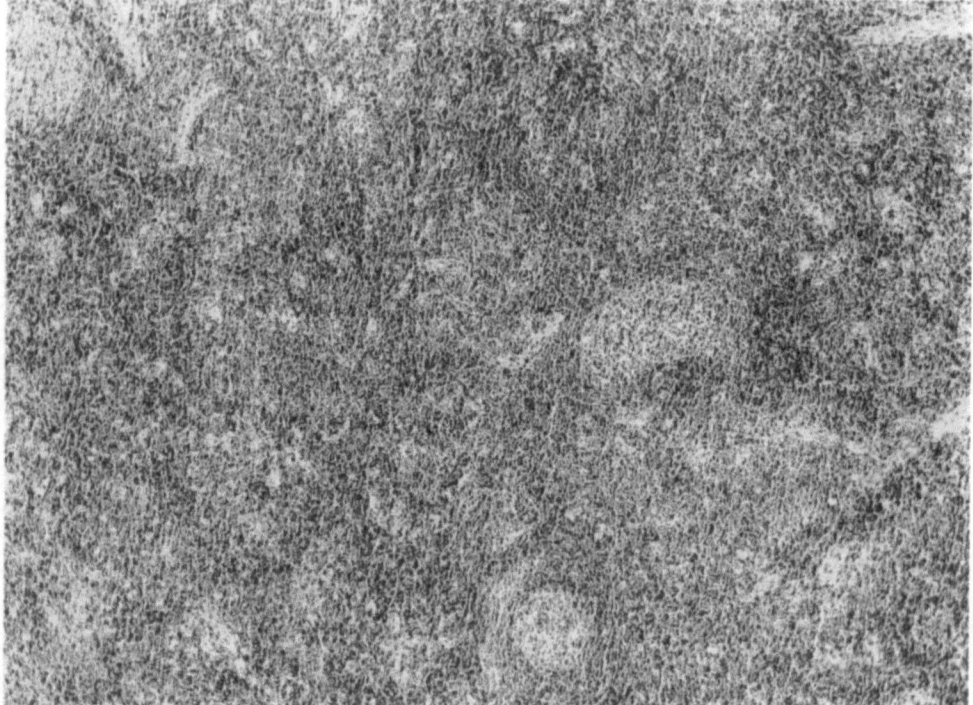

**Fig. 4.8.** Substantial obliteration of architecture with replacement of much of the follicular pattern by a mixture of lymphocytes and large, pale cells. The two largest pale areas were essentially normal germinal centres. H & E, × 62

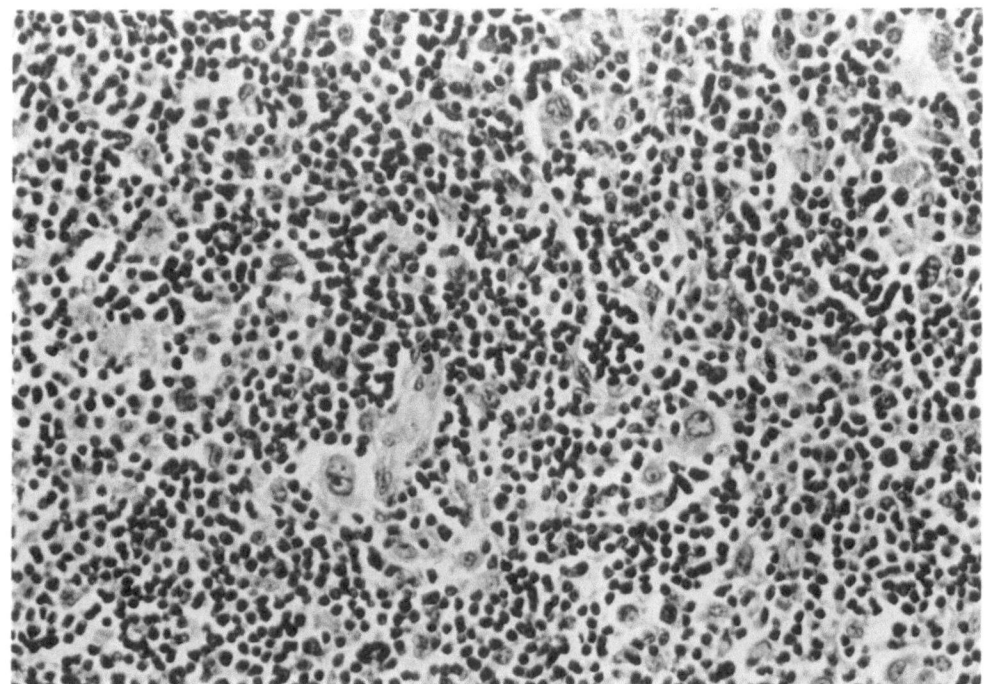

**Fig. 4.9.** Apparently normal lymphocytes predominate but there is an accompaniment of much larger, paler cells, some with notably large nuclei that make them at least candidate R-S cells. There is an acceptable 'mirror-image' cell at lower left centre. H & E, × 340

markedly polymorphic even though deeply pyknotic and thus bereft of fine detail. Many of these cells were large enough and aberrant enough to be acceptable as one-time R-S cells.

Within the limits set by the necrosis it seemed plausible to visualise the process as one whereby the node had gradually assumed the pattern of typical Hodgkin's disease, then rapidly undergone spontaneous regression. The diagnosis was given as 'Hodgkin's disease or a variant thereof'.

The affected area was irradiated and the swellings subsided, and the patient had no further related trouble before his death 4½ years later from a 'heart attack'. There was no necropsy and thus no means of knowing whether there was remnant disease internally or not. On the whole, however, it seems reasonable to interpret the evidence as indicating Hodgkin's disease which had the property of undergoing at least spontaneous remission if not resolution, i.e. an *appropriate diagnosis*.

### Case 4.4

F (50 years) complained of tiredness and loss of weight over some 5 months with night sweats and bilateral swelling of the neck for 2 weeks. Several nodes were palpable on both sides. No abnormality was found in throat, nose or ear. A 12 × 10 mm node was removed.

As shown in Figs. 4.10, 4.11 and 4.12, all normal architecture had disappeared. The node now consisted of a mass of aberrant polymorphic cells with many giant and multinucleated forms, and many, frequently aberrant mitoses. Eosinophil polymorphonuclears were scanty but otherwise the pattern had seemed abundantly to satisfy the criteria for a diagnosis of 'Hodgkin's sarcoma'. Serological investigations had seemed superfluous and were not suggested.

Within a few days of the biopsy the patient was feeling better and the lymph nodes gradually subsided. It was decided to withhold further treatment and to await events. There was no further trouble, no specific therapy of any kind was used, and the patient remains active and well 9 years later. By any standards this is puzzling. There must be continuing concern, with histology like this, that the condition will one day recur; but even if it does, this will have been a remarkable spontaneous remission.

Despite the later events, this still seems a

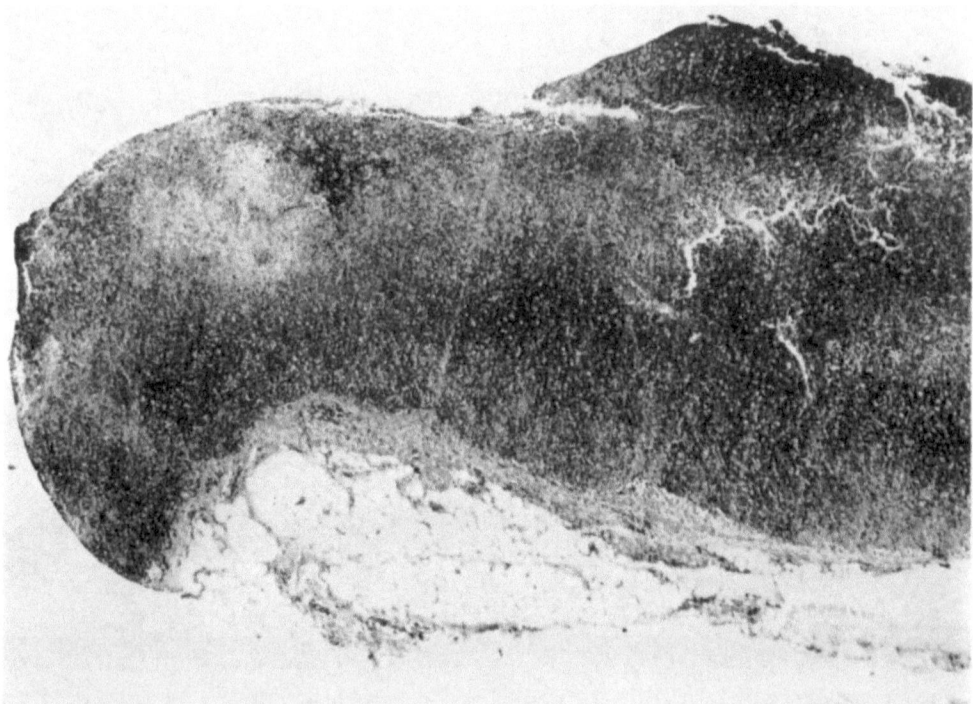

**Fig. 4.10.** No trace remains of normal architecture. The pale area at upper left is an area of fibrosis. H & E, × 26

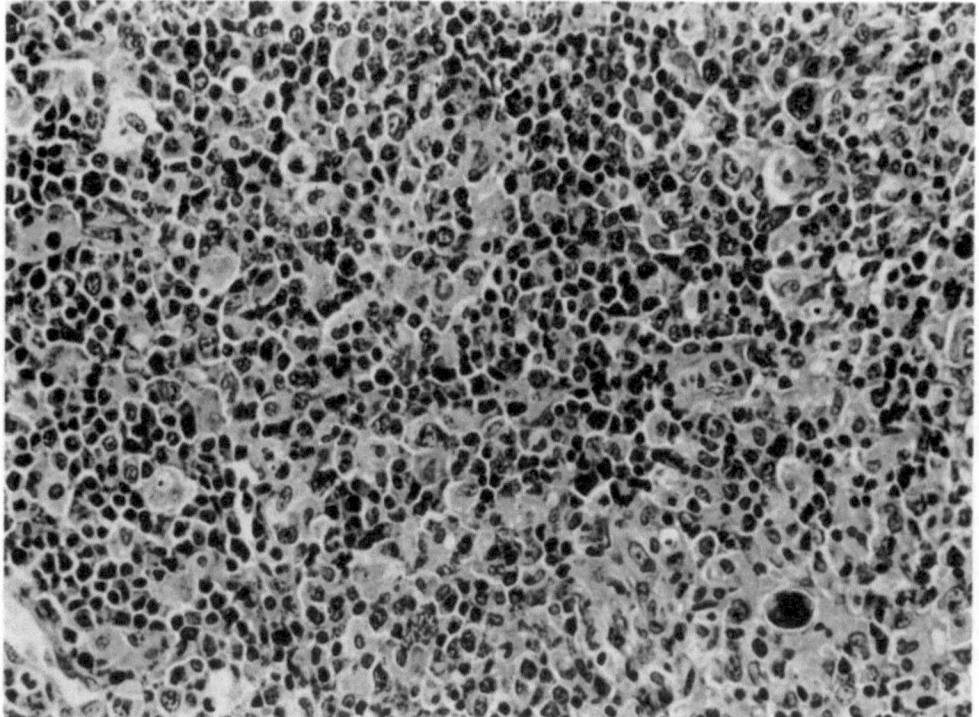

**Fig. 4.11.** An even mixture of smaller darker cells, sufficiently polymorphic to be lymphoblasts rather than lymphocytes, and much larger, paler cells of widely varying size and staining-intensity. H & E, × 340

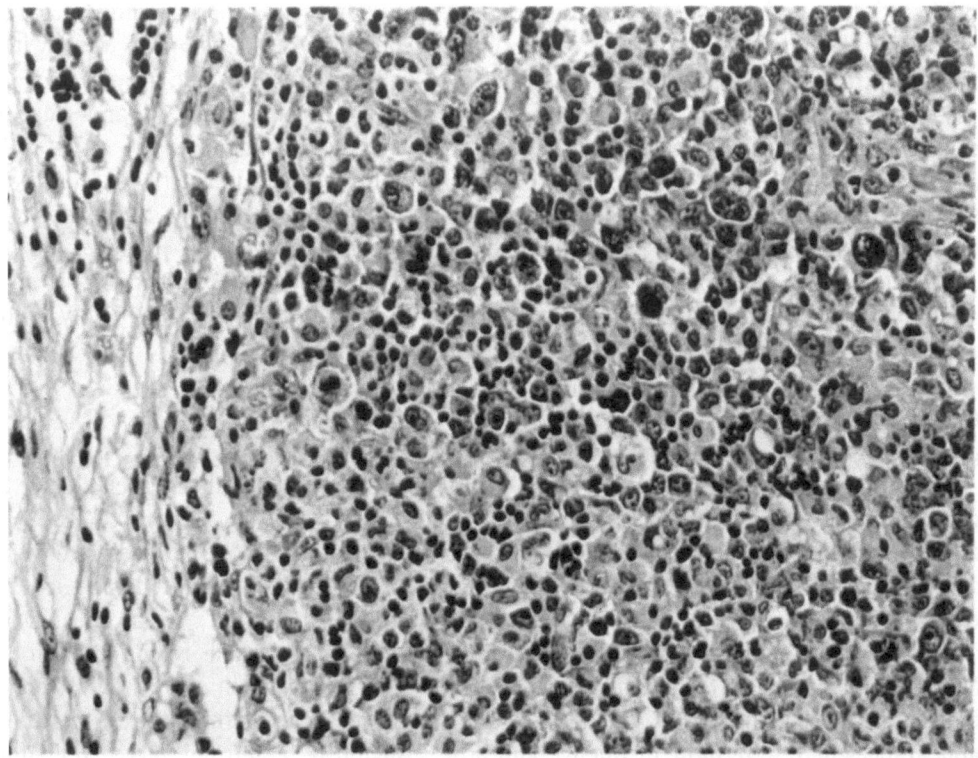

**Fig. 4.12.** This was the pattern along much of the lower concave surface shown in Fig. 4.10. The polymorphic cells seem to be permeating the capsule; the peripheral sinus at least is no longer clearly recognisable. The dark mass, upper right of centre, was an abnormal mitotic figure. H & E, × 340

wholly *appropriate diagnosis*. No doubt was entertained about its correctness at the time, and to that extent this was not in prospect a border-line problem. In retrospect, however, it appears all the more so year by year.

*Case 4.5*

M (23 years) with history of lump in groin for 1 year. Biopsy produced one node.

The node was large (25 × 10 × 10 mm) and uniformly whitish. There was loss of normal architecture to the extent that the pattern was broadly macrofollicular but not sheet-like. The 'follicles' were abnormal in having no germ centres but, instead, many aberrant large pale cells, frequently with two to five nuclei, mostly with prominent nucleoli, and occasionally in mitosis. There was no content of polymorpho-nuclears, eosinophil or neutrophil, and no significant degree of fibrosis. The appearances were reported as 'suggestive of an early form of lymphadenoma.'

The patient received radiotherapy and re-mained well for the next 12 years when he was seen as an outpatient complaining of pain in the loin for 2 weeks. Nodes were palpable in neck, axillae, and groins. Biopsy of a cervical node showed highly cellular malignant neoplasm considered from its cytology, with binucleate and multinucleate cells, and many cells in mitosis (often aberrant) to warrant diagnosis as 'Hodgkin's sarcoma'.

He received further radiotherapy but died 3 months later (no necropsy).

The original sections would probably now be diagnosed as lymphocyte-predominant Hodgkin's disease.

A *marginal under-diagnosis* despite which, however, the patient received appropriate therapy and then survived 12 years before dying from the disease.

*Case 4.6*

F (13 years) complained of painless swelling in left side of neck; she had a similar but smaller nodular swelling on the right side.

The 12-mm node was widely subdivided by fibrous bands that enclosed nodules of lymphatic tissue still for the most part retaining a follicular or, rather, in the absence of any normal germ centres, a pseudo-follicular pattern. Broadly, however, as seen in Fig. 4.13, the disturbance of architecture was considerable. The main abnormality at cellular level was the presence of clusters of large, pale, prominently nucleolated cells; binucleate forms were occasional, multinucleate forms extremely rare, and polymorphonuclears virtually absent. Mitotic activity amongst these large cells was prominent in many places (Fig. 4.14).

The appearances were held to be insufficiently characteristic to warrant a diagnosis of Hodgkin's disease, and serological investigations appropriate to an aberrantly 'reactive' node were recommended.

In the hope of establishing the diagnosis more firmly, a further node (from the other side of the neck) was removed 2 weeks later. The appearances here were more distinctive and now allowed a diagnosis of 'Hodgkin's disease' with fair certainty.

Despite radiotherapy and, 4 years later, chemotherapy, the disease progressed with gradual involvement of further groups of nodes, and the patient died, cachectic and anaemic, 7 years after initial diagnosis.

In retrospect, assessment of the first biopsy was ultracautious and probably a significant *under-diagnosis*. In practice, however, it was redeemed by the second biopsy 2 weeks later, and was thus therapeutically without consequence.

## Case 4.7

F (19 years) with supraclavicular swelling and paraesthesiae in the arm. A lobulated mass of tissue, 7 × 4 × 2 cm, was removed.

The features were regarded as those of 'early Hodgkin's disease'. It was unusual only in showing a considerable retention of follicular architecture though in even the best-preserved of the follicles the germ centres were populated by obviously abnormal large 'reticulum' cells, as was the surrounding mantle of lymphocytes.

The patient was treated by radiotherapy. She

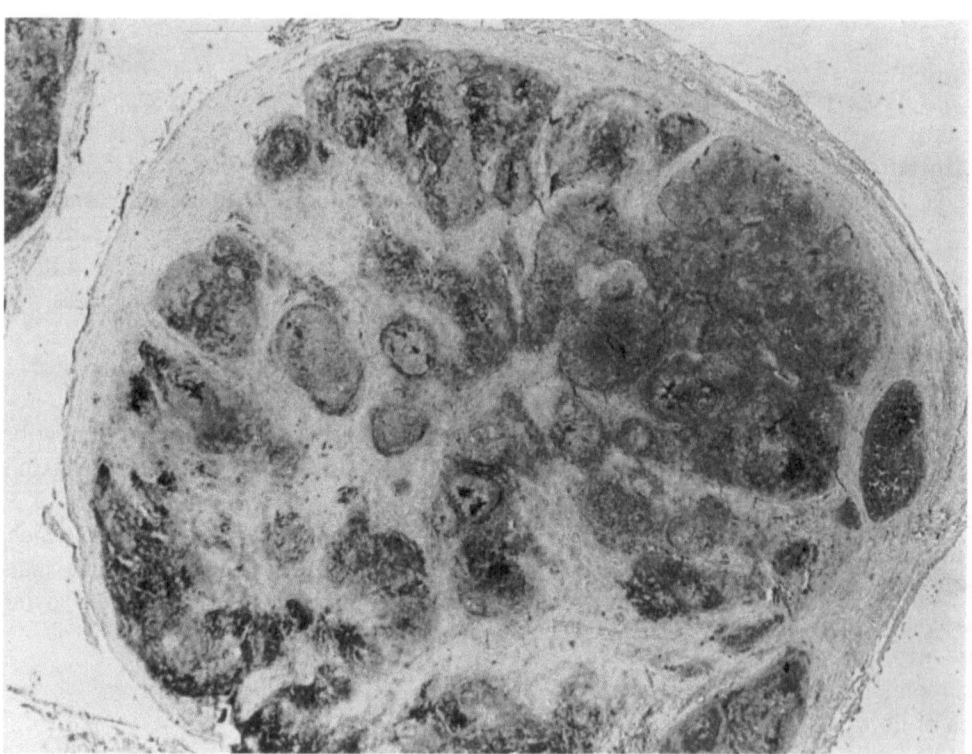

**Fig. 4.13.** An apparently sclerotic node. None of the foci of cells is a normal follicle. H & E, × 17

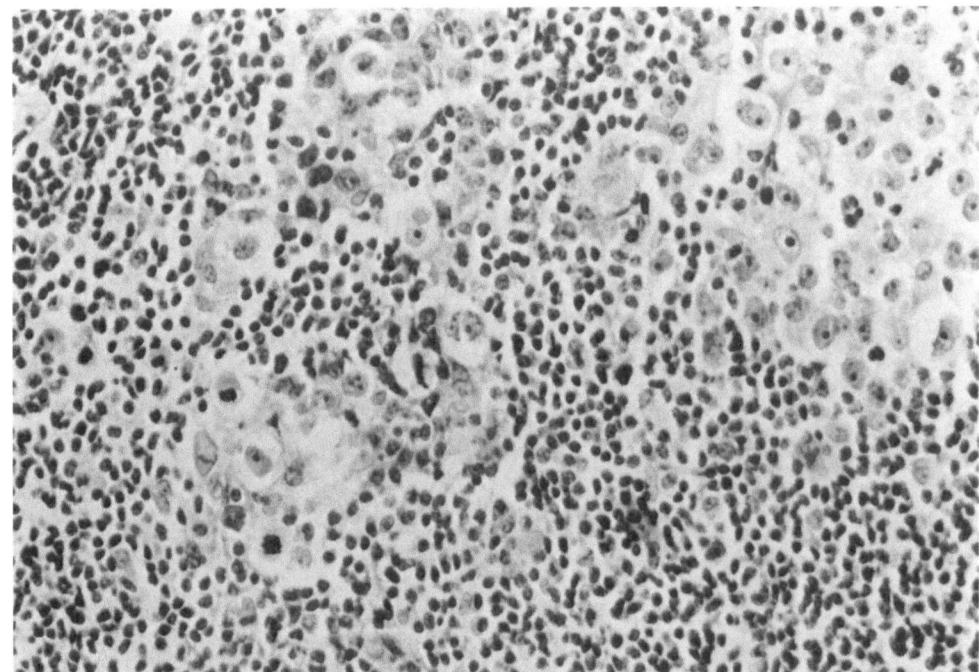

**Fig. 4.14.** Infiltration and replacement of the parenchyma by many large, pale cells with large, pale nuclei and prominent nucleoli. The incidence of mitoses is relatively high: there are two in the lower left quadrant and one at the upper right corner. Some of the cells are debatably, but none certainly, acceptable as R-S cells. H & E, × 340

remains well 12 years later, and it is hoped, has been cured.

Despite the uncertainty induced by the 12-year survival, this still seems an *appropriate* diagnosis.

### Case 4.8

M (47 years) with history of swelling in axilla for 6 months. Excision yielded two relatively large masses, 6 × 5 × 4 cm and slightly smaller, each containing discrete nodes up to 3 cm long.

There was total loss of normal architecture and replacement by the type of pattern seen in Fig. 4.15. This represents remnant lymphocytes (dark) being displaced and replaced by masses of eosinophilic cells (light) as shown in more detail in Fig. 4.16. The nuclei of these cells were relatively large and also pale but were a less striking feature than the voluminous cytoplasm which was, as just stated, notably eosinophilic. In all, the cells had a distinctly epithelioid appearance but did not have the focal or formal arrangement of tuberculoid granulomata. They did, however, occur sometimes in more aberrant forms as shown, for example, in Fig. 4.17, in which two multinucleated cells can be seen,

neither of typically Langhans type. Scattered around, also, are mononuclear cells with nuclei obviously larger than those of the pale cells. A cell of whatever variety in mitosis was rare. Eosinophil polymorphonuclears were present but scanty.

These features were worrying and considered possibly to represent an 'atypical form of Hodgkin's disease' but search was advised for any other possible cause. All investigations were negative, the patient appeared well and was 'kept under observation'.

Three years after removal of the axillary mass, a swelling developed in the left inguinal region. This was now much more distinctively Hodgkin's disease. Figure 4.18 shows cells that still had unusually much cytoplasm (still notably eosinophilic) and were now considered more acceptably R-S cells; aberrant mitotic forms, of which one is seen in Fig. 4.19, were relatively common. Radiotherapy was given but the condition progressed and the patient died with disseminated disease after a further 10 months.

(Whether aetiologically related or not, a cervical swelling appeared in the patient's son [aged 24] 1 year after the father's initial biopsy.

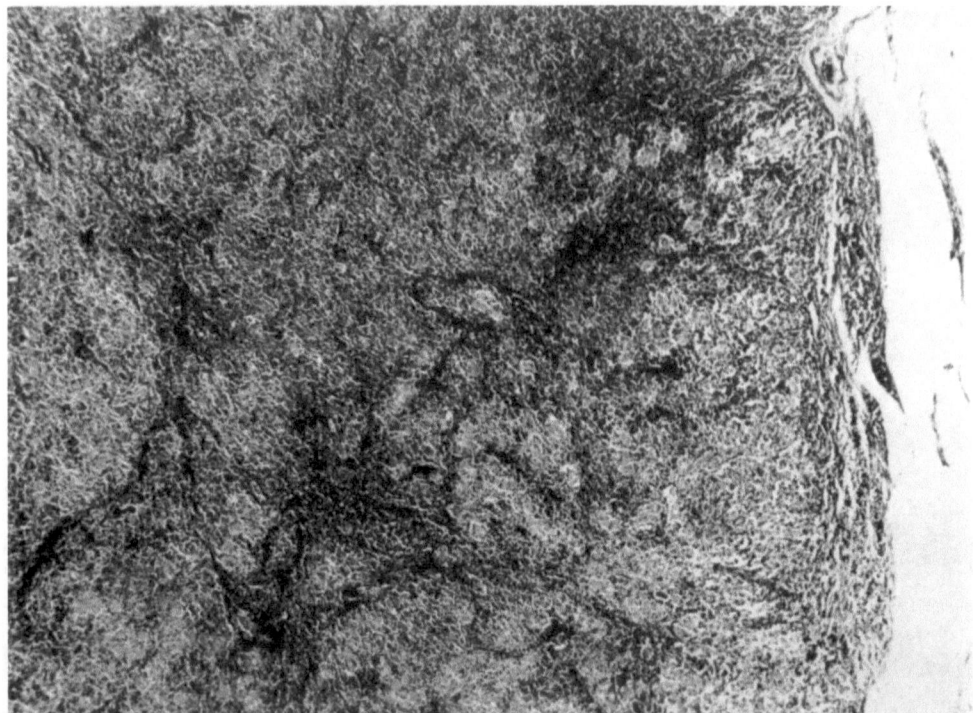

**Fig. 4.15.** Relatively massive replacement of the normal pattern by cells that appear pale here but had in fact an abnormally eosinophilic cytoplasm. Even so, they were otherwise similar to those illustrated in the two previous cases. H & E, × 60

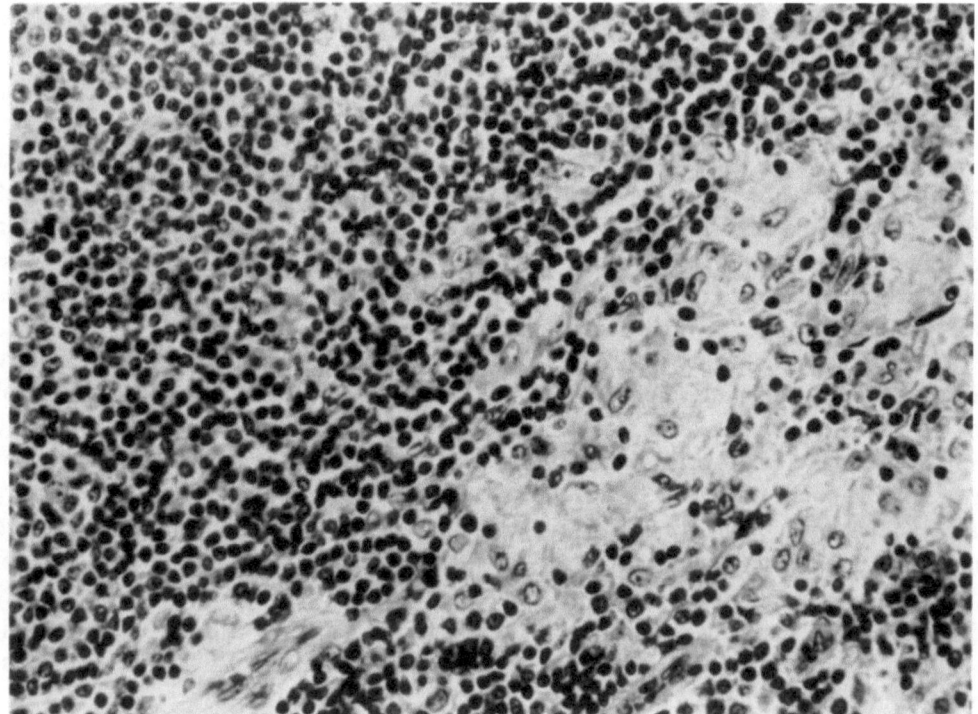

**Fig. 4.16.** Shows the ample cytoplasm of the paler cells and their manner of infiltration. Relatively little polymorphism is shown in this area. H & E, × 476

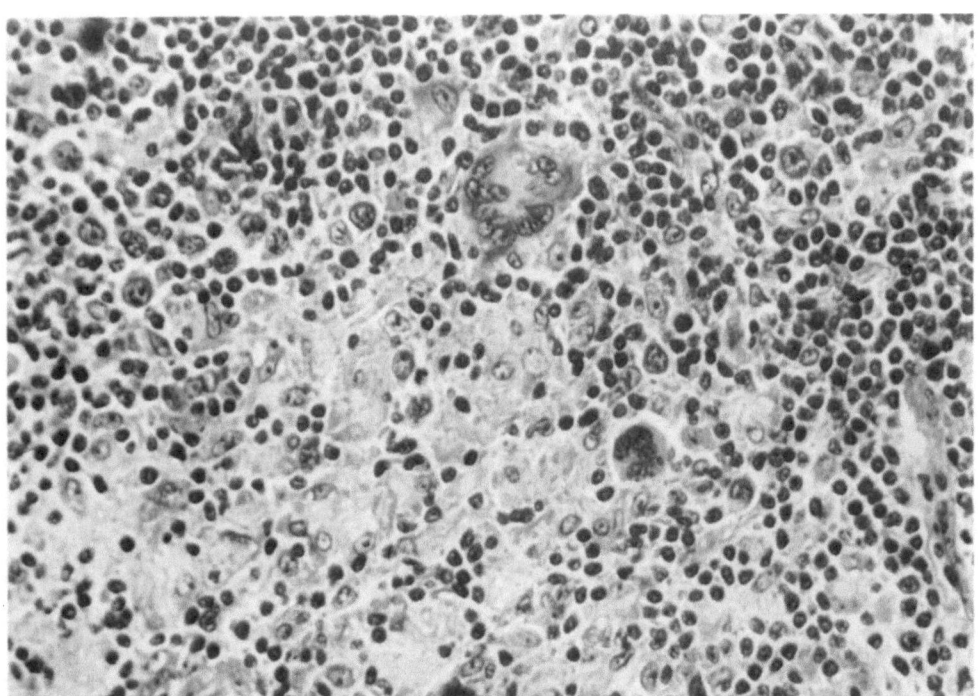

**Fig. 4.17.** Here there is a greater degree of polymorphism, due essentially to a variable increase in nuclear size among the pale cells and to the addition of multinuclear masses. None of these cells was in mitosis. H & E, × 476

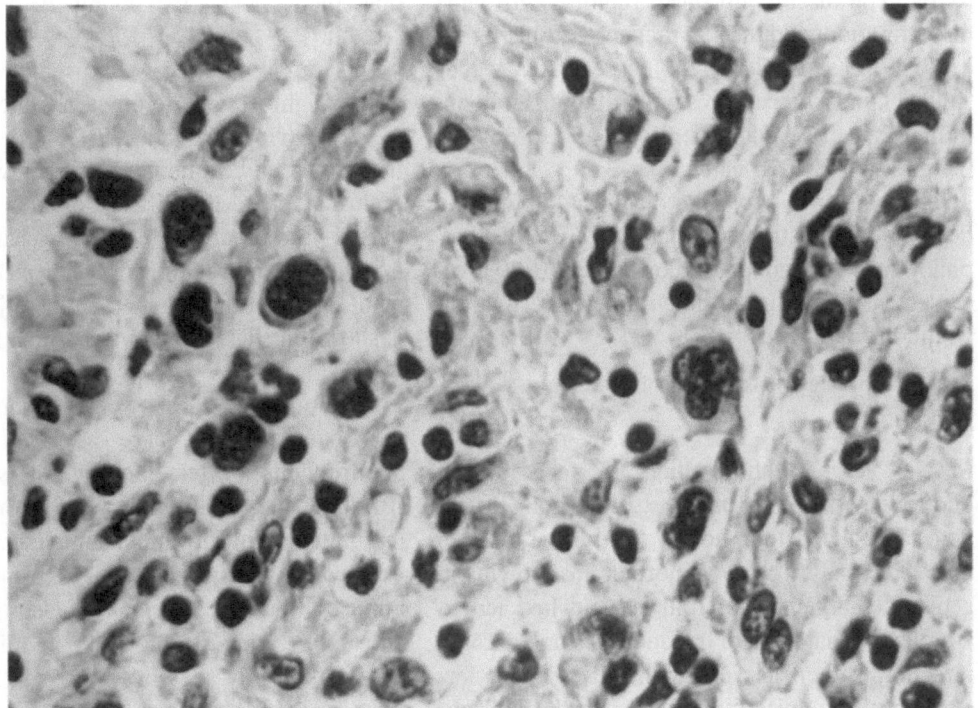

**Fig. 4.18.** The nucleocytoplasmic ratio of the aberrantly large cells is higher than hitherto, and the nuclei of some are more distinctly multilobular: most are acceptably R-S cells. H & E, × 952

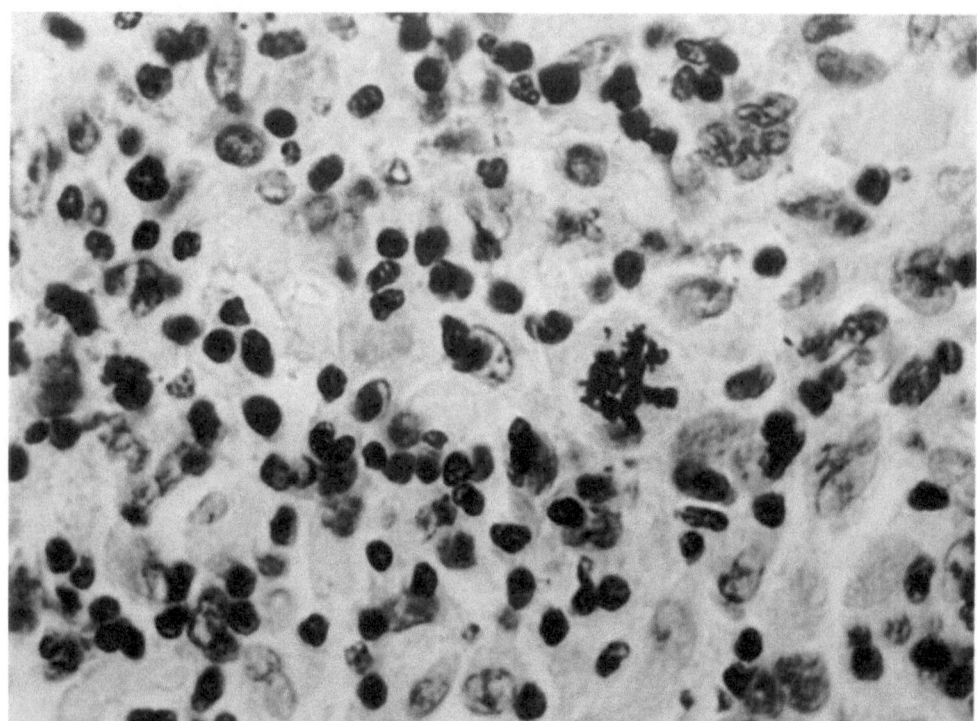

**Fig. 4.19.** Here there is less general polymorphism but there is one obviously aberrant mitotic figure. Similar aberrant figures were relatively common. H & E, × 952

This was typically Hodgkin's disease on microscopy. The disease advanced rapidly, with wide dissemination, and the son predeceased his father by 9 months. In Case 4.40 there was a rather similar concurrence of lesions in father and son, in that instance Hodgkin's disease and, probably, lymphosarcoma respectively).

This was an *appropriate* diagnosis though the degree of reservation was such that an 'expectant' policy only was adopted. Nowadays (1980), on evidence such as this, a much fuller investigation would have followed.

### Case 4.9

M (24 years) with swellings in neck, axillae and groins for some 3 months. Biopsy of cervical nodes produced four nodes, the largest 6 × 6 mm. The pattern was abnormal in showing a general enlargement of follicles and had led to a preferred diagnosis of 'reaction to some chronic infection' rather than Hodgkin's disease. In view of persisting clinical suspicion and the element of uncertainty in the pathological diagnosis, which was preferential rather than committed, an axillary node biopsy was performed. This provided a further four nodes; all were larger than the cervical, two being 20 × 15 mm in section.

All four nodes were abnormal; two appeared at first sight to have retained a follicular pattern, the other two to have lost it completely. In fact, the apparently follicular pattern was no more than that; these nodes were divided by bands of fibrosis into pseudo-follicles of varying size (Fig. 4.20). The more uniformly sheet-like replacement in the other immediately adjacent nodes is shown in Fig. 4.21, a view of the larger of the two.

Cytologically, all showed the same basic pattern consisting of large areas of apparently mature lymphocytes liberally interspersed with strikingly large pale cells, with correspondingly large nuclei and prominent nucleoli. These cells were only occasionally bi- or multinucleate; almost all had only a single nucleus and in some areas were remarkably often in mitosis, sometimes aberrantly so (Figs. 4.22, 4.23). In addition to this, many of the apparently mature 'background' lymphocytes were also in mitosis, so much so that, with the large clear cells subtracted, the nodes would have warranted diag-

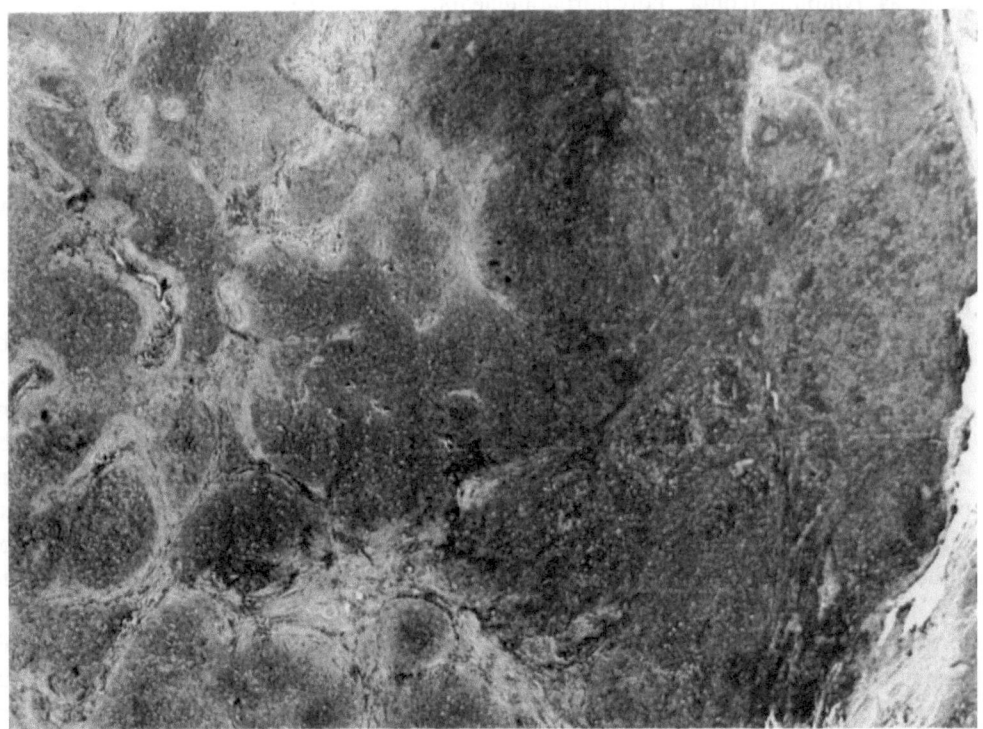

**Fig. 4.20.** Irregular subdivision of the parenchyma by bands of fibrous tissue of various sizes has produced a pseudofollicular pattern. H & E, × 12

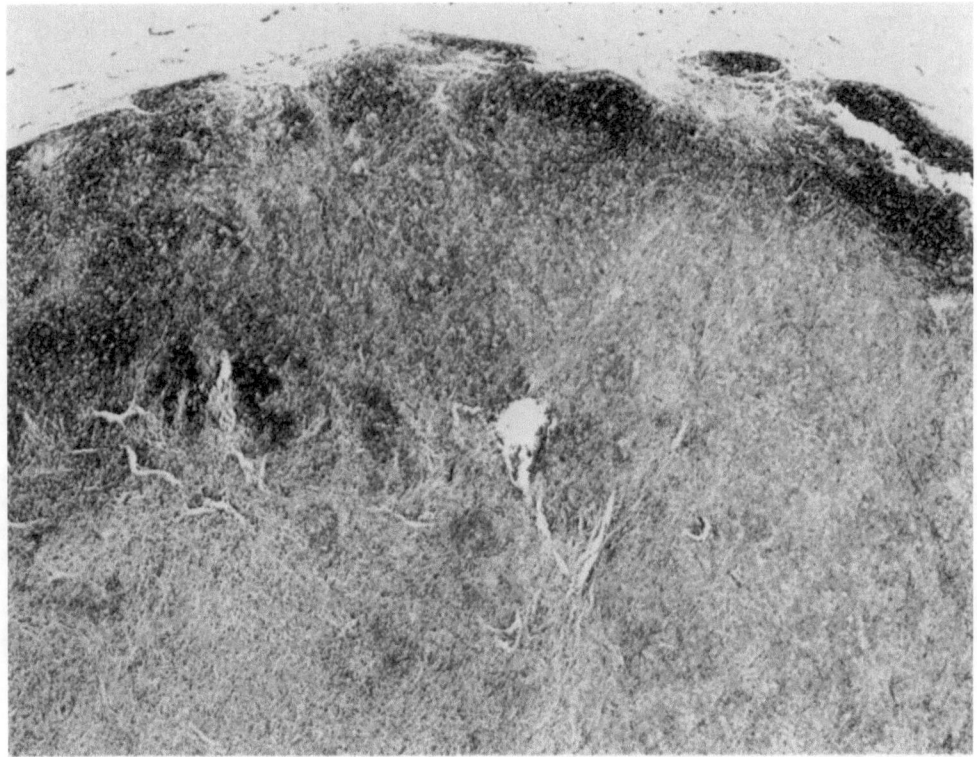

**Fig. 4.21.** In the other nodes, as here, there was a much more uniformly sheet-like transformation; hardly a trace of follicular pattern remains. H & E, × 12

nosis as lymphosarcoma. Polymorphonuclears, whether eosinophil or neutrophil, were almost wholly absent from all the nodes. Re-examination of the earlier sections, from the cervical nodes, showed that the same features were there also, though in much lesser degree.

The features described and illustrated were held now to justify diagnosis as 'atypical Hodgkin's disease' and the patient was treated by radiotherapy.

The patient was well 20 years later. For this reason, in doubting whether this really was a variant of nodular sclerosing Hodgkin's disease, we are simultaneously doubting whether, if that diagnosis is correct, the radiotherapy could possibly have achieved a cure. However, if the diagnosis is *not* Hodgkin's disease, it is very difficult to know what it is.

The first report was a marginal under-diagnosis: if both biopsies, of cervical and axillary nodes, are together considered as the initial biopsy, this was an *appropriate diagnosis*. Such doubt as remains is owed to the 20-year survival.

*Case 4.10*

M (75 years) admitted in a generally debilitated state with cough, anorexia and dysphagia, and found to have enlarged inguinal and axillary nodes. A node was removed from one inguinal and one axillary group; the larger was $3 \times 2 \times 2$ cm.

Nodes from both sites showed the same appearances, namely, total loss of normal architecture and replacement (at LP) by a uniform sheet of cells. At HP the population consisted predominantly of lymphocytes and reticulum cells with a generous infiltration by eosinophil polymorphonuclears. The reticulum cells were neither unduly large nor unduly bizarre but the range of size and shape was undoubtedly greater than in any ordinarily reactive node. Mitotic activity was also not unduly great, nevertheless it was greater than normal. A prominent accompaniment was widespread angio-endothelial proliferation in capillaries, quite similar to that familiar in gliomas.

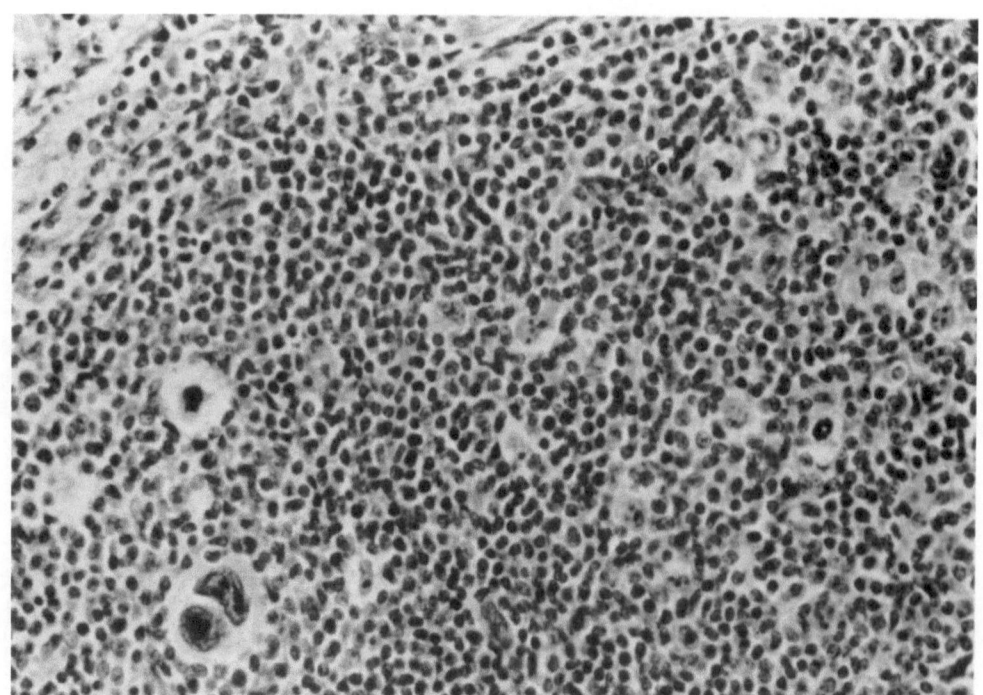

**Fig. 4.22.** Large aberrant cells in a background of generally uniform lymphocytes. The two pyknotic masses in the right half of the field, and the upper of the two in the lower left quadrant, represent cells in mitosis. H & E, $\times$ 340

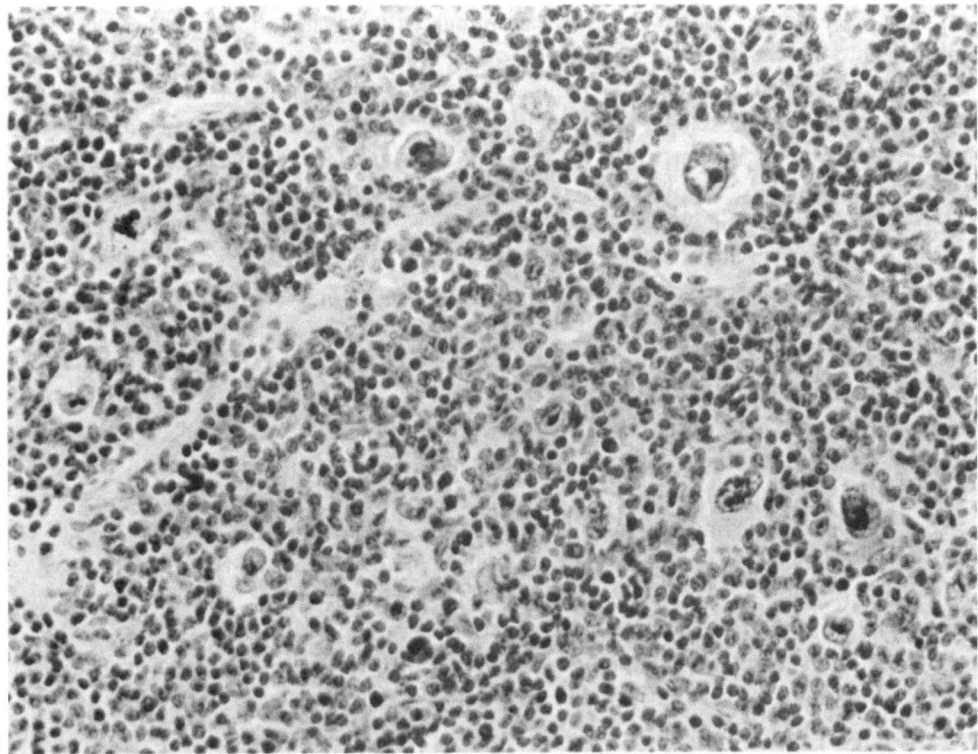

**Fig. 4.23.** There is an obviously greater degree of polymorphism here, due not only to the several monster nuclei but also to there being many cells morphologically intermediate between lymphocytes and larger cells with larger paler nuclei. The pyknotic mass at upper left corner is an aberrant mitotic figure, and of these there were many. Despite these appearances, and as mentioned in the text, the patient was well 20 years after radiotherapy. H & E, × 340

The blood picture was normal, the nodes contained no demonstrable organisms, and all investigations in search of an infective cause were negative. The most likely diagnosis was considered to be 'atypical Hodgkin's disease' even though not a single typical R-S cell had been seen.

The patient was never sufficiently well to leave hospital, and he died 7 weeks later. Necropsy showed enlargement of lymph nodes throughout and apparent infiltration of spleen and liver. Microscopy confirmed the presence in all these sites of tissue identical with that found on biopsy, and it had seemed right to let the diagnosis remain at 'atypical Hodgkin's disease'; in retrospect this still seems an *appropriate diagnosis* although, admittedly, those who regard the presence of R-S cells as a sine qua non for the diagnosis of HD would disagree.

*Case 4.11*

M (71 years) complained of general malaise and breathlessness. The left inguinal nodes were enlarged, and spleen and liver moderately enlarged to palpation. A single 10-mm node was removed.

The pattern of the node was substantially the same as that seen in Case 4.10. There were no true follicles, and only vaguely defined areas of greater cell density to give just a hint of a follicular pattern. Most of the cells were mature lymphocytes but there was a diffuse accompaniment of paler cells some just larger than others but none of the size, in respect of either nucleus or cytoplasm, of those illustrated for example in Case 4.9. These cells along with two other features, areas of early fibrosis and many eosinophil polymorphonuclears (four per hpf on average) were held to warrant diagnosis as 'atypical Hodgkin's disease'. There was minimal mitotic activity throughout, and none of the sheet-like character of a lymphosarcoma.

Three days after the biopsy the patient had a haematemesis requiring partial gastrectomy. The cause was a simple peptic ulcer. Neither it, nor the associated leucocytic infiltrate, indicated neoplasia, either carcinomatous or lymphomatous. No biopsy was taken from liver or spleen.

The patient was known to be alive 6 months later but had severe chronic bronchitis and congestive cardiac failure. Beyond that there was no trace but it seems likely that death would have been due to the cardiorespiratory lesions rather than anything lymphomatous. With its even lesser degree of polymorphism than the last case (4.10), this lesion was even more dubiously Hodgkin's disease. Overmuch significance had possibly been given to the general loss of pattern and the abundant eosinophil polymorphonuclears. Review strongly favours a reactive response, cause undetermined, rather than a neoplastic one, and to that extent this may be regarded as an *over-diagnosis*.

### Case 4.12

F (78 years) with a swelling on medial aspect of left elbow, first noticed after a fall on the elbow two months earlier. Excision produced two masses of fatty tissue, the larger 7 × 4 × 3 cm, both widely occupied by foci of firm white tissue. To judge from its size the mass seemed likely to have been present for much longer than 2 months.

The largest single nodule, in section, was 20 × 20 mm, and in only one area of 3 × 2 mm at the edge did a normal capsule and normal lymph nodal architecture remain. For the rest, the pattern was one of varying sized nodules of abnormal lymphatic tissue separated by bands of rather hyalinised fibrous tissue (Fig. 4.24). In some of these enclosed nodules there were acceptably normal germ centres. In others, the apparent germ centres altogether lacked phagocytic activity and had the rather cytologically uniform character of a follicular or giant-follicular lymphoma (though the lesion was certainly not of that variety). In yet others, the centres contained scattered large pale cells of clearly aberrant character (Fig. 4.25). In the

irregularly disposed extrafollicular substance of the nodules there were areas that would pass as simple reactive sinus histiocytosis and others acceptable as almost certainly lymphosarcoma, while sprinkled at random throughout were, again, the large pale cells either singly or in loose clusters of up to ten or thereabouts. No cells deserved the term giant-cell or R-S cell, mitotic figures were evident but few, and polymorphonuclears of whatever variety infrequent.

In all, therefore, the lesion showed a mixture of features that could be found individually in a wide range of malignant lymphomas. Collectively, they were considered to be best designated as probably an 'atypical Hodgkin's disease' though again the advice was given to search for evidence of any infective cause.

No further treatment was given, all further investigations were negative, and the patient remained generally well until her unrelated death 15 years later (aged 93). This lesion was received before nodular sclerosing HD had emerged as an entity. With its large clear cells at least candidates as 'lacunar' cells, the node probably is a mildly atypical form of this lesion, presumably restricted to one group of epitrochlear nodes, an unusual occurrence. At all events, the diagnosis suggested at the time was fair and *appropriate*.

### Case 4.13

M (20 years) with supraclavicular swelling present for 3 weeks. Biopsy produced a mass containing three nodes up to 15-mm across.

Appearances differed in the three nodes. In one (Fig. 4.26), the pattern was that of a diffuse and uniformly cellular 'lymphocytoma' with the addition of randomly scattered large, pale, mononuclear reticulum cells which had an appropriately large pale nucleus of frequently curious configuration. None, however, was a completely acceptable R-S cell. It was easy to believe, however, that with less adequate fixation they would have suffered cytoplasmic shrinkage and become, or at any rate closely simulated, the 'lacunar' cell of Hodgkin's disease (Fig. 4.27). Eosinophil polymorphonuclears were extremely few, and there was no fibrosis.

In the second node, all normal structure had disappeared. The population was one of roughly equal numbers of lymphocytes, reticulum cells

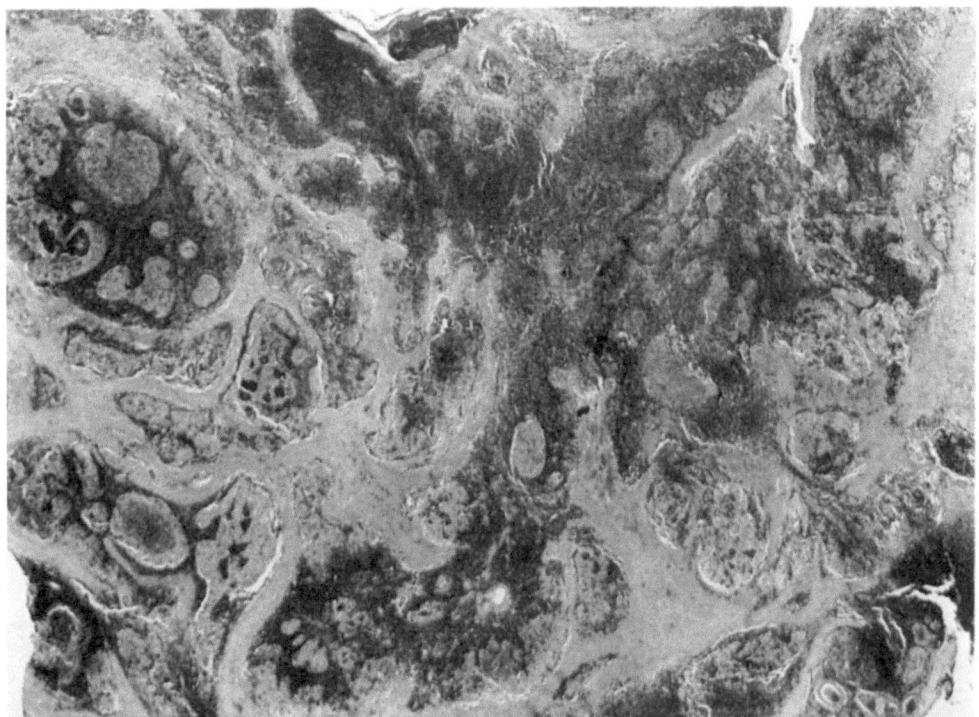

**Fig. 4.24.** The node is totally subdivided by bands of fibrous tissue. The more sharply circumscribed of the pale areas were persisting germinal centres. H & E, × 10

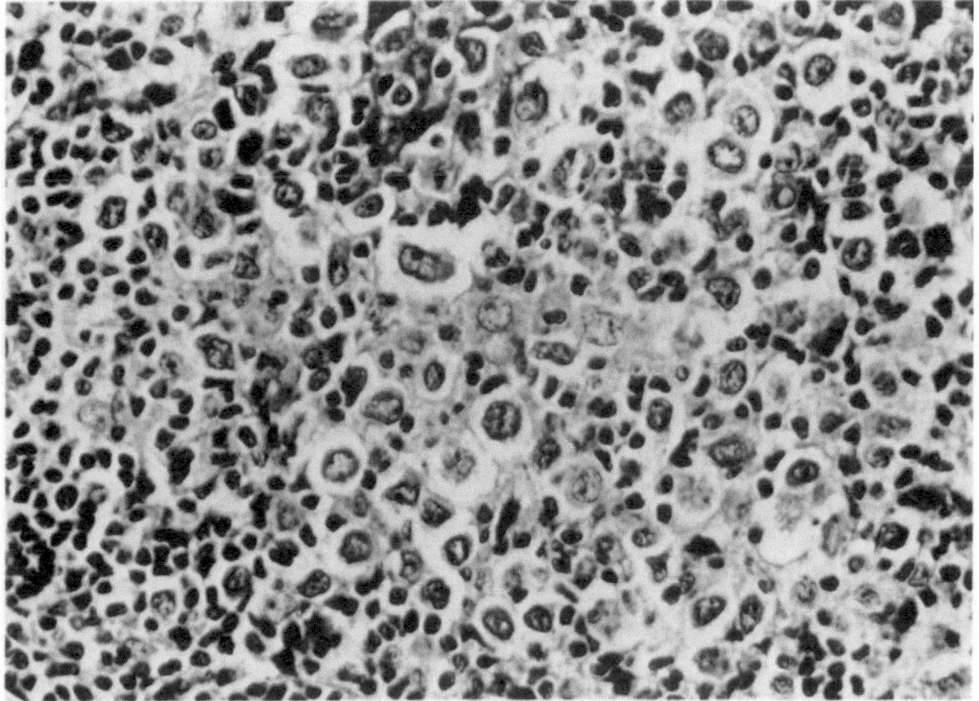

**Fig. 4.25.** Some of the paler foci consisted of this mixture of rather polymorphic lymphocytes, possibly lymphoblasts, and large pale cells with correspondingly large nuclei, also polymorphic. These are possibly 'lacunar' cells, which, with the undoubted sclerosis shown in the preceding figure, strongly suggest nodular sclerosing HD. H & E, × 520

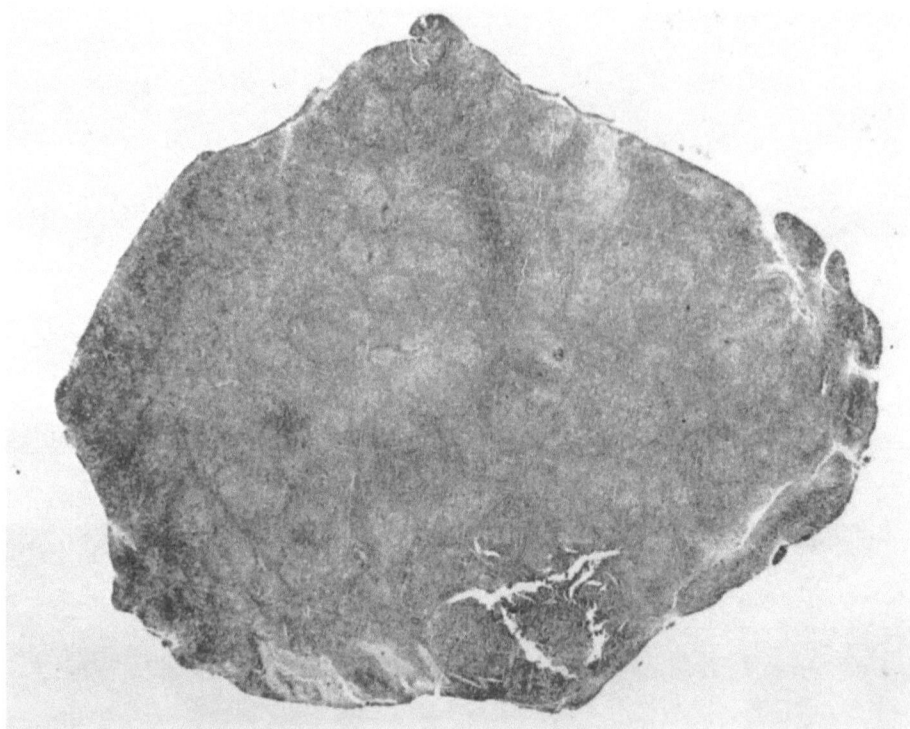

**Fig. 4.26.** An almost diffuse sheet of cells. The paler areas are due to loosening of the texture, not the remains of germinal centres. H & E, × 16

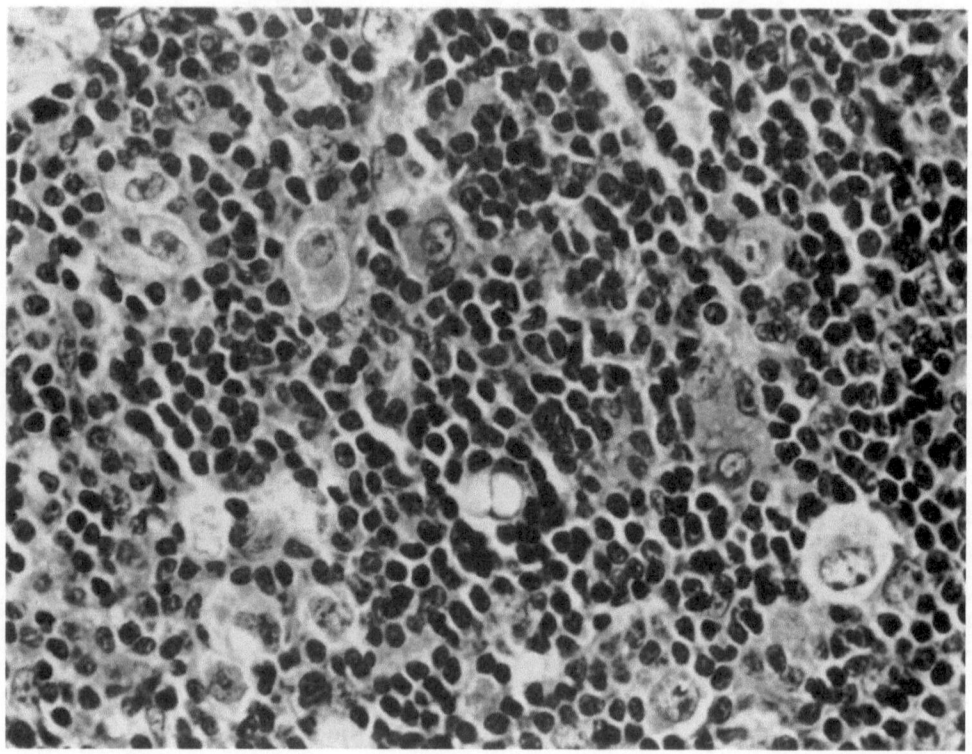

**Fig. 4.27.** Scattered pale foci contain larger cells with clear cytoplasm reminiscent of 'lacunar' cells. H & E, × 552

of essentially normal appearance, and eosinophil polymorphonuclears, i.e. a relatively massive influx of eosinophils. There were many such areas and they were separated, or perhaps one originally much larger area had been subdivided, by bands of partly hyalinised fibrous tissue (Fig. 4.28).

The third node showed some subdivision or break-up and a mixture of appearances of all the kinds just described.

It was considered not possible to decide firmly between a chronic inflammatory reaction and early Hodgkin's disease, and further appropriate investigations were advised. All were negative, and a fourth lymph node later removed from the same side of the neck showed appearances essentially the same as the most highly cellular member of the three originally examined.

Readmission was required 6 weeks later because of dysphagia caused by further increased swelling in the neck. The area was irradiated, the masses subsided and the patient was fully relieved. The same cycle was repeated 15 months later; submandibular swelling, irradiation, relief. However, recurrences of nodal enlargement throughout the neck and in the axillae continued despite further therapy, now also including chemotherapy; the patient became increasingly anaemic and cachectic and died 6 years after the initial biopsy.

There was no necropsy, so there is no knowledge whether the nodal cytology became any more diagnostic than it had been at the outset, but beyond reasonable doubt the patient died of a malignant lymphoma. In retrospect, instead of early Hodgkin's disease, and, even more so, of an inflammatory response, a preferable designation for the lesion would have been 'lymphoblastic lymphosarcoma'. However, despite its maturity of differentiation, it proved relatively rapidly fatal.

To the extent that a chronic inflammatory response was regarded as an equally likely cause of the histology, this was an *under-diagnosis*. At least, however, it led to a delay in treatment of no more than 6 weeks, a delay of probably little consequence.

### Case 4.14

F (57 years) with swelling in the neck found, on excision, to comprise four nodes from 8 to 15 mm in maximum dimension.

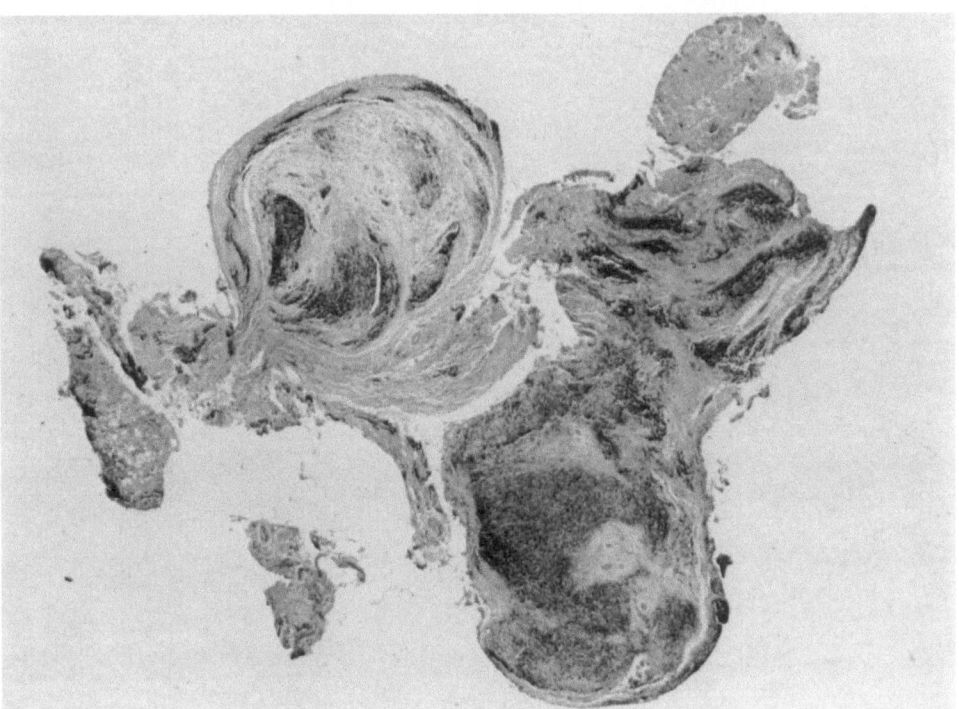

**Fig. 4.28.** An irregularly fibrotic node. It contained none of the large pale cells. The main abnormality was an abundance of eosinophil polymorphonuclears. H & E, × 16

There was a general loss of architecture and virtually total replacement of normal follicular pattern by areas of large pale cells lying among larger sheets of essentially normal lymphocytes (Fig. 4. 29). As shown in Figs. 4.30 and 4.31, the large pale cells had large pale nuclei that often contained a notably eosinophilic nucleolus: about 1 in 50 of the cells were binucleate or multinucleate. There were scanty polymorphonuclears and no fibrosis. The lesion was reported as a lymphoid neoplasm and designated 'atypical Hodgkin's disease'.

There was no recurrence in the neck following radiotherapy but 2 years later a mass appeared in the groin. Histologically it was essentially the same as the earlier lesion but now showed scanty eosinophil polymorphonuclears, an occasional cell acceptable as a R-S cell, and a little fibrosis. The patient died after a further 2 years with intractable pyrexia and, again, a mass in the right groin. Necropsy showed a 250-g mass of para-aortic nodes, splenomegaly (250 g) and bronchopneumonia. The necropsy sections have disappeared, so final detailed histological classification is not possible, but there

is no doubt in the least that the patient died from a 'malignant lymphoma' of some kind.

This was an *appropriate* diagnosis, at least at the time, some 20 years ago. There would be less hesitation now in firmly making the diagnosis Hodgkin's disease.

### Case 4.15

M (52 years) admitted for investigation of malaise and obvious loss of weight. He had been vaguely ill for some 3 years, with night sweats for 1 year. Examination showed enlarged cervical and axillary nodes. One was removed from the axilla.

As shown in Fig. 4.32, there was total loss of normal architecture. The general pattern is seen in Fig. 4.33 where much of the background is almost entirely hyalinised fibrous tissue. Probably half of the node was occupied by fibrous tissue; the rest had the higher cellularity seen at the right of this figure. In more detail, as in Fig. 4.34, the cytology was appreciably variable, including a scattering of abnormally large cells, approximately one such per 5 hpf, but with a few

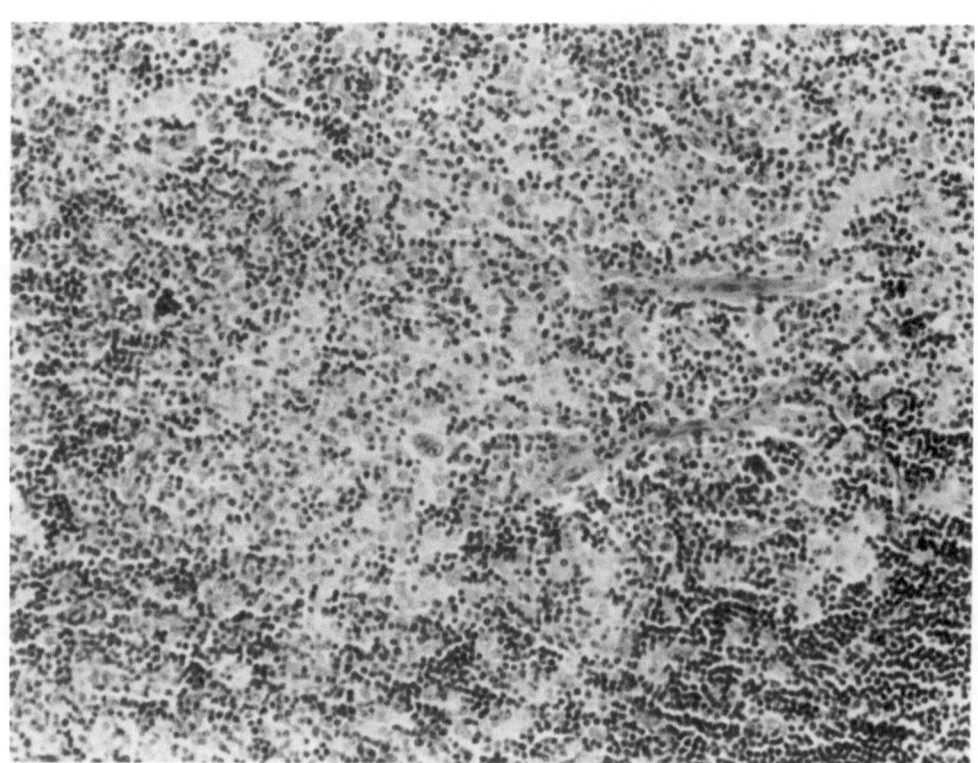

**Fig. 4.29.** A generally lymphocytic background relieved by areas of larger paler cells. H & E, × 221

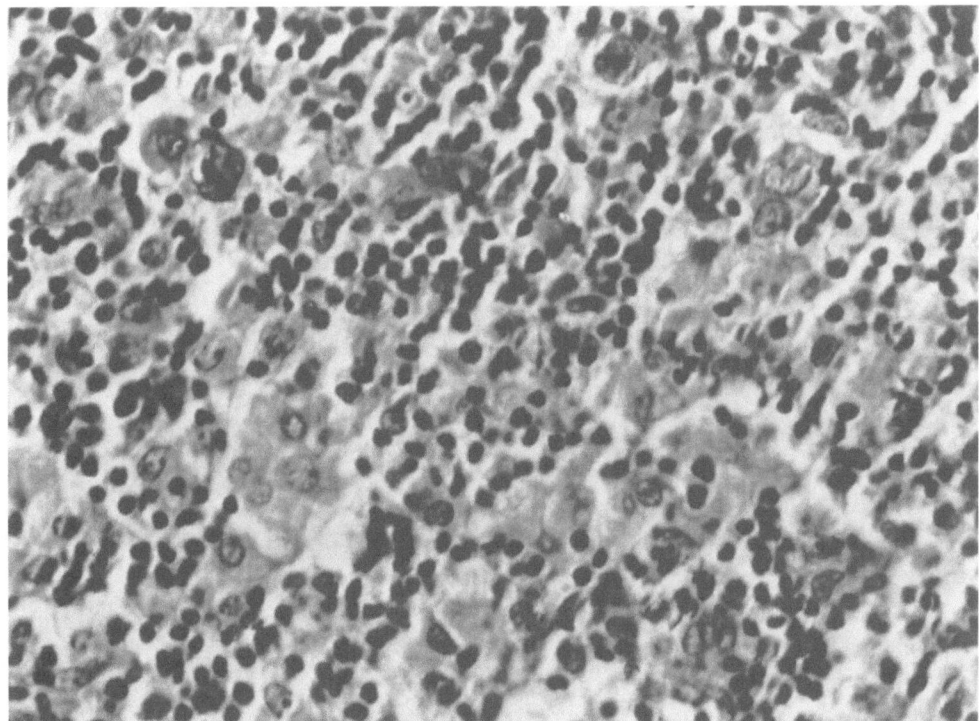

**Fig. 4.30.** The large cells have abundant, finely granular but rather pale cytoplasm. The example at top left corner is either multinuclear or has a multilobular nucleus. Nucleoli are frequently prominent. H & E, × 533

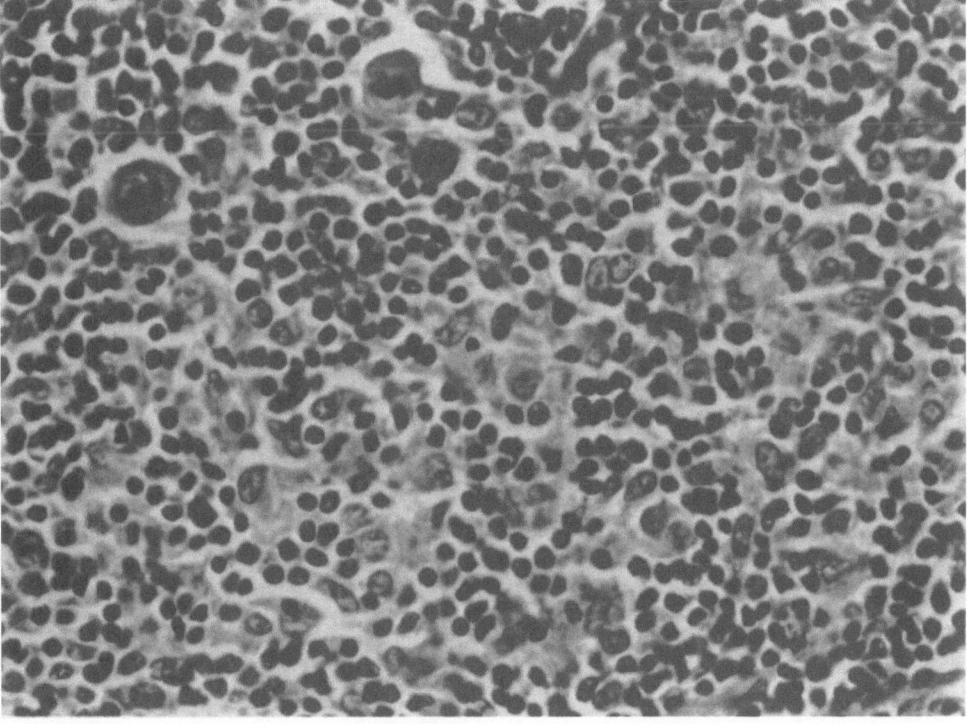

**Fig. 4.31.** Shows, top left corner, three of the largest cells; the uppermost is in mitosis. Just above right centre is a possible mirror-image cell. H & E, × 533

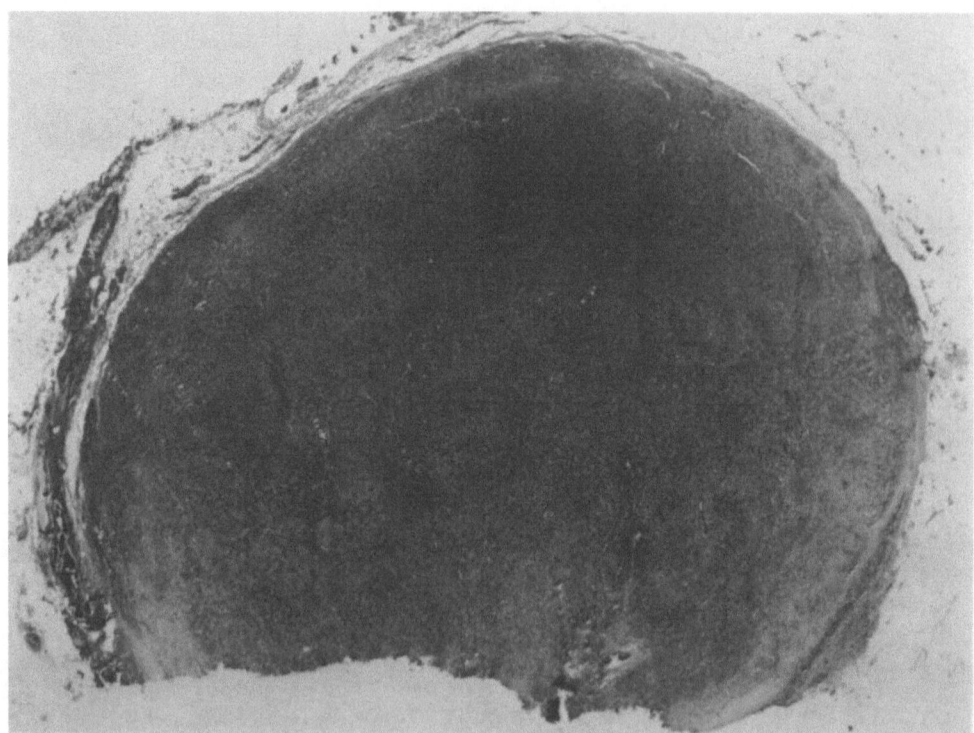

**Fig. 4.32.** A smooth sheet of cells totally devoid of formal pattern. Such pattern as there is was due to a degree of fibrosis (see text). H & E, × 13

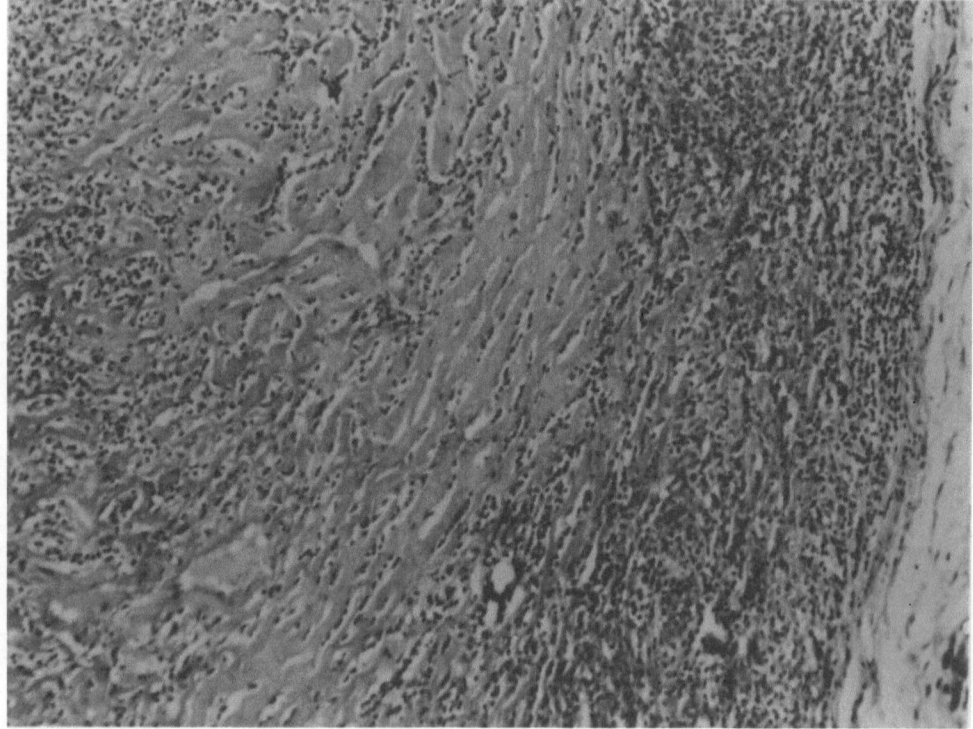

**Fig. 4.33.** Finely trabeculate collagen has been deposited in some areas and accounts for much of the pallor in the previous figure. H & E, × 131

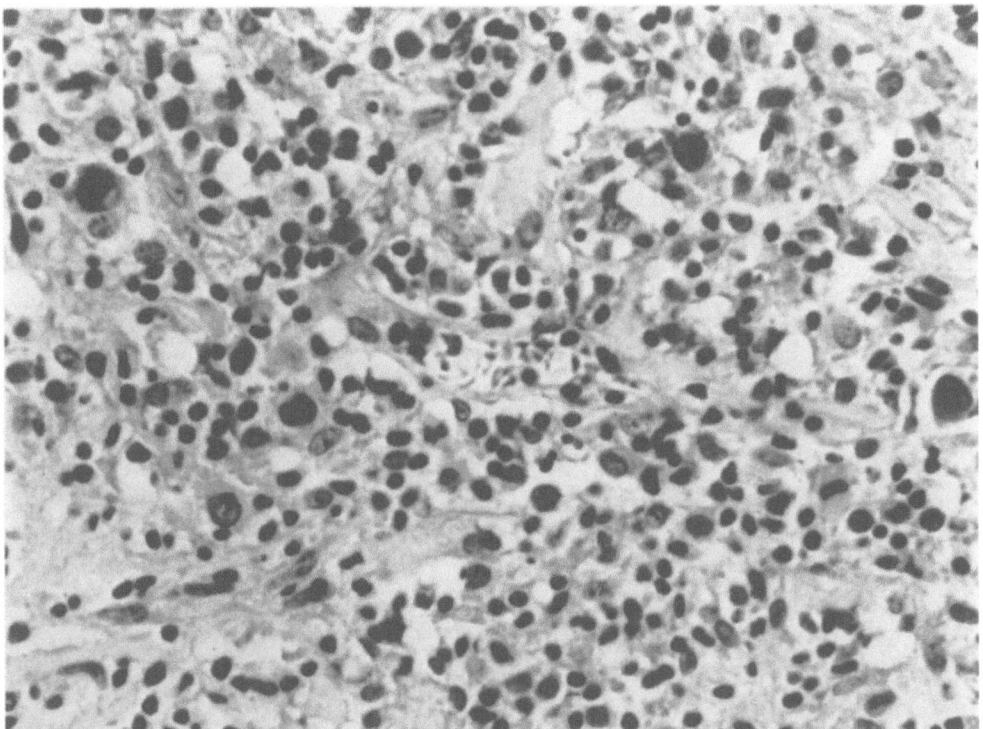

**Fig. 4.34.** Even without the four large pyknotic nuclei, the general picture is polymorphic and much more suggestive of a neoplastic than an inflammatory process. H & E, × 493

areas such as that illustrated where several lay relatively closely together. The cells were usually mono-, sometimes bi- and only rarely multinucleate. Eosinophil polymorphonuclears were absent.

Mitotic figures were quite numerous, and from their size were almost certainly the just-mentioned large cells in division. In view of the degree of fibrosis, which suggested the late stage of whatever the disorder might be, their frequency was rather a paradox.

The comment was made that the appearances could represent the end stage of Hodgkin's disease but that they could also be produced by some 'non-neoplastic reactive response'. The validity of this last opinion may now be doubted: it is difficult to believe that cells of this kind, with their mitotic activity, could represent other than a 'malignant lymphoma'.

The combined histological and clinical evidence was regarded as sufficiently diagnostic of a malignant lymphoma—probably Hodgkin's disease—to warrant radiotherapy, and this was started. Within 1 week, however, the patient became jaundiced and developed palpably en-larged liver and spleen. One week later he died. The lesions at necropsy, hepatosplenomegaly due to neoplastic infiltration and multiple lymph-adenopathy, were regarded as those of 'reticulum cell sarcoma'.

This, on review, appears a significant *under-diagnosis* to the extent that the possibility of some non-neoplastic condition should have received much less, preferably no, support. It made no difference in practice, however.

*Case 4.16*

F (62 years) with swellings in the left side of neck and left axilla, said to have been noticed for 1 week only. There were two nodes in the posterior triangle, the larger 20 × 15 mm, and one in the axilla.

There was virtually total loss of normal pattern. As shown in Fig. 4.35, the essential feature was massive replacement by sheets of relatively pale cells. They were pale by virtue of their nuclei being larger and more vesicular than the lymphocytes they were replacing (Fig. 4.36); they were also notably polymorphic and fre-

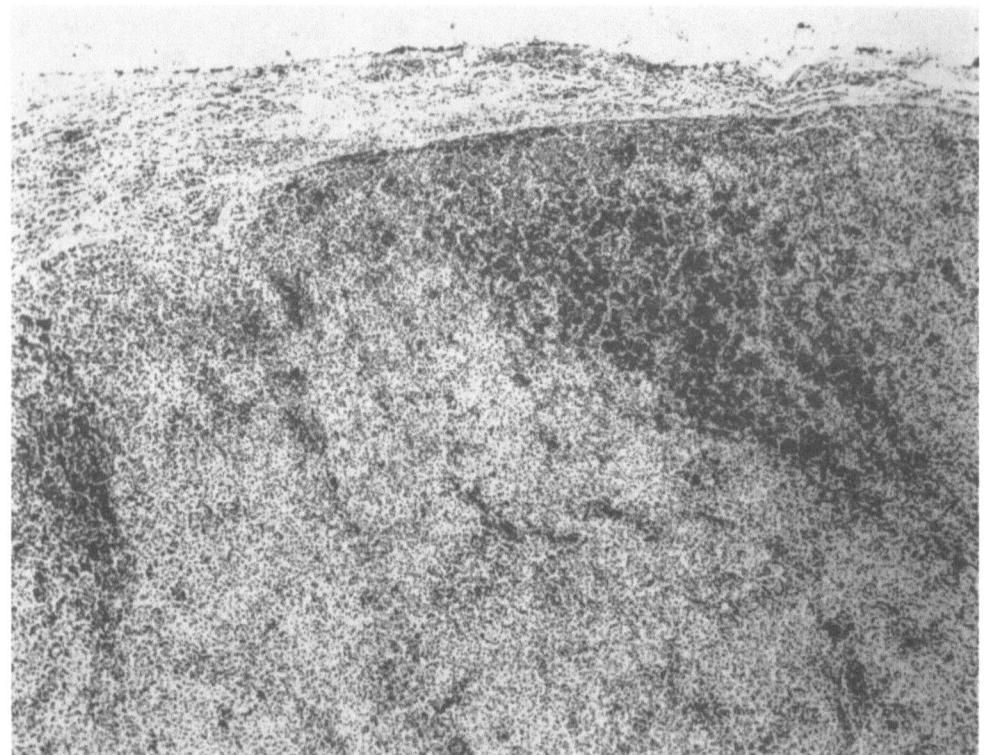

**Fig. 4.35.** Sheets of pale cells replaced much of the node. H & E, × 62

quently in mitosis. Besides these, but only very occasionally, there were giant nuclear forms as seen in Fig. 4.37. These were doubtless the reason for the histological report of '. . . very suggestive of Hodgkin's disease'. The blood picture was normal.

The patient had radiotherapy but within 5 months had developed nodal enlargement in both inguinal regions. The disease progressed with almost certainly abdominal involvement and led to death 10 months later (no necropsy).

In retrospect, the giant cells were so scanty (and eosinophil polymorphonuclears and fibrosis even more inconspicuous) that even the 'suggestion' of Hodgkin's disease seems difficult to sustain. A forthright diagnosis of 'reticulum-cell sarcoma' would have been more appropriate. However, even if there was an element of under-diagnosis here, the proper treatment was given, and designation of the lesion at the outset as RCS would have made no difference to the outcome.

A *marginal under-diagnosis* of no practical consequence, however, to the outcome.

*Case 4.17*

M (30 years) with swelling in neck gradually increasing over 6 months. The lesion was curetted. There were palpable nodes also in the other side of the neck and both axillae; the mediastinal shadow was broadened.

The material comprised some 20 fragments of soft whitish material, the largest 15 × 8 × 5 mm. It appeared to be basically lymphoid tissue transformed by massive reticulum-cell hyperplasia and heavy infiltration by neutrophil and, especially, eosinophil polymorphonuclears. Amongst these, as shown in Figs. 4.38 and 4.39, were not infrequent giant cells of bi- or multinucleate or multilobular character. In these figures, almost all the polymorphonuclear cells are of eosinophil type. The large cells were occasionally in mitosis and thought quite possibly to be R-S cells. There was no significant degree of fibrosis.

A firm choice could not be made between a 'granulomatous' or a 'malignant lymphomatous (probably Hodgkin's disease)' aetiology. The

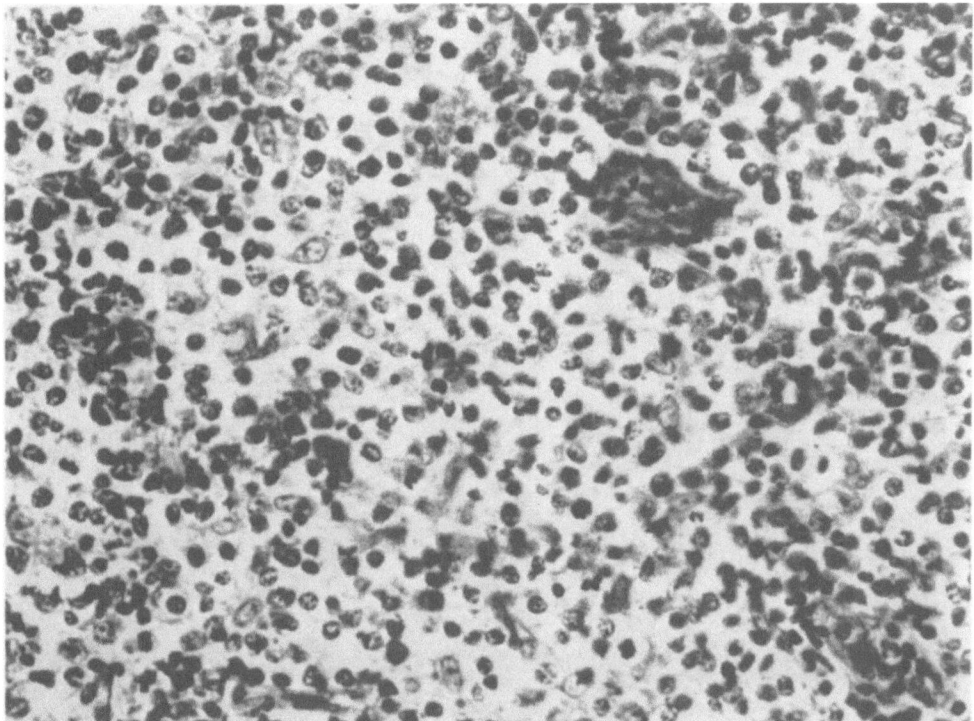

**Fig. 4.36.** The pale cells have almost invisible cytoplasm. There were four pyknotic mitotic figures in this area. H & E, × 476

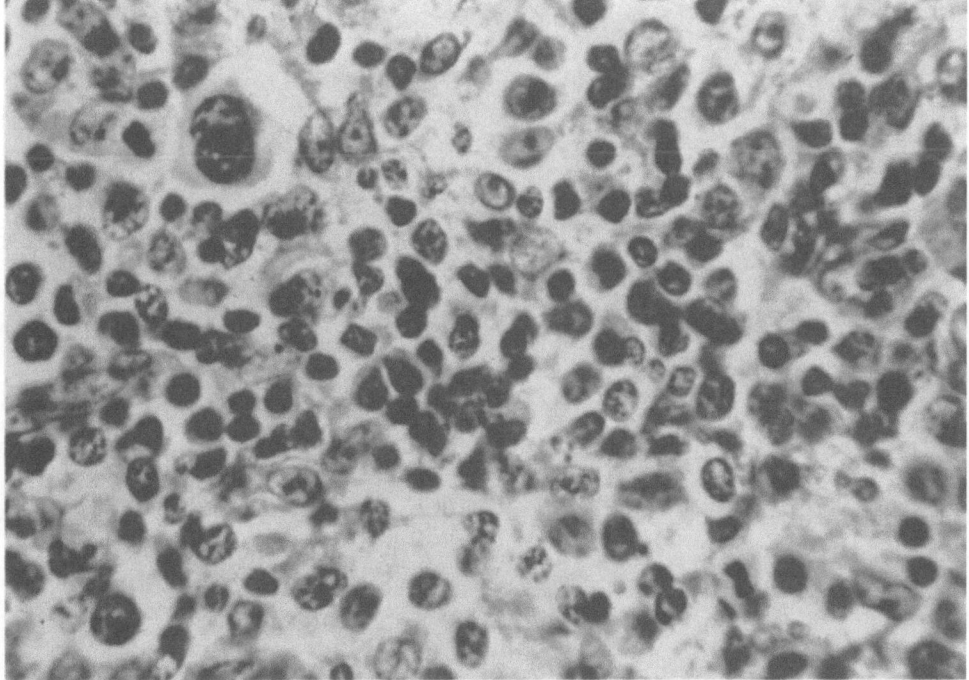

**Fig. 4.37.** Lymphocytes are greatly outnumbered by the pale cells. There are two mitotic figures, one top left corner beside the multilobular nucleus, one at lower right corner. H & E, × 952

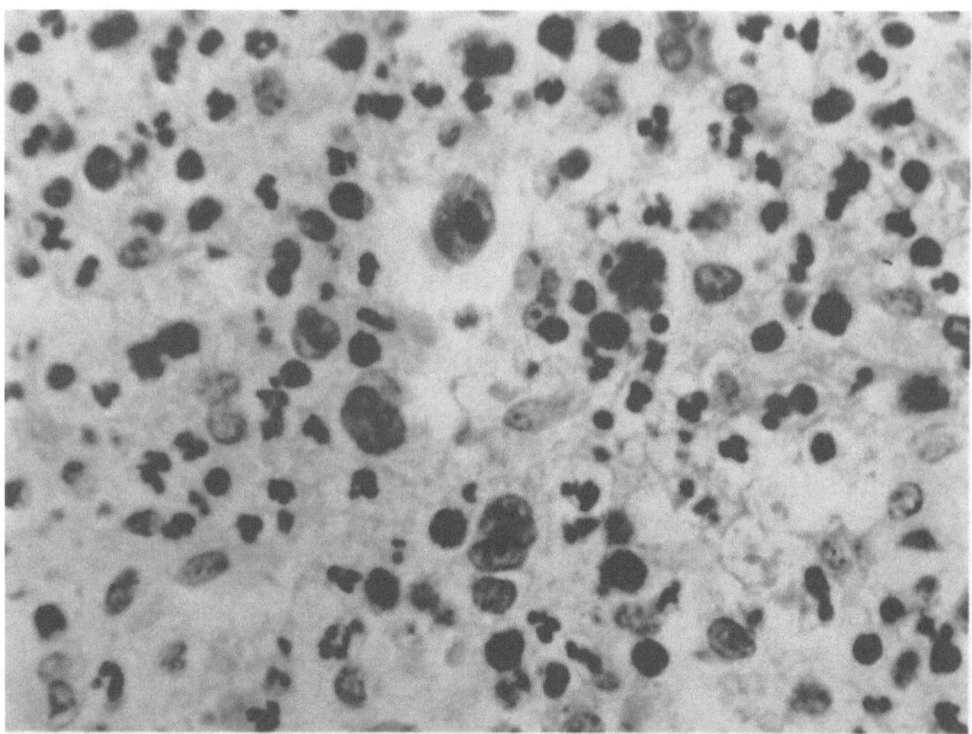

**Fig. 4.38.** This generally representative area shows many polymorphonuclears (all of eosinophilic type) and large cells with multilobular nuclei. H & E, × 952

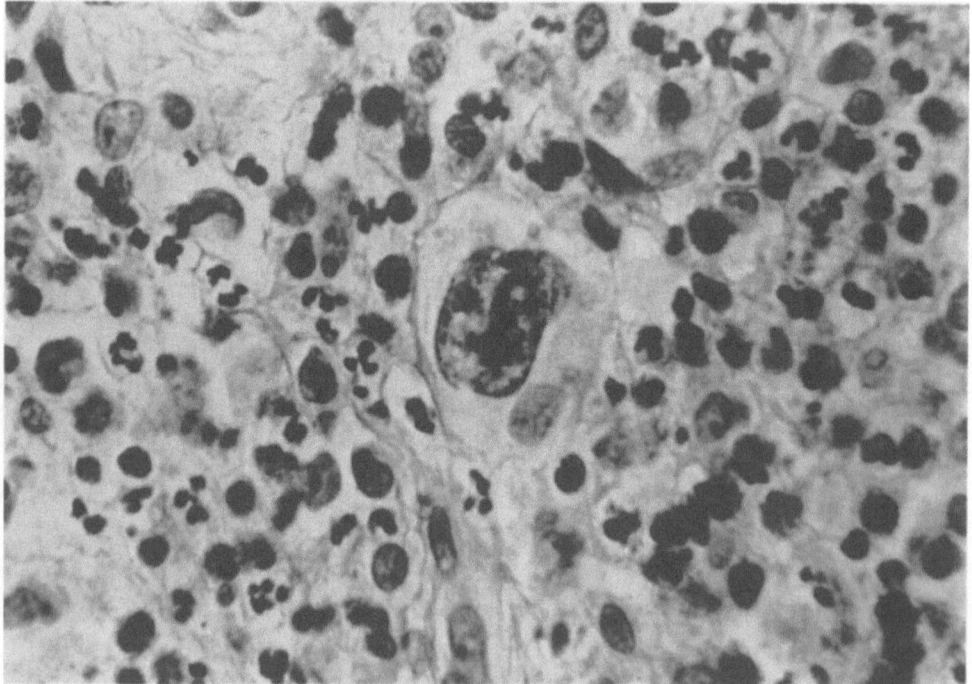

**Fig. 4.39.** An even larger cell with accompanying eosinophil polymorphonuclears again plentiful. Many of the cells, as in the previous figure, have finely granular cytoplasm. H & E, × 952

blood picture was normal. Treatment by radiotherapy was instituted.

After 6 months the mediastinal mass was larger, now displacing the trachea, and round cavities were present in both lungs, two on one side, one on the other. Bony architecture appeared normal throughout. Shortly after this, however, the patient developed another swelling, this time over the second right costal cartilage. Microscopically, this was identical with the original cervical lesion but showed also foamy lipid-laden macrophages in which cholesterol was amply demonstrable. Diagnosis now favoured the eosinophil granuloma/HSC group of disorders. Further radiotherapy was given. Three months later, one axillary mass was biopsied. The material from this is no longer on file but was reported as showing fewer eosinophil polymorphonuclears and many more 'foamy' macrophages.

The destructive lesions in the lungs slowly grew and within a few weeks destructive lesions were radiologically visible in the bones of the pelvis. The patient developed enlargement of spleen and liver, became increasingly jaundiced and died of bronchopneumonia 25 months after the onset of his illness: there was no necropsy. The final diagnosis preferred was 'Hand-Schüller-Christian disease'.

Still, in retrospect, this seems an *appropriate diagnosis*, the uncertainty at the time being overtaken by near-certainty on a second biopsy 6 months later.

## Case 4.18

M (18 years) with a lump on the back of his neck that had been growing over the past 6 months.

There was complete loss of architecture, though with little cytological aberrancy; the general appearance was that of a rather oedematous bag of mature lymphocytes. The only possibly significant abnormality was the presence of a very occasional cell with two or, even less commonly, three nuclei. The nuclei were not unduly large or polymorphic; there was no mitotic activity in these cells or elsewhere; and polymorphonuclears, whether eosinophil or neutrophil, were absent. The appearances were nevertheless held to indicate a 'primary neoplasm of lymphatic tissue, probably early Hodgkin's disease or lymphosarcoma'.

Despite the histological report, the restriction of the lesion to a single node was held to warrant an 'expectant policy'; no further treatment was given and the patient was well 15 years later. What may happen during the *next* 15 years remains to be seen but, so far at any rate, the lesion could be held to have been a 'benign lymphocytoma'.

The subsequent trouble-free 15 years in an untreated patient suggests that this was a marginal *over-diagnosis* albeit of no practical consequence. In retrospect, 'benign lymphocytoma' seems an appropriate term for the lesion even though this remains a debatable entity.

## Case 4.19

F (52 years) with recent enlargement of a swelling, said to have been present for 10 years, beneath the left side of the jaw. It was thought clinically to be a submandibular gland but excision yielded two oval masses, the larger 4 × 2 × 2 cm, each with a smooth, pale grey cut surface.

Appearances were essentially the same in both. Each was a lymph node that had suffered almost complete loss of normal architecture; something of a follicular pattern remained but, as in Case 4.6, absence of even a single normal germ centre made the term 'pseudo-follicle' more appropriate (Fig. 4.40). In some of these areas there were paler areas with a superficial resemblance to germ centres: in fact, the pallor was due to the presence of large cells with appropriately large nuclei, prominent nucleoli and voluminous eosinophilic cytoplasm of the type described earlier, as for example in cases 4.6 and 4.8. These cells were present not only in clusters but scattered at random singly or in twos and threes: about 1 in 500 was binucleate and a similar proportion in mitosis (Fig. 4.41). Multinucleate forms were rare; eosinophil polymorphonuclears rated on average two per hpf and were nowhere present en masse; neutrophils were scanty. There was no fibrosis.

The features as a whole were considered to be less than firmly diagnostic but certainly enough to warrant the term 'atypical Hodgkin's disease'. In view of the uncertainty, and the fact

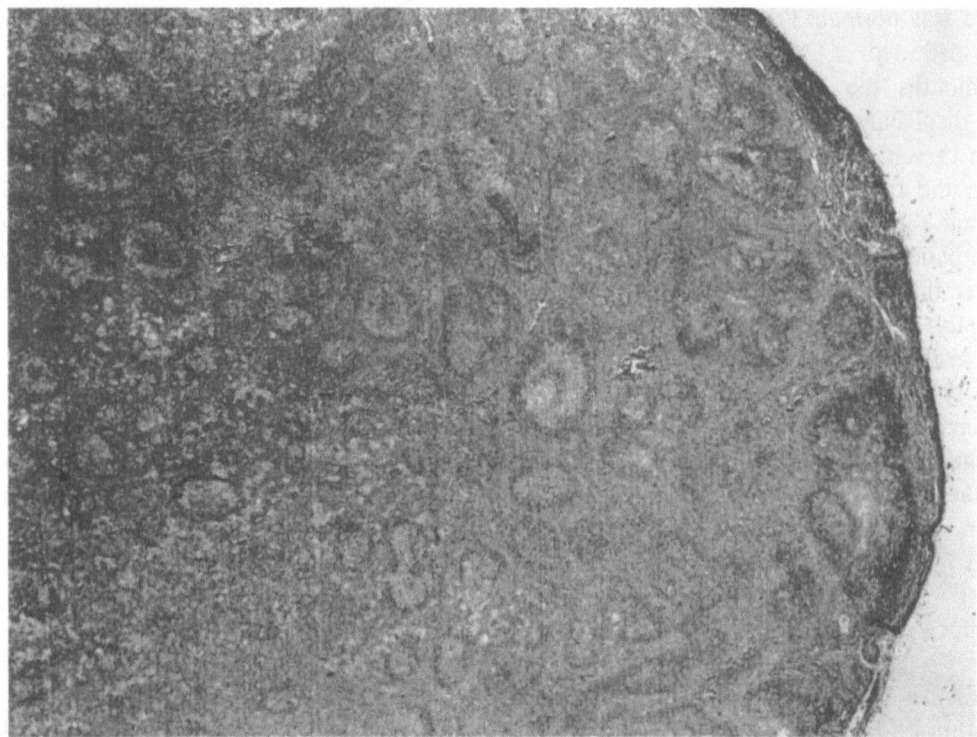

**Fig. 4.40.** A pseudo-follicular pattern throughout the whole node. None of the pale areas is a germinal centre, nor are any of the other circumscribed areas true follicles. H & E, × 13

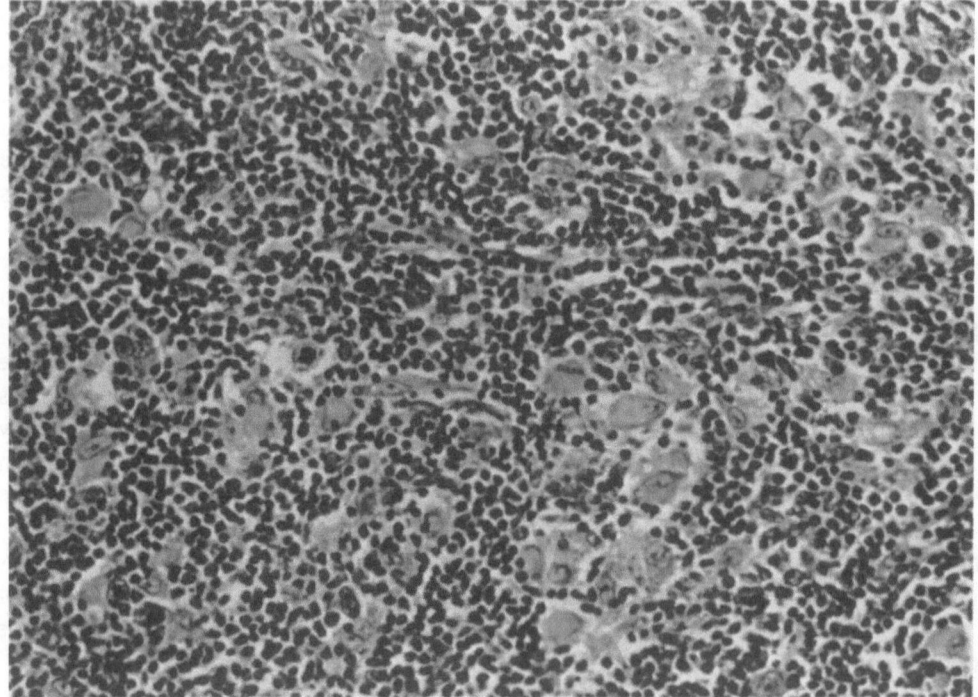

**Fig. 4.41.** The focal pattern in the previous figure was due to accumulations of cells of the kind shown here. All have a large volume of cytoplasm, large but not deeply staining nuclei and frequently prominent nucleoli. The pyknotic nucleus to left of centre is in mitosis. H & E, × 328

that these nodes not only appeared to be the only ones involved but had also been completely removed, it was considered reasonable to await further developments and do no more meantime.

There were no further developments for 13 years, when the patient, who had remained in good health during that time, reported with obvious enlargement of left supraclavicular nodes and a 3-cm mass in the uppermost part of the adjacent breast. The nodal tissue was now no longer recognisable as such but had the form of highly cellular sheets. Eosinophil polymorphonuclears were scanty, cells acceptable as R-S cells not seen, and fibrosis altogether absent. Primitive reticulum cells and lymphocytes were present in approximately equal number, the reticulum cells showing both considerable polymorphism and mitotic activity. The picture was now one of an unquestionably malignant undifferentiated neoplasm. Radiotherapy had little effect and the patient died within 12 months with disseminated disease.

Despite the prolonged latency and dormancy of the disease, the typical features of Hodgkin's disease did not emerge. It may be that the better designation would have been 'reticulum cell sarcoma' but even in retrospect this, one feels, would have been something of an over-diagnosis on the original material.

This was an *appropriate diagnosis*, to the extent at any rate that the lesion was diagnosed as a malignant lymphoma. Whether the 'expectant' policy adopted, nevertheless, was or was not appropriate is a matter of opinion. Whether therapy started after the first diagnosis would have been curative, we cannot know, but at least the patient resisted the lesion, untreated, for 13 years.

### Case 4.20

M (55 years) with nodule in cheek that had developed 'over the past few weeks'. It was totally excised and appeared on section as shown in Fig. 4.42.

The picture was one of mostly quite uniform cells of large lymphocytic or lymphoblastoid type, strongly suggesting a primarily lymphomatous lesion of some kind. In a few places, however, as shown in Fig. 4.43, there were small groups of cells of more primitive type with larger and sometimes double nuclei. The possibility of Hodgkin's disease was considered but the preferred and suggested diagnosis was a 'leukaemic infiltrate'.

Examination of the blood confirmed the existence of a 'chronic lymphatic leukaemia'. The patient died but not until 16 years later. The

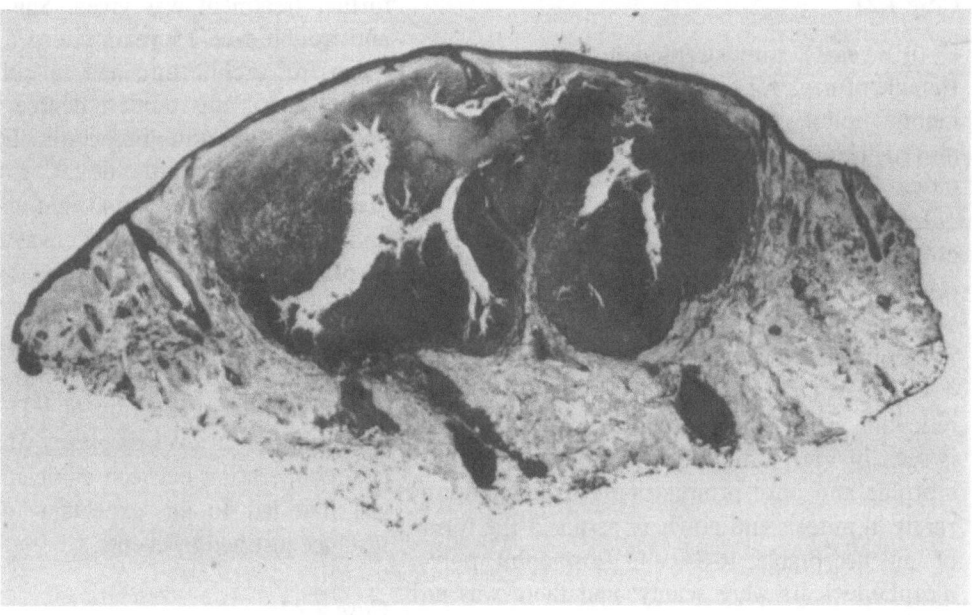

**Fig. 4.42.** A highly cellular nodule beneath the skin of the cheek and thus probably not originally a lymph node. H & E, × 12

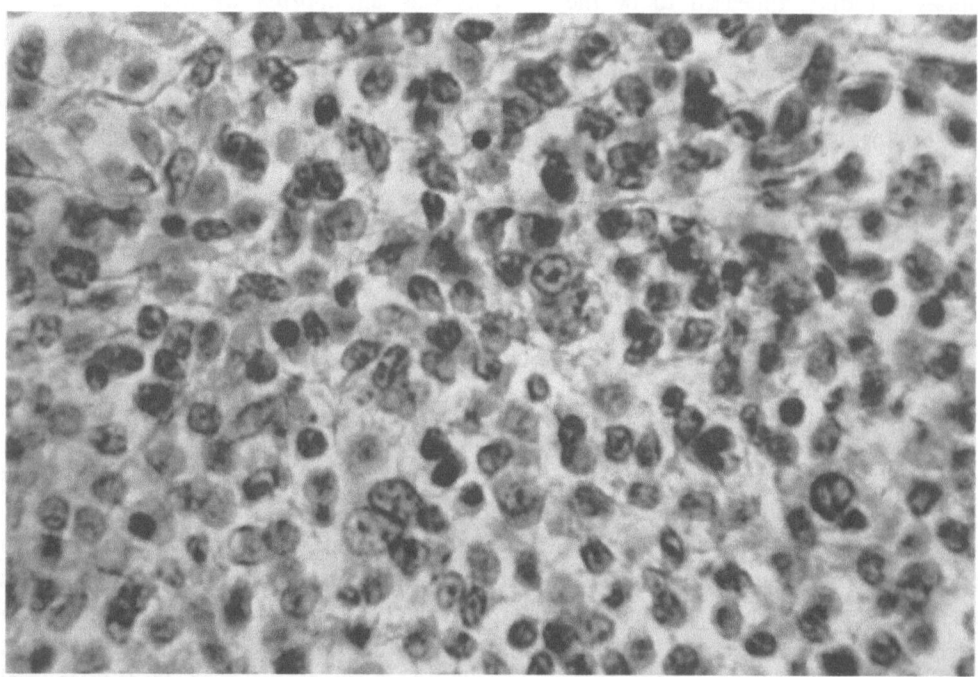

**Fig. 4.43.** The cells were larger than lymphocytes. Scattered cells, of which several appear here, were notably larger than those forming the general background and usually had conspicuous nucleoli. A possible mirror-image cell lies at lower left centre. H & E, × 952

large, apparently primitive, cells had not been the harbinger of either Hodgkin's disease or transformation to an acute leukaemic state.

An *appropriate diagnosis.*

### Case 4.21

F (19 years) with swelling in right posterior triangle of neck for some 8 weeks. Several freely mobile nodules were palpable. The mass removed included three discrete nodules, the two larger 15 × 8 mm in outline.

In approximately 50% of each node a generally normal follicular pattern, with germ centres, was retained. For the rest, the pattern was as shown in Fig. 4.44. The pale areas are not expanded germ centres but, as seen in Fig. 4.45, foci or sheets of rather loosely disposed reticulum cells. The morphology of these cells is seen in Fig. 4.46; they are moderately polymorphic and have prominent nucleoli but were rarely in mitosis and nowhere assumed the form of an acceptable R-S cell. Eosinophil polymorphonuclears were scanty, and there was no significant degree of fibrosis.

The loss of architecture and the polymorphism of the pale cells were of some concern. It was considered that the familiar problem of 'reactive' vs 'early Hodgkin's disease' could not be firmly answered.

No possibly causative local lesion was found, the patient remained generally well, and no further treatment was given. She was still well and trouble-free 15 years later.

Loss of architecture and reticulum cell polymorphism of this modest degree were, on this occasion at any rate, innocuous. Examination in retrospect leaves little doubt, as may be appreciated from Fig. 4.44, that the overgrowth and permeation of pale cells was a sinus histiocytosis as yet involving no more than some 50% of each node. The nodes were presumably 'reactive' but, as is so frequent, the cause was never established.

The significant mention of HD marks this as something of an *over-diagnosis* where, nevertheless, cooperation between clinician and pathologist had led to an 'expectant' policy, in this instance justified by events.

### Case 4.22

F (56 years) with pain and swelling in right groin for 1 month. She was otherwise well, no

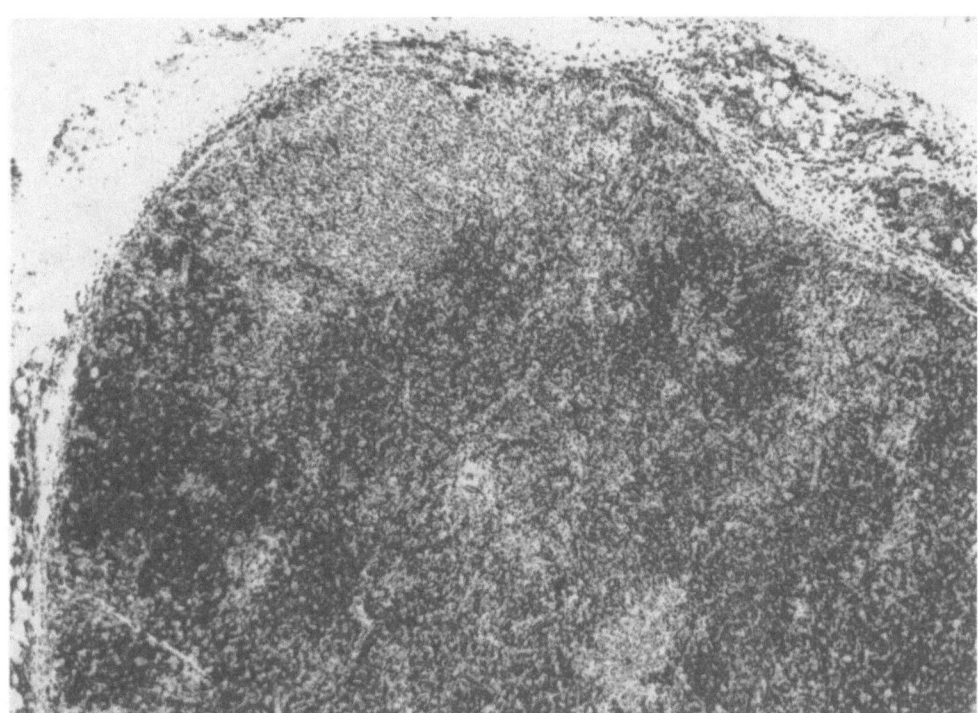

**Fig. 4.44.** A uniformly lymphocytic background interrupted by sheets of pale cells. H & E, × 60

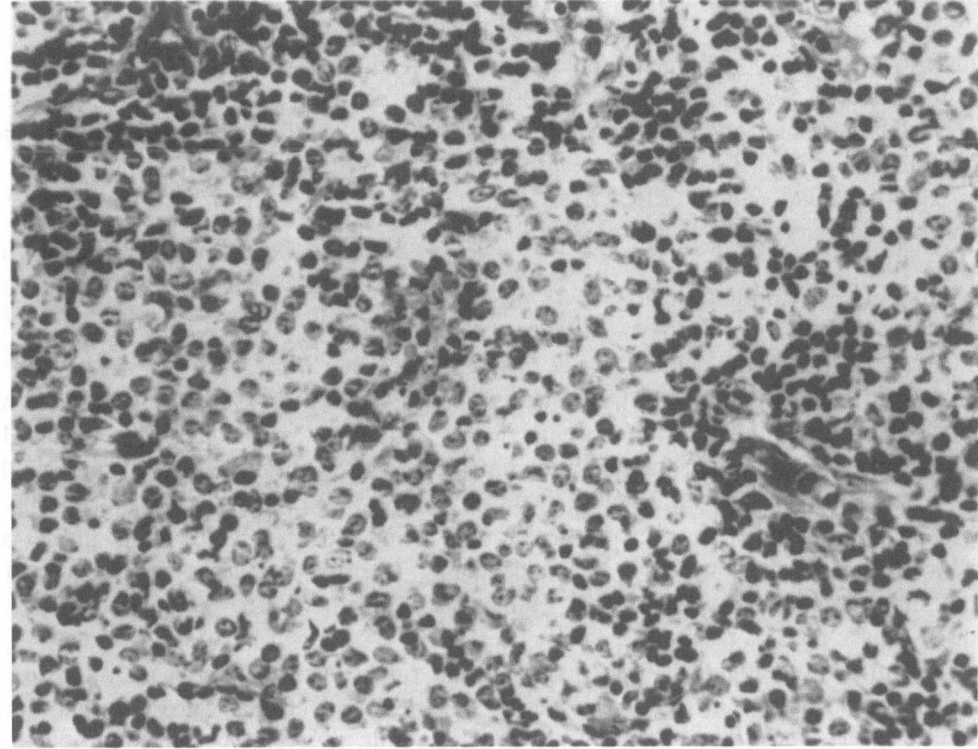

**Fig. 4.45.** The pale cells have much inconspicuous cytoplasm and notably polymorphic nuclei. H & E, × 493

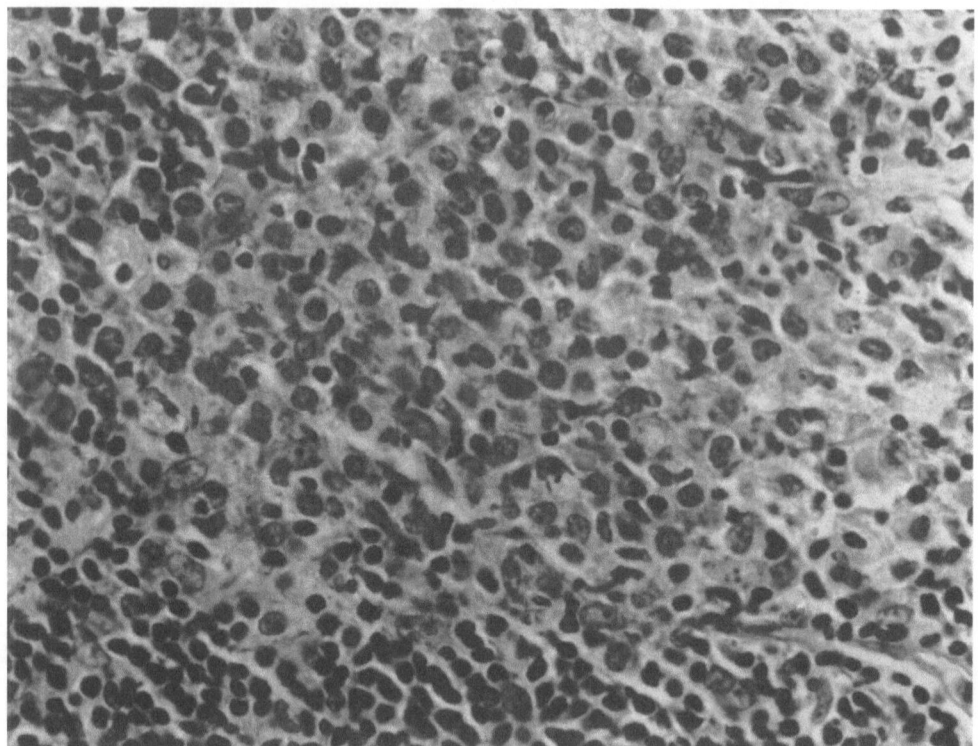

**Fig. 4.46.** The normal lymphocytes along lower edge emphasise the larger size and mildly polymorphic nuclei of the pale cells. Mitotic figures were scanty. H & E, × 553

other abnormalities were found, and the blood picture was normal. The fatty mass excised contained two large (20 × 10 mm) nodes.

As in Case 4.19, there was widespread loss of normal architecture and preservation in only a few areas, mainly just beneath the capsule, of a 'pseudo-follicular' pattern. Elsewhere the tissue consisted of an even mixture of lymphocytes, large pale cells with prominent nucleoli and eosinophil polymorphonuclears; in an average field the proportion of these was approximately 9 : 9 : 2. Although the pale cells were relatively large, and occasionally bi- or trinucleate, none could be used to illustrate a characteristic R-S cell. They were, however, frequently in mitosis to the extent of 1 figure per 2 hpf on average. It was uncertain whether the changes, which were in general more pronounced in one node than the other, represented an 'atypical Hodgkin's disease' or a 'reactive response', possibly allergic.

All further investigations were negative, no further treatment was given and the patient was well 8 years later. The uncertainty therefore remains. In view, however, of the 14-year latency shown by the lesion in Case 4.19, of rather similar morphology, the disease may not yet have run its course.

Review of the material leaves the reviewer still uncertain. This may be regarded therefore as an *appropriate* if still equivocal diagnosis.

CASE DATA II
? MALIGNANT LYMPHOMA OTHER THAN
HODGKIN'S DISEASE (TABLE 4.3)

*Case 4.23*

F (62 years) with 6 months' dyspepsia and gastric mass diagnosed on X-ray. The partially resected stomach showed marked thickening of the wall of the pyloric antrum (up to 15 mm) and enlarged nodes along the lesser curvature. The antral mucosa was congested and partly eroded.

As shown in Figs. 4.47 and 4.48, the mucosa and submucosa were widely and deeply infiltrated by mononuclear cells of varied morphology. Of four representative lymph nodes (the largest 10 × 6 × 4 mm) from the lesser curvature, one showed partial replacement by cells of the

**Table 4.3.** Eighteen cases of ? malignant (non-Hodgkin's) lymphoma.

| Case No. | Diagnosis on review | Treatment + or − | Outcome |
|---|---|---|---|
| *1 case under-diagnosed* | | | |
| 4.25 | Lymphosarcoma > follic. lymphoblastoma | − | Death @ 2 yr |
| *3 cases over-diagnosed* | | | |
| 4.23 | Plasmacytoma > lymphosarcoma | Gastrectomy | Unrelated death @ 8 yr |
| 4.24 | Lymphoid polyp > lymphosarcoma | Colostomy + radium | Alive @ 30 yr |
| 4.31 | Non-specific reactive > 'early Brill's disease' | − | Alive @ 16 yr |
| *14 cases appropriately diagnosed* | | | |
| 4.26 | Lymphosarcoma | − | Probable death @ 18 yr |
| 4.27 | Lymphosarcoma | + | Alive @ 9 yr |
| 4.28 | Reticulum cell sarcoma | + | Death @ 3 yr |
| 4.29 | ? SHML | − | Alive @ 20 yr |
| 4.30 | Metastatic carcinoma | − | Alive @ 13 yr |
| 4.32 | Non-specific reactive: cause known | − | Alive @ 10 yr |
| 4.33 | Non-specific reactive: cause known | − | Unrelated death @ 2 yr |
| 4.34 | Non-specific reactive: cause uncertain | + | Post-op. death |
| 4.35 | Still ambiguous: cause unknown | − | Alive @ 16 yr |
| 4.36 | Still ambiguous: cause unknown | − | Unrelated death @ 18 mo |
| 4.37 | Still ambiguous: cause known | − | Alive @ 15 yr |
| 4.38 | Still ambiguous: cause known | − | Alive @ 8 yr |
| 4.39 | Still ambiguous: cause known | − | Alive @ 6 yr |
| 4.40 | Still ambiguous | + | Alive @ 10 yr |

same aberrant type. These features were diagnosed as indicating 'lymphosarcoma'.

This case came to light only as the result of a surgeon colleague's remarking on the unexpectedly long survival of a former patient diagnosed as having had 'lymphosarcoma' of the stomach 8 years ago; she had, he learned, just died, a necropsy was to be performed, and he was interested.

The cause of death was bronchopneumonia after repair of a fractured femur. There was no neoplasm in or of stomach or lymph nodes in any area. Review revealed that the diagnosis should have been 'plasmacytoma' at the outset. This was an *over-diagnosis*: therapeutically it had little implication, prognostically it had much.

*Case 4.24*

M (17 years) with rectal bleeding and a feeling of 'something coming down'. A lobulate polypoid mass, 15 × 10 × 10 mm, of which Fig. 4.49 shows one half, was excised.

The mass consisted of mildly hyperplastic lymphoid tissue with prominent germ centres and rather unduly cellular stroma. As seen also in Fig. 4.49, the mucosa, though minimally ulcerated in a few places, was generally uninvaded and intact. The hypercellularity had been the main reason for the lesion's being diagnosed 'lymphosarcoma'; it was treated by radium implantation and colostomy; the rectum was not excised.

Review leaves little doubt that this was a 'benign lymphoid polyp' that would not today, with the lesion more widely familiar, be at much risk of diagnosis of lymphosarcoma. The patient was seen again 18 years later, when the colostomy prolapsed, and again within the past year, now 30 years since the original operation for the complaint of bleeding per rectum. Biopsy showed

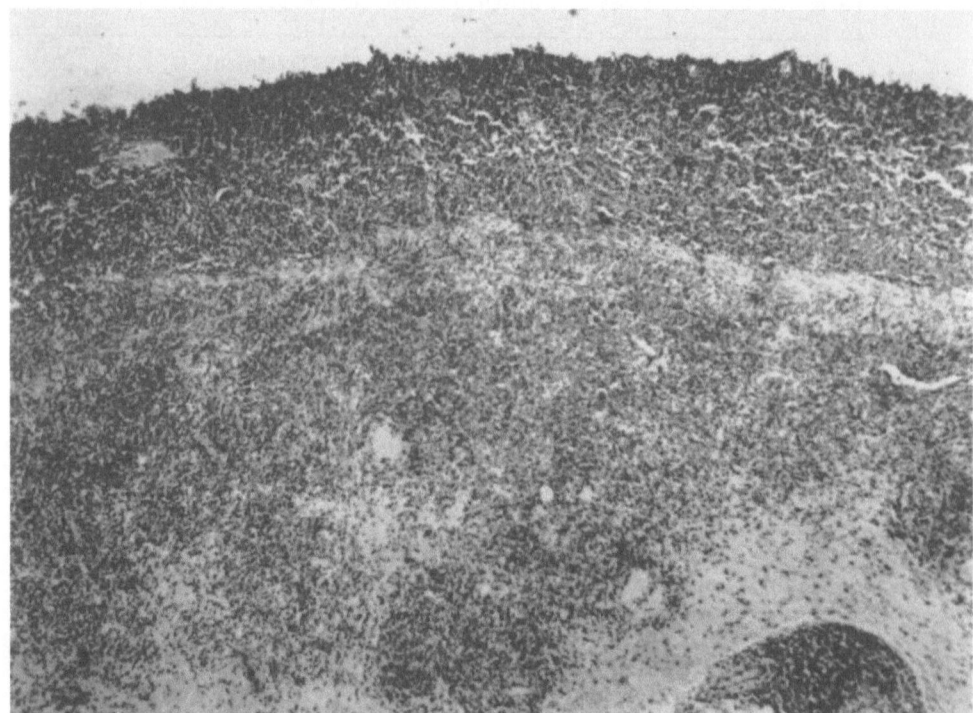

**Fig. 4.47.** The ulcerated surface and subjacent part of the highly cellular mass: the mucosa has disappeared. H & E, × 60

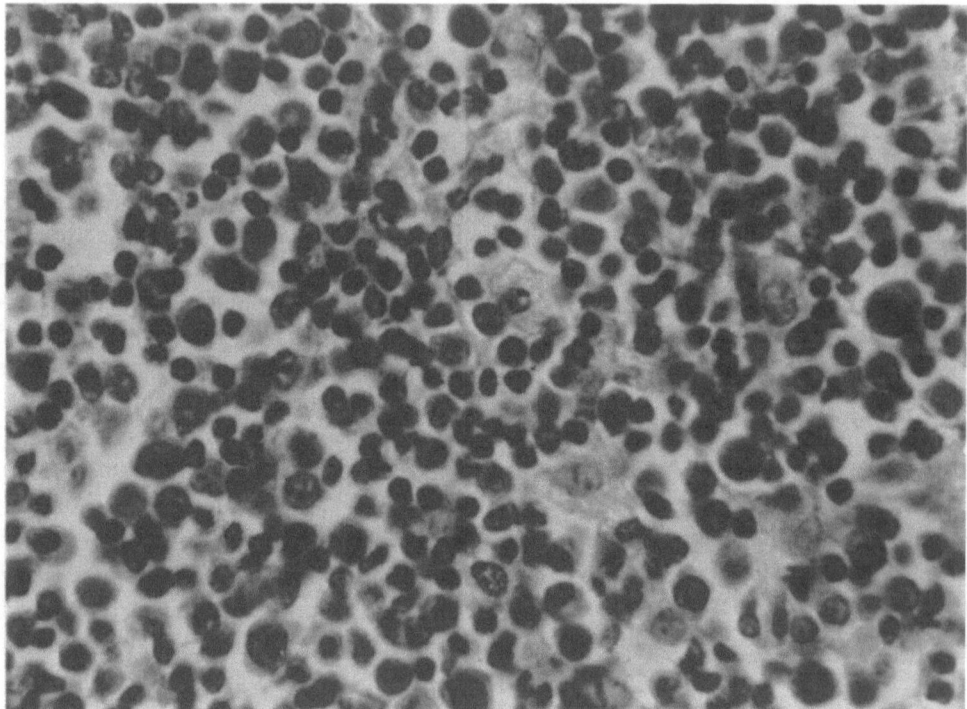

**Fig. 4.48.** The constituent cells are predominantly plasma cells, an occasional example (*right edge*) unusually large. H & E, × 952

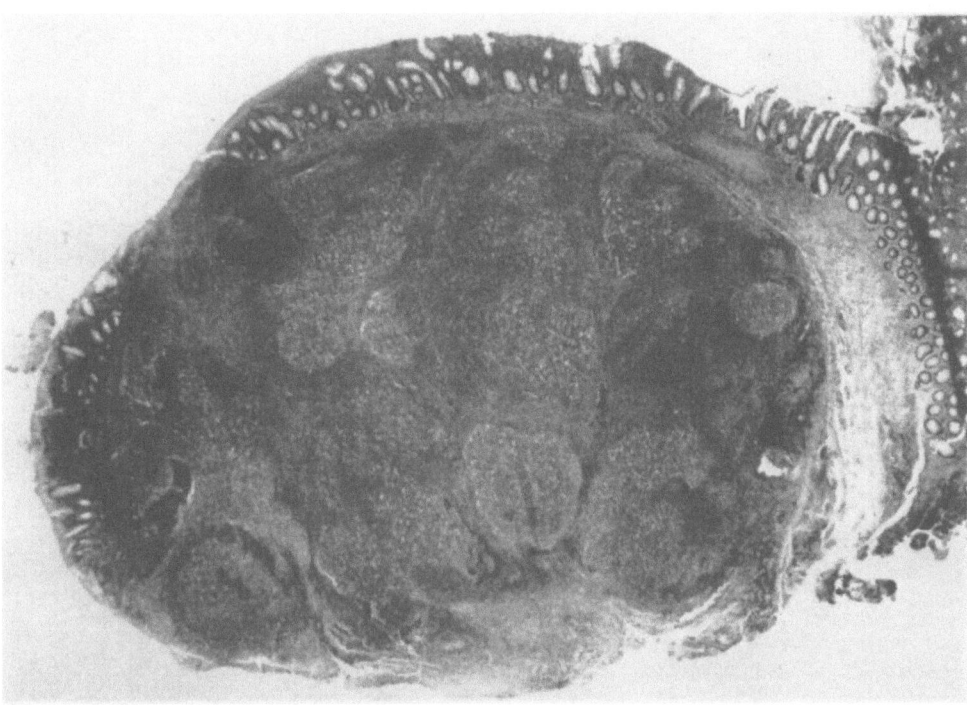

**Fig. 4.49.** The full extent of the partly ulcerated lymphoid polyp. H & E, × 9

a non-specific inflammatory reaction but there was also a degree of glandular aberrancy reported as 'disturbing'. The risk of a post-irradiation carcinoma clearly remains.

This was an obviously significant *over-diagnosis*.

### Case 4.25

M (59 years) with an initial complaint of 'vague indigestion' for a few months. Examination showed enlarged nodes in all palpable areas. An inguinal node was removed.

There was widespread and substantial loss of normal architecture but just a remnant trace of follicular pattern; this had been considered enough to justify a diagnosis of 'follicular lymphoblastoma'. However, the wide obliterating sheets of cells showed a significant degree of polymorphism and abundant mitotic activity, to the point where lymphocytic lymphoma now, in retrospect, seems a much preferable diagnosis. It was this cytology, no doubt, that had led to the original report's mentioning that this lesion was 'possibly more active than the majority of cases of this disease'.

The patient died 2 years later with widespread lesions. There was no necropsy but all evidence

supported the diagnosis of 'lymphosarcoma'. The pattern, in retrospect, would have been a misleading addition to any series of 'follicular lymphoblastoma'. A significant *under-diagnosis*.

### Case 4.26

F (39 years) with enlarged inguinal nodes (four nodes in a fatty mass, 4 × 2 × 2 cm) removed during repair of femoral hernia.

All the nodes examined retained at least a 'folliculoid' structure, best described, perhaps, as a giant follicular lymphoma without germ centres. Cell density was rather greater in the centre of the pseudo-follicles than at the edge, due essentially to subdivision of the parenchyma by narrow fibrovascular bands or septa (Fig. 4.50). The cells, essentially all mature lymphocytes, included a very occasional example much larger than the rest. These can be no more accurately named than just large 'reticulum' cells.

The lesion had been regarded as a form of giant follicular lymphadenopathy, to be regarded for practical purposes as a 'lymphosarcoma'. For whatever reason, no further treatment was given.

The patient was still well after 6 years but was then found to have bilateral enlargement of axillary and cervical nodes. One axillary node,

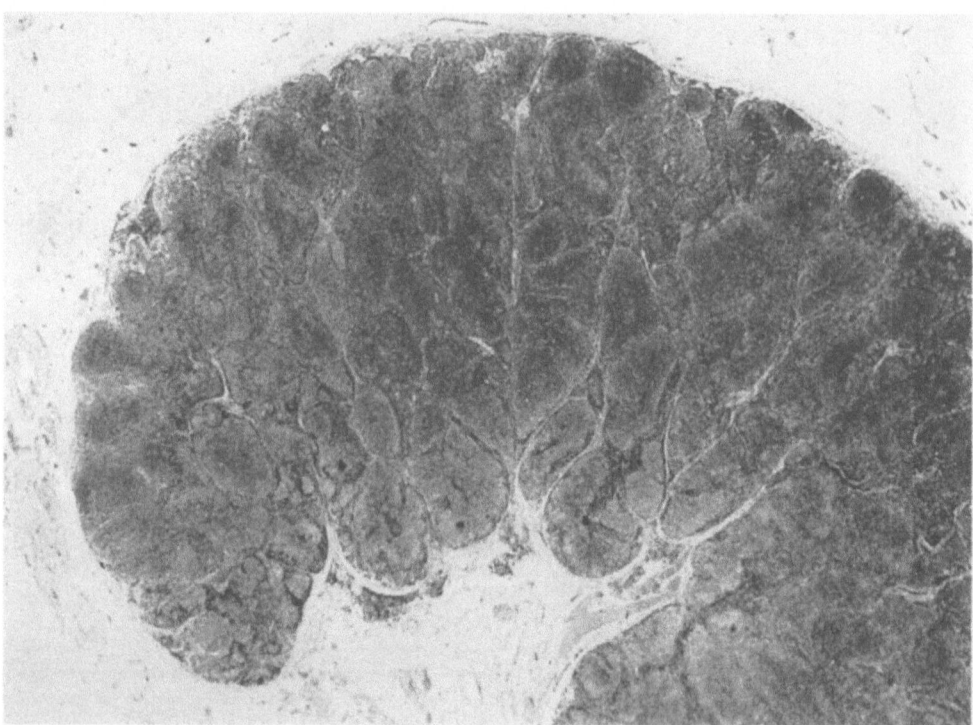

**Fig. 4.50.** The node retains something of a follicular pattern but less than the appearances here would suggest. There is appreciable subdivision or nodulation due to permeation by fine fibrous septa. H & E, × 12

20 × 15 mm, was removed. Sections showed only two points of difference from the original: (a) the 'pseudo-follicles' were rather larger than the original and the fibrovascular bands even narrower, (b) occasional pseudo-follicles had a central area of larger, paler cells, not enough to constitute a typical germ centre but at least closer to that than anything seen hitherto. Again, the lesion was diagnosed as 'for practical purposes, a lymphosarcoma', and again no specific treatment was thought necessary.

After a further 12 years, the patient developed increasingly severe diarrhoea with weight loss and melaena. An enlarged inguinal node (6 × 3 × 2 cm) was removed; others were still present in the other groin and both sides of the neck but not in the axillae. Microscopy showed the same broad pattern as before but, in detail, rather more individual cell polymorphism and mitotic activity. Over the 18 years to the present, the histological evidence had in effect changed from 'probably lymphosarcoma' to 'certainly lymphosarcoma'. The ultimate outcome is unknown but on the clinical evidence just described death probably followed not long after.

An *appropriate diagnosis* of a lymphosarcoma sustained, untreated, for 18 years.

### Case 4.27

F (51 years) with swelling in axilla for a few months. Excision produced a fatty mass containing an apparent 20-mm cyst filled with what seemed to be pultaceous pale green pus, and an 8-mm node.

The apparent pus was not pus but almost totally necrotic lymphatic tissue enclosed by a greatly thickened (up to 3 mm) fibrotic capsule in which there were small scattered foci of mixed lymphocytes and plasma cells. The structure appeared to be a completely 'infarcted lymph node'. It seemed plausible to associate the necrosis with the capsular sclerosis (which might have strangled the blood supply) but no reason was evident, in turn, for that, especially since the adjacent 8-mm node was structurally entirely normal. The patient was asked to return in 6 months.

Re-examination at this time showed enlargement of the nodes in the neck, groin and both axillae. A large inguinal node (30 × 25 × 20 mm) was removed; it had a smooth white fleshy cut surface.

Microscopy showed virtually total loss of architecture and replacement by sheets of lymphocytes among which were either individual or small clusters of large pale but notably eosinophilic reticulum cells (Fig. 4.51). These were rarely in mitosis, not unduly polymorphic, and nowhere to be designated giant cells (Fig. 4.52). Among the lymphocytes, however, mitoses were common: it was difficult to find a hpf that contained none; in most of the node, there were two to six per hpf. There appeared histologically still to be a possibility that the node could represent a reaction to infection of some kind but all investigations were negative. This fact, along with the high histological suspicion and the clinical findings, led to the decision that 'for practical purposes' the lesion should be regarded as a form of 'lymphosarcoma'. Treatment was started with radiotherapy and, 6 months later, chemotherapy.

During the next 2 years the patient had intercurrent illness including duodenal peptic ulcer and partial collapse of a lumbar vertebra, due apparently to simple osteoporosis, but has had no further trouble and remains well now at 9 years post-biopsy. The experience of this case combined with that of Case 4.3, where a large lymph node appeared to be totally infarcted, has engendered caution about the interpretation of not obviously explicable nodal necrosis; in these circumstances the possibility of a malignant lymphoma should always be considered.

The first diagnosis was straightforward and factually correct but the suspicious nature of the change was appreciated. The further biopsy was given an *appropriate diagnosis*. Lymphosarcoma probably was the correct diagnosis, and the patient possibly has been cured but, as Case 4.26 shows, even 9 years may not be long enough to substantiate this.

### Case 4.28

F (63 years) with swelling in the neck for 2 months. Biopsy yielded two nodes, the larger 10 × 10 × 6 mm.

The follicular pattern was reasonably well

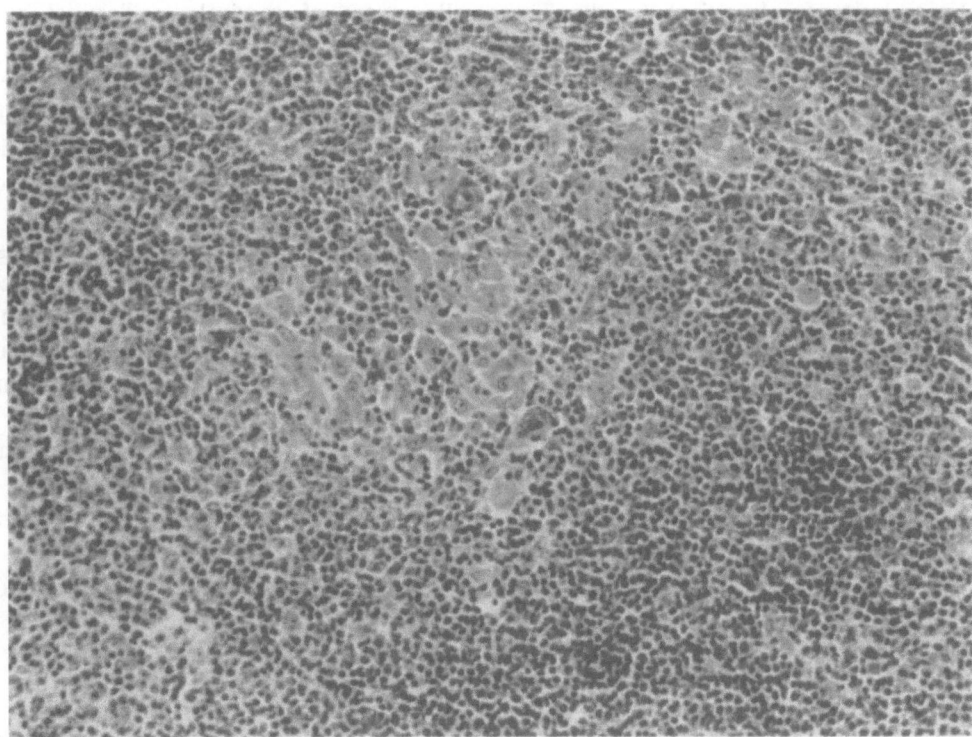

**Fig. 4.51.** Clusters of large pale cells dispersed among a uniformly lymphocytic background. H & E, × 221

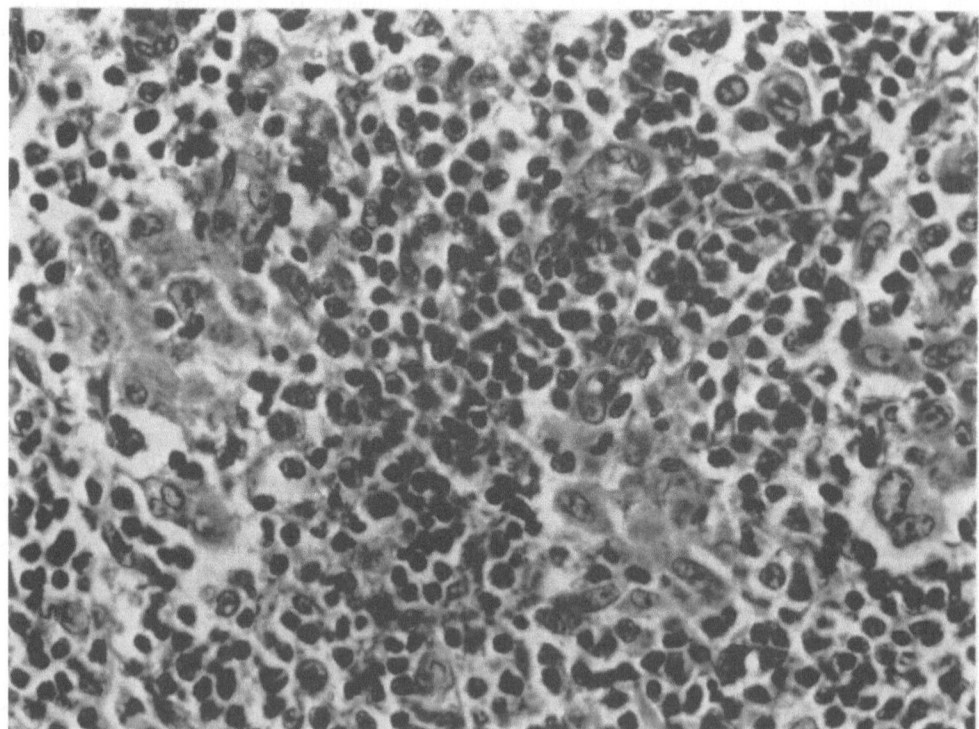

**Fig. 4.52.** The large pale cells have much cytoplasm and moderately polymorphic nuclei. At lower right edge is a possible mirror-image cell: in this, and in some others, nucleoli are conspicuous. H & E, × 533

preserved but obscured by a diffuse background hyperplasia of pale reticulum cells. These cells showed a slightly but definitely greater degree of polymorphism than normal, while an occasional cell was certainly larger and had a more irregular nuclear outline than in any non-specifically reactive node (Fig. 4.53). In one single 1-mm island, largely devoid of lymphocytes and of almost purely reticulum cell character, there were areas with up to five mitotic figures per hpf. This was the only such focus in a section containing in all some 200 mm² of nodal tissue. These features were disquieting but not considered evidence enough to justify a certain diagnosis of any form of malignant lymphoma. However, suspicion was such that radiotherapy was prescribed; that is, for practical purposes, the lesion was regarded as an 'early R-E sarcoma'.

An incidental histological feature was widespread angio-endothelial proliferation (Fig. 4.54) similar to that seen in Case 4.10.

The patient remained reasonably well for the next 3 years, then developed a rapid terminal illness with death just over 3 years after the initial biopsy. Necropsy showed massive enlargement of cervical, mediastinal and abdominal nodes with invasion of liver, one adrenal and one vertebra. Histologically, the tissue was highly cellular, polymorphic and abundantly mitotic. The most appropriate diagnosis was considered to be 'reticulum-cell sarcoma'.

Even in retrospect, a forthright diagnosis of RCS would scarcely have been justified on the original biopsy. Presumably, the condition was RCS at an early stage but the course of events taught little more than that, in some cases, even slight polymorphism of reticulum cells, with undue enlargement of some, and focal mitotic excess, even if rare, may represent a highly malignant lymphoma capable of totally anaplastic transformation within as short a period as 3 years.

An *appropriate diagnosis* on evidence still, in retrospect, equivocal.

### Case 4.29

M (51 years) with swelling in the groin that had increased gradually over the past 17 years. A 20-mm node was removed.

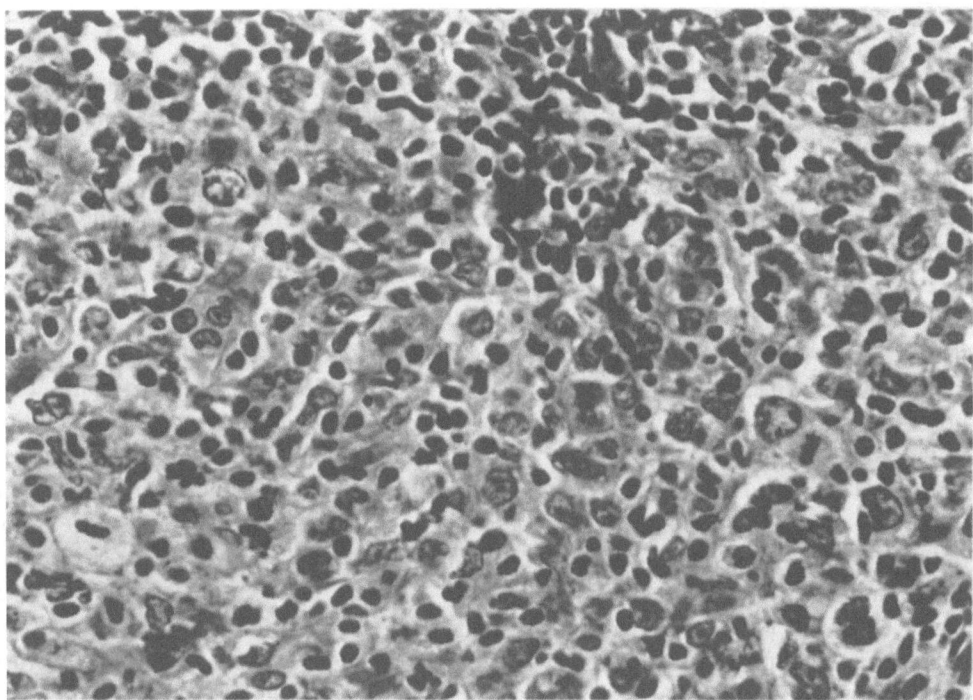

**Fig. 4.53.** Large cells with large and polymorphic nuclei outnumber lymphocytes in this area. Two cells are in mitosis, one at lower left corner, one in lower right quadrant near its upper edge. H & E, × 533

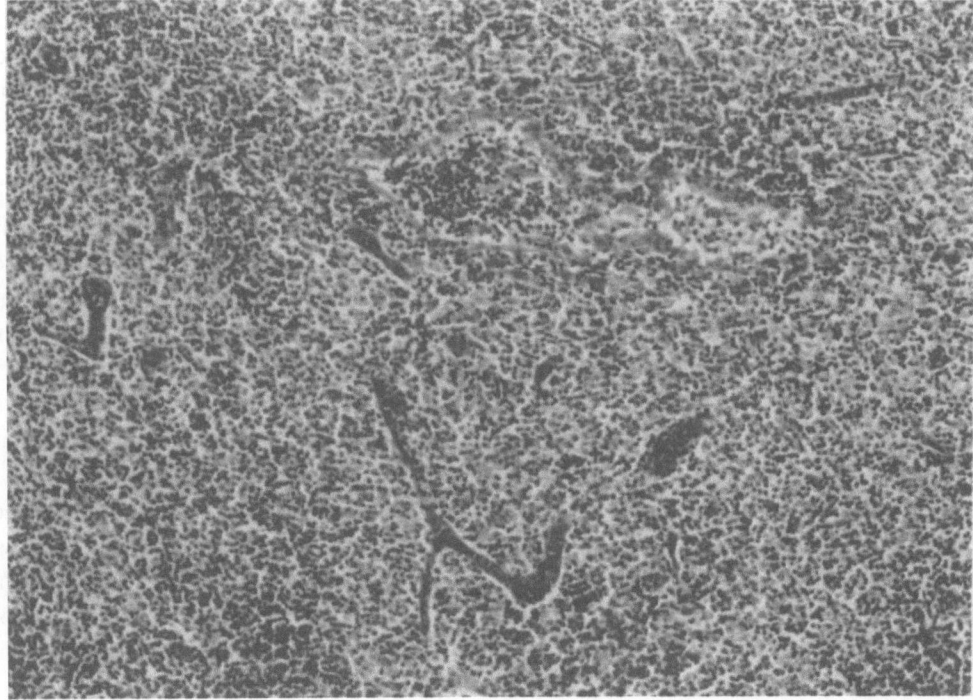

**Fig. 4.54.** Swelling of the endothelium has made prominent several vessels of capillary size, mostly in lower half of field, and also one, more probably a venous sinus, running transversely across the upper centre and to the right. H & E, × 136

The general follicular pattern was retained. The main abnormality was hyperplasia of the sinus reticulum cells, some unusually large. Scattered plasma cells and small accumulations of polymorphonuclears in some of the vessels helped to favour the diagnosis 'sinus reticulosis', possibly of infective origin rather than any neoplastic state.

Ten years passed until he was again referred to hospital with indigestion and loss of weight. Discovery of a duodenal ulcer led to gastro-jejunostomy; at the same time a $15 \times 10$ mm node was removed from the still-enlarged group in the groin.

The pattern was still substantially similar but there were now, in addition, many accumulations of large cells with prominent, rather dark nucleus and abundant eosinophilic, almost 'foamy' cytoplasm (Figs. 4.55 and 4.56); but for this foamy character they matched almost exactly the Hürthle cells of a thyroid. They were uniform and rarely, if ever, in mitosis (none was seen in several sections). The possibility of some thesaurosis such as Gaucher's disease was considered but no lipid could be demonstrated within the cells; also, no parasites or bacteria could be found. No firm diagnosis was offered.

A further 10 years passed, during which the patient had remained reasonably well; he was then examined for 'hoarseness'. The cause of this was uncertain but investigation revealed old tuberculous apical scarring; again an inguinal node biopsy was performed, and the appearances were again much as before. On this occasion, however, the features were thought to indicate 'reticulum cell medullary hyperplasia'.

The patient died 3 months later and there was no necropsy. We therefore do not know either the exact cause of death or the extent of the disease at that time. This, however, is of no great moment. The interest of the case lies in its demonstration of a lesion of lymph nodes of unusual histology that persisted for at least 20 years, and possibly for nearly 40. It may have been a variant of the entity described as 'sinus histiocytosis with massive lymphadenopathy' (SHML) by Rosai and Dorfman (1972).

This was given an *appropriate diagnosis* even if no more than essentially descriptive. The entity it probably is, SHML, had not then been identified, and there were no therapeutic implications.

*Case 4.30*

F (41 years) with a swelling at the angle of the jaw for 4 months. Excision showed it to consist of two nodes, 10 mm and 8 mm across.

The nodes were almost wholly replaced by strikingly large eosinophilic cells. Their nuclei also were large, not unduly polymorphic but frequently in mitosis, and often aberrantly so, but the cells owed their large size mainly to an abundance of cytoplasm. There seemed no doubt but that this was 'metastatic carcinoma with oncocytic features' but the question was raised originally whether the reticulum cells of a node could ever proliferate to this extent. That they can be large, abundant and eosinophilic is certain—they were so, for example, in the last case (4.29)—but proliferation to the extent present here seemed out of the question. Of possible primary sites for the lesion, salivary gland, thyroid, liver and nasopharynx seemed the likeliest but all investigations were negative.

To general surprise the patient remained well and required no medical attention for a further 4 years when she developed what was thought to be a sebaceous cyst on one temple. It was a carcinoma of the same eosinophilic type, some small lymphoid foci at the edge suggesting a one-time lymph node. Two months later she developed a 15-mm nodule above one eyebrow. This was again the same carcinoma, now invading the periorbital muscle, and systemic spread was the obvious expectation.

Nine years after this, that is, 13 years after the original biopsy, the patient is alive and well. As with the patient in Case 4.4, who had apparently unequivocal 'Hodgkin's sarcoma' and remains well, untreated, 9 years later, even if this eosinophilic carcinoma were to reappear and prove fatal, its behaviour will have been quite remarkable. The possibility of its being a melano-carcinoma (amelanotic) does exist. This is just acceptable histologically, while the behaviour, though still unusual, would be less unusual at any rate for a melanocarcinoma than for most other carcinomas. The possibility of its being a malignant form of lymph nodal sinus reticulosis or histiocytosis seems unlikely.

Despite the curious behaviour of the lesion, there is no reason to regard this as other than an *appropriate diagnosis*. The appearances may

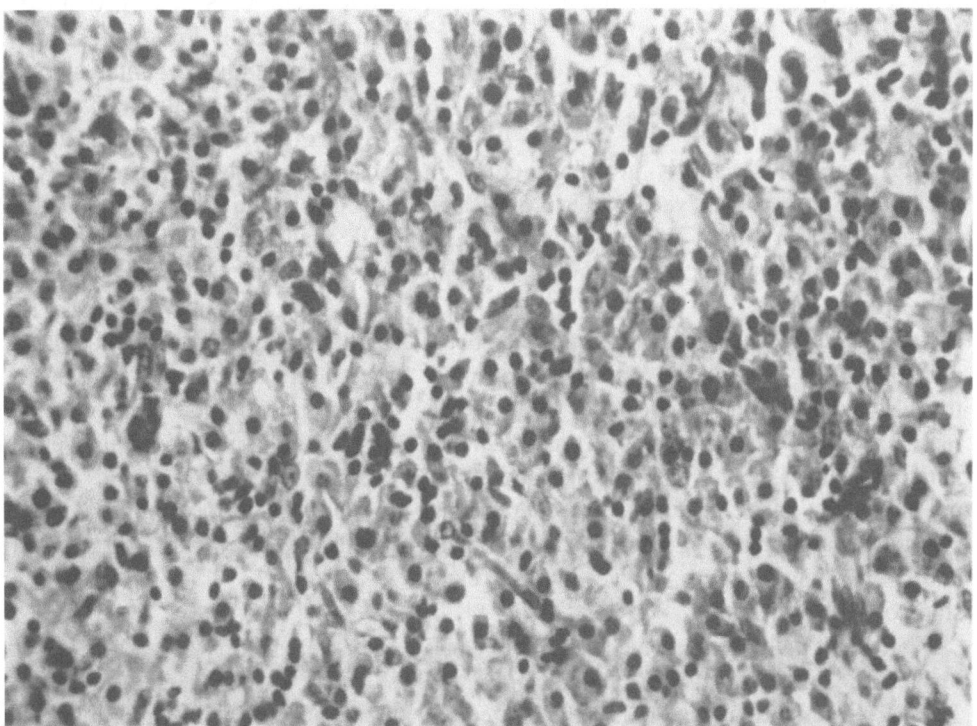

**Fig. 4.55.** Large pale and finely granular or foamy cells predominate. They were prominently eosinophilic and present in pulp as well as sinuses. H & E, × 272

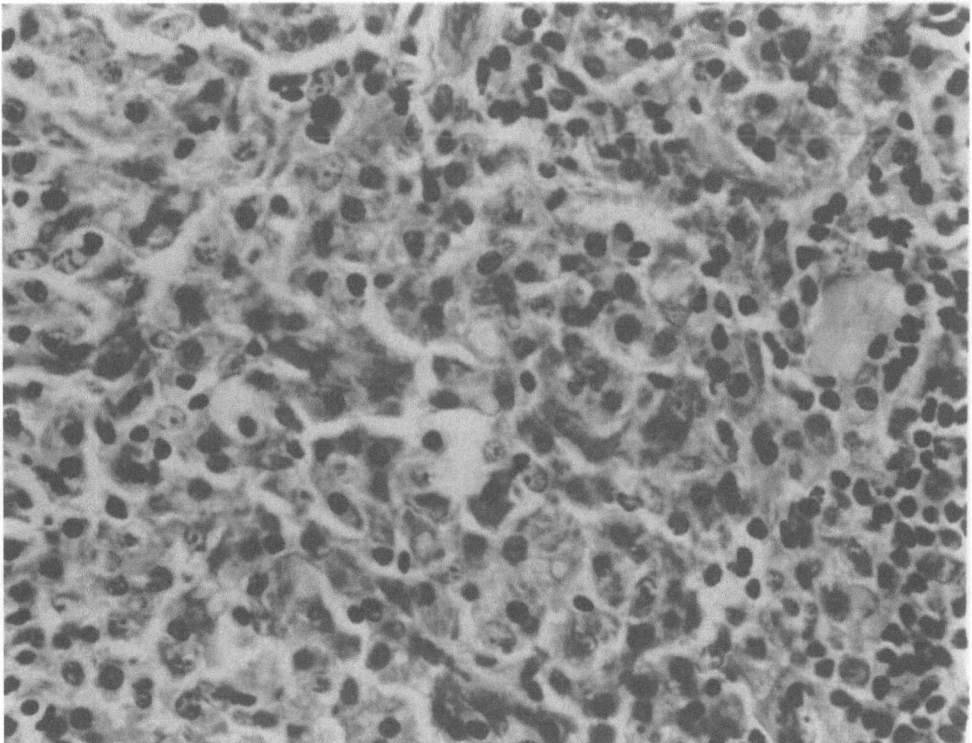

**Fig. 4.56.** The large size of the cells is owed to their volume of cytoplasm. The nuclei are generally uniform and little larger than the lymphocytes along the right edge. H & E, × 553

represent some entity as yet unfamiliar to all who have seen the sections.

### Case 4.31

F (29 years) with slowly growing nodule in neck, first noticed one year earlier: no lesion within mouth or throat to account for it. Exploration showed two nodes, 10 mm and 5 mm respectively.

Both nodes showed the same type of appearance, essentially an enlargement of germ centres to the degree that the 5-mm node, in a median section, was 70% occupied by three such expanded follicles. Their cells were moderately polymorphic and included quite numerous phagocytes and cells in mitosis. The appearances had been diagnosed as 'suggesting an early stage of Brill's disease'.

No further nodal enlargement developed, no further treatment was given, and all was well 16 years later. Almost certainly the node was 'reactive' but no reason for its hyperplasia emerged. Many, on recent review, again favoured 'reactive' as the explanation: the original opinion had thus probably been an appreciable *overdiagnosis* albeit one of no practical consequence.

### Case 4.32

M (14 years) with clinically acute appendicitis. Laparotomy showed a macroscopically normal appendix but also several large adjacent mesenteric nodes, i.e. 'mesenteric adenitis'.

Four nodes, the largest 12 × 10 × 8 mm, were received. Microscopically there was broad preservation of normal architecture with a generalised hyperplasia both at follicular level and at cellular level with a great increase in rather enlarged reticulum cells throughout. An occasional cell of this kind was notably larger than the rest and sometimes binucleate but none was morphologically acceptable as a R-S cell. Mitotic activity was widespread, the participating cells appearing to be almost all the paler reticulum-type cell rather than lymphocytes (maximum incidence in the most purely reticulum cell areas was two per hpf). This feature in particular had led to an expression of caution concerning prognosis although a strong preference was stated for a diagnosis of 'reaction to infection'. A suggestively epithelioid cast to some of the

large pale cells had prompted a search for tubercle bacilli but none had been found. Additional points of interest but uncertain significance are: (a) that capsular lymphatics contained quite numerous abnormally large cells of no diagnostic appearance. They were sometimes in mitosis and seemed likelier to be endothelial cells than transforming or transformed lymphocytes (cells exactly similar in site and appearance were seen in Case 4.39 [*see* Fig. 4.63], also, perhaps only by coincidence, in an inflammatory mesenteric node); (*b*) that the lymphoid tissue in the appendix itself was normal and seemingly wholly indifferent to whatever was stimulating the adjacent nodes.

The patient made a full recovery and was well at least 10 years later. An *appropriate* diagnosis.

### Case 4.33

F (50 years) with carcinoma of upper rectum. At resection, a mass of uncertain type was found in the concavity of the sacrum.

The mass was almost spherical and 4 cm in diameter. Microscopy showed it to be a single lymph node, and thus a relatively huge node. However, normal architecture was preserved to the extent that it contained abundant follicles, almost all with normal germ centres, of widely varying size. Throughout the whole of many sections there was no more to arrest attention than a very occasional pale reticulum cell larger than the others. Besides this, a few germ centres showed focal necrosis, and small clusters of plasma cells were common. All the evidence, positive and negative, identified this as a 'reactive lymph node'. Its very size, however, had caused much concern.

The patient died 23 months later with abdominal and hepatic carcinomatosis (source not identifiable at attempted palliative laparotomy 2 months before death) with no evidence of lymph nodal disease in superficial nodes.

It seems likely, therefore, that, despite its size, this was no more than a 'reactive node', instructive in showing just how large a node may be and yet not be neoplastic. I can recall a group of three nodes of similar size (also, as it happens, from the concavity of the sacrum) found in the course of a pan-hysterectomy where the surgeon could be convinced only with the greatest difficulty that they were not the seat of carcinoma metastatic from the cervix.

This was a correct and *appropriate diagnosis*: only the exceptional size of the node had caused suspicion.

### Case 4.34

M (50 years) with ischaemic (exertional) pain in left lower limb over a period of 6 weeks, pain and swelling of the limb for 4 days, and pain in the buttock for 3 days. There was obvious venous obstruction in the limb and a palpable mass in the LIF. Investigations showed obstruction of the iliac vessels and also ureter. Lymph nodes, none larger than 10 mm, were palpable in axillae and groins but the blood picture was normal. Two inguinal nodes were removed.

The follicular pattern was generally well preserved but what appeared to be greatly enlarged germ centres were in fact collections of loosely arranged, relatively large cells with abundant eosinophilic cytoplasm. They appeared similar to those, also hyperplastic, lining the sinuses and, thus, presumably reticulum cells; many contained a fine dusting of haemosiderin. Polymorphonuclears were few and mitoses scanty, and there were no giant cells. The appearances were regarded as disquieting but 'not neoplastic'. However, perhaps with the obstructing mass in the adjacent iliac fossa in mind, the opinion was given that the nodes might be 'draining a malignant neoplasm'.

This merest hint that a neoplasm might be somehow concerned was acted upon clinically with vigour to the extent that when, 1 week later, the Hb level fell rather suddenly to 50%, the pelvic mass was irradiated. Femoral nerve paralysis developed and 7 days later the patient suddenly collapsed and died. Necropsy revealed extensive retroperitoneal haemorrhage from a large ruptured aneurysm of the common iliac artery.

There was mild enlargement of nodes in the axillae and mediastinum; none was larger than 15 mm, and all showed prominent sinus reticulosis with almost complete absence of germ centres. In showing reticulum cell replacement of its germ centres, the originally biopsied node was atypical but the pattern may have owed something to its draining the aneurysm and containing so much iron. The spleen showed widespread reticulum cell hyperplasia but, rather unexpectedly, almost total atrophy of the lymphoid component.

On final review, the general conclusion was that the fairly generalised lymphadenopathy was probably a 'reaction to infection' of some kind. The patient was a farmer and toxoplasmosis seemed a possibility but only in retrospect. It is highly dubious whether the nodes carried any neoplastic threat, and, certainly, whatever lesion they may have been reflecting contributed nothing to the patient's death.

Even though the cause of the 'reactive' state remains unknown, and always will, this was an *appropriate diagnosis*. It is easy to say now that greater emphasis should have been laid on the need to explore the lower abdominal mass, and that no hint should have been given that the node might be 'draining' the area of a neoplasm; but that is hindsight. This was an unfortunately coincidental conspiracy of circumstances; it was also unfortunate that the pathologist knew in advance that the patient had a pelvic mass.

### Case 4.35

M (17 years) with swelling in side of neck for 10 weeks. General health good: blood picture normal. Two 10-mm nodes removed.

The general pattern was one of overall preservation of normal architecture with, however, some abnormality of the germ centres. These were unusually large and appeared often to be overflowing into or invading the adjacent parenchyma (Fig. 4.57). Also, their population of cells was unusually uniform; it consisted of sheets of cells slightly larger and paler staining than lymphocytes and was almost completely devoid of macrophages (Fig. 4.58).

This unusual uniformity and the permeation of the stroma by cells from the seemingly bursting germ centres had caused concern but the general retention of architecture was regarded as prognostically the most important feature. The final diagnosis was 'nonspecific reactive'.

All further investigations were negative, no further lymphadenopathy developed and the patient was well 16 years later. As in Case 4.31, no reason for the node's florid reaction ever emerged. This was an *appropriate diagnosis* on appearances still, on review, equivocal.

*Case 4.36*

M (82 years) with unilateral post-auricular and submandibular swellings. A 10-mm post-auricular node was removed.

There was some loss of pattern in that most of the follicles lacked germ centres, appeared to be 'melting' into surrounding parenchyma, and had produced many relatively large sheet-like areas. The cells retained the appearance of mature lymphocytes but were occasionally in mitosis. Firm decision whether the lesion was 'reactive' or 'early lymphosarcoma' was considered not possible. The blood picture was normal.

The patient died 18 months later from cardiac failure, and there was no necropsy. The nodes had remained virtually unchanged during this time, and further biopsy had seemed unnecessary. There is thus no way of knowing whether or not this was an early lymphosarcoma. In retrospect, the almost complete absence of sinus histiocytosis suggests a neoplastic rather than a reactive change.

An *appropriate diagnosis* on still equivocal evidence.

*Case 4.37*

M (16 years) with febrile illness, shadow at one apex, possibly a glandular mass in the mediastinum, and with enlarged left axillary and supraclavicular nodes of which one from each site was removed.

There was a widespread disappearance of follicles and replacement by sheets or clusters of pale eosinophilic cells with more cytoplasm and larger paler nuclei than the lymphocytes; they showed no significant polymorphism and were rarely in mitosis. Individually, they were quite comparable to the cells of a sinus histiocytosis but in one of the nodes certainly, and more so than in the other, the distribution of the cells was much more diffuse than in the 'usual' sinus histiocytosis. In view of the later-discovered aetiology, it is surprising that so few of the follicles that remained possessed a germ centre.

The changes were considered most probably

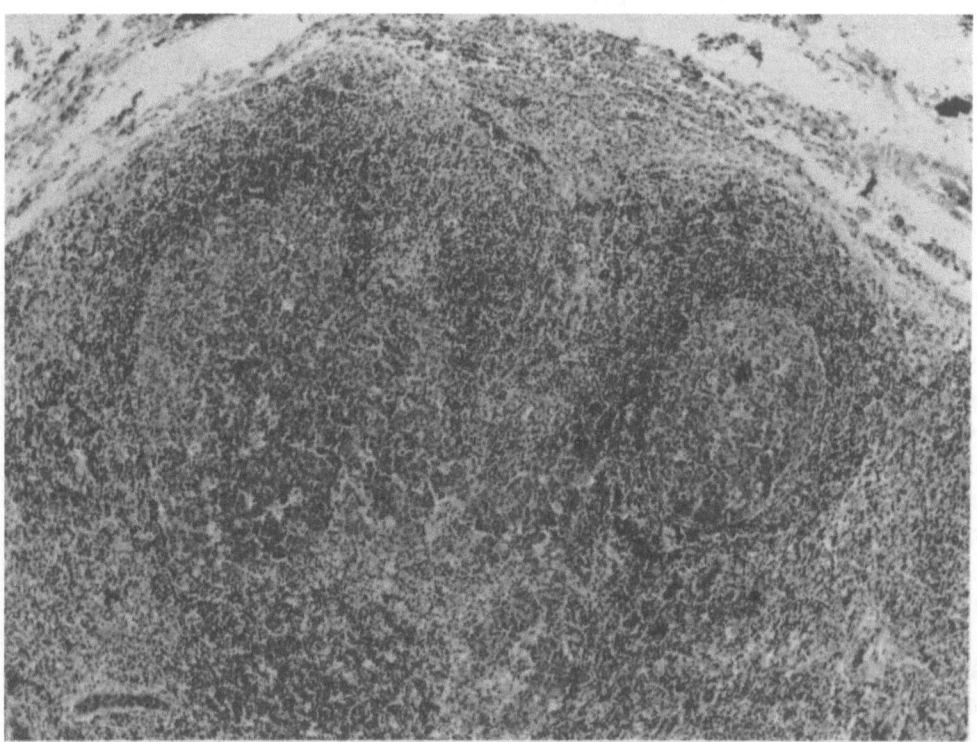

**Fig. 4.57.** The germinal centre at right is well circumscribed and normal. The lower margin of the much larger centre at left is poorly demarcated, the cells appearing to flow into the adjacent pulp. H & E, × 85

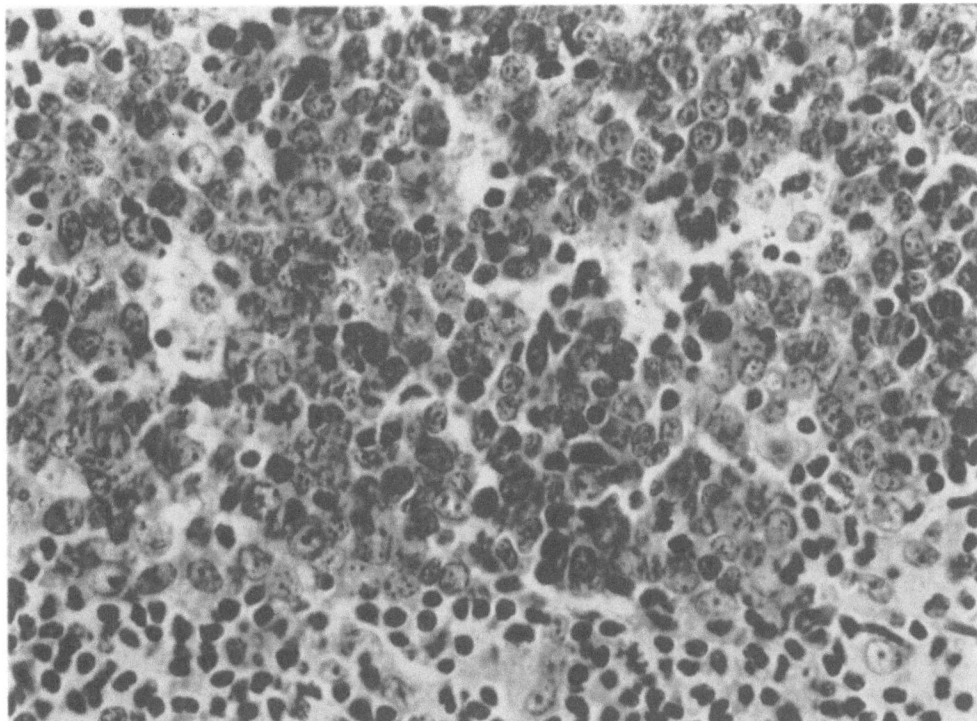

**Fig. 4.58.** The ill-defined edge of a germinal centre of which the constituent cells appear unduly large. H & E, × 553

'reactive' but an 'early malignant lymphoma' had been considered possible.

Uncertainty did not last long. Clinically, the signs and symptoms so strongly suggested pulmonary tuberculosis that chemotherapy had been started almost at once, and in advance of the lymph node biopsy. A further biopsy, this time of the affected area of lung, showed typically tuberculous features with many demonstrable AFB. These were clearly 'reactive' nodes (the patient was well 15 years later).

In so far as the possibility of a malignant lymphoma was raised at all, this was a marginal *over-diagnosis*, but, in so far as the histology still appears equivocal, it was an *appropriate diagnosis*.

*Case 4.38*

F (36 years) complained of a painful lump in the chest wall. A 10-mm nodule was excised.

Scarcely any trace of follicular pattern remained. Its place was taken by sheets of lymphocytes and moderately large pale reticulum cells in a proportion that varied according to area from about 10:1 to 2:1. The morphology of the cells is shown in Figs. 4.59, 4.60 which show also that the reticulum cells were frequently in mitosis, up to four per hpf in some places. Eosinophil polymorphonuclears were scanty and there were no multinucleated giant cells.

The blood picture was normal and uncertainty remained whether the abnormalities indicated a 'reactive or a neoplastic change'.

By the time the patient returned for routine examination and removal of sutures she had a well-developed typical eruption of herpes zoster within 10 cm of the normally healing incision. There was no further trouble and the patient was well 8 years later. With little doubt this was a 'reactive' node, reacting to the herpes virus.

This case was instructive in illustrating the extent to which normal architecture may be obliterated, and reticulum cells become enlarged, hyperplastic and mitotically active, yet not indicate malignancy. As in Case 4.37, where circumstances were so similar, the reported possibility of malignant lymphoma was something of an over-diagnosis. Even in retrospect, however, the histology still seems equivocal. To that ex-

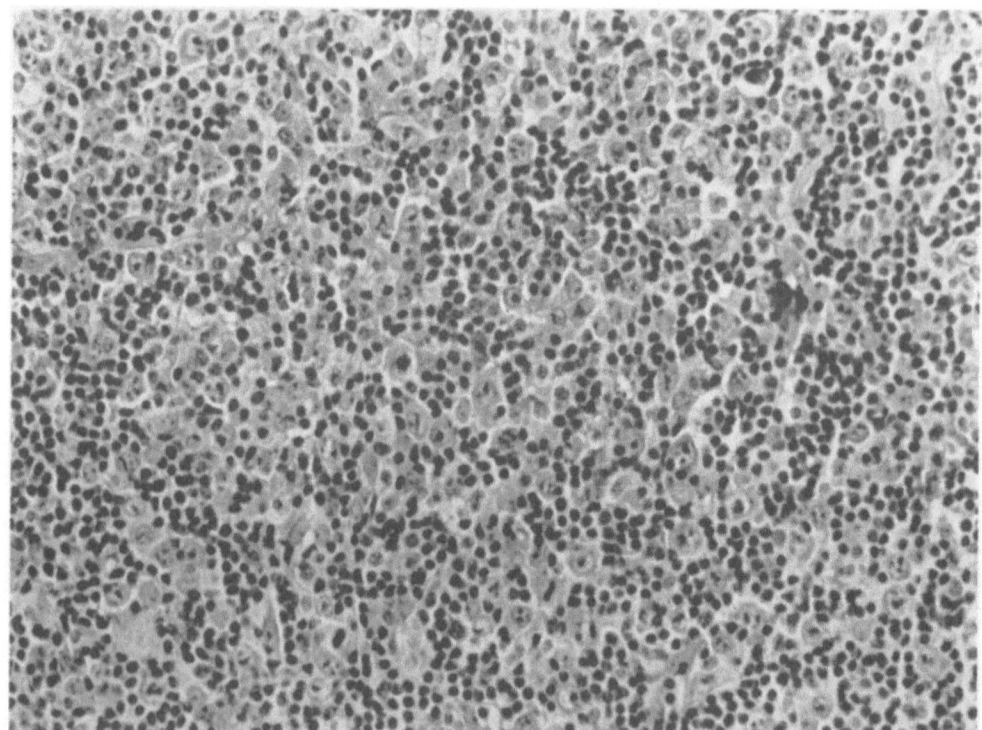

**Fig. 4.59.** A field representative of the whole node. Pale reticulum cells predominate. H & E, × 340

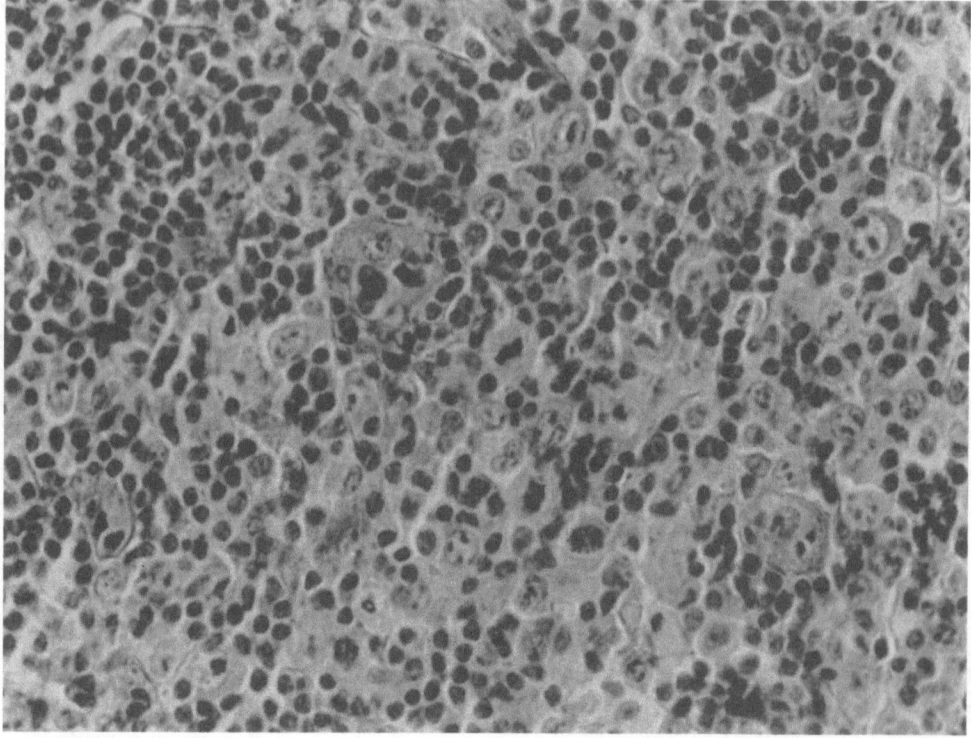

**Fig. 4.60.** The background cells are not only large with correspondingly large nuclei, but polymorphic and frequently in mitosis. There are four mitotic figures in the centre of the field, and many cells with prominent nucleoli. H & E, × 553

tent, the caution conveyed by the report was warranted and the ambivalent report itself *appropriate*.

### Case 4.39

M (44 years) with diarrhoea and pain with tenderness in RIF. The caecum and terminal ileum were thickened 'with skip areas', and the condition was believed to be Crohn's disease. The appendix and an adjacent 8-mm brownish mesenteric node were removed.

The node showed a broadly normal follicular architecture though germ centres were few (Fig. 4.61). The main and disquieting abnormality was the presence throughout the node of clusters or sheets of large pale cells, frequently in mitosis (up to four per hpf) and sometimes partly replacing the otherwise purely lymphocytic follicles (Fig. 4.62). As shown in Figs. 4.63 and 4.64, cells of possibly the same type were present also in capsular lymphatic channels. Similarly, they were partly replacing follicles in the otherwise normal appendix. No firm decision was considered possible whether the changes were 'reactive' or 'lymphomatous'.

All further investigations were negative, and, despite the high probability of his having Crohn's disease, the patient was known to be well 6 years later. Thereafter, he left the area and attempts to trace him have failed; no enquiries have been received on his behalf since then.

It is possible that the abnormality in the lymphatic tissue of both node and appendix was innocuous and no more than a reaction to the lesion, whatever its nature, in caecum and terminal ileum. It was, even so, a remarkably florid reaction, as closely simulating malignancy as the tissue in the preceding case (4.38) and equally demonstrating the degree of aberrancy that innocuously reactive cells may have to be allowed.

Even though indecisive, the diagnosis was *appropriate* to the extent that, in retrospect, the histology still seems equivocal. The likelihood that the lesion was a multifocal malignant lymphoma is probably slight.

### Case 4.40

M (22 years) with painless swelling in right submandibular region for 3 months. Exploration

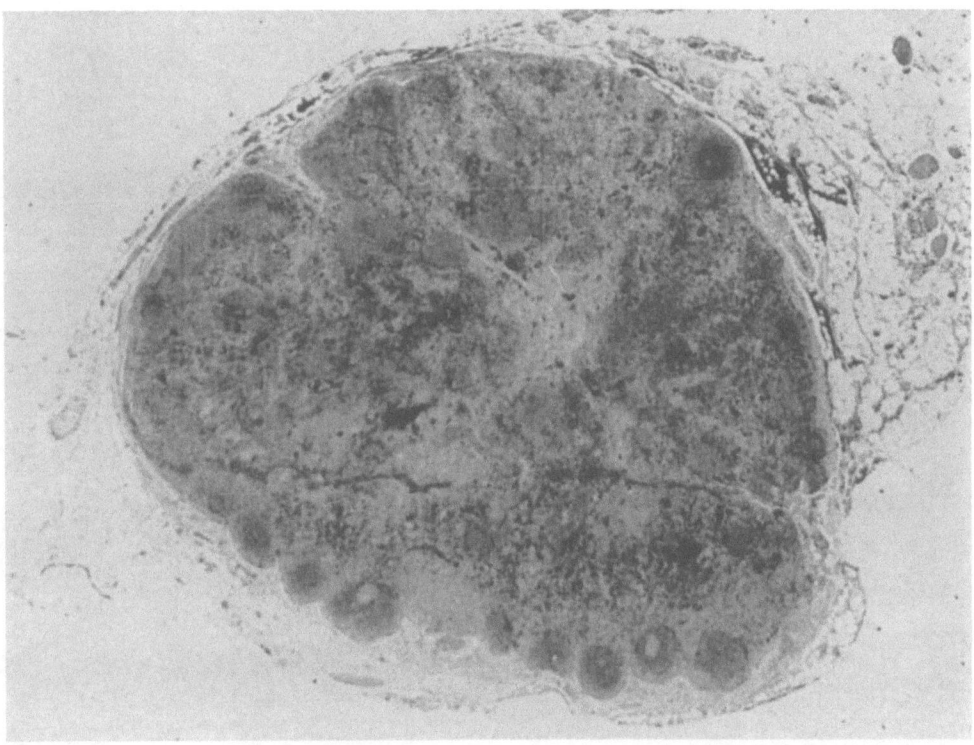

**Fig. 4.61.** The architecture is largely disrupted though a substantially follicular pattern is evident. There is appreciable fibrosis. H & E, × 17

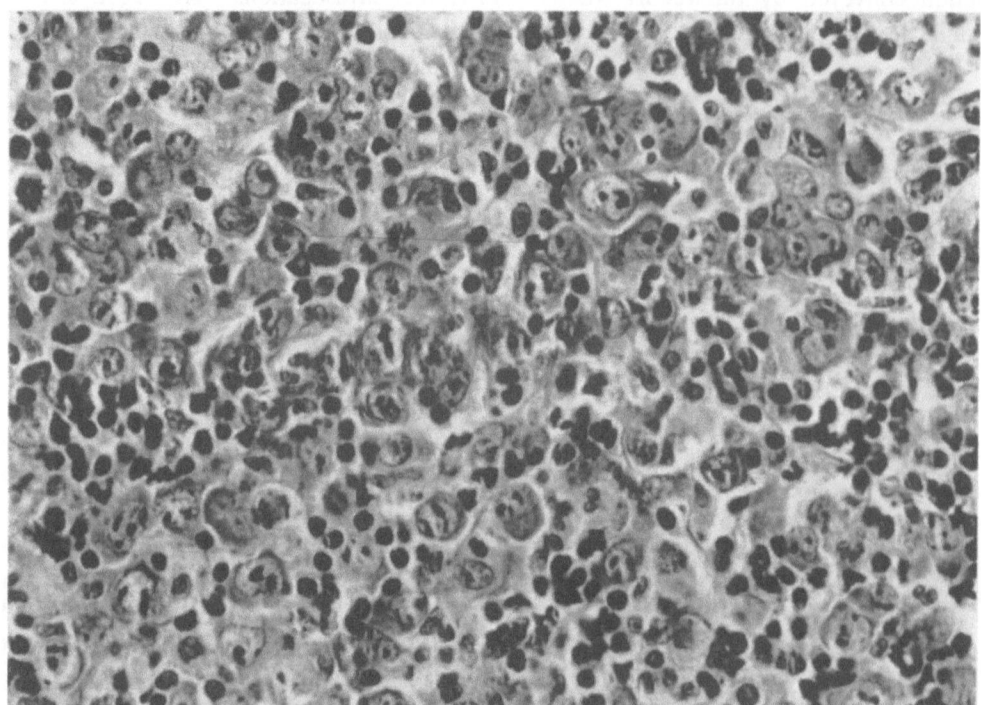

**Fig. 4.62.** There were many clusters of large polymorphic cells of this type: the nucleoli are frequently of irregular shape. The field contains four mitotic figures (a diaster lies near upper right corner, a metaphase plate near right edge of upper left quadrant) and is quite representative of the mitotic frequency in the polymorphic clusters. H & E, × 533

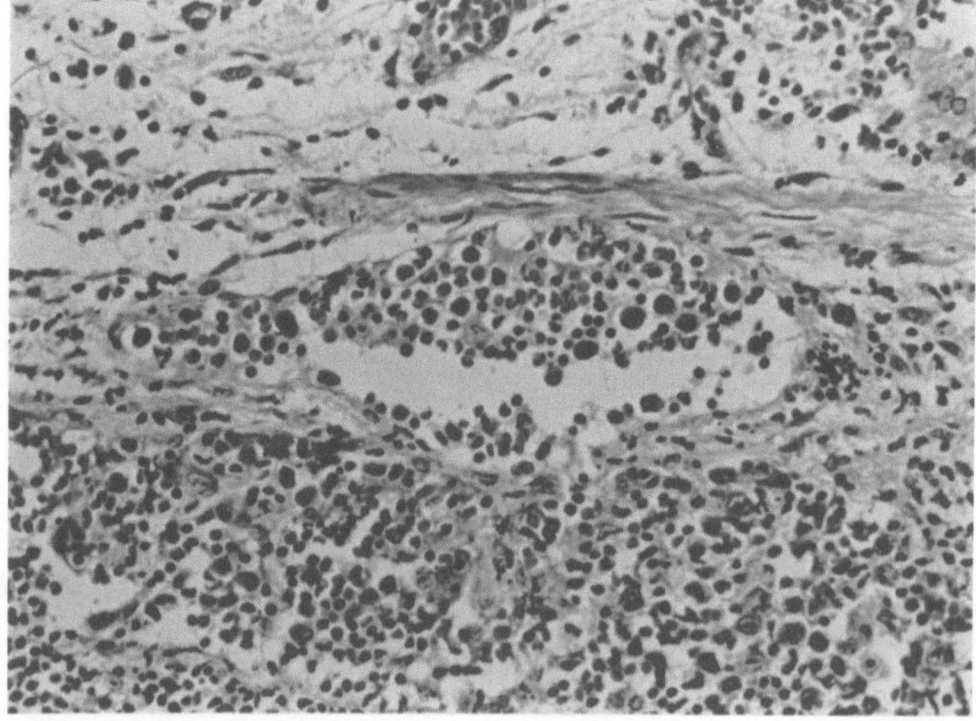

**Fig. 4.63.** An afferent lymphatic perforating the capsule contains mononuclear cells of widely varying size. H & E, × 340

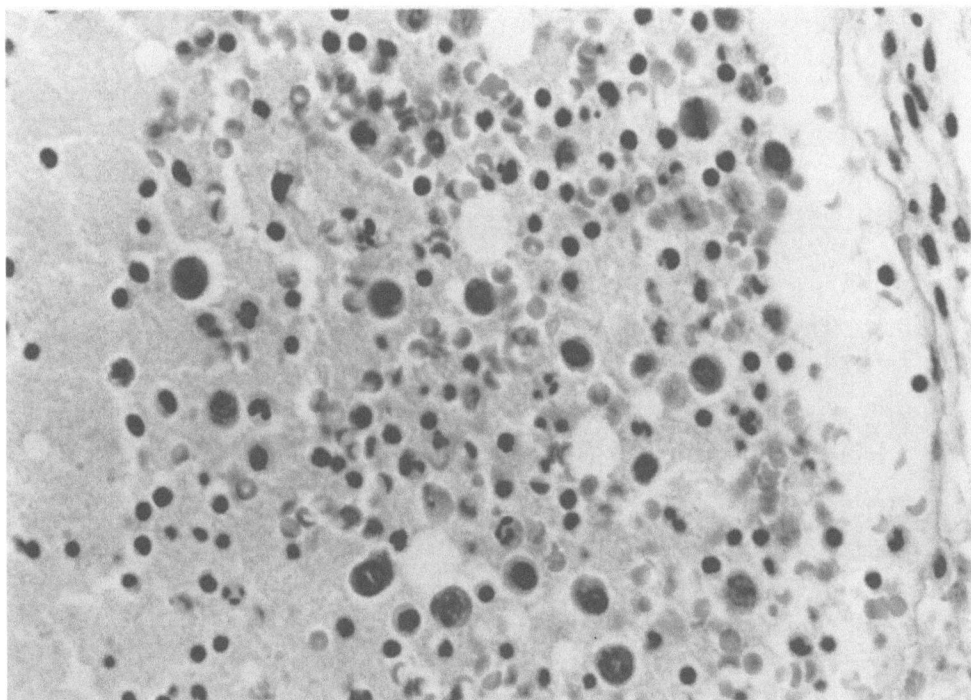

**Fig. 4.64.** A representative field of cells from within the lymphatic. They are unlike histiocytes and have a more plasmacytoid (or plasmablastoid) appearance: as seen at upper right corner, they were occasionally in mitosis. These cells, in some way transformed, may have comprised the abnormal population shown in Fig. 4.62. H & E, × 533

revealed a single relatively large node (20 × 15 × 10 mm).

Sections showed disturbance rather than loss of architecture. There was an abundance of follicles from 0.2 to 2.0 mm across. Most had normally formed germ centres yet the largest had none; the smallest consisted of little else (Fig. 4.65). Polymorphonuclears were rare and of neutrophil type. The follicles lacking a germ centre all contained a few scattered large pale reticulum cells of which some had a disquietingly large and sometimes lobular nucleus with prominent nucleolus (Fig. 4.66); occasionally others were in mitosis. In one area there was a 1-mm subcapsular linear granuloma with distinctive epithelioid cells and Langhans-type giant cells.

No micro-organisms were demonstrated, and the appearances were regarded and reported as not certainly diagnostic as between an 'inflammatory response or a lymphoma'. The recommended further investigations showed a normal blood picture and no serological abnormalities.

Re-examination after 3 months, as also recommended, revealed enlarged nodes in both axillae but not elsewhere. One of these showed follicular hyperplasia quite similar to the original, though with fewer of the follicles lacking germ centres and many fewer containing large pale reticulum cells. Again, the appearances were held to be nondiagnostic.

After a further 6 months the axillary nodes were still large but essentially ISQ; there were, again, enlarged nodes in the neck. Biopsy of both sites produced three nodes of which the largest (18 mm long, from the neck) now showed areas of loss of pattern caused by the mergence or melting of follicles with the production of larger solid sheets than had been seen hitherto. Although the cells were on the whole uniform, now almost all lymphocytes with scarcely any of the once-prominent aberrant reticulum cells, it was believed that the alteration had then to be taken to indicate transformation to 'lymphosarcoma'.

The patient was treated by radiotherapy, has been seen regularly, and remains well 10 years after the original biopsy.

Some doubt still remains whether this might

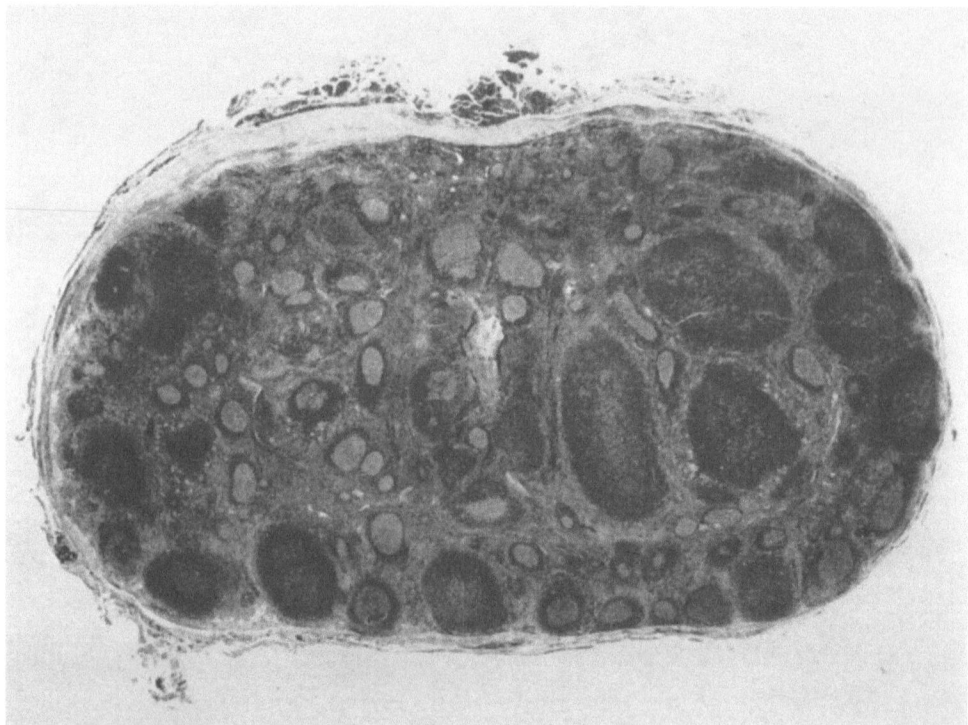

**Fig. 4.65.** An abundantly follicular pattern with follicles of widely varying size. Follicles with germinal centres are easily distinguishable. H & E, × 10

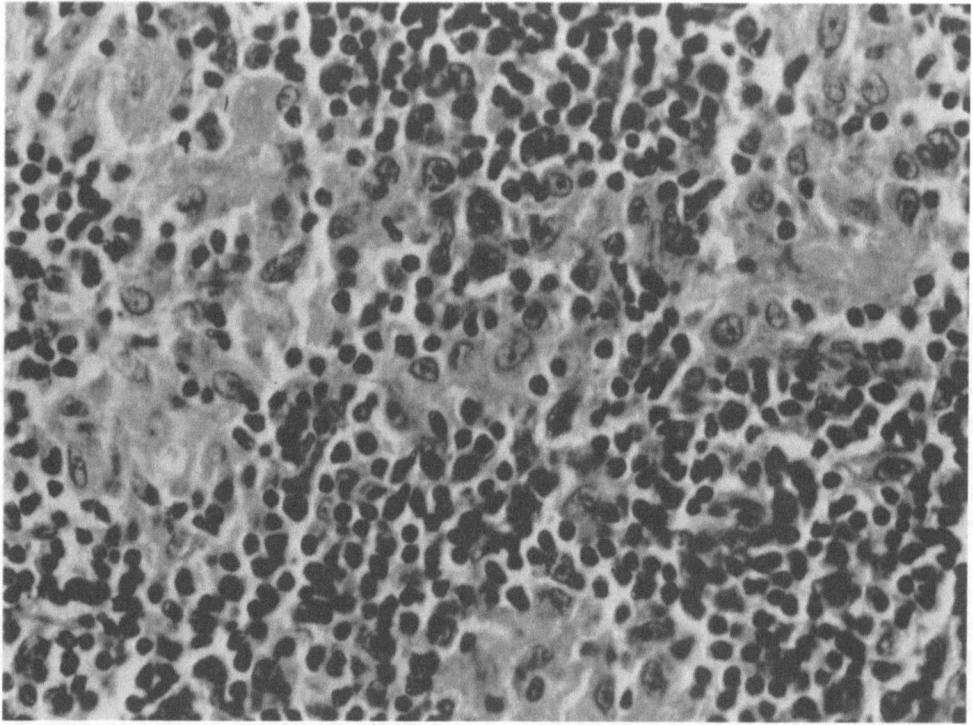

**Fig. 4.66.** The more solidly cellular areas contained clusters of pale cells with nuclei much larger than lymphocytes and mostly containing conspicuous nucleoli. They were not epithelioid cells. H & E, × 533

not have been an essentially reactive response to some undetected inflammatory/infective agent rather than truly a lymphosarcoma. An intriguing and possibly not unrelated factor is that 7 months after the initial biopsy the patient's father developed cervical gland enlargement that was histologically typical HD. He also was treated by radiotherapy and also remains well almost 10 years later.

It still seems proper to regard the original equivocal report as *appropriate*, especially since, even 3 years later, the histology in a further node was still less than certainly diagnostic. Again, bearing in mind the events in Case 4.26, the 10-year trouble-free survival may not yet be a sufficient guarantee of cure. In Case 4.8, it may be recalled, a father and son both developed and died from HD. A familial incidence such as this is not common but is well enough recognised. A possible lesson to be learned from these two examples is that, if one member of a family has an undoubtedly malignant lymphoma, equivocal histology in the node of another should also be regarded as those of a malignant lymphoma until proved otherwise.

The summarised data of the patients with ? non-H malignant lymphoma are shown in Table 4.3.

## COMMENTARY ON LOCAL SERIES

An attempt has been made with the 40 borderline cases as a whole to compare histological findings with the outcome, whether death or survival, in a search for prognostically useful correlations. To try to make the distinction as clear as possible, 'deaths' are cases where the patient did die of a ML; 'survivals' are cases where the patient received no specific treatment, in essence irradiation. The one case each of postoperative death, gastric plasmacytoma, leukaemic infiltration of skin, metastatic carcinoma and HSC disease have been omitted, as have the six cases of survival, possibly 'cures', where irradiation had been used. Patients dead of an unrelated cause have, however, been included with the 'survivals'. The numbers thus became, deaths 14, survivals 15.

Each case was then scored —, ±, + or ++ in respect of:

a) Preservation or loss of follicular architecture;

b) Preservation or loss of germ centres;

c) Presence and degree of sinus histiocytosis (SH);

d) Character of 'reticulum' cells:
   i) Degree of proliferation,
   ii) Nuclear pleomorphism,
   iii) Mitotic activity.

With numbers so small, the value of the analysis is limited but some possibly useful points did emerge:

1) There was total loss of follicular architecture in 6 of the 14 fatal cases but also in 5 of the 15 non-fatal cases.

2) Germ centres had been retained in only one of the fatal cases but in nine of the others (including two where the size of the centres varied widely).

3) Significant SH was present in none of the ML cases but present in six of the others (including two wherein the peripheral sinus did not participate).

4) Abnormal reticulum cell proliferation was present in all of the ML cases but also in all of the 15 others (almost by definition since this was a main reason for their being borderline lesions).

5) Nuclear pleomorphism and mitotic activity were equally prominent in both groups.

In all, therefore, the main conclusions on morphology are that, with borderline nodes, total or substantial loss of follicular architecture is of little prognostic help; that total loss of germ centres favours a neoplastic rather than an inflammatory reaction; that SH favours the reverse, an inflammatory rather than a neoplastic aetiology; and that a prominent degree of reticulum cell proliferation, pleomorphism and mitotic activity may be seen equally in neoplastic and in manifestly non-neoplastic lesions (e.g. the examples of herpes zoster and mesenteric adenitis).

As was shown in Table 4.1, there has been an almost equal tendency towards under-diagnosis and over-diagnosis, but, in detail, more particularly a tendency towards the under-diagnosis of HD. Lesions eventually proved to be MLs, HD in four of the eight, were initially diagnosed either only tentatively as malignant or as possibly not malignant. Review, in ignorance of the clinical outcome, suggests that greater emphasis should have been laid on the likelihood of malignancy at the outset, in at any rate these eight patients. Nevertheless, despite the histological hesitation, the mere expression of doubt in conjunction with the clinical findings had led to the use of appropriate or specific treatment in five of the patients. This illustrates a general point. Table 4.2 shows that, of the 22 '? HD' borderline patients, 11 received specific treatment. By contrast, of the 18 '? other lymphoma' patients (see Table 4.3), only five had received specific treatment. This difference suggests that, when histological doubt is expressed, the clinical factors as a whole determine the choice whether or not irradiation (and, nowadays, probably chemotherapy) is used. This assessment of evidence seems entirely right, and was on the whole in this series fully justified.

The tendency towards under-diagnosis may well have been real, even if unwitting, and there is a possible explanation. Whenever there is histological doubt, especially in the context of the malignant lymphomas, there is inevitably a reluctance to pronounce what is in effect a sentence of death even if treatment of the lymphomas probably is more effective nowadays than was the case a few years ago. The tendency to 'cling to hope' still widely prevails: the hope, that the lesion is really not a lymphoma, is expressed by the pathologist in his suggesting that a nonmalignant lesion is at least a possibility. This is not the only major factor. The very means whereby this better outcome is energetically sought, namely the diagnostic ordeal, may itself induce reluctance in the mind of the pathologist, consciously or unconsciously. The procedures now performed on a patient diagnosed as having HD (Kim and Dorfman, 1974), and possibly any other form of ML, are likely to include splenectomy and wedge or needle biopsies of liver; biopsies of bone marrow either by needle or removal of part of the iliac crest; biopsies of para-aortic, mesenteric and splenic hilar nodes; and lymphangiography as well as the later hazards of specific therapy, be it radiotherapy, chemotherapy or both. It is not surprising that the pathologist, aware of his fallibility and aware also of the totally different clinical implications of a marginal decision one way or the other way, tends to lean towards the lesser diagnosis. As mentioned in Chapter 1, perhaps this attitude is wrong; perhaps the pathologist should be totally uninfluenced by what he knows will be the clinical consequences of his diagnosis; perhaps so, but not all pathologists would agree.

## General Commentary

> The proportion of erroneous histologic diagnosis in cases diagnosed as Hodgkin's disease is higher than in almost any other neoplastic disease, varying from 15 to 47% in different series. (Franssila et al., 1977)

> Hodgkin himself was hardly silent before others began explaining what he really meant. The process has continued . . . (MacMahon, 1966)

Together, these quotations say much. All Hodgkin could have meant, without microscopy, was a particular kind of clinicopathological syndrome or entity. To what extent the entity as defined microscopically for the past many decades will be further reduced and refined by the recognition and removal of such lesions as immunoblastic lymphadenopathy (Lukes and Tindle, 1975) and the so-called Lennert lymphoma (Lennert et al., 1975; Editorial, 1976) remains to be seen, but without doubt, as diagnostic techniques evolve, debate on diagnosis and classification will extend. The same applies to the 'non-Hodgkin lymphomas'. Indeed, the position and prospect here are even more nebulous since HD possesses one feature, the Reed-Sternberg (R-S) cell, which, even if no longer as surely definable and diagnostic as once was believed, can at least be found or not found. There is no such marker for the non-Hodgkin type of lesion.[1]

### HODGKIN'S DISEASE

#### Reed-Sternberg Cell

The R-S cell is central to all the debate that surrounds HD. Tissues from a patient who has died from unquestionable HD will show lesions

---

[1] Hodgkin's disease is the last of the great eponyms, and no doubt it will stay until an aetiological agent is found. Its greatness is seen in its use in the negative sense, in defining the 'non-Hodgkin' lymphomas: distinction of this kind for a name is possibly unique (and scarcely diminished by Symmers's [1978] dismissal of the term as 'jargonic'!)

abounding in large aberrant cells of varied morphology, all acceptable as R-S cells. Matters are very different where a sprinkling of such cells, in a background of other aberrant cells—whether or not regarded as histiocytes, immunoblasts or reticulum cells—may be the only abnormality in a biopsied lymph node, for on the interpretation of these will depend whether the patient is diagnosed as having HD, with all that that entails, or not. For long the presence of this cell has been held to be a sine qua non for the diagnosis of HD, and this still seems a sound working principle. At the same time, even if it be true that 'all that is HD has R-S cells', the converse proposition that 'all that has R-S cells is HD' is certainly not true. Cells apparently indistinguishable morphologically from R-S cells have been seen in many lesions, including the angiomatous lymphoid hamartoma (Fisher et al., 1970), postvaccinial lymphadenopathy and, more importantly, infectious mononucleosis (Salvador et al., 1971; Tindle et al., 1972). Even without such cells, infectious mononucleosis is notorious as a producer of ambiguous histology, and appropriate serology is mandatory when this is so. Aids to the distinction between R-S cells and the pleomorphic 'immunoblasts' commonly characterising the nodal reaction to both infectious mononucleosis and toxoplasmosis are given in the especially helpful paper by Dorfman and Warnke (1974).

In view of the growing doubt about the specificity of the R-S cell, a systematic search for identical or closely similar cells was made by Strum and his colleagues (1970) in a wide variety of lesions, and the yield was great. Such cells were seen not only in infectious mononucleosis but also in rubeola, benign and malignant lesions of epithelial, stromal and lymphatic origin, including non-Hodgkin lymphomas (a substantial problem, to be sure), mycosis fungoides and myelomatosis; malignant fibroxanthoma and proliferative myositis; carcinomas of breast and lung, melanocarcinoma and a lymphocytic thymoma associated with myasthenia gravis. This is not to imply, of course, that the finding of such cells, which would then have to be designated pseudo-R-S cells, in, say, an otherwise straightforward carcinoma of breast or myelomatous focus, introduces HD as a serious diagnostic contender: it does, however,

diminish the diagnostic significance of structures that may often enough in the past have been accepted as R-S cells. Many guides to the recognition of the R-S cell have been offered (see, for example, Lukes et al., 1966; Franssila et al., 1967; Peckham and Cooper, 1969; Strum et al., 1970; Lukes, 1971; Taylor, 1974; and Azar, 1975) and their number emphasises how real the difficulty is. In his particularly well-illustrated contribution, Lukes (1971) concludes that a truly diagnostic R-S cell does exist, and that it may take one of three forms: (a) the so-called 'lacunar' cell that characterises nodular sclerosing HD, (b) the polyploid type as seen in the lymphocyte-predominant forms of HD, and (c) the pleomorphic variant found in the lymphocyte-depleted forms with sarcomatous morphology. An informative illustration in this paper, incidentally, shows how 'non-lacunar' the lacunar cell may be when fixed in Zenker's solution. According to the detailed studies of Anagnostou and his colleagues (1977), the lacunar cell and the R-S cell are the two possible end-products of a developmental sequence, namely, lymphocyte → transformed lymphocyte (immunoblast) → mononuclear 'Hodgkin' cell.

Increasingly, the R-S cell is being studied by newer techniques, as for example, the wide range of immunohistochemical procedures described by Curran and Jones (1978). Therefore, as the many pseudo-R-S cells are similarly investigated, we may expect to learn with diagnostic benefit whether they are simply morphological mimics or, indeed, in all discoverable respects identical. Until this happens, the true nature of the cell will remain debatable, whether an abnormal reticulum cell, a polyploid immunoblast (transformed lymphocyte whether of B or T type) or an abnormal histiocyte. In the opinion of Taylor (1974) and Azar (1975) the cell is a transformed lymphocyte, Azar adding that there seems to be ". . . no valid histochemical or ultrastructural evidence that it is a histiocyte". In the opinion of Curran and Jones (1978), on the other hand, the cell is probably ". . . a dendritic histiocyte of the type normally found in the lymphoid follicles". As with the cell ancestral to tumours of bone, search further back than this takes us within sight of cells emerging from the embryonic mesenchyme and shortly thereafter the zygote itself.

*Clinical Outcome*

The crucial test of histological accuracy in neoplastic pathology is the clinical outcome. If a patient is free of disease many years after the unequivocal diagnosis and treatment of a commonly malignant lesion, we begin to talk of cure, and cure will then be credited to the treatment used. The extent to which the patient's own defences contribute remains unknown but there is much to be said for the view that cancer is a systemic disease, like tuberculosis, and that, as with tuberculosis in the days before chemotherapy, the patient's defences are all-important. This, if true, creates immense difficulties, in turn, for assessments of cure, of prognosis and, ultimately, of diagnostic criteria; and especially is this so in the case of the malignant lymphomas where so often the putatively diagnostic histology is not unequivocal but equivocal.

However, there are many published accounts of long survival in apparently indubitable HD (and there might be as many with the non-Hodgkin lesions were they as definable as HD with unequivocal RS cells). Thus, Smetana (1969) gave details of 40 patients still alive more than 20 years after diagnosis from an original population of 388. The diagnoses had been confirmed on review, thus excluding the possibility earlier considered by the same author (Cohen et al., 1964) analysing the same group, that the long-lived patients might simply represent a wrongly diagnosed residuum. Of 402 patients reported by Lacher (1969), 90 survived more than 10 years, including some who almost certainly gained benefit from radiotherapy, with extensive symptomatic disease. In face of the fact that patients with constitutional symptoms are much likelier than those without to have multinodal and/or extranodal spread (Johnson et al., 1970; Cross and Dixon, 1971), these are impressive results. The view that systemic defences are mainly to thank was expressed by Chawla and his associates (1970), who gave an account of 58 patients with HD also surviving more than 10 years. This opinion is reinforced by the incidental finding by Strum and Rappaport (1971) of foci of HD in four patients who died from an unrelated cause more than 10 years after initial diagnosis: in their own words, "The finding of persistent Hodgkin's disease in long-term survivors, especially in those dying from

apparently unrelated causes, suggests that in some patients with Hodgkin's disease cure may in fact represent a state of equilibrium in which the host has come to terms with his disease". In contrast, however, a patient described by Wright (1975) had a trouble-free interval of 18 years, then died of the disease.

A broad survey of clinical outcome has recently been published by Aisenberg and Qazi (1976), who offer impressive evidence of improved survival-rates over the years in patients with all stages of HD. For the periods 1948–1964, 1965–1968 and 1969–1973, respectively, the survival rates at 5 years after diagnosis were 34%, 65% and 87%. There was no analysis of the series by age, sex or histological sub-group, only by clinical staging (the Ann Arbor classification: Carbone et al., 1971) when, as expected, the more widespread the disease, the worse was the prognosis. The histopathologist will naturally wish to know to what extent his subgrouping of the disease helps as a predictor: in comparison with clinical staging, as in the case of carcinoma of the breast, the contribution is small. Thus, in a study of 235 cases during the period 1948–1969, when the overall 5-year survival rate was 40% (and thus closely comparable with that of Aisenberg and Qazi), Patchefsky and his colleagues (1973) found patients with the lymphocyte-predominant (LP) and nodular sclerosis (NS) varieties to have a better 5-year survival rate, 60%, than those with the mixed cellularity (M) and lymphocyte-depletion (LD) varieties at 30% and 10% respectively.

However, the true significance, or lack of significance, of the histology is seen when analysed by stages; some combining of the subgroups was necessary. Within Stages I and II, the 5-year survival rate for LP and NS was some 70%, for M and LD, 30%. Within Stages III and IV, only LP at 50% was identifiable as prognostically less gloomy than the rest at approximately 20%. The authors of both these series make clear that improved survival rates do not necessarily imply improved cure rates, and indeed it seems wise still to be cautious in accepting claims of therapeutic success. Some of the difficulties were thoughtfully presented by Rapoport and his colleagues (1969) in their attempts to correlate the outcome with the use of chemotherapy. They point out that with four histological types of HD, four clinical stages, three age groups and two sexes there are 96 sub-groups, and to this one may add the element of uncertainty introduced into any series by the diagnostically borderline cases. These authors concluded, however, that, in comparison with an earlier series of patients treated by radio-therapy alone, chemotherapy probably did pro-long life. The nature of the response to treatment may itself be of some prognostic value in that those who suffer relapse within 2 years of initial therapy appear to have a worse prognosis than those who do not (Selzer et al., 1972).

### Invasion of Vessels

Invasion of blood vessels by the neoplastic tissue in HD has been considered as a feature of possibly predictive significance by some of the workers already mentioned (Rappaport and Strum, 1970; Strum et al., 1971). Elastica-staining of nodes was helpful in defining the presence of vessels, and with its aid invasion was found in approximately 6% of patients. These authors had little doubt that, within a given histological sub-type of HD, such invasion is prognostically ominous (histological sub-types have been found by Strum and Rappaport [1971a] to remain constant for many years: change, when it occurs, is usually towards a more aggressive form, seldom the reverse).

### Eosinophil Polymorphonuclear Cell: Granulomas

Another histological entity, the eosinophil poly-morphonuclear, has long figured as a component of HD histology yet has of late been largely neglected. An ultrastructural study of the cell in HD was reported by Kelényi (1969) who de-scribed extensive disruption and final disintegra-tion of the granules, greater in degree than that seen in nonspecific chronic inflammation, though this was of uncertain significance. The cell is not now given much diagnostic or prognostic im-portance. A similarly uncertain position is occupied by the epithelioid-cell granulomas occa-sionally seen in HD; they were found by Brincker (1970) in 6 of some 300 patients. This author offered various possible explanations for their appearance such as, for example, kinship with the sarcoid type of reaction sometimes present in nodes draining the area of a malignant

neoplasm, but concluded that no single explana-tion was consistent or valid. A higher incidence of granulomas was found by Kadin and col-leagues (1970), in 31 of 185 patients (in 18 of these 31 cases, the granulomas were found in tissues still free of HD). Here also the authors believed that no adequate explanation for the process was yet available.

### Focal Involvement of Nodes

The earlier-cited discovery by Strum and Rappa-port (1971) of focal nodal involvement by HD was retrospective and in a sense incidental. The same phenomenon, however, may be of signifi-cance prospectively, in relation to 'staging', and has been examined as such by Strum and Rappaport (1970a) and by Lukes (1971). The current practice of multiple biopsy for staging purposes has contributed much that is thera-peutically and prognostically valuable (though doubts have recently been raised by Griffin and his co-workers [1977] whether it need always be so extensive). Therefore, lesions are requiring to be recognised at an earlier stage of develop-ment than ever before: therefore, we should probably always make more than a single section from any lymph node (and enough to include suspicious areas in a serially sliced spleen) and be prepared to search for foci of HD of perhaps 1-mm diameter or less.

### Immunal Implications

It has long been clear that, in a disease causing at times such systemic disturbances as inter-mittent pyrexia, pruritus, eosinophilia and haemolytic anaemia, there must be demonstrable abnormalities in bodily tissues or products if only the techniques were available. Such tech-niques are now available in increasing number, and with them have come many observations on such features as the histochemistry and immuno-histochemistry of neoplastic and lymphoid cells (Braunstein et al., 1962; Curran and Jones, 1978) and their proliferative characteristics (Peckham and Cooper, 1969); the behaviour of immunoglobulins and lymphocytes (Amiel and Schneider, 1971; Lukes and Tindle, 1975; Stuart et al., 1977); and the proposal of related hypotheses on the nature of HD such as, for example, that of Order and Hellman (1972) who suspect a GVH reaction amongst T-lymphocytes.

As investigation spreads from the purely morphological to the more broadly immunological, so should further information become available on such broader matters as the interrelationships between HD and other diseases (the sarcoid type of reaction has already been mentioned), and its occurrence in childhood, pregnancy and within families, all of them areas wherein the pathologist may be approached for prognostic assistance.

The immunological and prognostic implications of the occurrence of herpes zoster in HD have been assessed by Wilson and his co-workers (1972). After commenting that herpes zoster is 20 times commoner among patients with HD than amongst the general population, they describe their own finding of herpes zoster in 31 (19%) of their 166 patients, all irradiated for HD. A possibly prognostic significance of zoster lay in the fact that those patients who developed it longer than 6 months after irradiation had a much higher incidence of recurrence of HD than those who developed it within 6 months of their treatment; immunosuppression by either the irradiation or the lymphoma or both seemed a likely explanation. Similar speculations are aroused by the findings in studies of HD in children. Thus, Newell and his colleagues (1970) were led to conclude, from a detailed comparison of many histological features, that HD in the child was significantly different from that in the adult and that the cellular response very possibly reflected ". . . fundamental differences in host response, by age, to the same etiology". In the series of 35 children studied by Strum and Rappaport (1970) the NS variety was by far the commonest (22 of the 35 cases) while none was seen with the LD variety: length of survival, when the paper was written, ranged from 3 months to almost 10 years.

### Pregnancy

The behaviour of HD during pregnancy has been assessed by Goguel and his associates (1969) in the case of 82 patients, 62 who were delivered, and 20 in whom the pregnancy ended prematurely by either spontaneous or therapeutic abortion. The outcome was better in patients already under treatment than in those as yet untreated: the advent of pregnancy during a period of relapse was an indication for termination. Pregnancies occurring after a 3-year remis-

sion were well sustained but the occurrence of pregnancy early in remission is likely to precipitate relapse. Experience suggested that active therapy, even chemotherapy, should be avoided during pregnancy; a point of general interest is that in all of the nine cases where vinblastine was repeatedly administered the infants were normal.

Further experience has been described by Holmes and Holmes (1978) who found that pregnancy was generally well tolerated by patients with HD, and also that neither the pregnancy nor the disease appeared to act adversely towards the other. Such dangers as there are reside in therapy, not only for a current pregnancy but, as McKeen and colleagues (1979) report, for a pregnancy that follows therapy.

### Hereditary Factors

A familial incidence of HD has been frequently reported. In the present series it was seen in a father and son (Case 4.8) and, in a somewhat related way, in the father of a man of 22 who very possibly had lymphosarcoma (Case 4.40). This last occurrence recalls the report of Creagan and Fraumeni (1972) who described a four-generation pedigree in which two siblings and a maternal aunt developed HD while several other members of the lineage developed such "disorders of an immune nature" as acute monocytic leukaemia, idiopathic thrombocytopenic purpura and Crohn's disease. The significance of familial incidence was considered at some length by MacMahon (1966) in his comprehensive review of the epidemiology of HD where, inter alia, he quotes without dissent an earlier opinion that the risk to close relatives of a patient with the disease of acquiring it themselves is some three times greater than applies to the general population. In all, however, he considered that the data then available were too "inadequate in both quantity and quality" to allow firm conclusions to be drawn.

### Non-Hodgkin Lymphomas

To some extent the non-Hodgkin lymphomas have already been considered, for, as MLs, they are the reciprocal of HD; the one group cannot be assessed without frequent reference to the other. The earlier notes, however, were necessarily concerned in the main with the nature and specificity of the R-S cell. What follows now is largely a selection from various published series of cases of non-H lymphoma of data which give useful guidance to prognosis. For an encyclopaedic account of the lesions the reader is referred to the volume by Lennert (1978).

It may be well to note here, as a possible pointer to future assessments of MLs, the recent description by Kim and his colleagues (1977) of 20 cases of 'composite lymphoma' as "... the simultaneous occurrence of distinctly demarcated foci of lymphoma having different histologic patterns in the same organ or mass". In 12 patients there were combined forms of non-H lymphoma; in the rest the combination was a non-H lymphoma and HD. A further ten examples have been analysed by van den Tweel and co-workers (1979) who have widened the concept to include "the occurrence of two different histologic types of lymphoma in one organ, or in two different organs at the same time, or during the course of the disease ...", and believe that the varied cellular patterns are "... better considered as different morphologic expressions of a single malignant cell type—the lymphocyte".

This interpretation, and the belief of Habeshaw and his colleagues (1979) that basically only two types of cell are ancestral to the non-H lymphomas, together comprise a notable return from 'splitting' to 'lumping'. To what extent such unifying concepts will simplify or diminish borderline problems for the routine histopathologist remains to be seen.

### 'Starry-sky' Appearance

The significance in nodes of the 'starry-sky' appearance (marked histiocytic phagocytosis), which is not peculiar to the so-called Burkitt lymphoma or even to MLs as a whole, was assessed by Oels and his co-workers (1968). The pattern was found in 18% of 85 immature or lymphoblastic sarcomas but in none of 100 mature or lymphocytic lesions, and was associated with a poor prognosis. The 5-year survival figures for patients with lymphoblastic sarcoma showing marked, moderate or no phagocytic activity were, respectively, nil, 12% and 31%.

### Nodular and Diffuse Lesions

A series of 405 cases of non-H lymphoma was analysed by Jones and his associates (1973) using in parallel the Rappaport classification (Rappaport et al., 1956) and the Ann Arbor scheme of clinical staging (Carbone et al., 1971). In general, the nodular lesions, whether poorly differentiated or well differentiated, and whatever the predominant cell type, were associated with significantly higher probabilities of survival than the diffuse lesions. In approximate and representative terms, derived from their data, the *nodular lesions* produced a mean survival probability of 0.6 at five years (from 1.0 to nil at 5 years for well-differentiated lymphocytic and histiocytic forms respectively); corresponding values for the *diffuse lesions* were 0.6 at only 1 year (from 0.3 to nil at five year for the poorly differentiated lymphocytic and undifferentiated forms respectively). In general, these figures substantiate, though more objectively and accurately, the impression of pathologists from the days before 'giant follicular lymphoma' and 'reticulum cell sarcoma' became outmoded terms, that the first group 'did well' and the second group 'did badly'.

According to these same workers, not all lesions that seem to be diffuse are so; some are nodular but recognisable as such only by reticulin staining. Also, in a retrospective review of cases originally diagnosed as RCS, only 55% were found to be lymphomas of the diffuse histiocytic variety, 25% were in fact nodular lymphomas; that is, the nodular lymphoma had been frequently under-diagnosed, and to that extent estimates of prognosis had been inaccurate. Higher degrees of nodularity had been found also by Patchefsky and his colleagues (1974) to be associated with better prognosis. Nodular fibrosis was not prognostically optimistic, nor, in general, vascular invasion prognostically pessimistic. Fibrosis in lymphomatous nodes had earlier been reported by others (Millett et al., 1969; Rosas-Uribe and Rappaport, 1972) as prognostically favourable, so the matter remains unsettled. The examples illustrated by Rosas-Uribe and Rappaport may comprise a separate sub-group; the subdivision by fibrous bands was such as to produce a picture closely simulating metastatic carcinoma.

Analysis of the behaviour of nodular lymphoma in 65 patients by Qazi and colleagues (1976) showed that, as so commonly applies, the clinical 'stage' of the disease is more important than the histological sub-type: patients with localised disease and disseminated disease had 5-year survival rates of, respectively 80% and 45% but, even so, few with even localised disease are ultimately cured. In general, patients aged less than 50 years (64% 5-year survival) fared better than those aged more than 50 years (34% 5-year survival). In the 18 patients who came to necropsy, the lesion in eight had ". . . converted to a diffuse pattern which was described as a pleomorphic reticulum cell sarcoma in two"; it had retained the pattern of a nodular lymphoma in the other ten. Treatment had appeared to have little effect. (Retention of nodular pattern had similarly characterised 25% of the cases coming to necropsy from the earlier series of 253 cases of 'follicular lymphoma' reported by Rappaport et al., 1956).

## Immunoblastic Lymphadenopathy

The lesion now known as immunoblastic lymphadenopathy (Lukes and Tindle, 1975; Rappaport and Moran, 1975; Editorial, 1975) is relatively well defined both morphologically and immunologically. With little doubt it is an entity but how specific an entity remains to be settled: its definition may not be easy since, as Lukes and Tindle point out, all cases so far have been treated as for ML. The disorder has a high mortality, yet remissions, with microscopically demonstrable involution of lesions, may occur in some patients in a way suggesting either an unusually favourable response to treatment or a significant tendency towards self-limitation. Therefore, even though the diagnosis may be made with fair assurance, prognosis is uncertain. Death is due in some cases to conversion of the lesion to a frank (immunoblastic) sarcoma, in others to infection, consequent on the almost invariably associated immunodeficiency in company with a diagnostically indicative polyclonal hyperglobulinaemia. In the experience of Meijer and his colleagues (1978), skin biopsy may at times be of great diagnostic value.

## Lennert Lymphoma

The disorder first described as a form of HD by Lennert and Mestdagh (1968), now the Lennert lymphoma, behaves as a ML and is characterised histologically by an abundance of appreciably epithelioid histiocytes and a polymorphous cellular infiltrate. R-S cells, however, are lacking.

In the opinion of Burke and Butler (1976), who describe 15 examples, the Lennert lymphoma is a lesion biologically mid-way between HD and immunoblastic lymphoma. It shares with the immunoblastic lymphoma certain clinical features such as allergies, polyclonal hyperglobulinaemia and a variale degree of immunoblastic proliferation, but lacks the vascular proliferation and amorphous interstitial precipitate. In the opinion of MacGillivray and MacIntosh (1978) it is a variant of lymphocytic lymphoma.

## LESIONS THAT MAY SIMULATE ML

Comment hitherto has concerned lesions firmly diagnosed as ML. To the patient with an equivocal lymph node, more important than the type of ML he might have is whether the lesion is ML at all: the extent to which abnormal tissue patterns in nodes are subject to over- and under-diagnosis as ML has already been noted. A list of conditions that may closely simulate ML is shown in Table 4.4, as also are some of their principal morphological features; some supplementary comments are added in the text. The table is offered as no more than an aide memoire, with the caveat that, depending on the stage and rate of evolution of the disease, the various morphological features in the vertical columns, as, for example, loss or preservation of a follicular pattern or germinal centres, vary greatly in degree, not only from patient to patient but also at different times in the same patient.

*Histiocyte/reticulum cell overgrowth* will, it is hoped, be self-explanatory. The phenomenon is present in some degree in almost every node abnormal enough to be worrying, and little purpose would be served here by entering the debate on the nature of these cells (the complexities were fully described by Gall, 1958: the newer immunological techniques may help to clarify them). *Abnormally large cells* refers particularly to scattered individual cells, not to the node mainly replaced by abnormally large cells as, for example, in a histiocytic lymphoma. The term has been used to embrace cells ranging in size from the Langhans giant cell to the binucleate cell that might or might not be a R-S cell. *Epithelioid cells* does not include those of manifestly tuberculoid follicular granulomas, for the manifestly tuberculous or sarcoid node will not often be confusing. However, as with all these morphological elements, there are degrees of expression to the point where, as Braylan and his colleagues (1977) have stressed, a widely epithelioid picture may so obscure an underlying ML (usually HD; the other MLs are less often concerned) as to make failure to diagnose a significant risk. The Lennert lymphoma mentioned earlier is a notably epithelioid-celled lesion and has to be remembered in this context.

*Necrosis* in nodes may be mainly focal or massive. Focal necrosis in company with an epithelioid-cell reaction will naturally raise the question of a tuberculous or other chronic necrotising granuloma. It is seen otherwise at its most extreme, with micro-abscess formation, in cat-scratch disease and the allied conditions. Massive necrosis, usually mediated by ischaemia, may have an obvious cause such as mechanical pressure; otherwise, malignant neoplasia, primary or secondary, must have a high place in any list of possible causes. Infarction may occur in nonmalignant nodes (five examples were reported by Davies and Stansfeld, 1972) but it seems sound, as a working rule, to regard widespread necrosis in a node as due to neoplasia until proved otherwise. Foci of still-viable cells around vessels or beneath the capsule can establish the diagnosis though several sections from different levels may have to be searched.

*Vascular proliferation*, either an increase in the number of small vessels or undue prominence of the endothelium or both, is a nonspecific appearance. Though common in the giant lymphoid hamartoma, and an apparently constant feature of 'immunoblastic lymphadenopathy', it may sometimes be seen in ML, in the non-H forms more often than in HD, but occurs also in inflammatory states, both specific, as in postvaccinial lymphadenitis (Dorfman and Warnke, 1974), and nonspecific (*see* Fig. 9.64 of Symmers, 1978). Its significance is unknown, and it is no guide to prognosis. The so-called vascular transformation of sinuses is mentioned later in the context of misleadingly prominent sinus-based tissue patterns.

*Fibrosis* of nodes was mentioned in relation to ML where its occurrence is variable and prognostically equivocal. It appears more constantly in some states than in others but has little significance. In company with fatty replacement of the parenchyma it is a common altera-

tion with age, well shown in almost any collection of nodes obtained at, for example, a Wertheim hysterectomy with pelvic clearance.

*Other features* are varied; one merits separate mention, the intra-, trans- and extracapsular extension of cells usually contained by the capsule, the so-called capsular transgression. This sometimes certainly abnormal occurrence may be of discriminant value but it is not peculiar to malignant neoplasia: quite normal nodes may sometimes show a deficiency of the capsule that allows lymphocytes to enter the surrounding fibrofatty tissue en masse. Mostly, in my own experience, transgression of diagnostic degree has been shown by a population of cells of a type that would of itself, whether inside a node or out, have raised seriously the question of neoplasia.

Particularly helpful analyses of lesions simulating ML have been given by Sieracki and Fisher (1970) and by Dorfman and Warnke (1974). These last observers, who, incidentally but commendably, emphasise that they have ". . . assiduously avoided utilizing the frozen section technique or needle biopsy . . ." divided the simulating lesions into four groups according to the type of structural disturbance produced: Table 4.4 has been constructed on the same basis. Thus, the four groups of Dorfman and Warnke, and the lesions numbered in the table that fall within these groups, are:

Follicular (nodular) pattern: 1, 2, 3, 4
Sinus pattern: 5, 6
Diffuse pattern: 7–11 inclusive
Mixed pattern: 12, 13, 14

No comment is offered on some of the lesions in Table 4.4, as, for example, the nonspecific reactive hyperplasia: the problem of distinguishing this disturbance from nodular lymphoma is widely familiar, and many authors over the years have presented the main points of difference in tabular form. Little more is given on some others than a reference to an informative publication. In many instances, the clinical circumstances will leave little doubt about the nature of a co-existent lymphadenopathy. At the same time, the clinical features must not be allowed to dominate, otherwise the patient with an enlarged node or nodes who has recently been vaccinated or who has chronic dermatitis or epilepsy will be at some risk of having their possibly co-existent ML under-diagnosed. To be sure, their

**Table 4.4.** Lesions of lymph nodes that may simulate a malignant lymphoma

| | Follicular pattern incr. + dim. − | Germinal centres incr. + dim. − | Histiocyte/reticulum cell overgrowth | | Abnormally large cells | Epithelioid cells |
|---|---|---|---|---|---|---|
| | | | Sinuses | Other | | |
| 1  Non-specific reactive hyperplasia | + | + | ± | | | |
| 2  Rheumatoid arthritis | + + | + + | + | | occasional multinucleate | |
| 3  Syphilis | | | | | | |
| a. Primary | + + | + + | ± | + especially paracortical | multinucleate giant cells | + paracortical |
| b. Secondary | + + | + + | | | multinucleate giant cells but fewer | + + fewer later |
| 4  Giant lymphoid hamartoma | | | | | | |
| a. hyaline-vascular | − | − | | | occ. large mononuclear | squamoid in follicle centres |
| b. plasma cell | + + | + + | | | occ. large mononuclear | |
| 5  SHML | ± | | + + | | histiocytes containing lymphocytes | |
| 6  Histiocytosis X | − | | + + | | occasional multinucleate | |
| 7  Lupus erythematosus | + early | | | | | |
| 8  Post-vaccinial adenitis Herpes zoster adenitis | + | + | ± | diffuse mottling | | |
| 9  Dermatopathic lymphadenitis | − | − | + + especially at periphery | | | |
| 10  Immunoblastic lymphadenopathy | − | − | + + | + + | + may be multinucleate | occasional cluster |
| 11  Drug-induced lymphadenopathy | ± | − | + | + | + may be multinucleate | |
| 12  Infectious mononucleosis | − | − | ± | + + | + may be multinucleate | occasional cluster |
| 13  Toxoplasmosis | + | + + | + 'monocytoid' | | occ. binucleate nucleoli few | + + ragged sheets |
| 14  Cat-scratch disease Lymphopathia venereum | ± | | ± | + focal > diffuse | | rarely |
| 15  Brucellosis | + | | + | + inter-follicular | occ. Langhans occ. others | − to + + |
| 16  Extra-medullary haemopoiesis | − | − | | | mega-karyocytes | |

| Other cells | Focal necrosis | Amorphous material | Vascular proliferation | Fibrosis | Other features | |
|---|---|---|---|---|---|---|
| | | | | | | 1 |
| plasma cells occ. neutrophils | | ± amyloid | + | | germinal centres may be over-run by lymphocytes | 2 |
| | | | | | | 3 |
| plasma cells + + | ± occ. massive | | arteritis + | | distinction between lesions of primary and secondary stages not sharp | |
| plasma cells ± | | | arteritis + + | + | | |
| | | | | | | 4 |
| plasma cells eosinophils | | | + + interfollicular | interfollicular ± calcification | sinuses absent | |
| plasma cells in sheets | | | + interfollicular | | | |
| plasma cells + eosinophils − | | | | | pericapsular fibrosis, histiocytes may be eosinophilic | 5 |
| eosinophils may be few | + or massive | | | | histiocytes markedly eosinophilic | 6 |
| plasma cells occ. + + | + wider later | + haematoxy-phil | | | occ. necrotising arteriolitis, ? cause of necrosis | 7 |
| mixed population | | | + | | | 8 |
| mixed population | | lipid melanin | | + | haemosiderin also may be present | 9 |
| mixed population | occasional small | + | + + | | capsular transgression | 10 |
| mixed population | − to + + | | ± | | capsular transgression | 11 |
| plasma cells + eosinophils few | | | occasionally + | | nucleolar differences from R-S cell | 12 |
| plasma cells + | occ. small c. neutrophils | | | | parasites demonstrable rarely | 13 |
| plasma cells + | + + micro-abscess | | | + later esp. in LV | late LV may appear 'gummatous' | 14 |
| plasma cells + neutrophils + eosinophils − | | | | | large atypical monocytes may closely simulate R-S cells | 15 |
| appropriate mixed population | | | | | | 16 |

ML will be diagnosed sooner or later but, with therapy ever improving, time is not to be lost. The pathologist who examines his sections initially 'blind' is the least likely to fall into this trap.

### Rheumatoid Arthritis

Rheumatoid arthritis may produce prominent follicular hyperplasia to the point where nodular lymphoma may be closely simulated, especially where, as has been reported by Nosanchuk and Schnitzer (1969), germinal centres may fuse and show a notable degree of the 'starry sky' appearance, and the capsule and perinodal fat may also be infiltrated.

### Syphilitic Adenitis

Syphilitic adenitis may likewise resemble a nodular lymphoma. This similarity was believed by Evans (1944) to hold particularly for secondary stage lesions, but more recent observers (Hartsock et al., 1970; Turner and Wright, 1973) found few if any sharp differences between the tissue changes in primary and secondary forms.

### Giant Lymphoid Hamartoma

The giant lymphoid hamartoma, an intrinsically benign mass of lymphoid tissue, occurs most commonly in the mediastinum, where it was first described by Castleman and his colleagues (1956), but may be found elsewhere (as, for example, in the retroperitoneum and neck [Lietz and Wanger, 1968]) and has been reported under several names. The clinical and radiological resemblance to a lesion of thymus is close; histologically the tissue is not thymus, but occasional foci of squamoid cells in the centre of lymphoid follicles may have a superficial and possibly misleading resemblance to Hassall's corpuscles. 'Angiofollicular lymphoid hyperplasia', a term sometimes used, emphasises the prominent vascularity of the lesion. 'Giant lymphoid hamartoma' is preferred by Symmers (1978) on the grounds that the mass lacks sinuses and is thus probably not a coalescent mass of intrinsically normal, if enlarged, nodes. The subdivision shown in Table 4.4 is that proposed by Keller and his associates (1972). The plasma cell form is not infrequently associated with such systemic disturbances as fever, malaise, anaemia and hyperglobulinaemia, suggesting in all a disturbance of immunoactive mechanisms (of still obscure nature). A recent example associated with refractory 'anaemia of chronic disorder' has been reported by Geary and Fox (1978).

### Sinus Histiocytosis

Sinus histiocytosis with massive lymphadenopathy (SHML), first described by Rosai and Dorfman (1972) and characterised, as the name suggests, by prominent hyperplasia of sinus histiocytes, may also be an expression of immunal disturbance. It has a protracted but generally benign course and requires to be distinguished histologically from the prognostically more serious Hand-Schüller-Christian and Letterer-Siwe varieties of histiocytosis X. A recent series has been reported by Lampert and Lennert (1976).

*Histiocytosis X* as an entity remains debatable but at least the term and its implications are familiar: accentuation of sinuses by the accumulation of large, minimally lipid-containing histiocytes is seen best in the early stages of its expression as Letterer-Siwe disease. Thereafter, the substance of the node becomes gradually replaced. Both here and in Hand-Schüller-Christian disease, the abundance of the cytoplasm and general lack of nuclear polymorphism and aberrancy in an otherwise puzzling node should suggest that the process is not truly neoplastic.

Sinus histiocytosis may be induced also by the absorption and storage of foreign substances as used, for example, in lymphangiography and in association with the 'depot' injection of drugs. The result is an *oleogranulomatous histiocytosis*. Recognition of the foreign material as such will usually be possible. Prominent sinus histiocytosis was seen in biliary duct lymph nodes (obtained at cholecystectomy) by Williams and Whittaker (1965) either alone or in combination with some or all of granulomata, giant cells or panhyperplasia in 22 of 80 patients. In one case the giant cells had raised the question of Hodgkin's disease: however, ". . . none showed mirror-image nuclear forms and the remainder of the node structure indicated a brisk reactive hyperplasia". Two of the nodes had shown appreciable fibrosis.

Sinuses may also be made unduly prominent by swelling of the endothelium, what Haferkamp and his colleagues (1971) have termed 'vascular transformation', in consequence of blockage of outflow of lymph, anastomotic shunting of blood into the sinuses and production of what these authors describe as "... a peculiar vascularized sinusoidal fibrosis". The two states just mentioned may coincide, as in the local case of a child whose porto-caval anastomosis had become occluded: many abdominal and retroperitoneal nodes showed an accumulation of lipid-laden histiocytes both within sinuses with swollen endothelium and also throughout the pulp. As reported by Rywlin and co-workers (1966), the fibrosis accompanying vascular transformation may be simulated by the angiomatoid and spindle-celled pattern produced in nodes by *Kaposi's sarcoma*. These authors also give a warning that, because of the commonly associated leucocytic infiltration, the condition may be mistaken for either a plasmacytoma or a non-specific chronic inflammatory response. The involvement of nodes in Kaposi's sarcoma in the complete absence of lesions in the skin has been reported by Bhana and his associates (1970).

### Lupus Erythematosus

The description by Moore and his colleagues (1957) of changes in lymph nodes in *lupus erythematosus* has been mentioned already. An earlier account was that by Fox and Rosahn (1943).

### Postvaccinial Lymphadenopathy

Postvaccinial lymphadenopathy is associated with a focal or diffuse 'mottled' hyperplasia of activated lymphocytes (immunoblasts) to the point where, in the diffuse forms, HD may seem possible. In 20 such examples reported by Hartsock (1968), ML had been diagnosed in nine, and, in six of the nine, HD. The misleading element is the appearance that some or most of the presumably immunoblastic cells may have. Confusion with classical R-S cells may be unlikely but confusion with the mononuclear cells of HD, the 'Hodgkin' cell to some, is certainly possible. For this reason, Hartsock has particularly advised that a diagnosis of HD should not be based on mononuclear cells of this type. Two

further points are relevant: (a) the fact of a recent vaccination may be overlooked, (b) nodal response of this kind may be stimulated not only by vaccinia but by many other vaccines, for example, diphtheria, influenza and tetanus, and possibly by all: in view of this varied aetiology it is not surprising that the response to herpes zoster is morphologically so similar. There is sometimes a suspicion that the enlargement of a node in association with zoster may be a response, not to the virus but to secondary infection in the skin: in local Case 4.38, at any rate, this was not sustained; the node was removed before the vesicles had appeared.

### Dermatopathic Lymphadenopathy

Dermatopathic lymphadenopathy (Jarrett and Kellett, 1951) occurs by definition in association with an eruption of the skin, most commonly exfoliative but of a wide variety. The histological changes, initially a widening of the sinuses then an invasion or occupation of the peripheral pulp by foamy macrophages, produce a pattern that is often suggestive even under a $\times$ 10 magnification. A potentially confusing situation may arise if, as sometimes happens, a causal exfoliative dermatitis has itself been caused by a ML. A first-biopsied node may show the dermatopathic picture, and a later-biopsied node, fortuitously, the ML.

### Immunoblastic Lymphadenopathy

As described by Lukes and Tindle (1975) immunoblastic lymphadenopathy shows a 'morphologic triad': proliferation of arborising small vessels, prominent immunoblastic proliferation, including plasmacytoid and plasma cells, and the interstitial deposition of an amorphous acidophilic material (nature still uncertain). Even without the systemic and immunological disturbances that act as diagnostic pointers, these morphological characteristics make a strongly suggestive combination. The main clinical features of the lesion were mentioned earlier (p. 130).

### Drug-induced Lymphadenopathy

Drug-induced lymphadenopathy may show a wide range of histological abnormality, from moderate but polymorphic and mitotically active reticulum cell hyperplasia with plasma cell accompaniment and perhaps focal necrosis, through increasing cellularity and polymorphism to a pattern diagnostic of ML, most commonly HD of mixed cellularity. The drug usually concerned is hydantoin or a related anticonvulsant; so, the possibility remains that drugs of this type may on occasion be truly carcinogenic and directly responsible for the ML. The lesser degrees of structural change regress with stoppage of the drug, the more advanced degrees may not; on one reported occasion (Gams et al., 1968) the nodes regressed when the drug was stopped but later reappeared as a fatal ML. In the experience of these authors, ". . . no consistent clinical or histologic criteria existed to differentiate benign from malignant lymphoid reactions". Drugs other than anticonvulsants may produce at least the lesser degrees of histological disturbance. In practice, therefore, and as is probably a routine procedure already, any report on a node of equivocal pattern should include an enquiry about intake of drugs. A similarly pseudo-lymphomatous reaction in subcutaneous tissue and adjacent skeletal muscle has been reported (Wilden and Scott, 1978).

## Infectious Mononucleosis

With its immunoblastic hyperplasia, mitotic activity, cells so like R-S cells, and general polymorphism, infectious mononucleosis is perhaps the most notorious of the ML-simulators, to a degree, still, where over-diagnosis as HD is a significant risk. Certainly, biopsy of a node is not often likely to be the first investigation performed on a patient later known to have IM but it may be; the danger of over-diagnosis is then real. One cannot do better here than reproduce the conclusion of Symmers (1978) that the diagnosis cannot be made by histology alone, that histology may suggest the possibility but that only serological and haematological investigations can establish the diagnosis. This authoritative opinion will be widely endorsed for its directness and lack of ambiguity. Its implication is that any node of pleomorphic cellularity with a pattern less than unequivocally diagnostic of HD should not be diagnosed as HD. It also demonstrates that histological information gained in retrospect may on occasion be quite unreliable

for use in prospect. There have been many accurately descriptive accounts of the appearances in nodes in known IM, yet attempts to translate them into criteria for positive diagnosis have failed: 'compatible with' is a long way from 'diagnostic of'. The difficulties were well described by Salvador and his colleagues (1971).

## Toxoplasmosis

Like IM, toxoplasmosis can rarely be diagnosed histologically with total assurance; it equally demands serological investigation. However, the nodal disturbance, if not wholly specific, is usually less suggestive of a ML than is that of IM. Besides prominent follicular and germ centre overgrowth, ragged-edged sheets of various sizes of epithelioid histiocytes are a constant feature with more, and often paler, cytoplasm than in most granulomatous lesions; they are described by Sieracki and Fisher (1970) as 'incomplete granulomas'. The conjunction of this feature with prominent sinus histiocytosis, in which the cells may resemble blood monocytes, helps to distinguish toxoplasmosis from at any rate tuberculosis and sarcoidosis which rarely show sinus histiocytosis. Histologically descriptive accounts have been given by Stansfeld (1961) and, with an assessment of the value of serological testing, Dorfman and Remington (1973).

## Cat-scratch Disease and Lymphopathia Venereum

Cat-scratch disease and lymphopathia venereum may show identical lesions in nodes, typically, in the early stages, micro-abscesses with a surrounding of rather epithelioid histiocytes sometimes in palisaded pattern. In time, with increasing necrosis, the micro-abscess becomes the well-known stellate abscess, still termed 'abscess' though the content is likely by then to be necrotic debris rather than pus. The histiocytic reaction may become so hypercellular and polymorphic as to suggest ML. This was so in a comparable local case, not of cat-scratch disease (and not in the present series) but of 'mesenteric adenitis' of probably Yersinial aetiology where, besides focal suppuration, the nodes showed a striking degree of mitotic, and aberrantly mitotic, activity. 'Mesenteric adenitis', unspecified, has almost as many causes as 'lymphadenitis' unspecified; the Yersinial form (*Yersinia enterocolitica* or *Y. pseudotuberculosis*) may show changes entirely similar to those produced, though usually in more superficial nodes, by cat-scratch disease.

### Brucellosis

Many years ago brucellosis was recognised as a condition able to produce changes in nodes indistinguishable from HD; an early publication was that of Rabson (1939). The histological similarity may be close but soon there were claims that differentiation was possible; a table of discriminant criteria was produced by Gall and Page (1945). The problem, as so often in this context, involves decision whether or not a large cell in a generally immunoblastic background is a R-S cell; and again, only immunological or serological evidence may be diagnostic.

### Metastatic Carcinoma

Metastatic carcinoma, in particular melanocarcinoma, was added to the lesions in the last three of their four groups by Dorfman and Warnke who commented that, however produced, the sinus pattern in which the sinuses are distended by abnormal cells may closely resemble the 'malignant histiocytosis' described by Rappaport (1966) and by others since (*see*, for example, MacGillivray and Duthie, 1977). The distinction between metastatic carcinoma and ML may indeed be difficult, especially where a pharyngeal carcinoma has spread to cervical nodes. Here at least, however, the position is in one sense straightforward; the patient has a malignant neoplasm. Diagnostically and prognostically, a more insidious state may be produced by what Dorfman and Warnke aptly call the 'deceptively bland' and histiocyte-like appearance of metastatic mammary carcinoma within sinuses (this recalls the comparable mimicry of histiocytoma produced by mammary carcinoma when metastatic to the eyelid as reported by Hood et al., 1973). The danger of under-diagnosis here is obvious, as is the danger of over-diagnosis represented by the later-mentioned occasional presence of naevus cells beneath the capsule.

Rarely, metastatic carcinoma may also be simulated by the presence in nodes, most commonly pelvic or inguinal, of endometriosis (*see* chapter 10), and, as mentioned in connection with carcinoma of the breast, of epithelial inclusions or cysts of nonspecific character (*see* Garret and Ada, 1957). The essentially normal cytology of structures of these kinds should serve to minimise the risk of overdiagnosis as glandular carcinoma.

### Lymphomatoid Granulomatosis

Lymphomatoid granulomatosis is rare, relative to the entities in Table 4.4, and has not been included. It deserves mention nevertheless as a pseudo-lymphomatous process that appears sometimes to be successfully treatable (with steroids). It occurs predominantly in the lungs (see Chapter 9) and is a destructive proliferative lesion characterised by infiltration of the tissues by polymorphic histiocytes, lymphocytes and plasma cells: similarity to Wegener's granulomatosis may be close. A full account of 152 cases has been given by Katzenstein and her associates (1979).

To the extent that the lesions in Table 4.4 may simulate a ML, they are technically pseudo-lymphomas. However, since each is positively diagnosable as not ML but some other condition, they are rarely given the name. 'Pseudo-lymphomas' in the usual sense are either masses of hyperplastic lymphoid tissue or inappropriately dense accumulations of inflammatory cells. They occur most commonly in the gastrointestinal tract and lung but have been described in most tissues. Whatever their site, the diagnostic difficulty has the same basis, namely, the degree of confidence with which the pathologist can identify a mainly lymphocytic/histiocytic (or plasma cell) population as hyperplastic or inflammatory rather than ML (or plasmacytoma). Lesions of this kind at various sites either have been mentioned or will be mentioned in other chapters as may be appropriate.

The limitations of histology and cytology in the interpretation of borderline problems in lymph nodes are severe but they are generally acknowledged, and to the extent that they are acknowledged the likelihood of over-diagnosis and under-diagnosis diminishes. Ancillary aids to diagnosis are many, and available with varying dependability for more than half of the conditions listed in Table 4.4. The pathologist has some responsibility here to suggest to the clinician such further investigations, mostly serological, as may be available. In others of the conditions, such as the postvaccinial and dermatopathic forms of lymphadenitis, study of the clinical data, again with perhaps a helpful enquiry from the pathologist, may resolve doubts raised by the histology. Techniques of investigation along immunological lines are already supplementing histological assessment but it will be long before they supplant it. The newer techniques may narrow the zone of uncertainty between what is and what is not ML but they will not abolish it for they, too, will find their own zones of uncertainty. Whether or not a patient has a ML, as with many other cancers, is far from being a simple 'yes/no' question.

Investigations of this kind, and the implications of current research into the nature of malignant lymphoproliferative lesions, have been reviewed in broad perspective by Hansen and Good (1974). The survey is informative and includes also, in useful tabular form, an indication of the interrelationships between the essentially morphological classifications of the malignant lymphomas (Rappaport et al., 1956; Gérard-Marchant et al., 1974) and the basically immunological and functional classification of Lukes and Collins (1975). At the outset, Hansen and Good rather severely underestimate such diagnostic capacity as the morphologist does have, limited though it be. They state that, "The absolute histological criteria of malignant disease in the tissue must include obliteration of normal lymph node architecture, invasion of the lymph node capsule, and alterations in morphology or clear morphological or cytological evidence of neoplasia of proliferating cells." One feels bound to say that if pathologists waited until all these criteria were fulfilled, few patients would be diagnosed as having ML until they were dead; and even then there would still be nodes only partly involved. However, none will differ from their further opinion that ". . . precise definition of lymphoproliferative malignant disease remains difficult". The extent to which the clinical pathologist can overcome, or will hope to overcome, the difficulties has been the subject of this chapter.

## Conclusions

1) In borderline nodes:
   a) Total loss of follicular architecture may be as common in lesions that progress to fatal ML as in those that regress.
   b) Retention of germinal centres is commoner in nonmalignant lesions than in those that progress to unequivocal ML.
   c) Prominent sinus histiocytosis is commoner in benign lesions.
   d) Prominence of 'reticulum' cells is per se ambivalent.
   e) Nuclear polymorphism and undue mitotic activity are also per se ambivalent.

2) Cells resembling R-S cells may be found in many lesions not Hodgkin's disease. The 'lacunar' type is probably the most nearly diagnostic form: however, type of fixation largely determines how 'lacunar' the cell will be. Immunohistochemical techniques offer promise of greater diagnostic specificity.

3) Prognosis in HD depends on the clinical stage rather than the histology but, of histological subgroups, the lymphocyte predominant is the least unfavourable.

4) The aetiology and significance of HD-associated granulomas remains uncertain.

5) Removal of nodes for purposes of 'staging' HD reveals hitherto unfamiliar patterns of focal involvement. Diagnostically, the size of the borderline problem is inversely proportional to the size of the focus involved.

6) The 'starry sky' appearance is not peculiar to the Burkitt lymphoma.

7) Nodular (non-H) lymphomas are prognostically more favourable than diffuse lymphomas: accurate distinction may be aided by reticulin staining. Diffuse lesions may simulate metastatic carcinoma, and vice versa.

8) The epithelioid-celled Lennert lymphoma may be a lesion biologically midway between HD and immunoblastic lymphadenopathy. Both these recently described lesions are associated, inter alia, with hyperglobulinaemia. Their full prognostic implications have yet to be assessed.

9) Many lesions involving nodes may simulate ML histologically. A table of 16 such states (Table 4.4) is given. Not all are equally important diagnostically. The most significantly simulant are drug-induced adenopathy, infectious

mononucleosis, brucellosis and metastatic carcinoma.

10) The term 'pseudolymphoma' is usually applied mainly to reactive overgrowths of lymphoid tissue or inappropriately dense infiltrations of inflammatory cells in tissues other than lymph nodes.

# References

Aisenberg AC, Qazi R (1976) Improved survival in Hodgkin's disease. Cancer 37: 2423–2429

Amiel JL, Schneider M (1971) Etudes immunologiques dans la maladie de Hodgkin. Bull Cancer (Paris) 58: 9–20

Anagnostou D, Parker JW, Taylor CR, Tindle BH, Lukes RJ (1977) Lacunar cells of nodular sclerosing Hodgkin's disease. An ultrastructural and immunohistologic study. Cancer 39: 1032–1043

Azar HA (1975) Significance of the Reed-Sternberg cell. Hum Pathol 6: 479–484

Bhana D, Templeton AC, Master SP, Kyalwazi SK (1970) Kaposi sarcoma of lymph nodes. Br J Cancer 24: 464–470

Braunstein H, Freeman DG, Thomas W, Gall EA (1962) A histochemical study of the enzymatic activity of lymph nodes: III Granulomatous and primary neoplastic conditions of lymphoid tissue. Cancer 15: 139–152

Braylan RC, Long JC, Jaffé ES, Greco FA, Orr SL, Berard CW (1977) Malignant lymphoma obscured by concomitant extensive epithelioid granulomas. Report of three cases with similar clinicopathologic features. Cancer 39: 1146–1155

Brincker H (1970) Epithelioid-call granulomas in Hodgkin's disease. Acta Pathol Microbiol Scand [A] 78: 19–32

Burke JS, Butler JJ (1976) Malignant lymphoma with a high content of epithelioid histiocytes (Lennert's lymphoma). Am J Clin Pathol 66: 1–9

Carbone PP, Kaplan HS, Musshoff K, Smithers DW, Tubiana M (1971) Report of the Committee on Hodgkin's disease staging classification. Cancer Res 31: 1860–1861

Castleman B, Iverson L, Menendez VP (1956) Localized mediastinal lymph-node hyperplasia resembling thymoma. Cancer 9: 822–830

Chawla PL, Stutzman L, Dubois RE, Kim U, Sokal JE (1970) Long survival in Hodgkin's disease. Am J Med 48: 85–92

Cohen BM, Smetana HF, Miller RW (1964) Hodgkin's disease: Long survival in a study of 388 world war II army cases. Cancer 17: 856–866

Coppleson LW, Factor RM, Strum SB, Graff PW, Rappaport H (1970) Observer disagreement in the classification and histology of Hodgkin's disease. J Natl Cancer Inst 45: 731–740

Cottier H, Turk J, Sobin L (1973) A proposal for a standardized system of reporting human lymph node morphology in relation to immunological function. J Clin Pathol 26: 317–331

Creagan ET, Fraumeni JF (1972) Familial Hodgkin's disease. Lancet II: 547

Cross RM, Dixon FWP (1971) A combined clinical and histological assessment of survival of patients with Hodgkin's disease. J Clin Pathol 24: 385–393

Crum ED, Ng ABP, Tsoa L-1, Kellermeyer RW (1974) Hodgkin's disease. Survival and histological classification in a general medical center 1952–1971. Am J Clin Pathol 61: 403–411

Curran RC, Jones EL (1978) Hodgkin's disease: An immunohistochemical and histological study. J Pathol 125: 39–51

Davies JD, Stansfeld AG (1972) Spontaneous infarction of superficial lymph nodes. J Clin Pathol 25: 689–696

Dawson PJ, Cooper RA, Rambo ON (1964) Diagnosis of malignant lymphoma. A clinicopathological analysis of 158 difficult lymph node biopsies. Cancer 17: 1405–1413

Dorfman RF (1974) Classification of non-Hodgkin lymphomas. Lancet II: 961–962

Dorfman RF, Remington JS (1973) Value of lymph-node biopsy in the diagnosis of acute acquired toxoplasmosis. N Engl J Med 289: 878–881

Dorfman RF, Warnke R (1974) Lymphadenopathy simulating the malignant lymphomas. Hum Pathol 5: 519–550

Editorial (1969) The Hodgkin maze. Lancet II: 728–729

Editorial (1973) Epidemiology of Hodgkin's disease. Lancet II: 647–648

Editorial (1974) Follicular lymphomas. Lancet I: 1088–1089

Editorial (1975) Immunoblastic-cell proliferations. Lancet I: 260–261

Editorial (1975a) Blind alleys in the Hodgkin's maze. Lancet I: 556–557

Editorial (1976) The Lennert lymphoma. Lancet II: 507

Editorial (1979) Looking at lymphomas. Lancet I: 306–307

Evans N (1944) Lymphadenitis of secondary syphilis: Its resemblance to giant follicular lymphadenopathy. Arch Pathol 37: 175–179

Fisher ER, Sieracki JC, Goldenberg DM (1970) Identity and nature of isolated lymphoid tumors (so called nodal hyperplasia, hamartoma, and angiomatous hamartoma) as revealed by histologic, electron microscopic, and heterotransplantation studies. Cancer 25: 1286–1300

Fox RA, Rosahn PD (1943) The lymph nodes in disseminated lupus erythematosus. Am J Pathol 19: 73–99

Franssila KO, Kalima TV, Voutilainen A (1967) Histologic classification of Hodgkin's disease. Cancer 20: 1594–1601

140    Lesions of Lymph Nodes

Franssila KO, Heiskala MK, Heiskala HJ (1977) Epidemiology and histopathology of Hodgkin's disease in Finland. Cancer 39: 1280–1288

Gall EA (1958) The cytological identity and inter-relation of mesenchymal cells of lymphoid tissue. Ann NY Acad Sci 73: 120–130

Gall EA, Page SG (1945) Intermittent fever with lesions simulating those of Hodgkin's disease. Am J Clin Pathol 15: 431–445

Gams RA, Neal JA, Conrad FG (1968) Hydantoin-induced pseudo-pseudolymphoma. Ann Intern Med 69: 557–568

Garret R, Ada AEW (1957) Epithelial inclusion cysts in an axillary lymph node. Report of a case simulating metastatic adenocarcinoma. Cancer 10: 173–178

Geary CG, Fox H (1978) Giant lymph node hyperplasia of the mediastinum and refractory anaemia. J Clin Pathol 31: 757–760

Gérard-Marchant R, Hamlin I, Lennert K, Rilke F, Stansfeld AG, Unnik, JAM van (1974) Classification of non-Hodgkin's lymphoma. Lancet II: 406–408

Goguel A, Helpt-Eppinger M, Teillet F, Weil M, Jacquillat C, Bernard J (1969) Maladie de Hodgkin et grossesse. Nouv Rev Fr Hematol 9: 581–600

Griffin T, Gerdes A, Parker R, Taylor E, Hafermann M, Taylor W, Tesh D (1977) Are pelvic irradiation and routine staging laparotomy necessary in clinically staged IA and IIA Hodgkin's disease? Cancer 40: 2914–2916

Habeshaw JA, Catley PF, Stansfeld AG, Brearley RL (1979) Surface phenotyping, histology and the nature of non-Hodgkin lymphoma in 157 patients. Brit J Cancer 40: 11–34

Haferkamp O, Rosenau W, Lennert K (1971) Vascular transformation of lymph node sinuses due to venous obstruction. Arch Pathol 92: 81–83

Hall CA, Olson KB (1956) Prognosis of the malignant lymphomas. Ann Intern Med 44: 687–706

Hansen JA, Good RA (1974) Malignant disease of the lymphoid system in immunological perspective. Hum Pathol 5: 567–599

Hartsock RJ (1968) Postvaccinial lymphadenitis. Hyperplasia of lymphoid tissue that simulates malignant lymphomas. Cancer 21: 632–649

Hartsock RJ, Halling LW, King FM (1970) Luetic lymphadenitis: A clinical and histologic study of 20 cases. Am J Clin Pathol 53: 304–314

Holmes GE, Holmes FF (1978) Pregnancy outcome of patients treated for Hodgkin's disease. A controlled study. Cancer 41: 1317–1322

Hood CI, Font RL, Zimmerman LE (1973) Metastatic mammary carcinoma in the eyelid with histiocytoid appearance. Cancer 31: 793–800

Iversen OH, Sandnes K (1971) The reliability of pathologists. A study of some cases of lymph node biopsies showing giant follicular hyperplasia or lymphoma. Acta Pathol Microbiol Scand [A] 79: 330–334

Jarrett A, Kellett HS (1951) The association of generalized erythrodermia with superficial lymph-adenopathy (lipomelanic reticulosis). Br J Dermatol 63: 343–362

Johnson RE, Thomas LB, Chretien P (1970) Correlation between clinicohistologic staging and extra-nodal relapse in Hodgkin's disease. Cancer 25: 1071–1075

Jones SE, Fuks Z, Bull M, Kadin ME, Dorfman RF, Kaplan HS, Rosenberg SA, Kim H (1973) Non-Hodgkin's lymphomas IV. Clinicopathologic correlation in 405 cases. Cancer 31: 806–823

Kadin ME, Donaldson SS, Dorfman RF (1970) Isolated granulomas in Hodgkin's disease. N Engl J Med 283: 859–861

Katzenstein A-LA, Carrington CB, Liebow AA (1979) Lymphomatoid granulomatosis. A clinico-pathologic study of 152 cases. Cancer 43: 360–373

Kelényi G (1969) Eosinophile Leukocyten in den Geweben I. Veränderungen der eosinophilen Leukocyten bei Lymphogranulomatose. Virchows Arch [Cell Pathol] 2: 297–310

Keller AR, Hochholzer L, Castleman B (1972) Hyaline-vascular and plasma-cell types of giant lymph node hyperplasia of the mediastinum and other locations. Cancer 29: 670–683

Kim H, Dorfman RF (1974) Morphological studies of 84 untreated patients subjected to laparotomy for the staging of non-Hodgkin's lymphomas. Cancer 33: 657–674

Kim H, Hendrickson MR, Dorfman RF (1977) Composite lymphoma. Cancer 40: 959–976

Kreyberg L, Iversen OH (1959) Early diagnosis of malignant conditions in lymph nodes. Br J Cancer 13: 26–32

Lacher MJ (1969) Long survival in Hodgkin's disease. Ann Intern Med 70: 7–17

Lampert F, Lennert K (1976) Sinus histiocytosis with massive lymphadenopathy. Fifteen new cases. Cancer 37: 783–789

Lennert K (1978) Malignant lymphomas other than Hodgkin's disease. In: Uehlinger E (ed) Histology, cytology, ultrastructure, immunology. Springer, Berlin Heidelberg New York (Handbuch der speziellen pathologischen Anatomie und Histologie, vol 1/3B)

Lennert K, Mestdagh J (1968) Lympho-granulomatosen mit konstant hohem Epithelioidzellgehalt. Virchows Arch [Pathol Anat] 344: 1–20

Lennert K, Mohri N, Stein H, Kaiserling E (1975) The histopathology of malignant lymphoma. Br J Haematol [suppl] 31: 193–203

Lennert K, Stein H, Kaiserling E (1975a) Cytological and functional criteria for the classification of malignant lymphomata. Br J Cancer [suppl II] 31: 29–43

Lietz H, Wanger F (1968) Über das benigne Lymphom. Angiofollikuläre Lymphknotenhyperplasie. Dtsch Med Wochenschr 93: 1191–1194

Livesey AE, Sutherland FI, Brown RA, Beck JS, MacGillivray JB, Slidders W (1978) Cytological basis of histological typing of diffuse Hodgkin's disease. Demonstration of an implied misnomer in the terminology of the Rye classification. J Clin Pathol 31: 551–559

Lukes RJ (1971) Criteria for involvement of lymph node, bone marrow, spleen, and liver in Hodgkin's disease. Cancer Res 31: 1755–1767

Lukes RJ, Butler JJ (1966) The pathology and nomenclature of Hodgkin's disease. Cancer Res 26: 1063–1081

Lukes RJ, Collins RD (1974) Immunologic characterization of human malignant lymphomas. Cancer 34: 1488–1503

Lukes RJ, Collins RD (1975) New approaches to the classification of the lymphomata. Br J Cancer [Suppl II] 31: 1–28

Lukes RJ, Tindle BH (1975) Immunoblastic lymphadenopathy: A hyperimmune entity resembling Hodgkin's disease. N Engl J Med 292: 1–8

Lukes RJ, Butler JJ, Hicks EB (1966) Natural history of Hodgkin's disease as related to its pathologic picture. Cancer 19: 317–344

Lukes RJ, Craver LF, Hall TC, Rappaport H, Ruben P (1966a) Report of the nomenclature committee (from Symposium on "Obstacles to the control of Hodgkin's disease"). Cancer Res 26: 1311

MacGillivray JB, Duthie JS (1977) Malignant histiocytosis (histiocytic medullary reticulosis) with spindle cell differentiation and tumour formation. J Clin Pathol 30: 120–155

MacGillivray JB, MacIntosh WG (1978) A case of Lennert's lymphoma. J Clin Pathol 31: 560–566

McKeen EA, Mulvihill JJ, Rosner F, Zarrabi MH (1979) Pregnancy outcome in Hodgkin's disease. Lancet II: 590

MacMahon B (1966) Epidemiology of Hodgkin's disease. Cancer Res 26: 1189–1200

Meijer CJLM, Scheffer E, Lauw GP, Smit AFD, Ottolander GJ den (1978) Skin biopsy in angioimmunoblastic lymphadenopathy. Lancet I: 771–772

Millett YL, Bennett MH, Jelliffe AM, Farrer-Brown G (1969) Nodular sclerotic lymphosarcoma. A further review. Br J Cancer 23: 683–692

Moore RD, Weisberger AS, Bowerfind ES (1957) An evaluation of lymphadenopathy in systemic disease. Arch Intern Med 99: 751–759

Newell GR, Cole SR, Mietinnen OS, MacMahon B (1970) Age differences in the histology of Hodgkin's disease. J Natl Cancer Inst 45: 311–317

Nosanchuk JS, Schnitzer B (1969) Follicular hyperplasia in lymph nodes from patients with rheumatoid arthritis. A clinicopathologic study. Cancer 24: 343–354

Oels HC, Harrison EG, Kiely JM (1968) Lymphoblastic lymphoma with histiocytic phagocytosis ("starry sky" appearance) in adults. Guide to prognosis. Cancer 21: 368–375

Order SE, Hellman S (1972) Pathogenesis of Hodgkin's disease. Lancet I: 571–573

Patchefsky AS, Brodovsky H, Southard M, Menduke H, Gray S, Hoch WS (1973) Hodgkin's disease. A clinical and pathologic study of 235 cases. Cancer 32: 150–161

Patchefsky AS, Brodovsky HS, Menduke H, Southard M, Brooks J, Nicklas D, Hoch WS (1974) Non-Hodgkin's lymphomas: A clinicopathologic study of 293 cases. Cancer 34: 1173–1186

Peckham MJ, Cooper EH (1969) Proliferation characteristics of the various classes of cells in Hodgkin's disease. Cancer 24: 135–146

Qazi A, Aisenberg AC, Long JC (1976) The natural history of nodular lymphoma. Cancer 37: 1923–1927

Rabson SM (1939) Pathologic anatomy of human brucellosis. Am J Clin Pathol 9: 604–614

Rapoport A, Cole P, Mason J (1969) Correlates of survival after initiation of chemotherapy in 142 cases of Hodgkin's disease. Cancer 24: 377–381

Rappaport H (1966) Tumors of the hematopoietic system. Atlas of tumor pathology, sect III, fasc 8. Armed Forces Institute of Pathology, Washington, D.C.

Rappaport H, Moran EM (1975) Angio-immunoblastic (immunoblastic) lymphadenopathy. N Engl J Med 292: 42–43

Rappaport H, Strum SB (1970) Vascular invasion in Hodgkin's disease: its incidence and relationship to the spread of the disease. Cancer 25: 1304–1313

Rappaport H, Winter WJ, Hicks EB (1956) Follicular lymphoma. A re-evaluation of its position in the scheme of malignant lymphoma, based on a survey of 253 cases. Cancer 9: 792–821

Rosai J, Dorfman RF (1972) Sinus histiocytosis with massive lymphadenopathy: A pseudolymphomatous benign disorder. Analysis of 34 cases. Cancer 30: 1174–1188

Rosas-Uribe A, Rappaport H (1972) Malignant lymphoma, histiocytic type with sclerosis (sclerosing reticulum cell sarcoma). Cancer 29: 946–953

Rywlin AM, Recher L, Hoffman EP (1966) Lymphoma-like presentation of Kaposi's sarcoma. Three cases without characteristic skin lesions. Arch Dermatol 93: 554–561

Salvador AH, Harrison EG, Kyle RA (1971) Lymphadenopathy due to infectious mononucleosis: Its confusion with malignant lymphoma. Cancer 27: 1029–1040

Selzer G, Kahn LB, Sealy R (1972) Hodgkin's disease. A clinicopathologic study of 122 cases. Cancer 29: 1090–1100

Sieracki JC, Fisher ER (1970) Diagnostic problems involving nodal lymphomas. Pathol Annu 5: 91–124

Smetana HF (1969) Hodgkin's disease: A follow-up study of patients surviving more than twenty years after the original diagnosis. J Pathol 98: 231–240

Stansfeld AG (1961) The histological diagnosis of toxoplasmic lymphadenitis. J Clin Pathol 14: 565–573

Strum SB, Rappaport H (1970) Hodgkin's disease in the first decade of life. Pediatrics 46: 748–759

Strum SB, Rappaport H (1970a) Significance of focal involvement of lymph nodes for the diagnosis and staging of Hodgkin's disease. Cancer 25: 1314–1319

Strum SB, Rappaport H (1971) The persistence of Hodgkin's disease in long-term survivors. Am J Med 51: 222–240

Strum SB, Rappaport H (1971a) Interrelations of the histologic types of Hodgkin's disease. Arch Pathol 91: 127–134

Strum SB, Park JK, Rappaport H (1970) Observation of cells resembling Sternberg-Reed cells in conditions other than Hodgkin's disease. Cancer 26: 176–190

Strum SB, Hutchison GB, Park JK, Rappaport H (1971) Further observations on the biologic significance of vascular invasion in Hodgkin's disease. Cancer 27: 1–6

Stuart AE, Williams ARW, Habeshaw JA (1977) Rosetting and other reactions of the Reed-Sternberg cell. J Pathol 122: 81–90

Symmers WSC (1968a) Survey of the eventual diagnosis in 600 cases referred for a second histological opinion after an initial biopsy diagnosis of Hodgkin's disease. J Clin Pathol 21: 650–653

Symmers WSC (1968b) Survey of the eventual diagnosis in 226 cases referred for a second histological opinion after an initial biopsy diagnosis of reticulum cell sarcoma. J Clin Pathol 21: 654–655

Symmers WSC (1978) The lymphoreticular system. In: Systemic Pathology, 2nd edn. Churchill, Edinburgh, pp 504–891

Taylor CR (1974) The nature of Reed-Sternberg cells and other malignant "reticulum" cells. Lancet II: 802–807

Tindle BH, Parker JW, Lukes RJ (1972) "Reed-Sternberg" cells in infectious mononucleosis? Am J Clin Pathol 58: 607–617

Turner DR, Wright DJM (1973) Lymphadenopathy in early syphilis. J Pathol 110: 305–308

Tweel JG van den, Lukes RJ, Taylor CR (1979) Pathophysiology of lymphocyte transformation. A study of so-called composite lymphomas. Amer J Clin Pathol 71: 509–520

Wilden JN, Scott CA (1978) A pseudolymphomatous reaction in soft tissue associated with phenytoin sodium. J Clin Pathol 31: 761–764

Williams G, Whittaker JS (1965) Diagnostic problems in biliary duct lymph nodes. J Clin Pathol 18: 43–46

Wilson JF, Marsa GW, Johnson RE (1972) Herpes zoster in Hodgkin's disease: Clinical, histologic and immunologic correlations. Cancer 29: 461–465

Wright CJE (1975) Death from Hodgkin's disease after 18 years' complete remission. Cancer 36: 1132–1137

# 5 Lesions of the Soft Tissues

Prognostic problems posed to the pathologist by overgrowths of the soft tissues and skeletal system are many. Their cause, and the possible consequences of their solution, are easy to state. The normal mesenchymally derived cell is ubiquitous and has many forms, and its reacting and neoplastic equivalents have many more. The neoplastic may be virtually indistinguishable from the non-neoplastic, reactive or reparative, and the malignant neoplastic from the benign neoplastic; while even lesions that are unanimously acceptable as histologically malignant may behave in a quite unpredictable way. Nowhere in the histopathology of tumourous growths is there such nebulous nosology, and the array of terms is bewildering. In practical terms, the pathologist faces a considerable risk of both under-diagnosing and over-diagnosing: with many of the lesions commonly sited in a limb, and amputation still perhaps the only hopeful treatment, the consequences of a wrong diagnosis may be grave.

Preceding chapters have cited series of neoplasms of various kinds where retrospective review has produced many revised diagnoses; for example, a lymph node once diagnosed as showing Hodgkin's disease now regarded as innocent. The same holds for reviews of lesions originally regarded as sarcomas in soft tissue and in the skeletal system. With these tissues, however, there is a twofold difference: (a) lesions of intermediate malignancy exist, such as the fibromatoses, that infiltrate and recur but almost never metastasise, which have few counterparts in epithelium and lymphatic tissue, and (b) many forms of spindle-celled overgrowth, sometimes highly aberrant, have been found by patient observation to be not sarcomas but, to general surprise, benign, i.e. morphologically 'pseudo-sarcomas'.

Amongst series of cases subjected to diagnosis on review was that of Pritchard and his colleagues (1974) in which, of 330 lesions diagnosed originally as fibrosarcoma, 113 were later excluded 'because of . . . a revised diagnosis': of these 113, 79 were some other form of malignant neoplasm, the remaining 34 presumably benign (in retrospect, a diagnostic false-positive rate of 34/330 or just over 10%). A series of 50 'soft tissue sarcomas' was analysed by Dahl (1976), and of these 32 were re-diagnosed as atypical fibroxanthoma. Reports of the over-diagnosis of skeletal lesions as sarcomas are less common but individual instances of the over-diagnosis of osteosarcoma are not rare (in one such case described by Kahn and his associates [1969] the patient refused the recommended disarticulation of a lower limb and was well 6 years after curettage of the osteolytic femoral lesion later re-diagnosed as an aneurysmal bone cyst). One of the few series identifying such instances is that wherein McKenna and co-workers (1966) reviewed their cases of sarcomas of the osteogenic series. The total with adequate clinical and pathological data was 657: the diagnosis was changed to a malignant lesion of some other kind in 67, to a non-malignant lesion in 32 (a diagnostic false-positive rate of 5%). In all, the amount of over-treatment that results from over-diagnosis of this kind is probably not great. The impression gained from a modest reading of the literature, and from general enquiry and experience, is that amputation is rarely used as first treatment for a lesion diagnosed as a fibrosarcoma or indeed any other type of sarcoma of the soft tissues, and even the recurrent lesion has to be particularly extensive or destructive before this is done. Local excision is almost always given every chance. In the occasional case, amputation (or some comparably radical procedure such as removal of an eye or carotid vessels) is what in retrospect might have saved the patient's life but to minimise the slender risk of metastasis by always amputating would be quite unacceptable. With lesions in bone, again the risk of over-treatment is probably small: it is hard to believe that a responsible pathologist would not, when in doubt, minimise the risk by seeking the help of a colleague or colleagues with specialist experience.

## Local Series

In comparison with the number of problems raised by epithelial overgrowths as a whole in the local series, those raised by comparable lesions of the soft tissues, a total of 36, have been few. In view of the much greater amount of soft tissue there is in the body than epithelium, this may be surprising but only until we consider overall figures for mortality from carcinomas and sarcomas. In the UK, for example, taking into account notified malignant neoplasms of the gastrointestinal tract only, deaths registered in England and Wales in 1973 were 39,300: for all malignant neoplasms of 'connective and other soft tissue' the figure was 309 (Registrar General, 1973). The number of cases identified in the local series as presenting a borderline problem was 36: in 9 of these the original diagnosis had been sarcoma of some form. For comparison, during the same period the number of patients, including the above 9, diagnosed in the same hospital as having a nonvisceral, soft-tissue sarcoma was 51 (these included 10 of indeterminable type, and 3 where the question 'carcinoma or sarcoma?' could not be answered). The broad nature of the problems is shown below.

### SUMMARISED TOTALS

### Fibroblastic Lesions

In 15 patients the lesions were basically fibroblastic. In two, the lesions were under-diagnosed: in Case 5.2, the pattern was found on review to be characteristically that of a dermatofibrosarcoma protuberans (DFSP) rather than a 'cellular

fibroma' but even correct identification at the time would have made no significant difference to the treatment: in Case 5.15, recurrent growth within 4 weeks of a mass on the leg of a 12-year-old girl was certainly fibrosarcoma whereas the original lesion had been diagnosed as, again, a 'cellular fibroma'. Even on review, the original lesion still seems borderline and, as such, is quite unlikely to have led at the time to amputation even if the preferred diagnosis had been fibrosarcoma. A further recurrence virtually demanded below-knee amputation, and there has been no trouble since. This is in keeping with the generally better prognosis that fibrosarcoma has in children than in adults.

Two lesions were over-diagnosed. In Case 5.17, a nodule of plantar fibromatosis was diagnosed as fibrosarcoma. The advice offered simultaneously with the diagnosis, namely, that excision might prove adequate treatment, informed the surgeon that the lesion was one of marginal malignancy; it also proved sound. The over-diagnosis in Case 5.22 was minimally significant in practice. Warning that the myxoid lesion could well recur was (now recognisably) needless; it was an area of nodular fasciitis.

The diagnosis in four cases was inappropriate but innocuously so. Two 'myomas' and a 'neuro-naevus' are now identifiably of the dermatofibroma/histiocytoma family. The fourth lesion, a markedly polymorphic but mitotically inactive spindle-celled mass, now seems much more appropriately diagnosable as a degenerative myoma.

The remaining lesions were correctly diagnosed but had all given rise to some prognostic concern, as, for example, with a recurrent dermatofibrosarcoma, recurrent digital fibroma, a persistently progressive desmoid, and a haematoma-sarcoma.

### Synovial Lesions

In 8 of the 12 cases comprising this group, the problem was essentially that caused by nodular synovitis, its certain recognition and its implications. None had led to amputation, of even a digit, and there have been no sequelae even with one (Case 5.5) where excision was almost certainly incomplete. Case 5.6 gave a useful lesson on how mitotically active such tissue may be yet still be innocuous. This observation cannot be allowed general relevance; it means only that in nodular synovitis the allowance to be given to mitotic activity can be generous.

The lesion in Case 5.29 showed quite fortuitously that immediate amputation is not always mandatory to save life from a synoviosarcoma. The 3½-year interval between initial biopsy and amputation was owed solely to the fact that the lesion in the popliteal fossa was thought very possibly to be metastatic carcinoma: as became clear eventually, the pattern was an expression of the carcinomatoid moiety of the pseudo-carcinosarcomatous differentiation that most synovial sarcomas show somewhere.

In Case 5.30 a lower limb had to be lost. The initial diagnosis was villo-nodular synovitis, and there is no reason on re-examination of the sections to doubt the correctness of this. However, tissue removed later was held to show synoviosarcoma. This sequence of events would in many circumstances lead to amputation but in this particular patient, even without the change in diagnosis, the limb could not, for simple anatomical reasons, be saved. The patient's continued survival in good health adds to a suspicion that the monstrous synovial overgrowth was a basically benign villo-nodular synovitis throughout.

The patient in Case 5.31 whose lesion of foot was either a synoviosarcoma or, more probably, an extra-skeletal Ewing's sarcoma-like tumour, as described by Angervall and Enzinger (1975), is still alive 12 years after a below-knee amputation. Whichever of the two diagnoses is correct, his survival (with neither radiotherapy nor chemotherapy) is equally unexpected since, of the 35 affected patients traced by Angervall and Enzinger, 22 had died of the neoplasm. Even if anatomically practicable, which it was not, and despite the favourable outcome with the synoviosarcoma in Case 5.29, local excision would have been discouraged on this occasion: the below-knee amputation was optimum treatment, and the patient was spared the rigours of chemotherapy.

### Fatty Lesions

There were two liposarcomas in the series. One, Case 5.28, was initially under-diagnosed as a 'myxoid fibroma'. There was a double mistake here. First, such fatty tissue as was present in the original biopsy was not abundant and was accepted as no more than that expected in subcutaneous tissue; it is even yet difficult to identify it as certainly part of the neoplasm. Second, the mitotic incidence was underestimated. As noted later, the incidence would have been better assessed in terms of mitotic figures per hundreds of cells, not per tens or hundreds of hpfs. Even if the lesion had been diagnosed as sarcoma, it is doubtful, in view of the general reluctance to amputate as first treatment, whether the possibly life-saving amputation would have been carried out after the first biopsy. It no doubt would have been carried out when the lesion recurred 2 years later but by that time the inguinal nodes were already widely involved.

The second case, Case 5.32, was a retroperitoneal lesion of characteristically recurrent type. It probably did shorten the life of the patient; nevertheless she achieved 78 years.

### Reparative Lesions

Reparative reactions caused two of the seven over-diagnoses, one (Case 5.25) comprising exuberant tissue that grew at the site of removal of a prolapsed lumbar disc 3 weeks earlier, the other (Case 5.35) similarly exuberant tissue that appeared 13 months after excision from beside the tibio-fibular joint of a synovial cyst or 'ganglion'. At least in the first case the paravertebral mass, even if regarded as neoplastic, was regarded as benign (though, in retrospect, it would have been a strange neurilemmoma that grew so large in 3 weeks). The mass was considered to have been excised in toto, and an expectant policy was adopted, correctly as events turned out. In the second case, despite the preferred diagnosis of synoviosarcoma, the borderline nature of the decision and discussion about this with the surgeon led again to an expectant policy, again justified by later events. Extruded material of synovial origin or association does at times appear to stimulate a significantly desmoplastic and mitogenic activity.

In Case 5.23, a lesion believed to be essentially reparative, was an area of proliferative myositis. However, since trauma sometimes seems certainly concerned in the genesis of this condition and is difficult to exclude with assurance in all others—unless a cause is seen as obvious as the *Trichinella spiralis* mentioned by Enzinger and Dulcey (1967)—the diagnostic error here was an imprecision semantic rather than patho-logically significant.

Insofar as myositis ossificans may be regarded as a reparative reaction, the single example that caused concern (Case 5.24) may be included in this group. Only familiarity with the varied tissue patterns of the lesion can minimise the risks of over-diagnosis as a sarcoma.

### Other Lesions

Two of the remaining lesions were malignant mesenchymomas. The first (Case 5.26) was initially under-diagnosed as a 'cellular lipo-myxoma' and killed by metastasis 5½ years later. The first recurrence, within 6 months, was diagnosed as sarcoma, and it is difficult to under-stand now why amputation was not performed then or, if not then, why not after either of the further recurrences 3 years and 4 years later. Perhaps the patient was utterly adamant in refusal; at any rate, the ultimate decisions were jointly those of surgeon and patient.

The second patient (Case 5.27) was fortunate in having a pelvic malignant mesenchymoma of restricted malignancy. Its recurrence 4 years after excision was discovered at routine follow-up examination: further excision, this time supple-mented by radiotherapy, has gained 8 years trouble-free survival to date.

The lesion in the remaining patient (Case 5.33), a 'granular cell myoblastoma', was not per se dangerous but stimulated a warning of possi-ble recurrence because of seemingly inadequate removal. Its nonrecurrence supported the view that, as with most such lesions, the mass was not neoplastic but degenerative.

Review has yielded:
Underdiagnoses, 4
Overdiagnoses, 7
Inappropriate diagnoses, 5
Appropriate diagnoses, 20
The 36 cases regrouped in this way comprise Table 5.1.

### Case Data

### Case 5.1

M (47 years) with mass that had grown slowly on anterior abdominal wall over the past 6 years, now 4 × 3 × 3 cm.

The lesion was reported as a "cellular fibroma, the deep aspect of which extends to the line of excision". As shown in Figs. 5.1 and 5.2, it had the typically storiform pattern of a 'dermato-fibrosarcoma protuberans' (DFSP). Mitoses were extremely few.

The lesion recurred and was 9 × 7 × 7 cm when further excised 10 years later. Micro-scopically it was virtually identical with the initial mass. The patient died after a further 7 years, without recurrence, from an unrelated cause.

This was a marginal *under-diagnosis*, marginal to the extent that the likely transection of the lesion had at least been reported. Had this been acted upon, and immediate re-excision been performed, there might not have been a recurrence.

### Case 5.2

M (12 years) with a lump on the volar aspect of the upper forearm, noticed during the past 4 months. It was excised, 18 × 10 × 10 mm, and found to be a highly cellular, pleomorphic, spindle-celled neoplasm.

The whole of the mass, with overlying skin, is seen in Fig. 5.3. It had been cleared by the line of resection around the left margin, though by barely 1 mm in the fixed and processed prepara-tion, but had been transected along the lower margin. The area of greater density, in the centre, indicates the area of highest cellularity.

Figure 5.4 shows the general spindle-celled character with, in this area, something of a fasciculate pattern but nowhere was it distinc-tively storiform. In the central area the cells were more crowded and, as seen in Fig. 5.5, showed a marked polymorphism (nuclear diam-eter varying by a factor of 4); mitotic figures in this area were numerous with a maximum in-cidence, in places, of 3 per hpf (Fig. 5.6).

The lesion was diagnosed as 'dermatofibro-sarcoma' with a comment on the probable in-completeness of excision.

The area of the lesion was further excised 3 weeks later; the excised mass included skin, with an original well-healed scar, and a thin layer of skeletal muscle on the deep surface. Microscopy of a central 10 × 8 × 5 mm nodule showed recurrent or remnant sarcomatous tissue.

There has been no further trouble and the

**Table 5.1.** Thirty-six cases of equivocal lesions of soft tissues.

| Case No. | Diagnosis on review | Treatment | Outcome |
|---|---|---|---|
| *4 cases under-diagnosed* | | | |
| 5.1 | DFSP > 'cellular fibroma' | Excision × 2 | Unrelated death @ 7 yr |
| 5.15 | Fibrosarcoma > 'highly cellular fibroma' | Excision × 2: amputation | Alive @ 22 yr |
| 5.26 | Malignant mesenchymoma > 'lipomyxoma' | Excision: amputation | Death @ 6 yr |
| 5.28 | Liposarcoma > 'myxoid fibroma' | Excision: re-excision + r/th | Death @ 5 yr |
| *7 cases over-diagnosed* | | | |
| 5.8 | Nodular tenosynovitis > osteoclastoma | Excision, probably incomplete | Alive @ 9 yr |
| 5.9 | Nodular tenosynovitis > 'myxoid fibroma' | Excision | Alive @ 8 yr |
| 5.17 | Plantar fibromatosis > 'fibromyxoma' | Excision + r/th: re-excision | Alive @ 12 yr |
| 5.22 | Nodular faciitis > 'fibromyxoma' | Excision | Alive @ 9 yr |
| 5.25 | Reparative > neurilemmoma | Excision | Alive @ 8 yr |
| 5.30 | Nodular synovitis > synoviosarcoma | Excision: amputation | Alive @ 11 yr |
| 5.35 | Reparative > synoviosarcoma | Excision | Alive @ 9 yr |
| *5 cases inappropriately diagnosed* | | | |
| 5.3 | Dermatofibroma > neuronevus | Excision, incomplete | Alive @ 22 yr |
| 5.4 | Dermatofibroma > myoma | Amputation (phalanx) | Alive @ 16 yr |
| 5.7 | Histiocytoma > myoma | Excision, probably incomplete | Alive @ 5 yr |
| 5.23 | Prolif. myositis > reparative | Excision | Alive @ 8 yr |
| 5.34 | Myoma > fibroma | Excision | Alive @ 12 yr |
| *20 cases appropriately diagnosed* | | | |
| 5.2 | Dermatofibrosarcoma | Excision × 2 | Alive @ 8 yr |
| 5.5 | Nodular tenosynovitis | Excision, probably incomplete | Alive @ 10 yr |
| 5.6 | Nodular tenosynovitis | Excision | Alive @ 12 yr |
| 5.10/5.14 | Nodular tenosynovitis | Excision | Alive 12 to 20 yr |
| 5.16 | Neurofibrosarcoma | Excision + r/th | Alive @ 11 yr |
| 5.18 | Fibrosarcoma | Amputation | Alive @ 20 yr |
| 5.19 | Recurrent digital fibroma | Excisions + partial amputation + r/th | Stabilised @ 20 yr |
| 5.20 | Fibromatosis | Excision × 2, still ? complete | Alive @ 6 yr |
| 5.21 | Desmoid tumour | Many excisions | Death @ 12 yr |
| 5.24 | Myositis ossificans | Excision | Alive @ 11 yr |
| 5.27 | Mesenchymoma | Excision: re-excision + r/th | Alive @ 12 yr |
| 5.29 | Synovial sarcoma | Excision, amputation | Alive @ 13 yr |
| 5.31 | Synovial sarcoma (still some doubt) | Amputation | Alive @ 12 yr |
| 5.32 | Liposarcoma | Multiple excisions | Death @ 24 yr |
| 5.33 | Granular cell myoblastoma | Excision, probably incomplete | Alive @ 11 yr |
| 5.36 | Neurofibroma, later fibrosarcoma | Excision × 2 | Alive @ 14 yr |

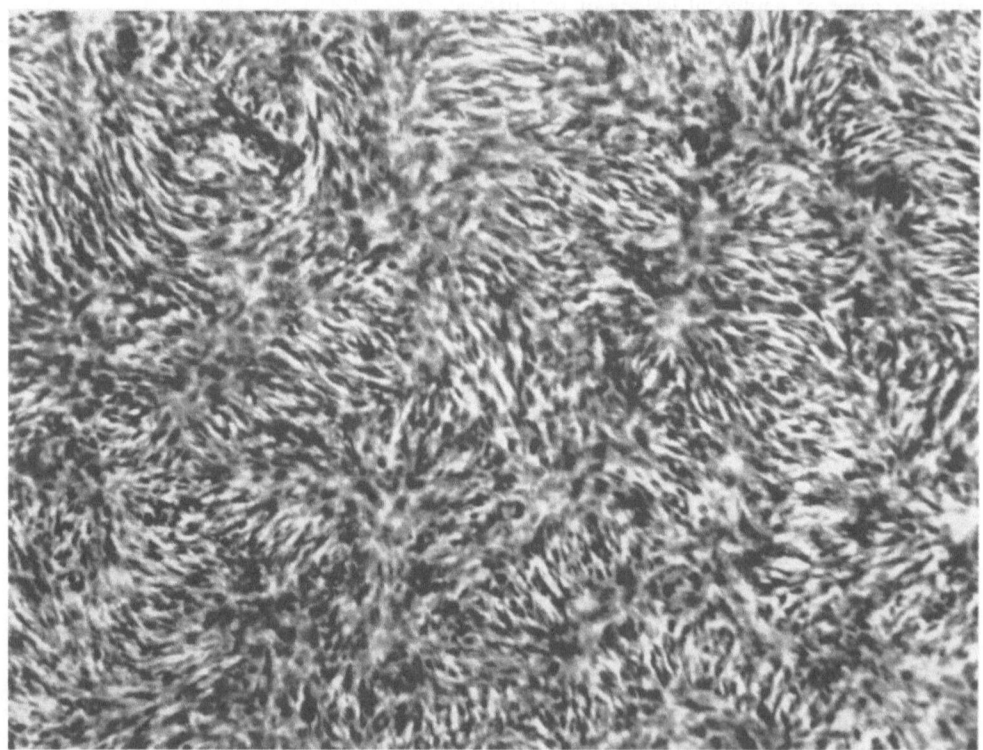

**Fig. 5.1.** The typically whirligig or storiform pattern of DFSP. H & E, × 246

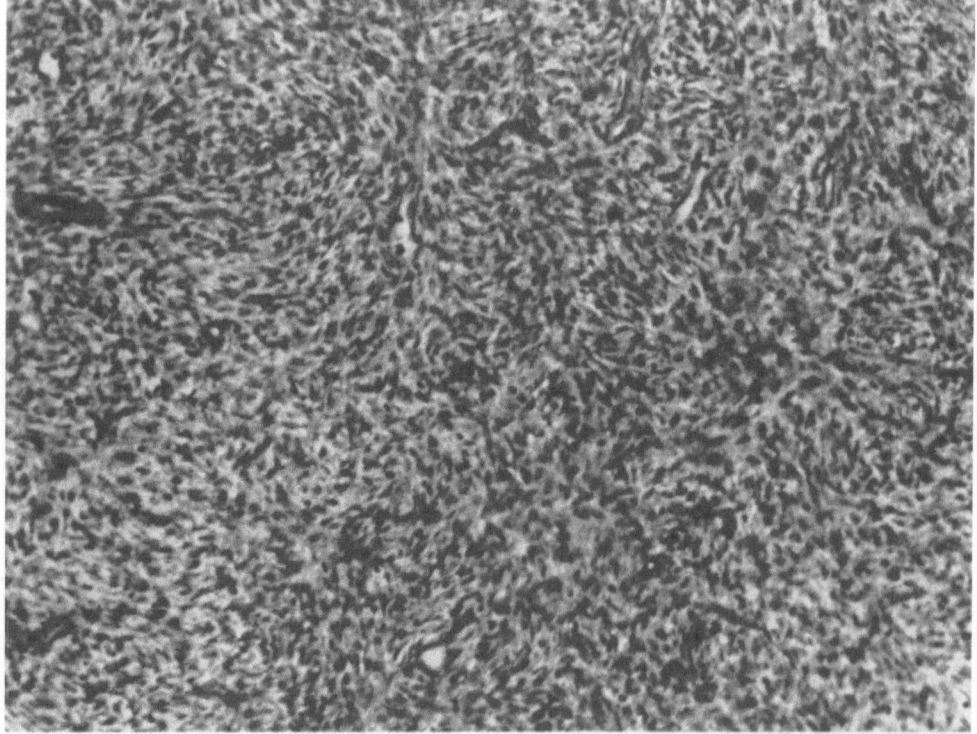

**Fig. 5.2.** Another area from the same lesion as Fig. 5.1 where a storiform pattern is hard to discern. Had sampling been inadequate, only diagnostically uncertain tissue such as this might have been seen. H & E, × 246

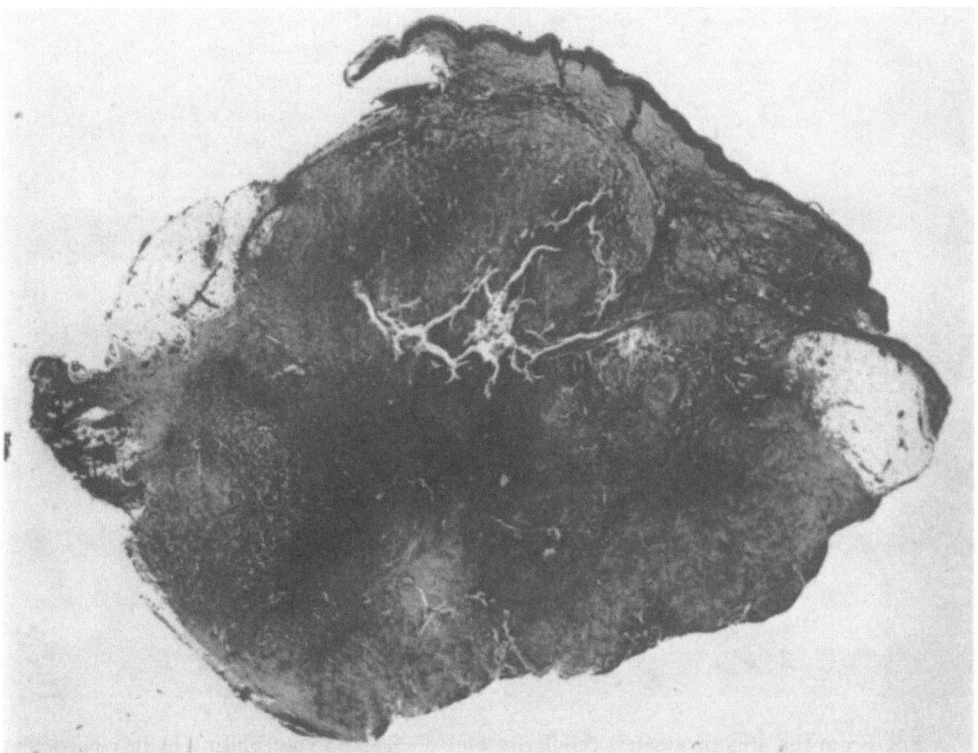

**Fig. 5.3.** A mass of highly cellular tissue, transected along the lower edge. H & E, × 10

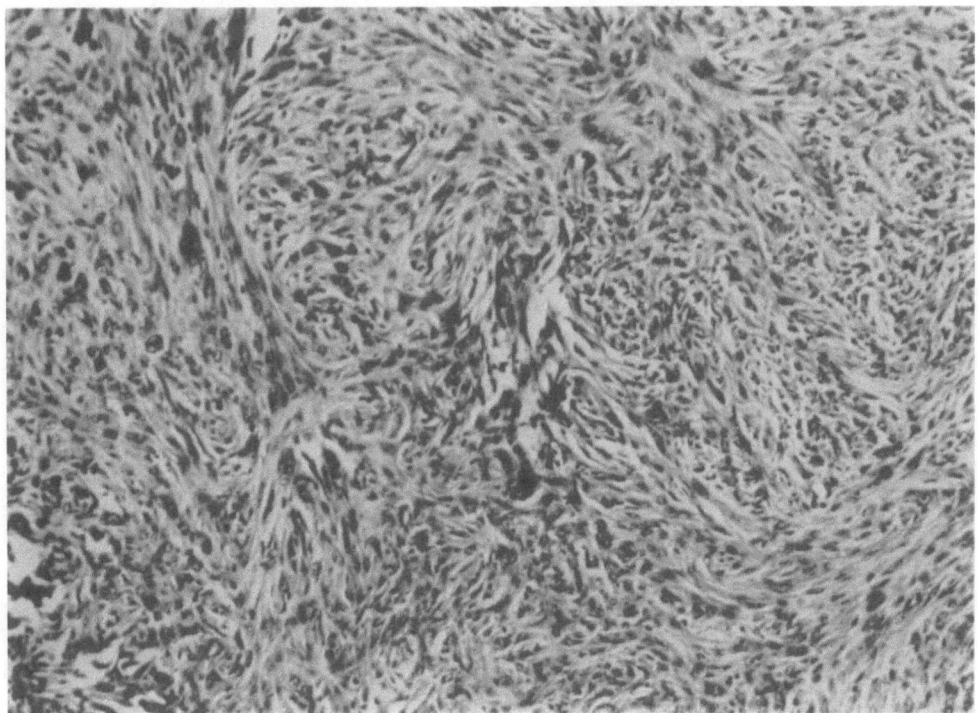

**Fig. 5.4.** The cells are of spindle form and have a notably fasciculate though not classically storiform pattern. H & E, × 140

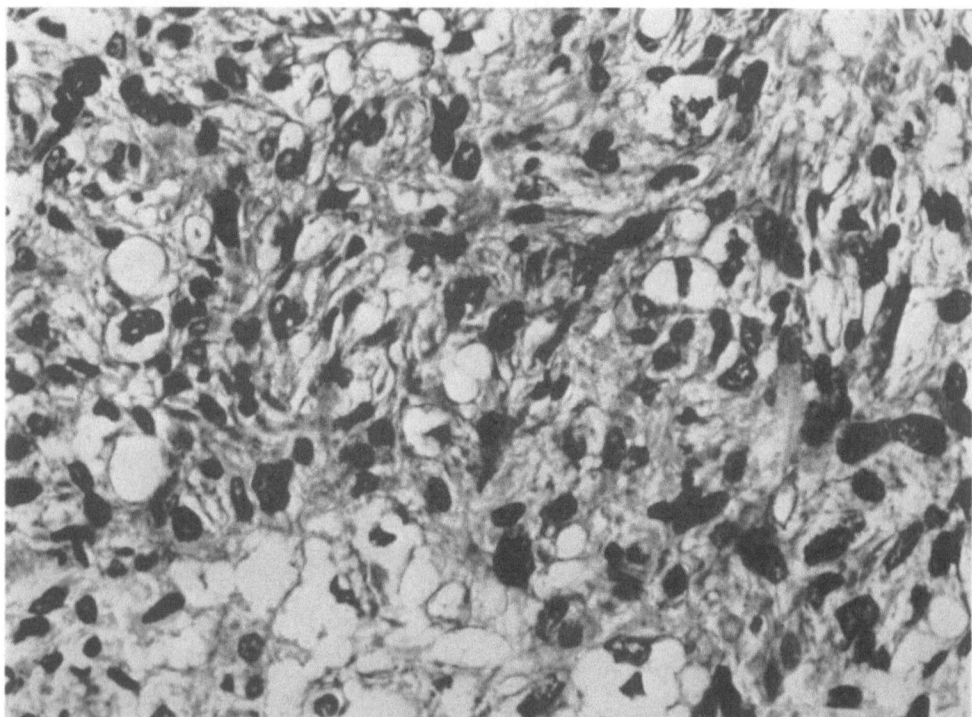

**Fig. 5.5.** From the area of greatest cellularity and nuclear polymorphism: in this particular field the growth was mildly myxoid. H & E, × 476

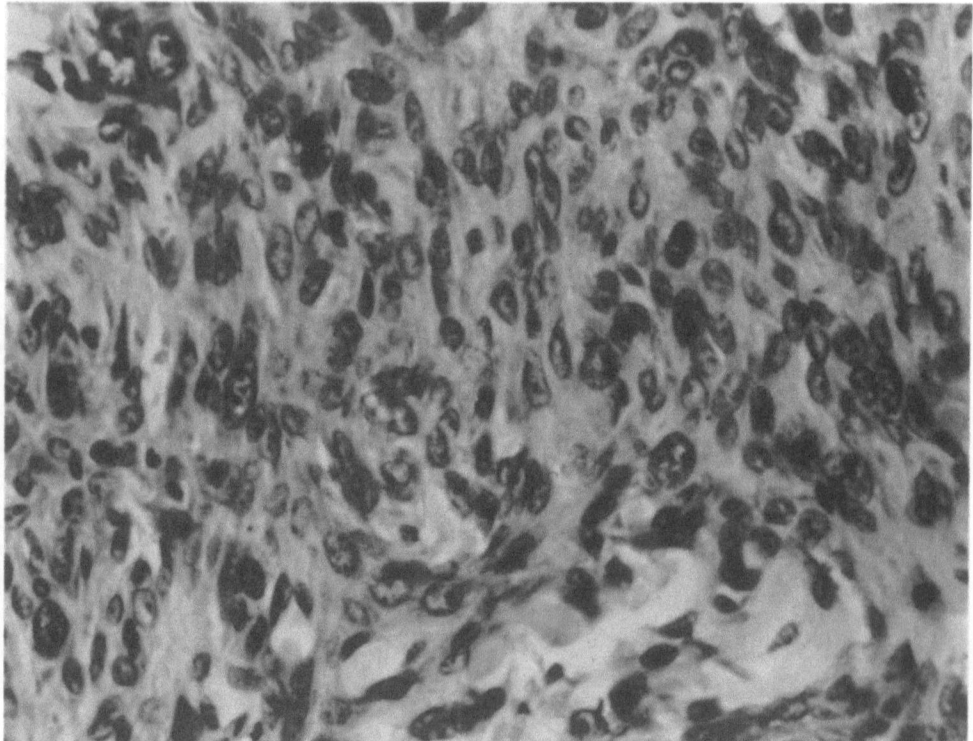

**Fig. 5.6.** The cells here are less hyperchromatic but still vary much in size. There is a mitotic figure in lower right-hand corner. H & E, × 493

area of involvement remains healthy 8 years later. It seemed clear that, at the time of the first operation, whatever tissue had been left in situ had not had the form of a 10 × 8 mm nodule: there had therefore been an appreciable degree of new growth during the short interval to the second operation. Any expressed hope that any remnant tissue would have regressed would have been unfulfilled.

*Pace* the relationship of lesions of this kind to the 'histiocytoma', the diagnosis may reasonably be regarded as *appropriate*. The absence of a typically storiform pattern was possibly the reason why the nodule was not diagnosed as DFSP.

### Case 5.3

M (16 years) with a diffuse swelling in skin over posterior aspect of shoulder. It was excised and formed a central thickening in a 4 × 2 cm ellipse of skin 4 mm deep.

Initial sections across the summit of the swelling showed a rather gyriform spindle-celled mass extending from the deep line of resection to, and

seemingly blending with, the basal layer of the epidermis. The epidermis here was relatively pale-staining, hyperkeratotic and flattened. By contrast, sections from beyond the summit of the swelling showed an entirely normal epidermis with sharply defined basal layer (Figs. 5.7, 5.8). The blending of spindle-cells and basal-cells was so intimate (Fig. 5.9) as to suggest the possibility of spindle-celled naevus, and a form of 'neuro-naevus' was suggested as the likeliest diagnosis. For his interest and comments, a section had been sent to the late Dr Pierre Masson who replied that the lesion was in no respect a naevus but a 'recurrent dermatofibrosarcoma of Darier'.

As in the previous case (Case 5.2) only the lack of a fully-developed storiform pattern stands in the way of diagnosis as a DFSP; some might still consider this a proper diagnosis, others prefer dermatofibroma or fibrous histiocytoma. At any rate, the original diagnosis was *inappropriate*.

Despite the evident transection of the mass on its deep surface there was no recurrence; the area was trouble-free 20 years later.

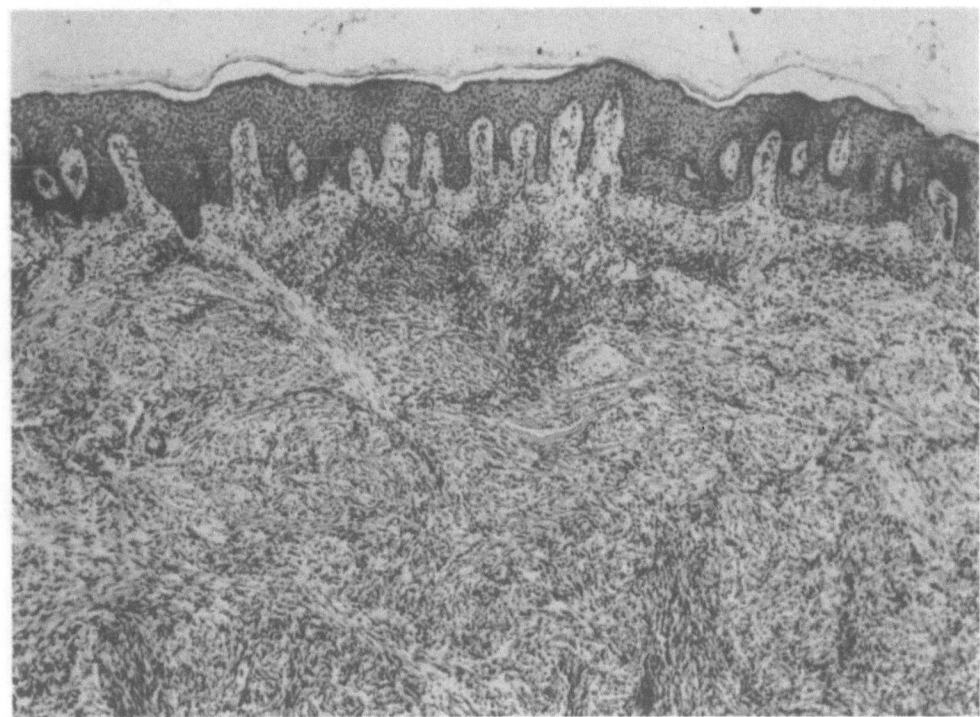

**Fig. 5.7.** Part of a quite highly cellular spindle-celled overgrowth covered by essentially normal epidermis. H & E, × 60

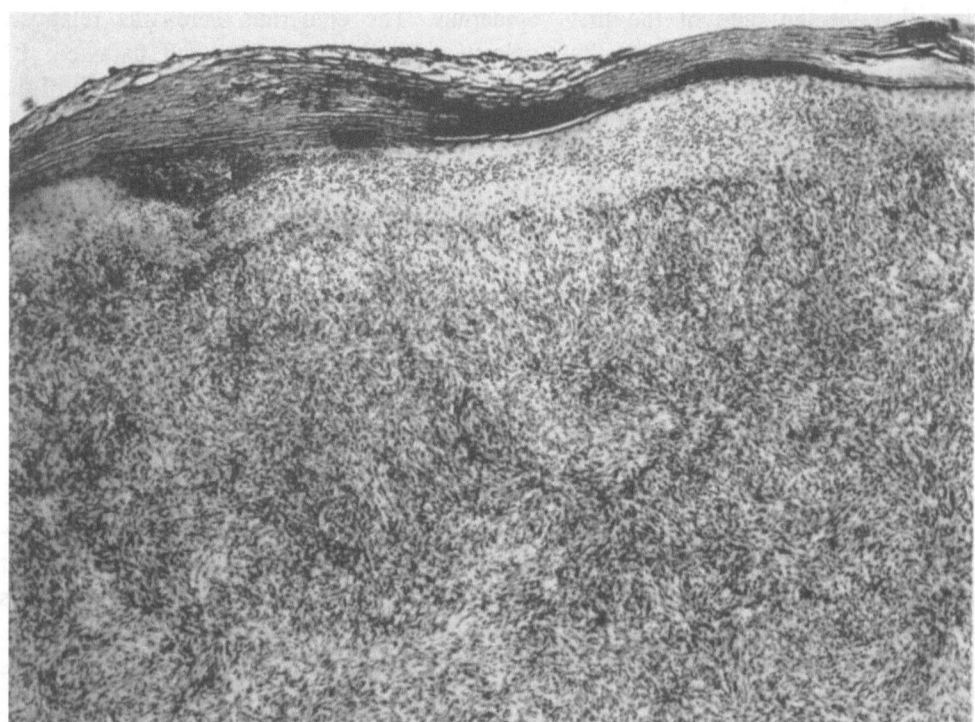

**Fig. 5.8.** In an adjacent area, the basal layer of the epidermis merges almost indistinguishably with the spindle-celled tissue. H & E, × 60

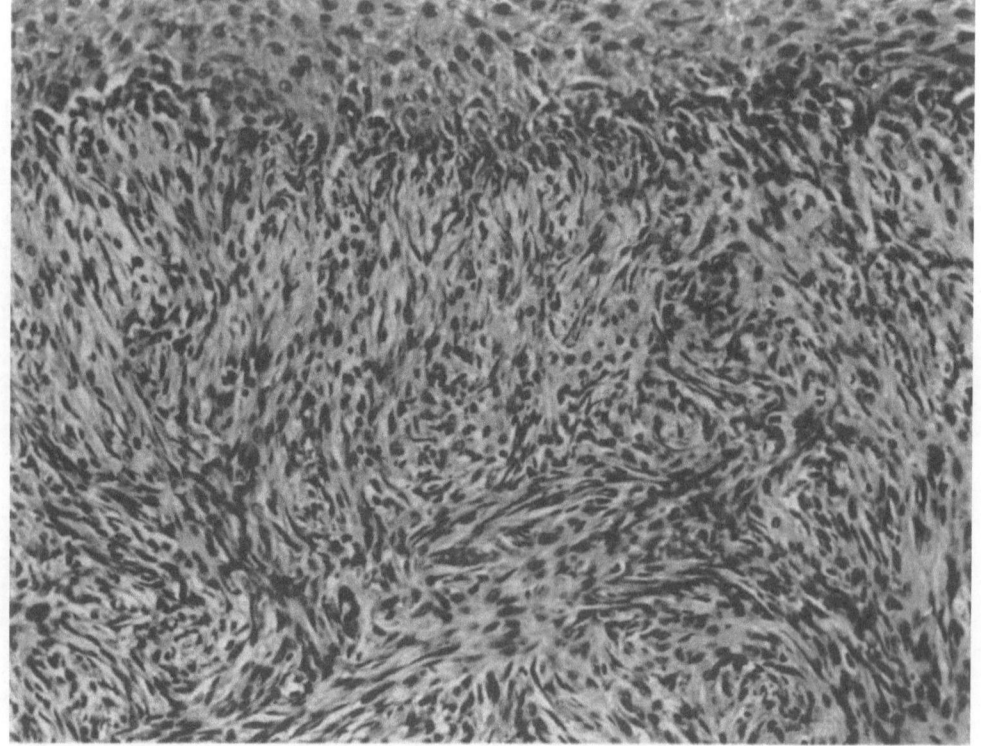

**Fig. 5.9.** The smooth mergence of basal epidermis and fibroblastic mass. H & E, × 238

The unusual overlying epidermal change would seem to be but one of the expressions of abnormal behaviour epidermis may show when covering a histiocytoma. In his examination of 457 dermal histiocytomas, Schoenfeld (1964) found "some tendency toward atypical epidermal proliferation" in as many as 231. Such changes may closely simulate, inter alia, seborrhoeic keratosis, keratoacanthoma and even basal-cell carcinoma.

*Case 5.4*

M (32 years) with painful swelling beneath left ring finger-nail, which had increased over previous 10 months. The nail was raised by an obvious mass that also protruded forwards and occupied much of the pulp of the distal phalanx. Clinically, the mass appeared obviously neoplastic and amputation was performed through the metacarpo-phalangeal joint.

Dissection showed the mass, firm and white, to be 15 × 10 × 5 mm, lying as an oval disc between the nail bed and phalangeal bone, and projecting beyond the end of the nail (Fig. 5.10).

The lesion was a fasciculate spindle-celled growth (Fig. 5.11) mildly polymorphic and mitotically active to the extent of approximately 1 figure per 6 hpf; no certainly aberrant forms were seen. The feature that caused most concern was the almost total infiltration of the bone by the neoplasm (Fig. 5.12): this highly invasive capacity had obviously been countered by the amputation but its significance vis-à-vis metastasis remained uncertain. The lesion was diagnosed as a 'myoma cutis'.

The patient has remained trouble-free for 16 years. Despite the highly infiltrative character of the lesion, and the consequent opportunity at any rate for metastasis, metastasis had not occurred. To that extent diagnosis of the lesion as benign was justified. However, recent examination of further sections has shown occasional multinucleated giant cells of typically Touton type. This feature, in conjunction with the almost storiform pattern in some areas, suggests that the lesion was rather a dermatofibroma or 'fibrous histiocytoma'. The original diagnosis was thus probably *inappropriate* but innocuously so.

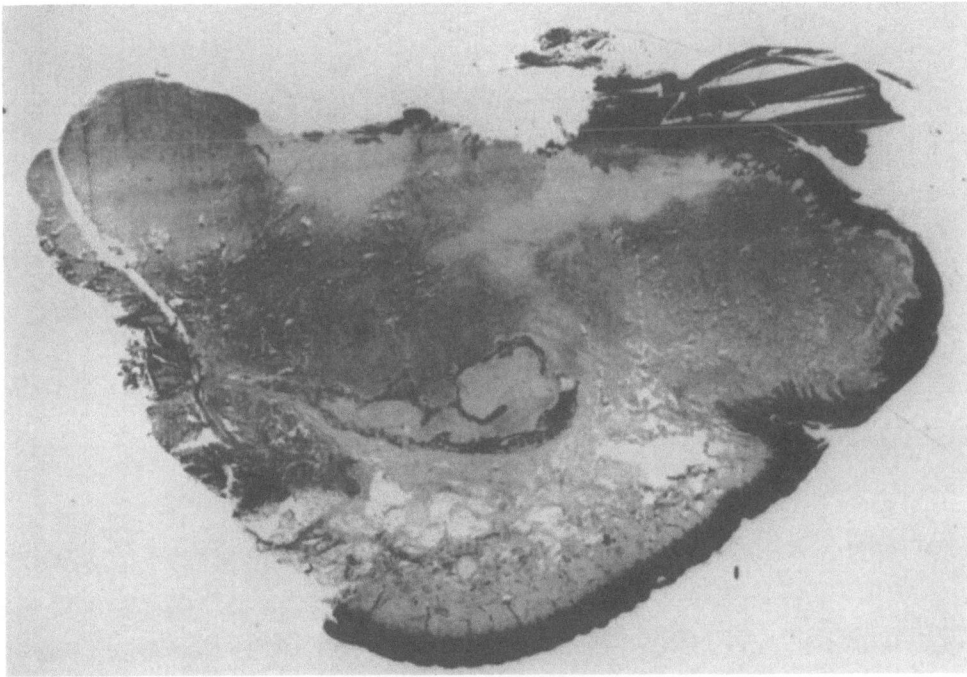

**Fig. 5.10.** An oval mass of highly cellular tissue lying between the splintered remnants of nail (*above*) and the normally thick digital epidermis (*right* and *below*). Part of the phalangeal bone lies in the centre. H & E, × 7

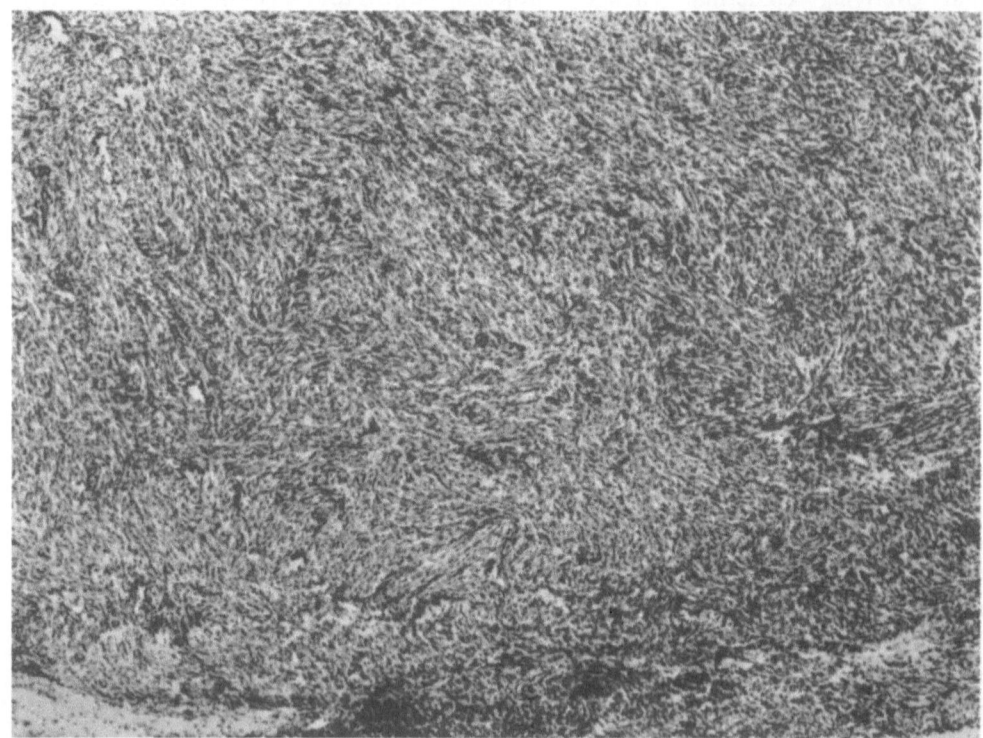

**Fig. 5.11.** The general highly cellular, fasciculate pattern. H & E, × 62

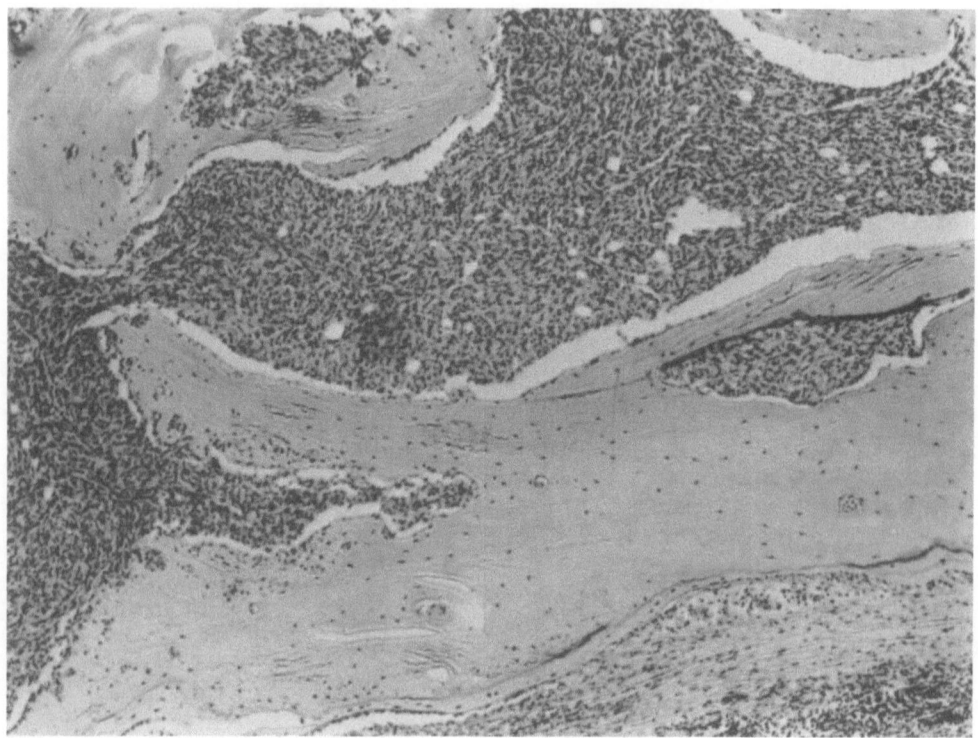

**Fig. 5.12.** Extensive permeation of bone by the neoplasm. H & E, × 62

### Case 5.5

M (37 years) with painful nodule on medial side of sole, clinically a localised thickening of the plantar fascia. The mass was poorly defined but apparently completely removed by the excision of a block of tissue 5 × 2 × 2 cm. Dissection showed a moderately well-circumscribed central nodule, clearly demarcated from skeletal muscle on one side, and gradually merging with the plantar fascial fibrous tissue on the other (Fig. 5.13).

The mass was quite highly vascular. In Fig. 5.14, virtually all the lumina belong to blood vessels. The degree of cellularity varied but was relatively high focally, when the cells were notably polymorphic and, as seen in Fig. 5.15, mitotically active. Scanty multinucleated giant cells were also present.

The true nature of the lesion was uncertain as was the prognosis in terms of risk of local recurrence (the question of sarcoma did not arise). There were morphological features of both angioma and 'nodular tenosynovitis ('giant-cell tumour of tendon sheath')' and the second of these was the diagnosis made.

It was doubtful if excision had been complete but there was no further trouble; the patient was known to be well and quite without disability 10 years later. The diagnosis was *appropriate* even if nowadays there might be a preference for 'fibrous histiocytoma'.

### Case 5.6

F (32 years) with painful locking of right knee over past 18 months. A 4 × 4 × 2 cm mass of tissue was removed from the joint capsule.

The lesion was clearly a so-called 'giant-cell tumour of tendon sheath' (fibrous histiocytoma etc.). It was highly cellular with its cells infiltrating widely into surrounding fat (Fig. 5.16). Multinucleated giant cells were frequent (Fig. 5.17) as were deposits of haemosiderin. Thus far there was no problem. What did cause concern was the high cellularity of the tissue and, in particular, its high rate of mitotic activity. In the most cellular areas, mitoses had an average

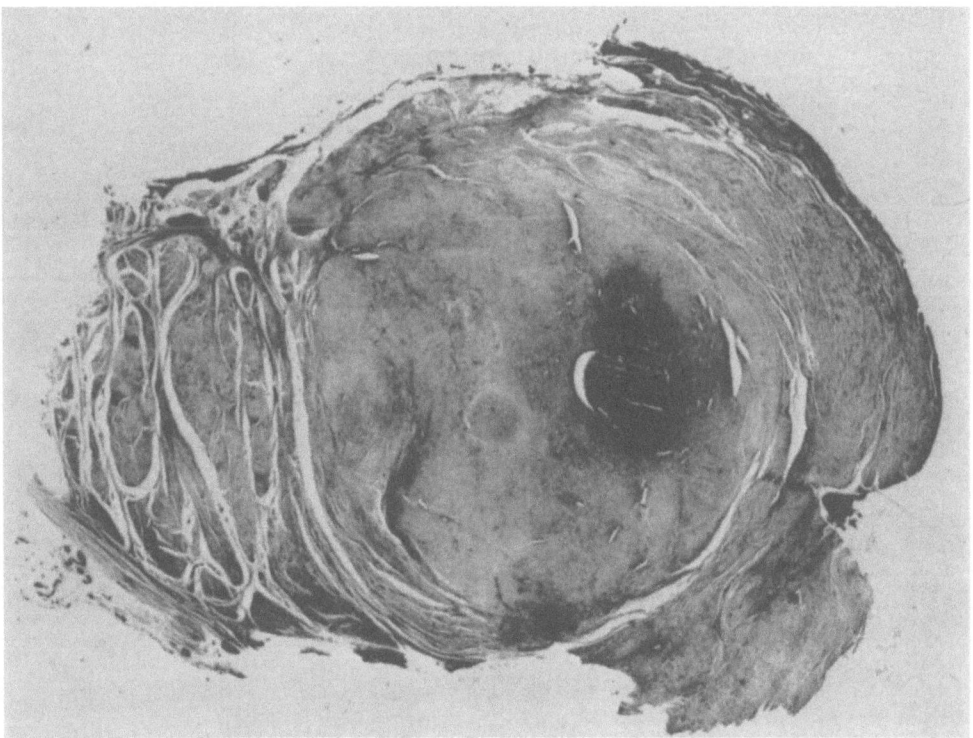

**Fig. 5.13.** A nodule of tissue lying between plantar muscles (*left*) and plantar fascia (*right*). H & E, × 12

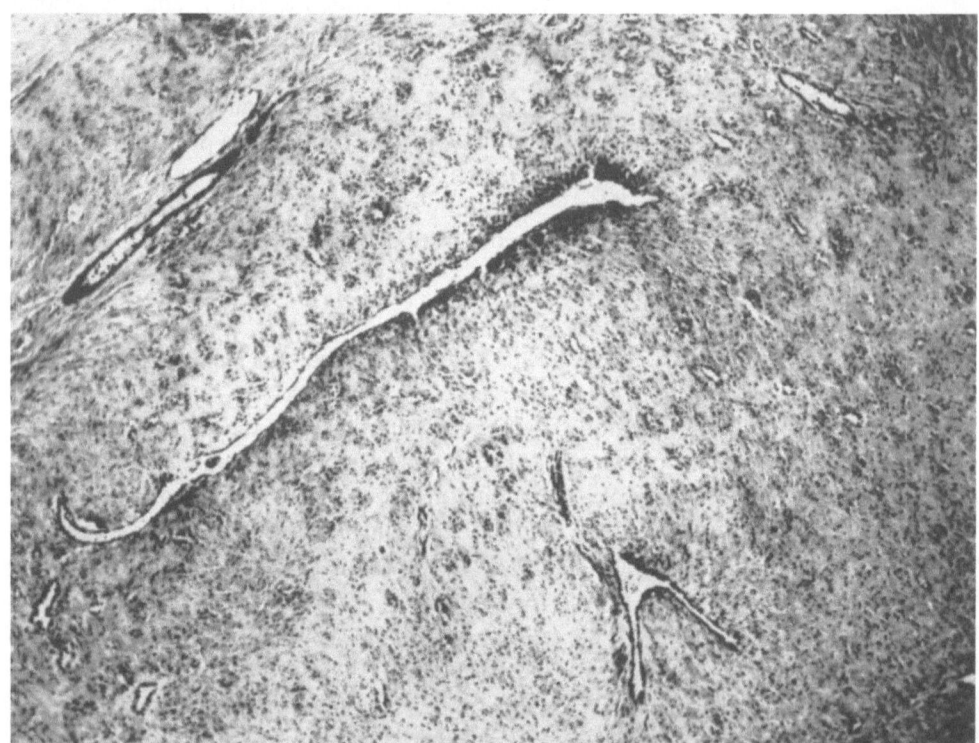

**Fig. 5.14.** An area where numerous vascular channels are producing an angiomatoid pattern. H & E, × 62

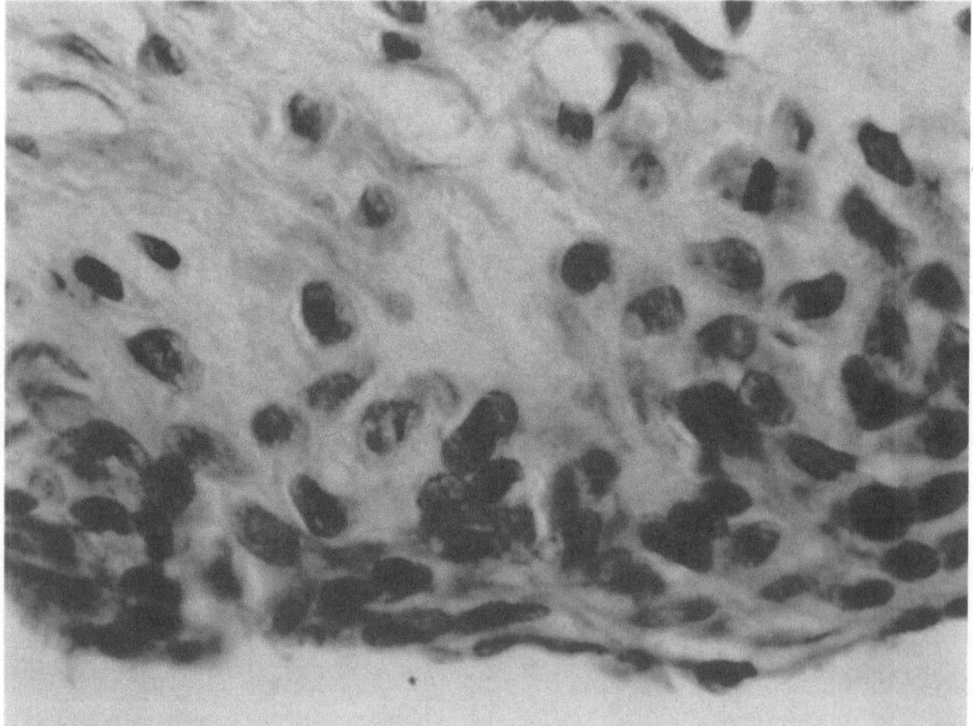

**Fig. 5.15.** Rather hyperchromatic cells adjacent to the lumen of a vessel. A cell at top right-hand corner is in mitosis. H & E, × 985

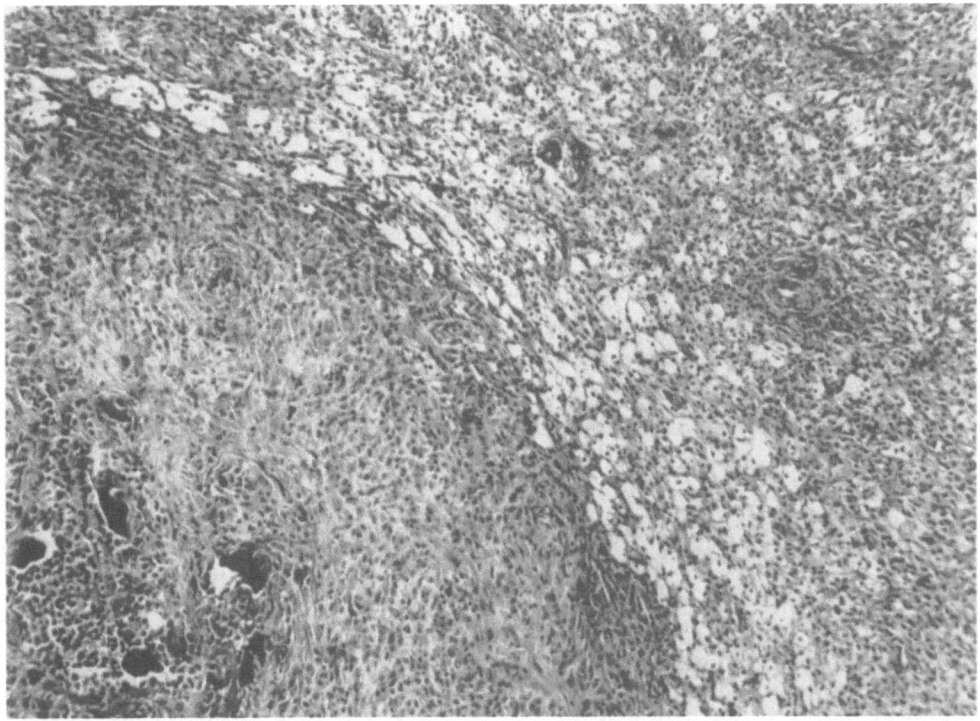

**Fig. 5.16.** Part of the edge of what was diagnosed as a 'giant-cell tumour of tendon sheath'. The degree of infiltration of its constituent cells into surrounding fatty connective tissue is high. H & E, × 62

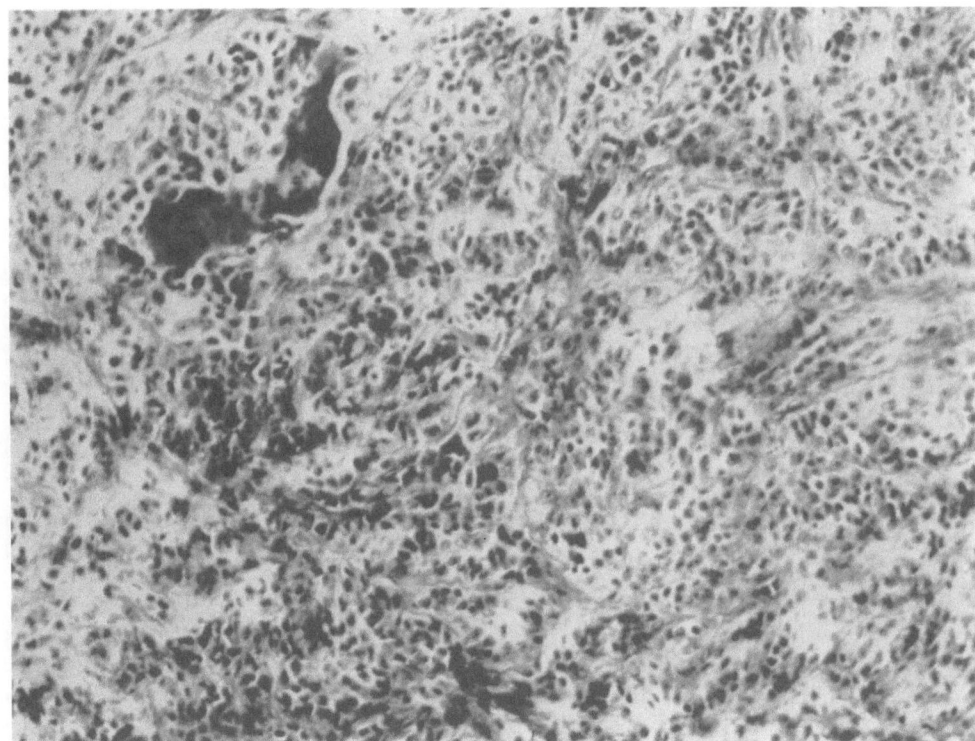

**Fig. 5.17.** Two large multinucleated cells (*top left*) amongst a rather polymorphic, moderately dense population of cells. H & E, × 123

frequency of 1 per 2 hpf while individual hpf showing two or three mitoses were easy to find; in addition, as shown in Fig. 5.18, aberrant forms were also easy to find.

No further treatment was advised or given though the high cellularity and mitotic activity prompted a warning that recurrence was possibly likelier to occur in this case than with most such lesions.

There were no complications, and the knee has remained trouble-free for at least 12 years.

The diagnosis was *appropriate* and not in doubt: what was uncertain was the significance of so much, and sometimes such aberrant, mitotic activity. On the evidence of the outcome here, lesions of this kind may show a great deal of activity and still be safely regarded as wholly benign.

### Case 5.7

M (35 years) with a 10-mm nodule on volar aspect of wrist for 'less than a year'.

The lesion was a typically spindle-celled 'nodulus cutaneus'. The cells were uniform and only occasionally in mitosis (1 per 20 hpf). It

had been reported as a 'myoma cutis', incompletely removed and thus representing some risk of recurrence. However, despite a complete absence of giant cells and haemosiderin, the presence of scattered foam cells makes 'histiocytoma' much the likelier diagnosis.

There was no further treatment, and no regrowth during the next 5 years at any rate: such remnant tissue as there was had regressed. The original diagnosis was *inappropriate* but innocuously so.

### Case 5.8

F (33 years) with a hard 25 × 15 × 10 mm swelling over palmar aspect of distal phalanx of thumb which had existed for many years, but recently had shown more rapid growth. Full excision was attempted. The nodule was adherent to both tendon sheath and periosteum.

Transection of the mass showed mottled pale pinkish tissue with a flake of (phalangeal) bone at one edge. Histologically, in generally descriptive terms, it was a 'chondromatous giant-cell tumour'.

A representative area is shown in Fig. 5.19.

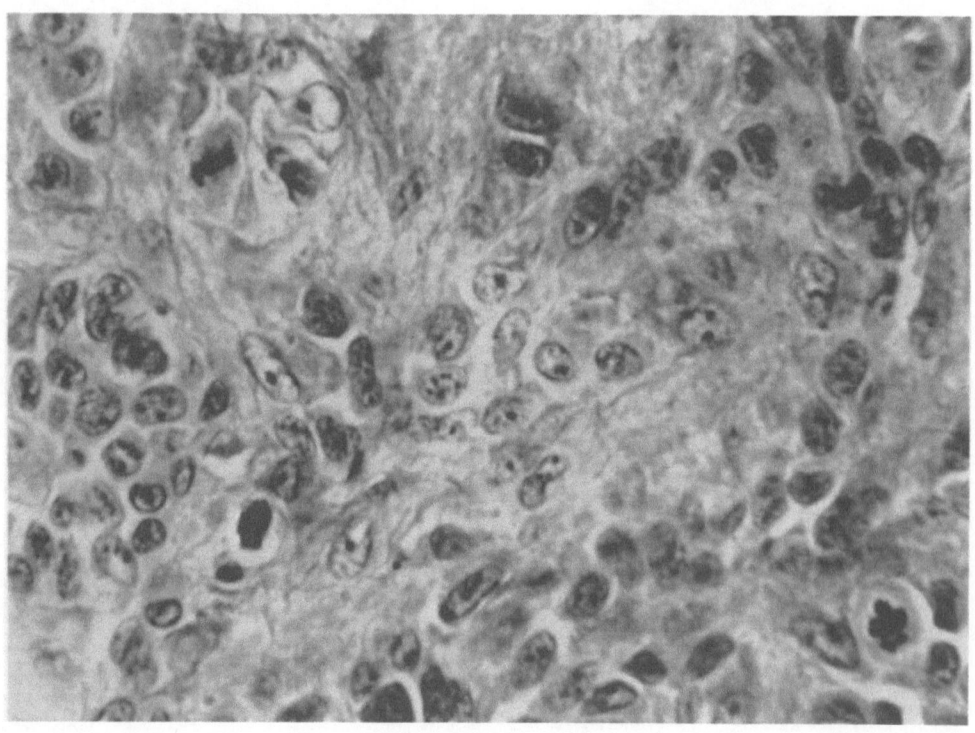

**Fig. 5.18.** There is appreciable polymorphism of the cells: 3 are in mitosis (2 in *left half* of field, 1 at *lower right-hand corner*). The lower right-hand figure is aberrant. H & E, × 845

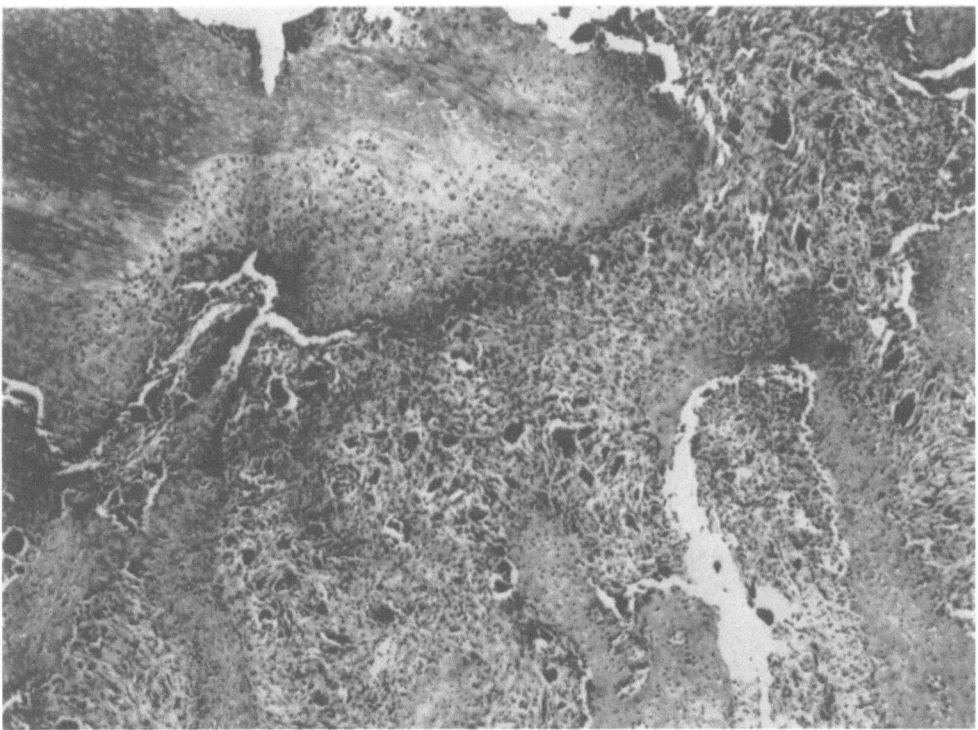

**Fig. 5.19.** A generally polymorphic picture composed of a mass of cartilage (most of *top left* of field) with adjacent quite highly cellular tissue containing multinucleated giant cells and osteoid trabeculae. H & E, × 62

The relatively uniform mass, top left, is cartilage. Elsewhere is a mixture of part-cartilaginous, part-osteoid trabeculae roughly outlined by giant-cells and a background of stromal tissue of relatively high cellularity. Similar features are shown in Fig. 5.20 with the edge of a zone of cartilage at right, and giant-cells and stromal tissue elsewhere. A typical giant-cell is seen in Fig. 5.21 where there is also, in the centre, a mitotic figure. In the more cellular areas, up to five mitoses, none aberrant, were present per hpf. Several representative sections raised serious doubts whether excision had been complete.

The diagnosis considered the most reasonable at the time was 'chondromatous osteoclastoma' but the precise designation seemed less important than the assessment of prognosis. The factors that weighed most heavily here were the apparent incompleteness of excision and the striking degree of mitotic activity in the most highly cellular foci scattered throughout the stroma. The advice given was that recurrence was probable.

No further treatment was given; no recurrence developed, and the thumb was fully functional when the patient was last seen 9 years after the excision. Either the opinion that excision was incomplete was wrong or any remnant tissue must have regressed despite its relatively high mitotic capacity.

In all, it seems likely that this was basically a 'nodular tenosynovitis' that had undergone extensive cartilaginous metaplasia. Little weight can be given to its adhesion to the tendon sheath; a mass of whatever kind in that restricted site could hardly do other than become adherent at an early stage. Further, behaviour of this kind, in particular absence of recurrence, would have been quite unusual had the lesion really been an osteoclastoma. This was an *over-diagnosis*.

### Case 5.9

F (22 years) with swelling over flexor surface of middle finger which had been apparent for 3 months. The excised mass was firm, fibrotic and 12 × 8 × 7 mm, described clinically as having been 'fixed to tendon sheath'.

The pattern, descriptively, was that of a 'myxoid fibroma', and thus it was diagnosed. Its general form, varying from paucicellular to quite

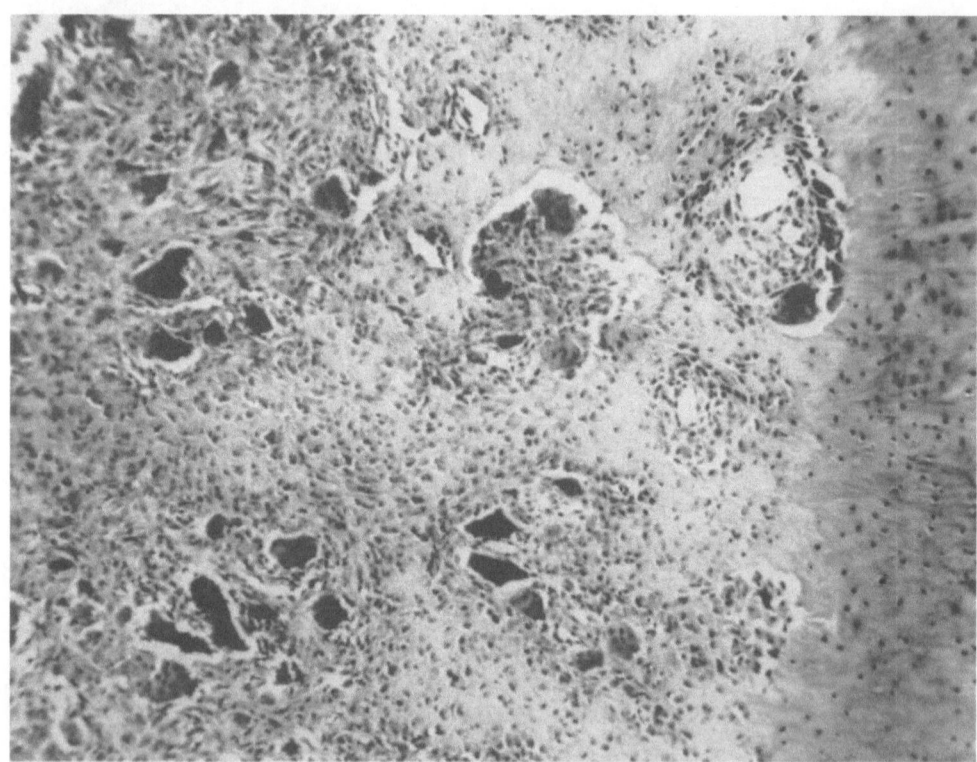

**Fig. 5.20.** Typical tissue adjacent to structurally normal cartilage (*right*). H & E, × 123

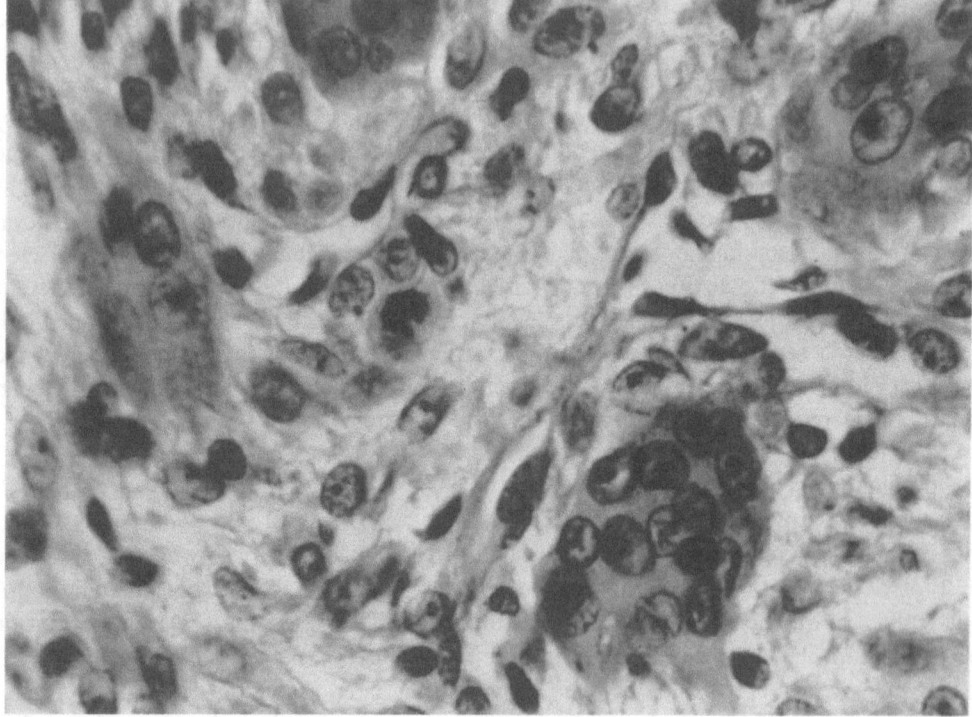

**Fig. 5.21.** Shows one multinucleated giant cell of average size and three smaller ones; also, just left of centre, a cell in mitosis. H & E, × 985

highly cellular, is shown in Figs. 5.22 and 5.23. Earlier experience with a somewhat similarly myxoid lesion that had unexpectedly metastasised induced a cautious report that, while metastasis was probably unlikely in the present case, local recurrence remained a distinct possibility.

Nothing further was done, the area healed well and was still trouble-free for at least 8 years thereafter. In retrospect, and when reassessed in company with the other similar lesions in this series, the lesion was almost certainly an instance of 'nodular tenosynovitis'. The original diagnosis, with its expressed concern, was an appreciable *over-diagnosis*.

### Cases 5.10–5.14

These five cases were all examples of 'nodular tenosynovitis', four on the palmar aspect of a digit, one in the popliteal fossa, all characterised by an impressively high cellularity and degree of mitotic activity. In each, areas could be found with mitoses as frequent as 4 per hpf: though none was frankly multipolar, many were acceptable as 'normal' only by generous allowance.

In all five a warning was given about liability to recurrence. None of the patients, however, received any further treatment and none suffered recurrence within periods of 12–20 years. In all, the diagnosis was *appropriate*.

### Case 5.15

F (13 years) with tender nodule on ankle over past 6 months. When exposed it was some 2 × 1 × 1 cm and infiltrating surrounding tissue.

The lesion was a highly cellular, spindle-type growth. The decision was straightforward, sarcoma or not, fibroma or fibrosarcoma? The cells were not unduly polymorphic, and mitoses, none aberrant, were no more numerous than 1 per 20 hpf. The lesion was diagnosed as 'highly cellular fibroma'.

Within 4 weeks the lesion had regrown to become a mass as large as before; that is, it had achieved within 4 weeks what had earlier taken 6 months and probably longer. The histology of the recurrent mass now left no doubt: mitoses were as many in places as 6 per hpf, and some were aberrant: the tissue was diagnosed as 'fibrosarcoma'.

It was hoped that the second excision would prove curative but it did not. The mass had again grown to the same size 8 months later, and below-knee amputation was performed. However, the patient has had no further trouble and is well, married and with a family, 24 years later.

In one respect, on review, this was, of course, an *under-diagnosis*: the lesion twice recurred and was eliminated only by amputation. On the other hand, despite the ample opportunities over some 15 months, metastasis did not occur. Biologically, the lesion appears to have been a rapidly growing fibroblastic neoplasm but only locally aggressive or malignant; to that extent, this was a rather qualified under-diagnosis.

### Case 5.16

M (14 years) with 5 × 3 cm painless nodule slowly increasing in size for the past 3 years over the upper inner aspect of the leg. The excised mass was 4 × 2 × 2 cm, firm and yellowish-white.

The lesion was spindle-celled, fasciculate rather than whorled, widely traversed and subdivided by bands of hyalinised collagen, poorly demarcated around much of its edge, and infiltrating muscle at one point (Fig. 5.24).

With allowance for plane of section, the nuclei, as shown in Fig. 5.25, were relatively uniform. Mitoses were scanty, at no more than 1 per 20 hpf, and not aberrant. Nuclei of a vacuolated or ballooned appearance, as seen in the centre of the figure, were relatively common (this figure gives a fair impression of their frequency); their significance is uncertain.

The lesion was diagnosed as a sarcoma, probably 'neurofibrosarcoma'.

The area was irradiated but not further excised, and all has remained well during the 11 years since then. The factor that almost certainly determined diagnosis as 'sarcoma' was the frankly infiltrative invasion of skeletal muscle. It seems reasonable on this basis to regard the diagnosis as having been *appropriate*.

### Case 5.17

M (18 years) with history of painless lump on sole of foot, gradually increasing over past 12 months to present size of 2 × 2 cm. The mass was excised; it was firm and elastic, yellowish-

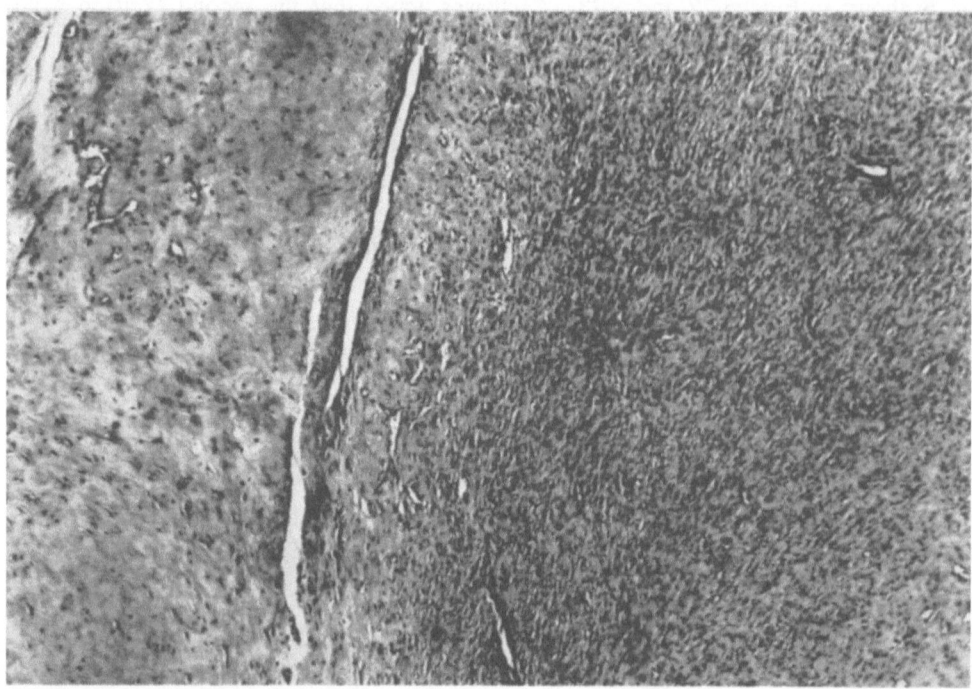

**Fig. 5.22.** Most of the mass had the highly cellular composition seen in right half of this field. As on left, elsewhere it was less highly cellular but more vascular and in places almost myxoid: the tissue here is closely similar to that in part of the plantar mass shown in Fig. 5.14. H & E, × 60

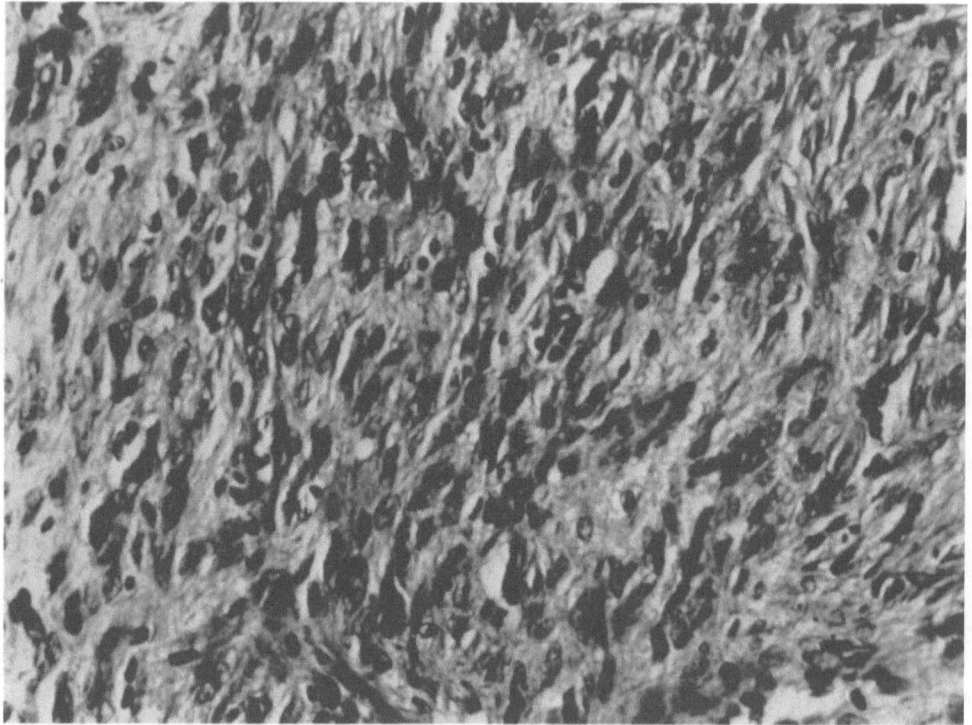

**Fig. 5.23.** The highly cellular tissue that comprised most of the lesion. H & E, × 374

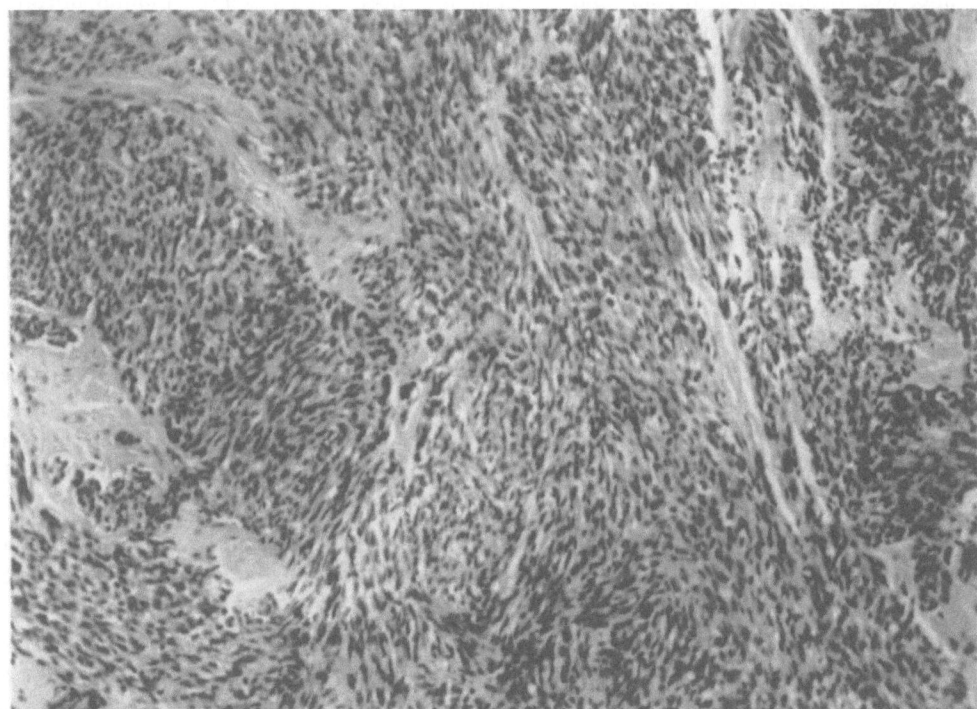

**Fig. 5.24.** A highly cellular mass, fasciculate but not storiform. The paucicellular areas at left of the field are foci of skeletal muscle which was widely infiltrated. H & E, × 123

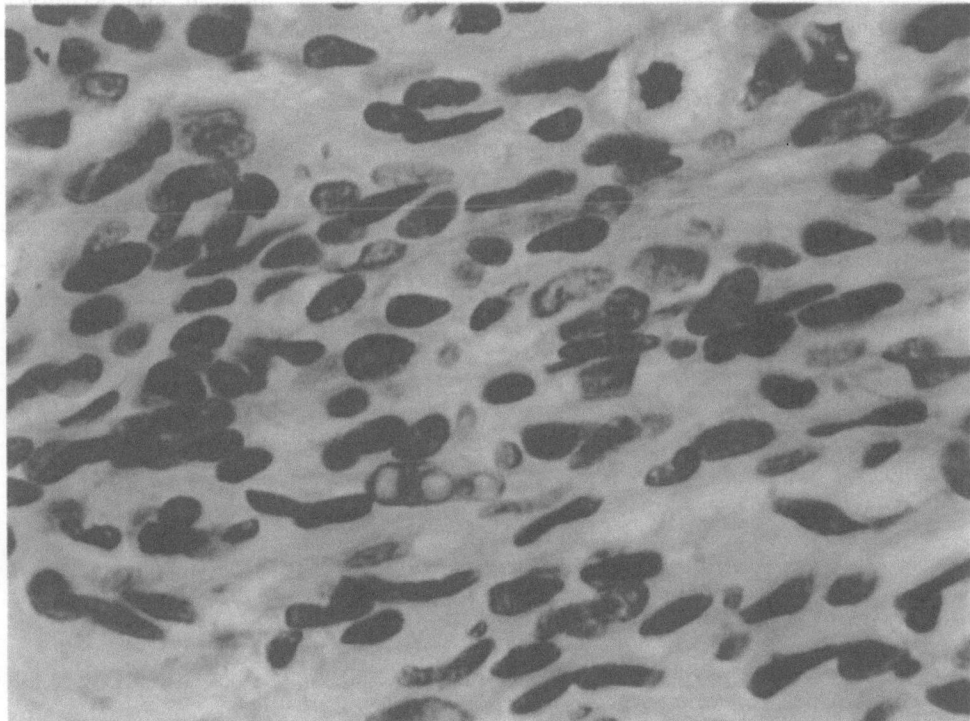

**Fig. 5.25.** The nuclei were particularly clearly defined and mildly hyperchromatic. Neither at this magnification nor overall, as in Fig. 5.24, does the tissue have the 'tissue-culture-like' appearance of a nodular fasciitis. There is a mitotic figure near top right edge. H & E, × 985

white, well demarcated in some places, shading imperceptibly into surrounding tissue at others.

The abnormal tissue was of spindle-celled character, varying in cell-density in keeping with the general disposition as shown in Fig. 5.26. It varied also in the amount of mitotic activity but in the most highly cellular area there was an incidence up to 1 mitotic figure per 3 hpf; none, however, was aberrant. The degree of maximum cellularity is shown in Fig. 5.27.

The lesion was clearly sarcomatoid; was it sarcomatous? The diagnosis given was '. . . sarcoma (probably fibrosarcoma) . . . ', with a suggestion that complete local excision could well be adequate treatment. The excision was followed by irradiation.

The lesion recurred 17 months later and was again excised. Histologically it appeared essentially identical to the original. There has been no further trouble during the succeeding 12 years.

This was probably an instance of *overdiagnosis* but at least in conveying the diagnosis 'sarcoma' the pathologist had simultaneously advised that local eradication could be curative. After one recurrence, received in the laboratory with concern, this opinion was justified. In retrospect, the better term would probably have been 'highly cellular plantar fibromatosis', but at all events, the satisfactory outcome has shown that, despite a local recurrence, tissue as highly cellular and mitotically active as this may have little or no metastasising capacity.

### Case 5.18

M (13 years) with a swelling that had reappeared in the upper inner thigh. The initial swelling, some $10 \times 8 \times 6$ cm, had followed a blow 12 weeks earlier, was diagnosed as a haematoma, and had been successfully aspirated 4 weeks after the injury. It largely subsided after the aspiration but recurred 6 weeks later and was explored by open operation.

The material received comprised four fragments of haemorrhagic fleshy tissue, the largest $4 \times 3 \times 2$ cm.

The components of the material were blood clot, granulation tissue, abundant haemosiderin and large pigment-free areas of what was morphologically a highly cellular spindle-celled sarcoma. The cells were disposed in swirling swathes and bands as shown in Fig. 5.28. In detail, as seen in Fig. 5.29, they were relatively small and uniform, and occasionally in mitosis. Points of possible significance, in retrospect, are

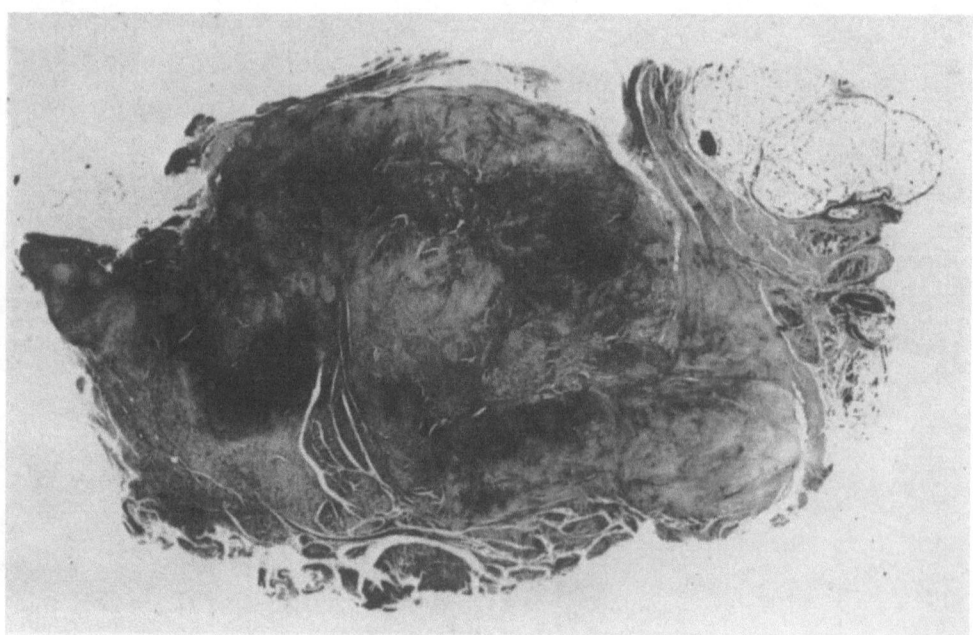

**Fig. 5.26.** A plantar nodule of varying density in proportion to the cellularity. It merges with muscle below but is relatively well demarcated above. H & E, × 10

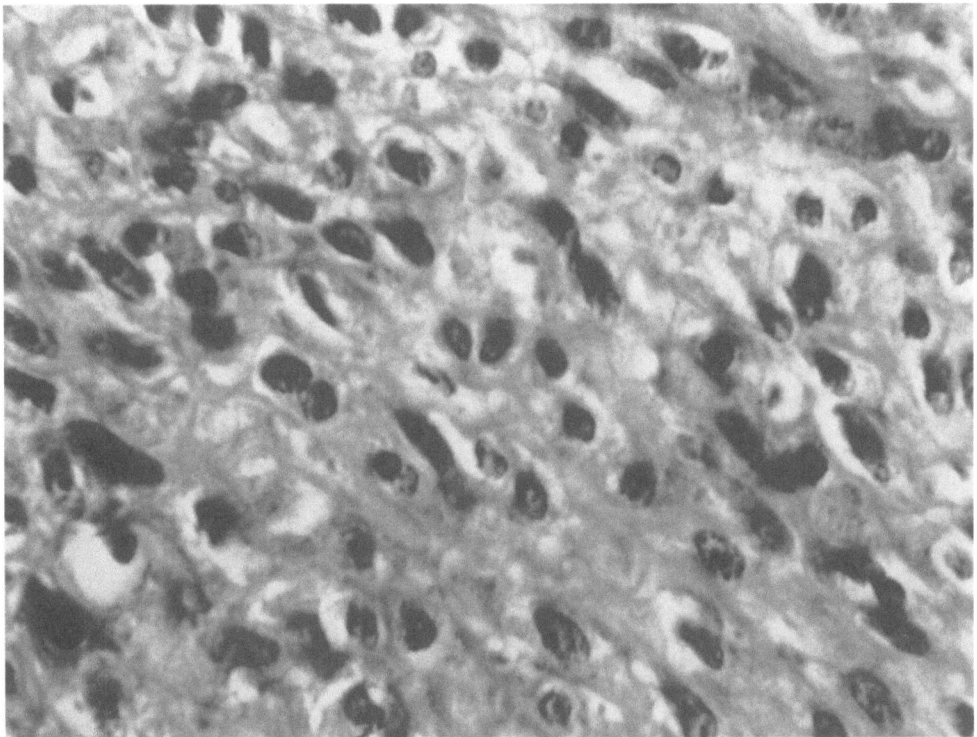

**Fig. 5.27.** At most, as seen here, it was moderately highly cellular. The lesion recurred but was cured by a further excision. Designation as a sarcoma was at least a partial over-diagnosis. H & E, × 985

that all mitoses seen appeared normal and that their incidence, no more than 1 per 20 hpf, was appreciably less than seemed appropriate to such highly proliferative tissue.

The gravity of the lesion was obvious; amputation was clearly in question. There seemed little alternative to a diagnosis of 'fibrosarcoma' but further opinions were sought. None suggested otherwise, and one senior colleague wrote that he ". . . would be content to use this lesion to teach my students about spindle-cell sarcoma". However, favourable experience with a somewhat similar lesion in the pectoralis major of a young man (Lendrum, 1948) led another colleague to suggest that the surgeons be invited to explore fully the possibility of local resection in the double hope that metastasis had not yet occurred and that the leg could be saved.

However, exposure of the lesion 11 days later found the mass so large and so situated—it was 18 × 8 × 6 cm, poorly encapsulated, occupied the upper third of the adductor compartment, and extended into the obturator muscles—that local removal would have entailed excision of at least all the adductor muscles and, thus, a useless limb. With obviously neoplastic tissue almost within the obturator foramen, hindquarter amputation seemed the only safe course, and this was done.

The patient adapted well to his prosthesis and remains fit and active 20 years later. With so relatively good an outcome, when the probability of metastasis had seemed so high, all those concerned in the original assessment resolved that on any such future occasion the initial recommendation must be local excision. There remains some uneasiness that this perhaps was an over-diagnosis. True, consciences were salved to some extent by the fact that even if the lesion had been dogmatically diagnosable as of a non-metastasising character, which it could not, there was, for anatomical reasons, no way of avoiding amputation; but that does not allay all the anxiety. Had the lesion been equally extensive but exciseable, in, say, one of the lower vastus muscles, and amputation had been performed, the worry about over-diagnosis would have remained to this day. Even so, with such

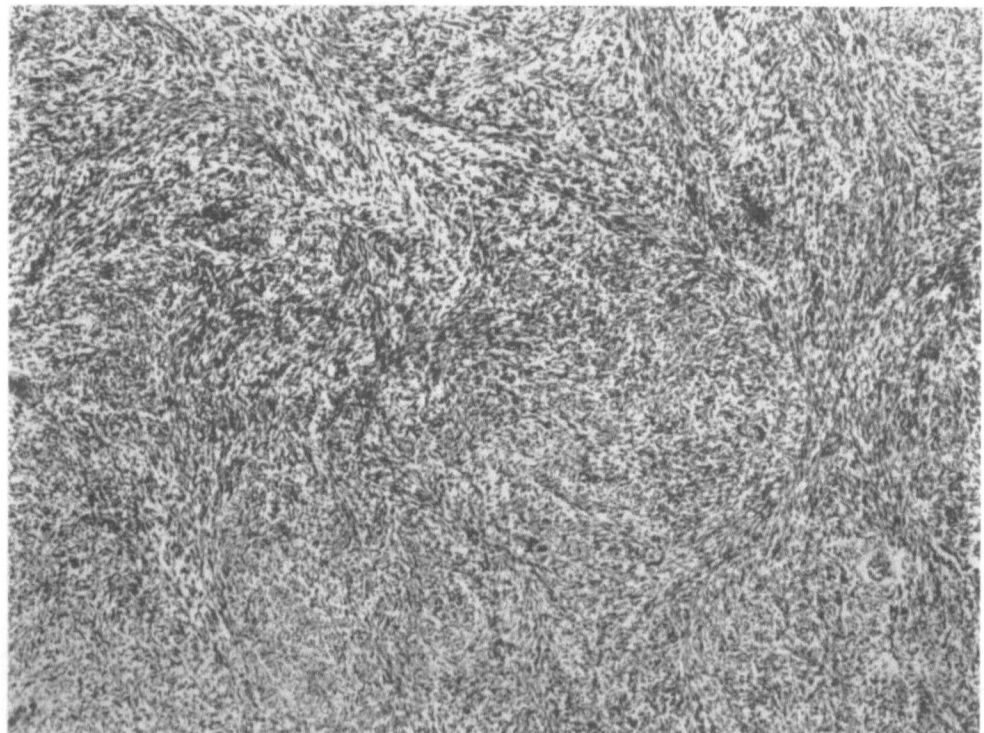

**Fig. 5.28.** The highly cellular tissue obtained at the excision of the apparently recurrent haematoma. There was much haemosiderin amongst it. H & E, × 62

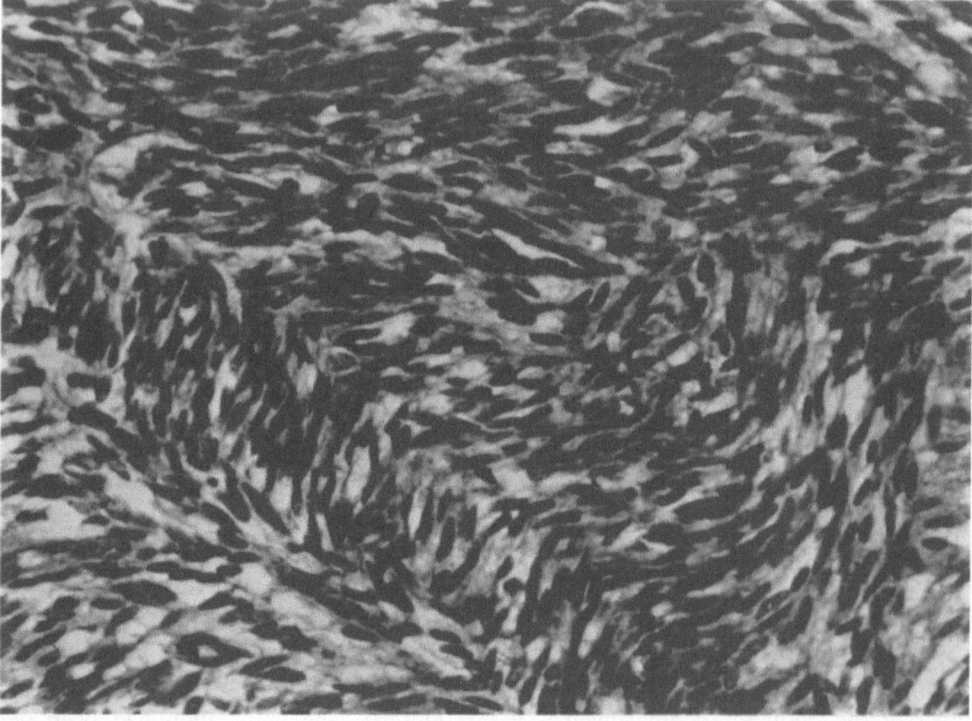

**Fig. 5.29.** This degree of cellularity and the not infrequent mitoses made the diagnosis of fibrosarcoma inescapable. H & E, × 374

unanimity of histological opinion, the diagnosis was entirely *appropriate*.

A note on haematoma-sarcoma is included in the General Commentary on this section.

## Case 5.19

M (15 months) with nodules on fingers of left hand, first noticed at age 6 months. Histologically the nodules showed a fibromatous or fibromatoid character. Frequent recurrences over the next 6 years required repeated treatment by, at various times, local excision, partial amputation and irradiation. The condition appeared then to stabilise; the child was now aged 7 years and had had partial amputation of the middle, ring and little fingers.

This appeared to be typically 'recurrent digital fibroma.' Figure 5.30 shows one of the early recurrent masses immediately beneath and flattening the epidermis. Its moderately highly cellular character is seen in Figs. 5.31 and 5.32. It was nowhere more highly cellular than this in any of the many pieces of tissue received over the 6 years, and showed only very scanty mitoses.

Eosinophil cytoplasmic inclusions of the kind first described in such lesions by Reye (1965) were prominent in the tissue excised on the earlier occasions but almost wholly absent from that obtained 6 years later.

The outcome, or at any rate a later occurrence, was not only unexpected, but unusual.

The boy, now a school-boy of 16, was seen again 10 years after the last excision of tissue from the already partly-amputated fingers with a large (4 × 3 cm) haematoma on the dorsum of the afflicted hand; it had apparently followed a trivial injury, a glancing blow from a hammer. The appearance and bulging character of the mass caused concern and biopsy was arranged. By the time this was performed, 3 days later, there was swelling and haemorrhagic discolouration of almost the whole of the forearm.

Microscopy of two pieces of tissue (the larger 20 × 5 × 5 mm) taken from the region of the original haematoma showed material of alarmingly high cellularity and mitotic activity, to the point where sarcoma was seriously considered. In practice it was decided, meantime at any rate, to designate it 'sarcomatoid' and, in view of its highly cellular and vasoformative character, to recommend irradiation. However, during the 3

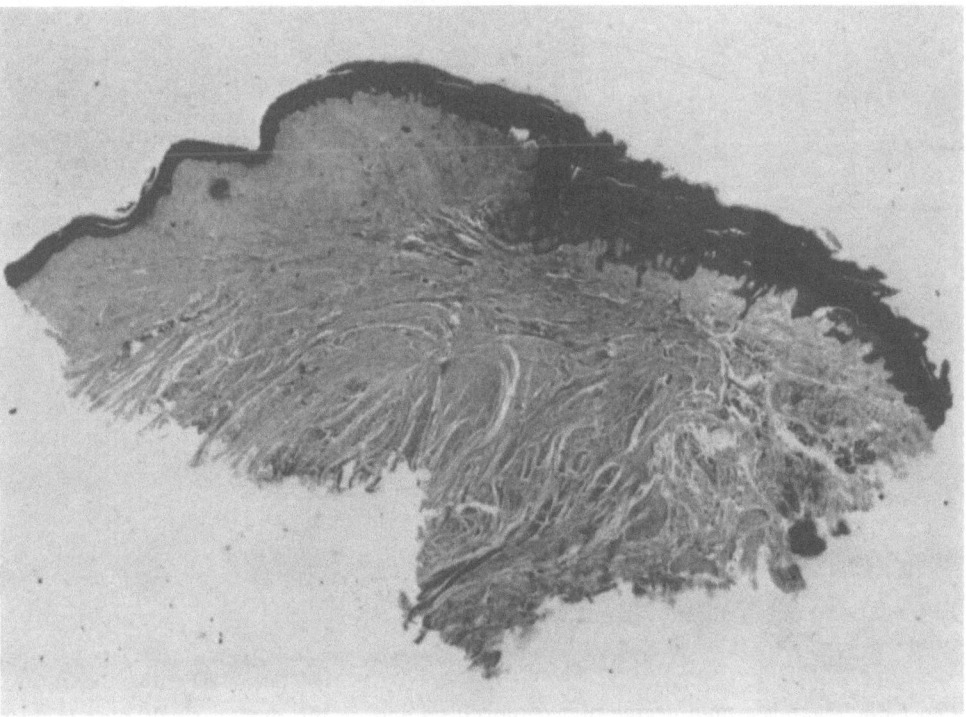

**Fig. 5.30.** To left, an area of recurrent fibroma lies within the dermis and is flattening the epidermis. H & E, × 14

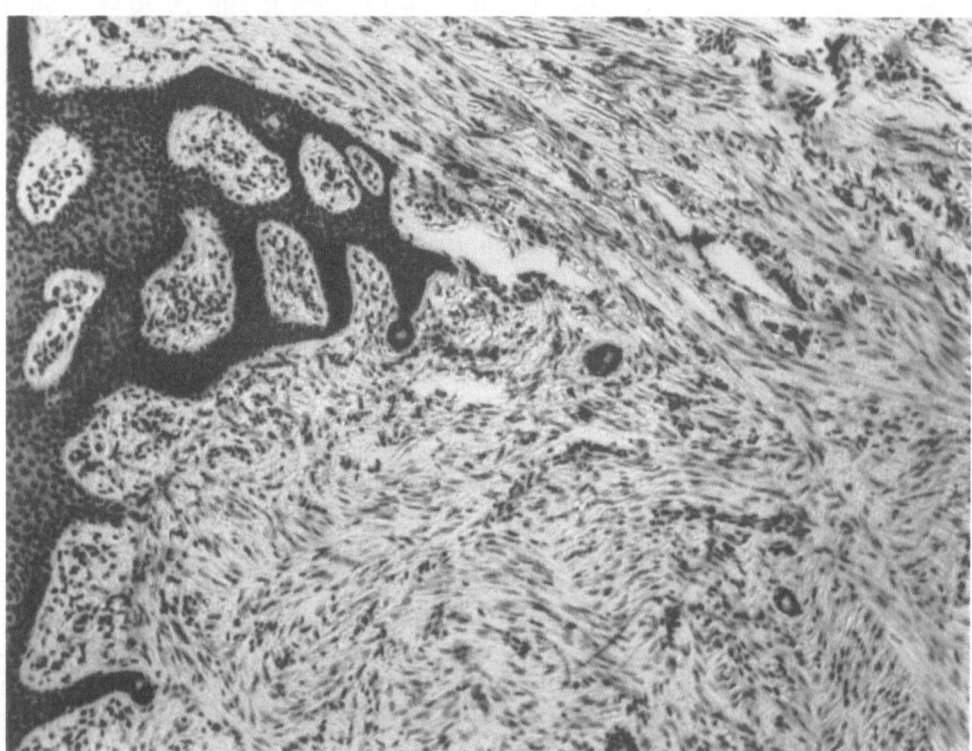

**Fig. 5.31.** The recurrent fibroblastic overgrowth is only moderately highly cellular but permeates the whole of the dermis. H & E, × 123

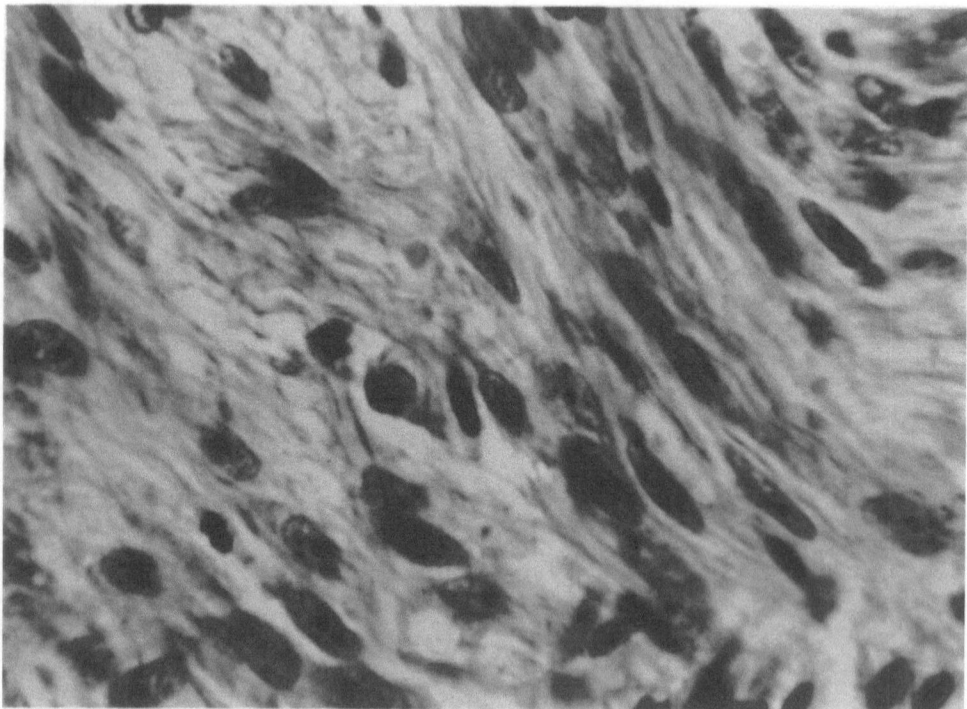

**Fig. 5.32.** There is a mild degree of polymorphism and, in this area, a single mitotic figure (*lower left corner*). The original tissue and that seen on all subsequent occasions was essentially the same. H & E, × 952

days between the biopsy and receipt of the histological report, the haemorrhagic swelling in the forearm had increased and now reached the antecubital fossa. The possibility of sarcoma still remained, therefore the decision was taken to perform a further biopsy from the swollen haemorrhagic tissue just distal to the antecubital fossa. This showed only extravasated blood and mild cellulitis with no features to indicate malignancy. After irradiation and symptomatic treatment the condition subsided and has remained trouble-free for the 5 years between then and now.

The main cause for concern was whether this was a granulation tissue sarcoma akin to that described by Dawson and McIntosh (1971), but events showed it was not. Emotional factors were involved and there is some possibility that the original injury, perhaps with later additions, was self-inflicted. Be that as it may, the exuberance of the reparative tissue response does raise the question whether those who develop recurrent digital fibromatosis in childhood may not have a form of 'connective tissue diathesis' such that tissue of this kind is unusually prone to respond atypically and excessively to any future insult.

The original diagnosis was *appropriate*. In the opinion of Kauffman and Stout (1961) the recurrent digital fibroma of children is a form of histiocytoma.

### Case 5.20

M (12 months) with mass in thigh (4 × 2 × 2 cm).

Sections from the mass showed a ramifying plexiform spindle-celled structure with ill-defined edges. It contained many small nerve-bundles but 'fibromatosis' seemed as suitable a term as 'neurofibromatosis'. Adequacy of excision was doubtful and likely recurrence predicted. Further excision was performed 4 weeks later when an 8 × 4 × 3 cm skin-covered mass again showed wide permeation by neurofibromatoid bands, and still there were areas where adequacy of excision was doubtful.

No further treatment was given and there was no regrowth of the mass during the next 6 years. Such persisting remnants as there may have been, and almost certainly there were some, had presumably regressed. The diagnosis was *appropriate*.

### Case 5.21

F (33 years) para. 3, with a painful swelling beside the umbilicus that had increased over the past six months. At operation, the mass was firm, white and 15 × 4 × 2 cm, apparently entirely within the rectus muscle of which, to achieve clearance, a large portion had been removed.

In all respects, this was a typical 'desmoid tumour', neither hypercellular nor unduly mitotically active.

The patient suffered repeated recurrences until, 10 years later, virtually the whole of the anterior abdominal wall was involved. During this time, a pregnancy had to be terminated and sterilisation performed. Death occurred during the 12th year after the original diagnosis but details of the terminal events could not be obtained. The diagnosis was *appropriate*, and obviously so.

### Case 5.22

M (12 years) with pain and slight swelling over posterior aspect of left hip present for 3 weeks. Exploration showed much of the posterior aspect of the hip-joint occupied and enveloped by yellowish-white myxoid tissue closely adherent to but not penetrating the joint capsule and partly surrounded by the piriform and obturator muscles. Total removal was attempted.

The abnormal tissue was at the least myxomatoid or fibro-myxomatoid. Its degree of cellularity and vascularity varied with the amount of myxoid matrix. Mitoses were few and not aberrant. Its infiltrative capacity was high and there was extensive permeation of the many fragments of skeletal muscle included among the excised material. A portion of joint capsule was similarly infiltrated.

The lesion was reported as a 'fibromyxoma (myxoma)', likely to recur but not to metastasise.

No further treatment was given and the patient was known to be well and trouble-free 9 years after the operation.

It is difficult to believe that, with as extensive and apparently infiltrative a lesion as this, every abnormal cell had been removed and that this was the reason for cure; the remnants presumably regressed. Almost certainly the lesion is an example of the pseudo-sarcomatous or 'nodular fasciitis' described by Hutter and his colleagues

(1962) and by others. Insofar as the original diagnosis implied a neoplasm, and a neoplasm likely to recur, it was an *over-diagnosis*.

### Case 5.23

M (53 years) with a 6-month history of painful, hard swelling in upper lateral thigh. X-ray of femur and pelvis normal. The mass, 6 × 4 × 2 cm, excised from substance of vastus lateralis, was brown with patchy red/yellow mottling, and had the general appearance of skeletal muscle.

The lesion was broadly characterised by patchy destruction of muscle and an associated hyper-cellular reaction, though even in the areas of greatest destruction and cellularity the sarcolem-mal sheaths remained largely intact (Fig. 5.33). Amongst the proliferating cells, mitotic figures were moderately numerous (1 per 10 hpf on average): was the lesion neoplastic or reparative?

The process appeared to be, first and in its most extreme form, one of coagulative necrosis of the muscle fibres: with this went loss of striation and shrinkage and loss of sarcolemmal nuclei; second, lysis of sarcoplasm to the point where the sarcolemmal tunnels were completely empty of muscle substance and even nuclei. In less severely affected areas, generally around the edges of the totally necrotic foci, the fibres had commonly 'rounded-up' to form clearly identi-fiable muscle giant cells (Fig. 5.34) in company with a striking proliferation of apparently histio-cytic and sarcolemmal cells. This degree of proliferation with its mitotic activity and co-existent giant cells formed a notably hyper-cellular and hyperplastic picture. Leucocytic infiltration was of only moderate degree; of those cells that were present, eosinophil polymorpho-nuclears predominated (but not enough to war-rant the term 'eosinophil granuloma').

The lesion was finally reported as probably benign and essentially *reparative*.

No further treatment was given, and the pa-tient was trouble-free 8 years later. The lesion was almost certainly an example of 'proliferative myositis'. The original diagnosis was adequate for practical purposes but *inappropriate* in failing to identify the lesion as an entity already de-scribed at the time.

### Case 5.24

F (17 years) with a complaint of pain and swelling in region of the shoulder. Examination showed a smooth 4 × 3 × 3 cm mass over the outer part of pectoralis major. There was no evidence of bony involvement either clinically or radiologically. The swelling had been present for 4 weeks and was associated with a blow to the region some 3 weeks before that.

The mass consisted of variably cellular, but over wide areas highly cellular fibroblastic, tissue amongst which were many osteoid or bony trabeculae at all stages of differentiation (Fig. 5.35). The trabeculae were mostly well covered by osteoblastic cells. Multinucleated cells of seemingly osteoclastic type were present but few and scattered (Fig. 5.36).

Although the diagnosis favoured, and reported, was 'myositis ossificans', some concern was caused by the degree of cellularity and mitotic activity in many places. In areas such as that at the upper left-hand corner of Fig. 5.35, the fibroblastic/osteoblastic cells formed almost un-broken sheets, while hpf containing up to three mitotic figures were easy to find. Figure 5.36 shows such an area and includes also one of the relatively infrequent osteoclast-like cells. Despite the cellular activity the prognosis was regarded as good.

The patient, to date, has had no further trouble for 11 years, and the function of the pectoralis major was in no way impaired. The diagnosis was correct and *appropriate*. The significance of such hypercellularity and mitotic activity as was present here is the subject of later comment.

### Case 5.25

M (37 years) with severe backache recurrent 3 weeks after removal of a prolapsed lumbar disc. Exploration of the operation site showed an extradural mass of soft pinkish tissue.

The character of the tissue is shown in Fig. 5.37. It is a highly cellular spindle-type over-growth including, or at any rate surrounding, occasional small islands of bone. In some cases this appeared to be new bone; elsewhere there were foci of destruction of bone. As shown in

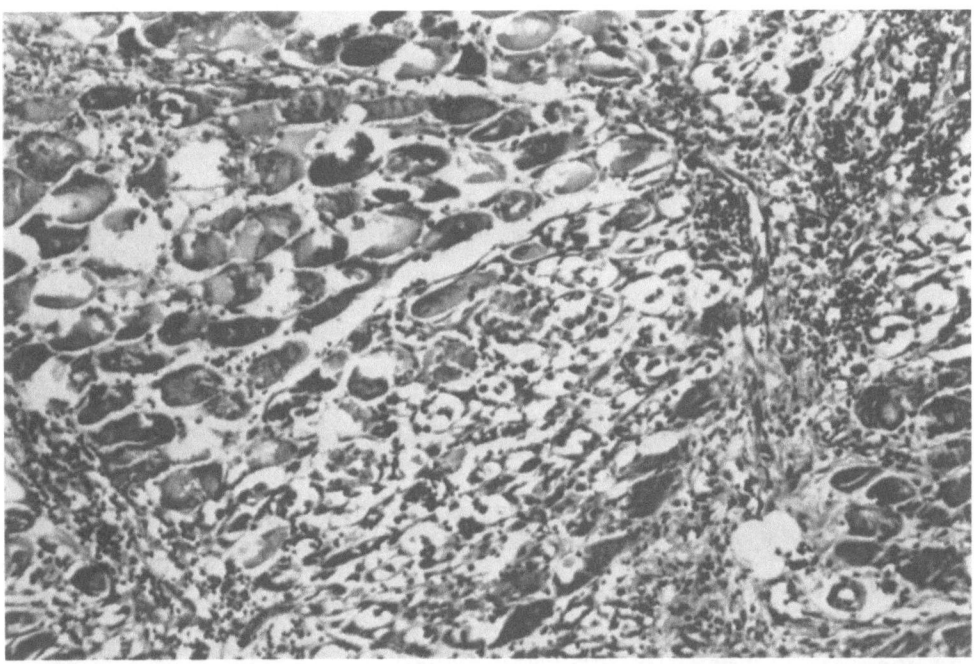

**Fig. 5.33.** Many of the skeletal muscle fibres show changes from mild vacuolation to almost total lysis. Where lysis has been complete, only empty sarcolemmal tubes remain. There is leucocytic infiltration (*top right-hand corner*) but less than expected with so much destruction of tissue. H & E, × 140

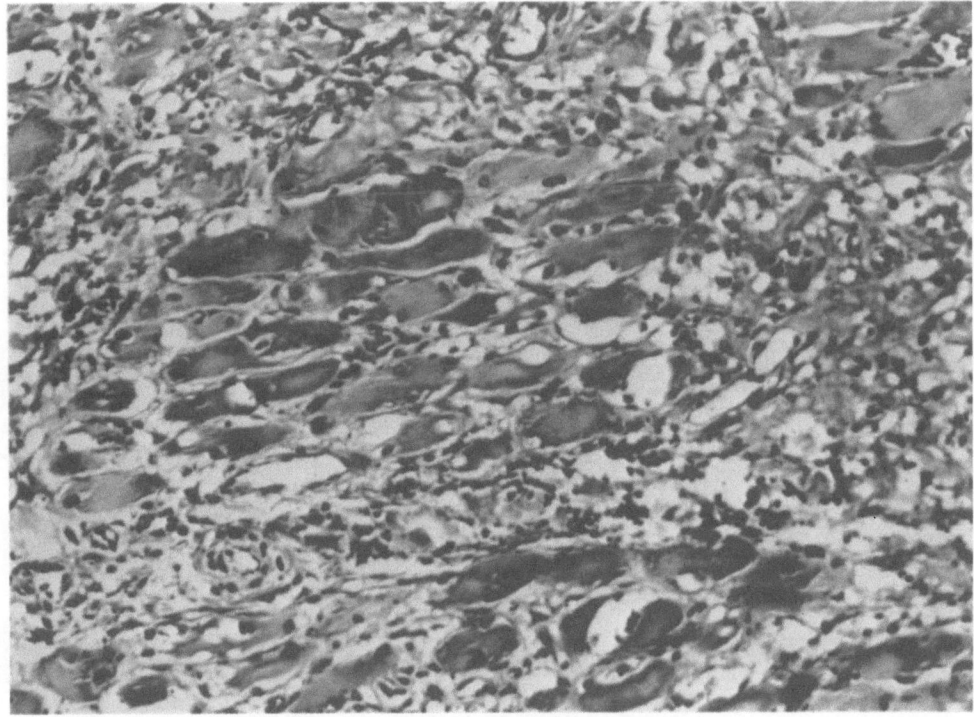

**Fig. 5.34.** The multinucleated masses here are clearly 'muscle' giant-cells. Empty or near-empty sarcolemmal tubes are again evident. H & E, × 229

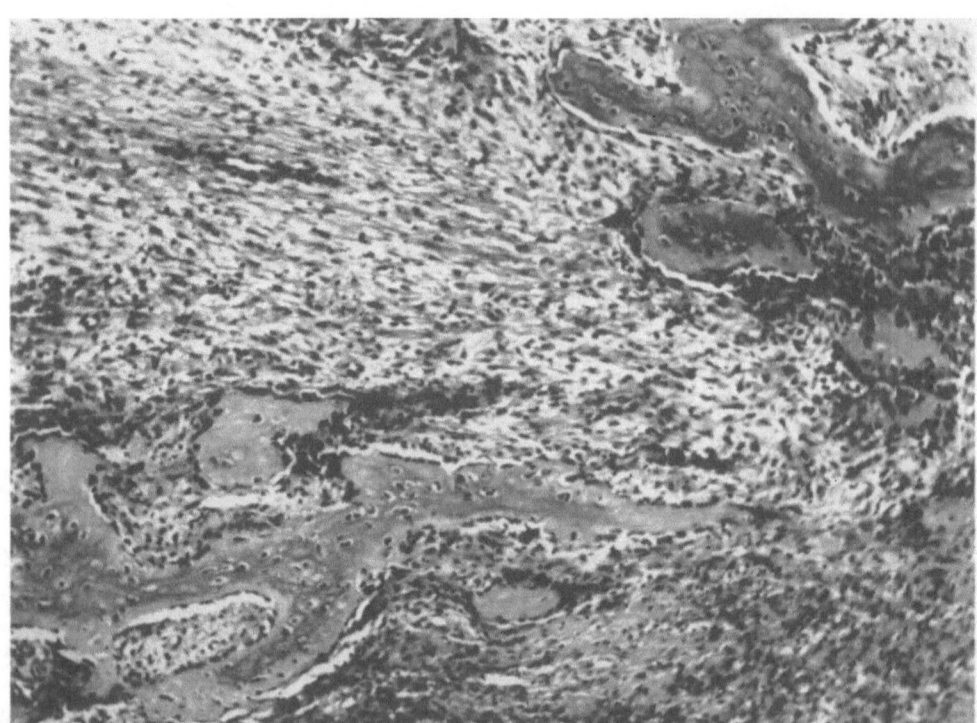

**Fig. 5.35.** A mixture of variably cellular fibroblastic tissue and bony trabeculae. H & E, × 119

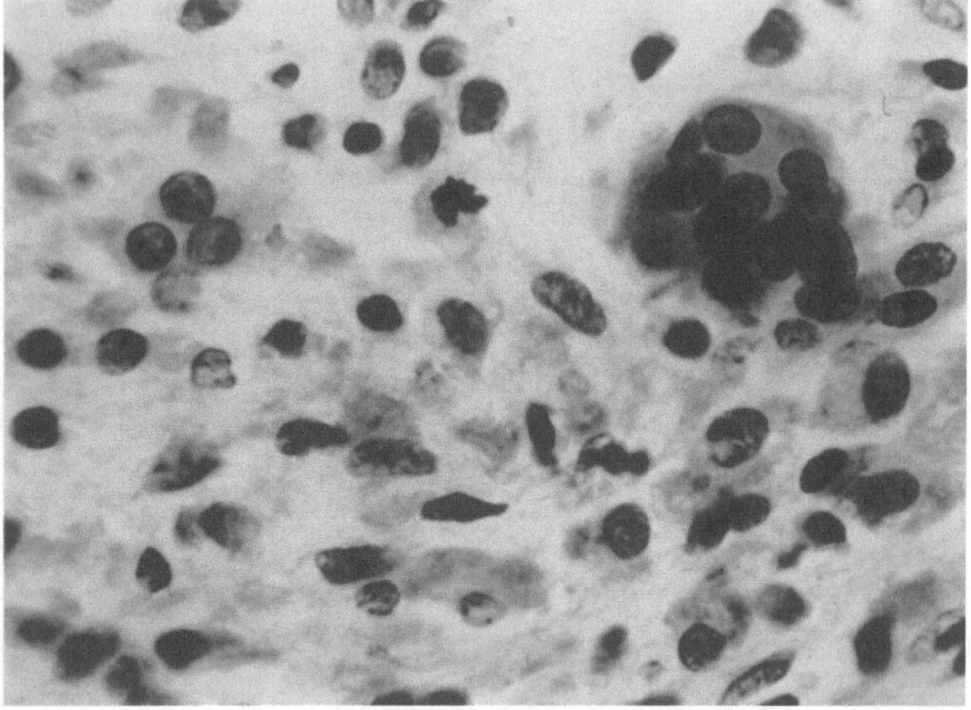

**Fig. 5.36.** An area that contains a multinucleated giant-cell, three mitotic figures (one *upper centre*, two of roughly oblong contour, *slightly below* and to *right* of this), and a mixture of nuclei, only some spindled and probably fibroblastic. H & E, × 952

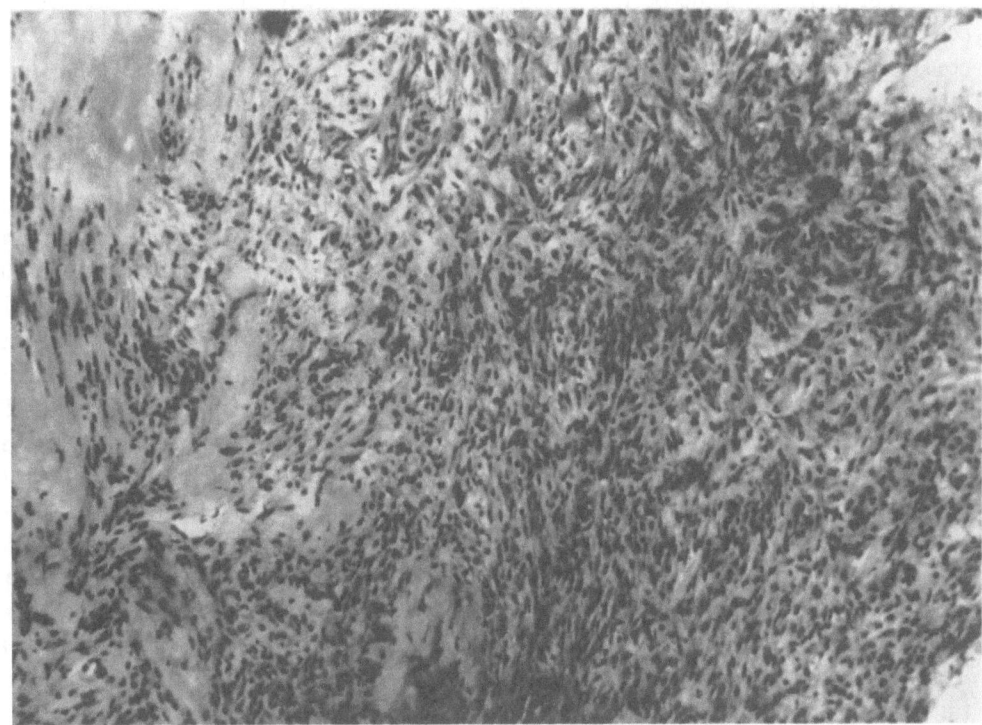

**Fig. 5.37.** Highly cellular fasciculate tissue in association with (*top left-hand corner*) an area of amorphous substance, probably extruded nucleus pulposus. In some such areas, osteoid transformation was occurring (*below and to right*). H & E, × 119

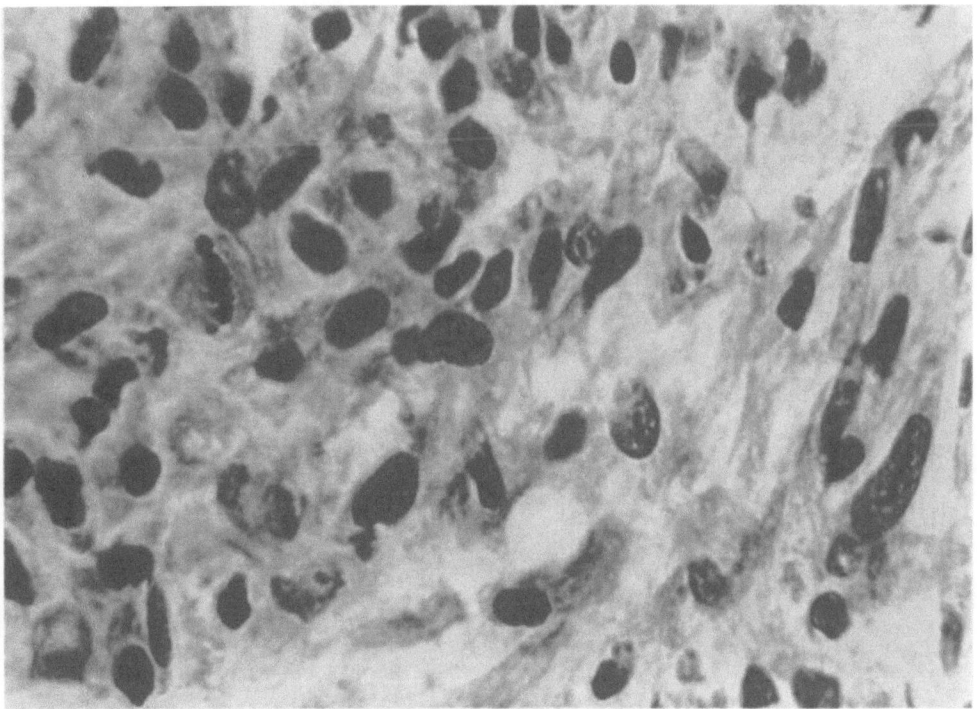

**Fig. 5.38.** This degree of polymorphism and scattered mitoses (*upper left*) caused concern but appears in retrospect to have been part of a reparative reaction only. H & E, × 952

Fig. 5.38, there was some polymorphism of the cells and occasional mitoses. The tissue was considered to be neoplastic and most probably 'neurilemmoma'.

The abnormal tissue was excised so far as possible, the area healed well, and the patient remains trouble-free 8 years later.

Almost certainly this was not a neoplastic growth but an unusually exuberant reparative reaction. A later, somewhat similar occurrence in another patient has led to a suspicion that extravasated disc substance (nucleus pulposus) may have a highly 'irritant' or fibroplastic effect. This was an *over-diagnosis*.

### Case 5.26

F (41 years) with swelling on dorsum of foot; excised (3 × 1 × 1 cm) + irradiation; recurred within 6 months; further excision and irradiation. Three years and 4 years later she had two further excisions. Reappearance of the mass led to a below-knee amputation, 5½ years after the initial treatment.

The morphology of the first-excised tissue is shown in Figs. 5.39, 5.40 and 5.41. It was moderately highly cellular, for the most part lacking any particular pattern, especially beneath the fairly well-defined capsule (Fig. 5.39) but notably fatty in some places (Figs. 5.40, 5.41). Mitoses averaged 1 per 2 hpf and the diagnosis suggested was 'lipomyxoma'.

Figure 5.42 shows part of the first recurrence. The pattern had changed considerably and was now a combination of much more highly cellular, markedly vasoformative (upper right) and almost chondroid (lower left) tissue. Mitotic figures were now much more numerous and averaged 2 per hpf in some areas. The tissue was now regarded as sarcomatous. Tissue removed later, however, again showed more of a fibrolipomyxoid pattern than an angiochondroid, and mitoses were never again so abundant.

Four months after the amputation, the patient had a haemoptysis, and chest X-ray showed a shadow regarded as probably a metastasis. Shortly thereafter, she developed a mass in the abdominal wall (not removed because it appeared to be regressing at one stage), then a cerebral haemorrhage, also probably due to metastasis. This was the final episode and she died within days of the haemorrhage.

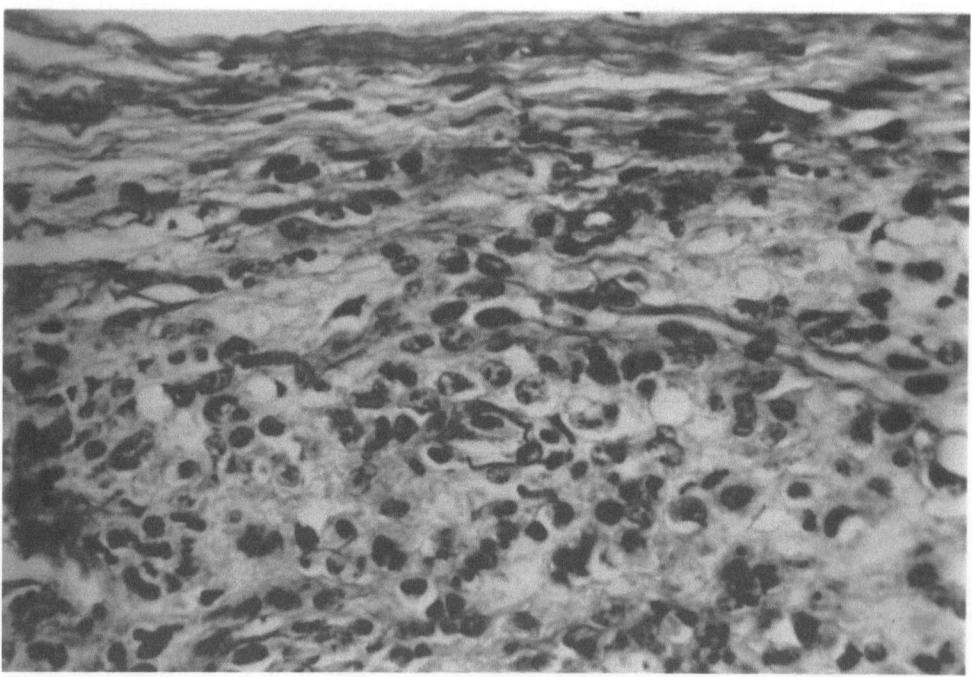

**Fig. 5.39.** Beneath a fairly well-defined compressed capsule or pseudo-capsule the cellular neoplastic tissue has no particular pattern but the nuclear character suggests a cell-type other than fibroblastic. H & E, × 476

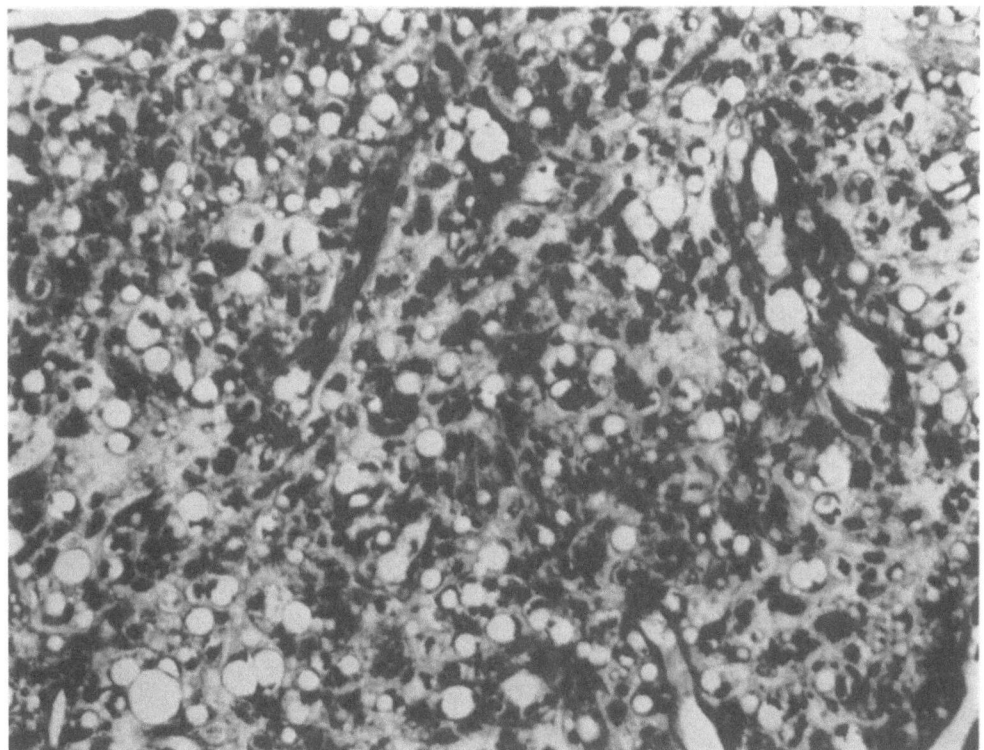

**Fig. 5.40.** The tissue here is of predominantly fatty but partly myxoid pattern. H & E, × 246

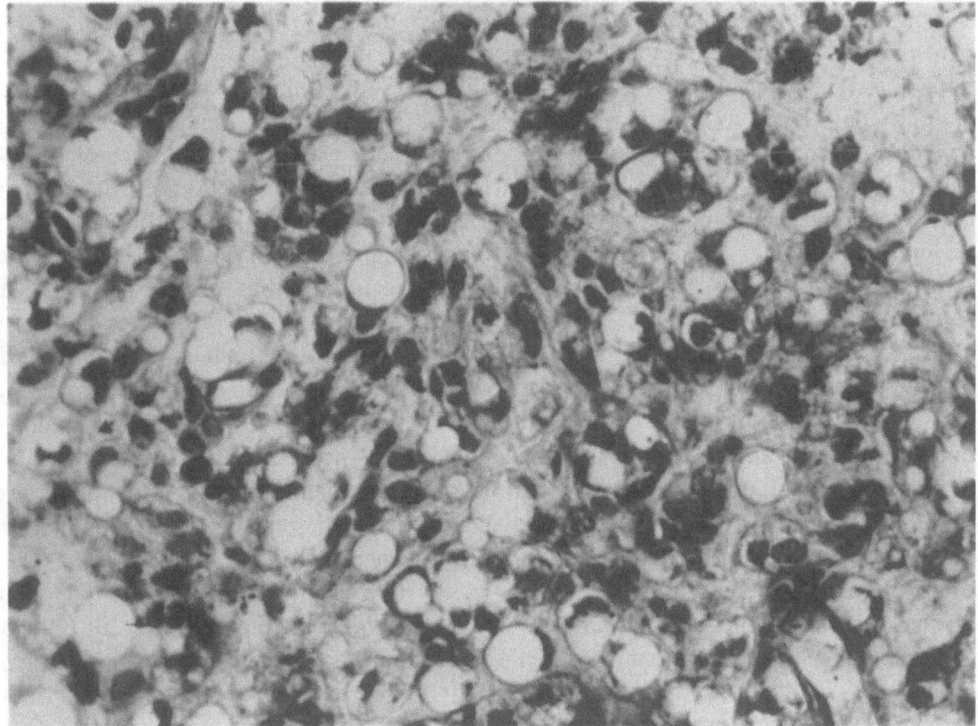

**Fig. 5.41.** An area such as this, where there is appreciable nuclear polymorphism, would contain on average one mitotic figure. H & E, × 476

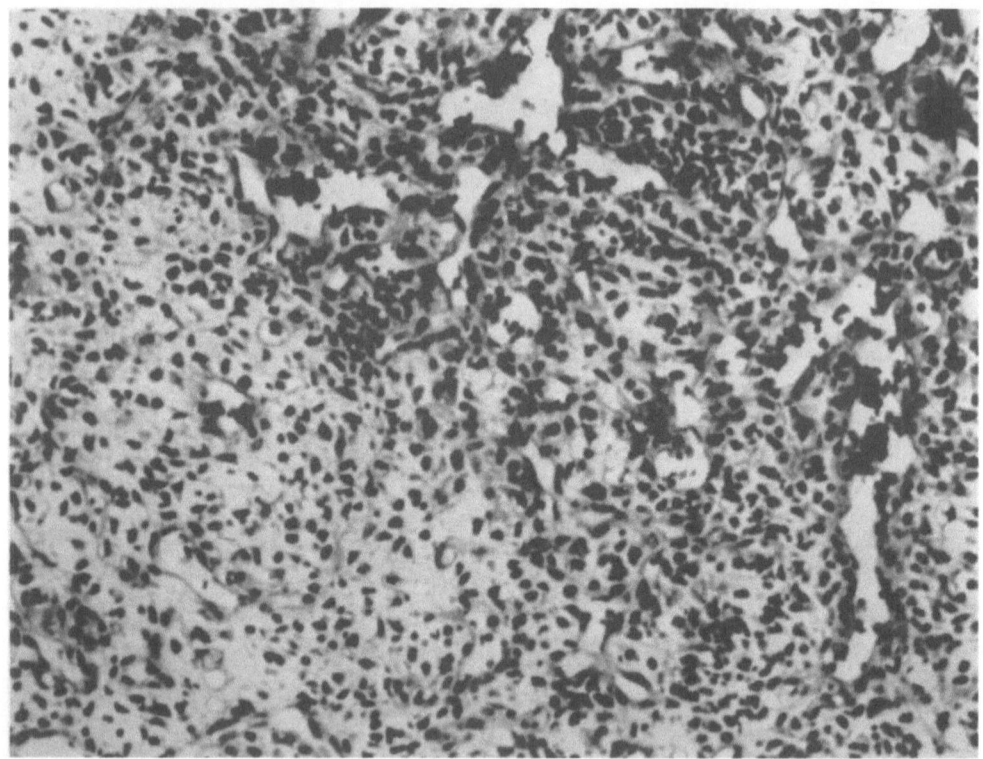

**Fig. 5.42.** Most of the upper right half of the field consists of notably angiomatoid tissue: the lower left half resembles primitive or rather myxoid cartilage. H & E, × 246

The diagnosis here should have been 'malignant mesenchymoma'. This entity was not at the time of original diagnosis as generally familiar as now but, even so, re-examination of the original sections leaves no doubt that the lesion should have been identified as a sarcoma, however descriptive the actual term used. This was an *under-diagnosis*.

### Case 5.27

F (39 years) with a pararectal mass found during operation for uterine prolapse; further operation showed a retroperitoneal origin. When removed it was a whitish-pink myxoid mass, 700 g and 35 × 13 × 3 cm, centrally cavitated along half its length with three smooth polypi projecting into the cavity.

The general histological pattern was fibromyxomatous but there were scattered foci where, individually, differentiation was suggestively angiomatous, myomatous, lipoblastic or histiocytic with aggregates of lymphoid tissue here and there. It was diagnosed as a (retroperitoneal) 'mesenchymoma'; recurrence was considered probable.

At routine examination 4 years later, the patient having remained well in the interim, a mass was felt in the Pouch of Douglas. This was of the same type as the original lesion. Removal was this time followed by irradiation. It is perhaps too soon, even yet, to say that all risk of recurrence has passed but at least the patient remains well 8 years after the last episode, and the diagnosis still appears *appropriate*.

The question of the part played by the irradiation arises. On the first occasion, the patient was not irradiated and suffered recurrence 4 years later. On the second occasion, she was irradiated and has been trouble-free for 8 years since then. One wonders whether, had irradiation been used on the first occasion, recurrence would have happened at all. Obviously we can only speculate but from this sequence of events an instructive point emerges. Enquiry why irradiation was not used initially elicited the reply, "because the condition was benign"; that is, despite a mention of liability to recurrence, the term 'mesenchymoma' had not sufficiently conveyed to the clinicians the connotation of malignancy that it should. This matter is considered later.

## Case 5.28

M (36 years) with mass behind tendo Achillis for past year; excised, 12 × 5 × 4 cm with mucoid cut surface.

The pattern was predominantly that shown in Fig. 5.43, relatively widely-separated round, oval or spindle cells in a mucoid matrix but with occasional areas (Figs. 5.44 and 5.45) where there is greater cellularity due both to the presence of thin-walled but well-endothelialised vessels and to a generally greater density of nondescript mesodermal cells. Fat cells can be seen in these last two figures; they were nowhere more abundant than this. Mitotic figures were present but normal and no more frequent than 1 per 8 hpf.

The lesion was diagnosed as a 'myxoid fibroma', and the opinion given that local recurrence was a strong possibility (it was poorly encapsulated) but metastasis, at this stage at any rate, unlikely.

Two years later the lesion recurred, but now associated with a mass in the ipsilateral inguinal region. Tissue from both areas was virtually identical with that seen originally; it was no more aberrant or mitotically active than before. All that was grossly recognisable was removed by the surgeon.

There was again recurrence at the ankle after a further 2 years; on this occasion irradiation gave much initial improvement but within a year neuritic pains in the legs betrayed neoplastic tissue around the lumbar spine. Within a few months there was involvement also of the cervical spine, quadriplegia, and death. Necropsy showed neoplastic masses in para-aortic nodes, vertebrae and ribs, and within the pelvis. Figure 5.46 shows tissue obtained at necropsy; the lesion had become much more highly cellular and pleomorphic in many areas but was notably fatty in others, the whole picture now warranting diagnosis as 'liposarcoma'. The term originally used was an *under-diagnosis*. Review of the first sections indicated that more attention should have been paid to the frequency of mitotic figures. This was thinly cellular tissue: had the population of cells been more dense, the in-

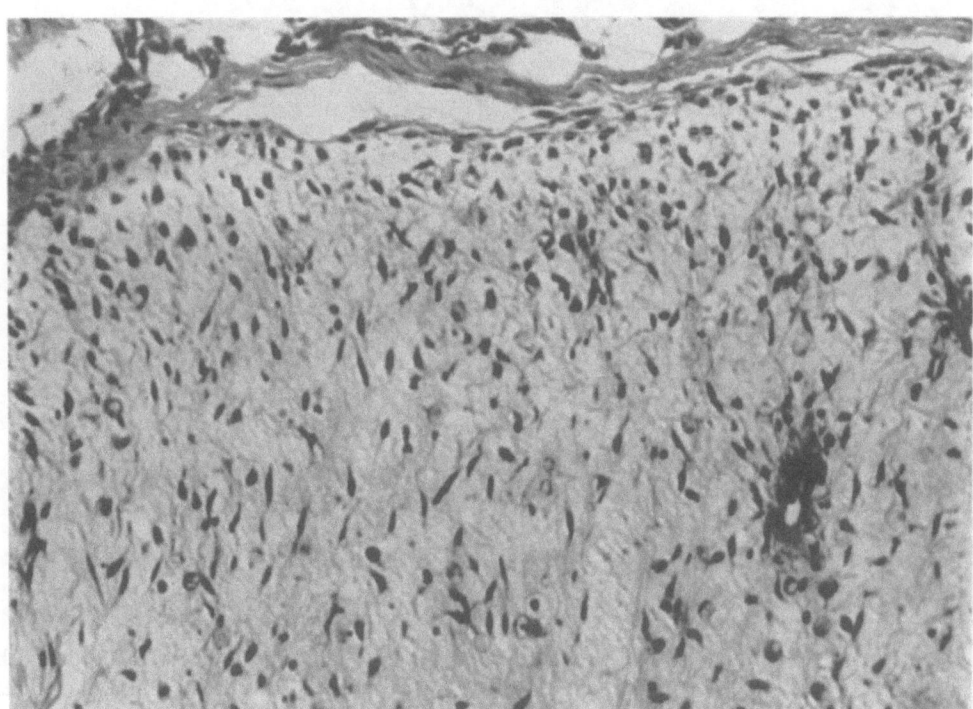

**Fig. 5.43.** Shows the pattern diagnosed as 'myxoid fibroma': it characterised most of the neoplasm. H & E, × 238

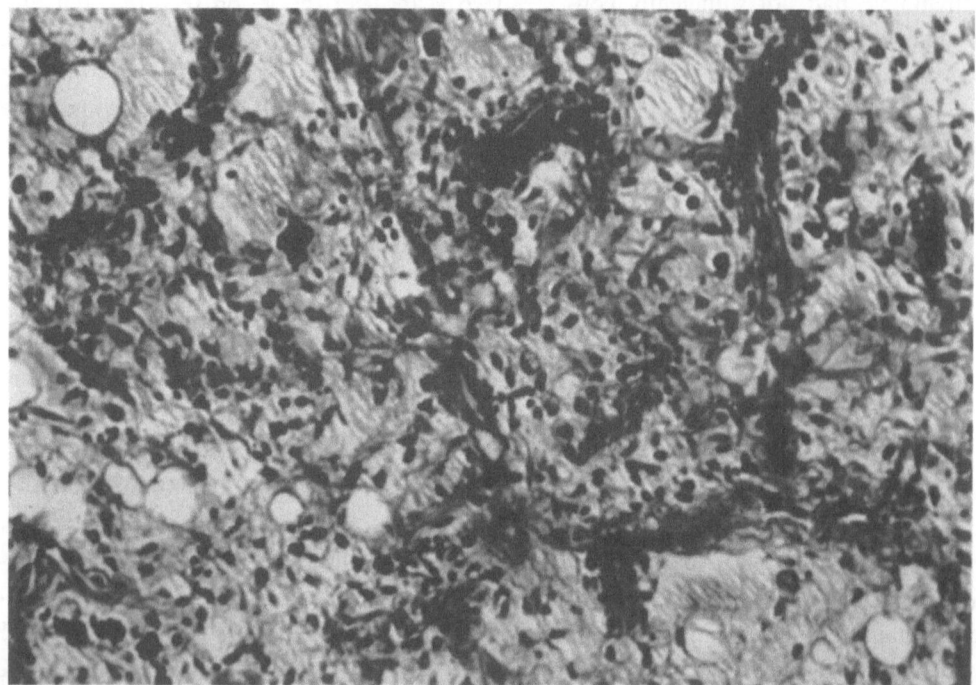

**Fig. 5.44.** In places such as this there was higher cellularity due partly to prominent vessels but partly also to background cells with round or oval, not spindle-shaped, nuclei, some of which belong to fat cells. H & E, × 246

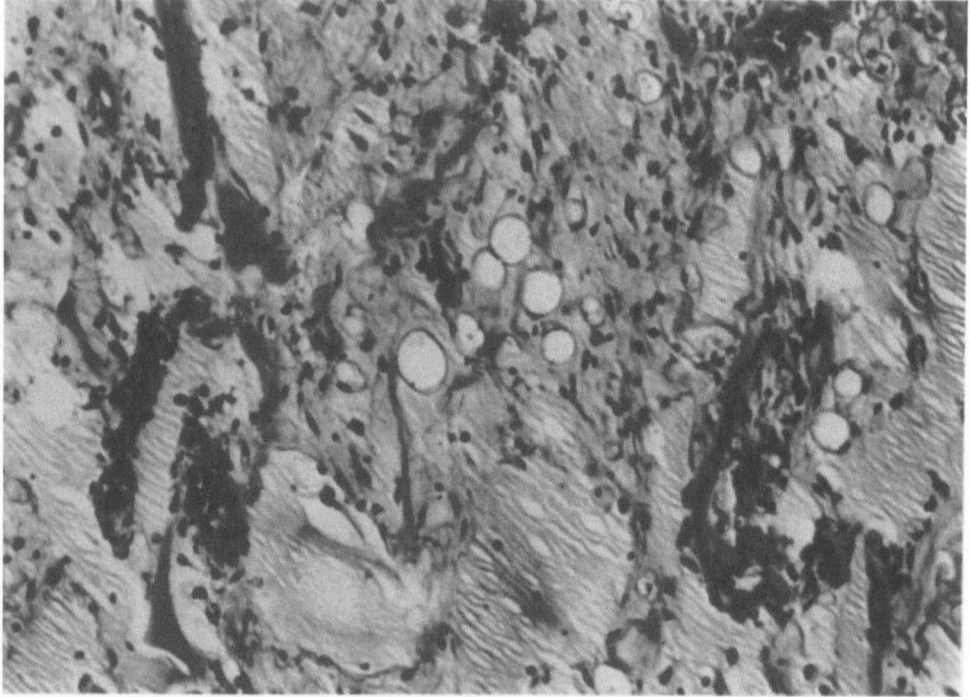

**Fig. 5.45.** There is much myxoid substance here, also prominent fat cells. Some cells, such as at top left-hand corner, had an intermediate appearance that seemed to link the obvious fat cells with those of undifferentiated appearance in the background. Mitotic figures were relatively few; however, had the cells been as closely packed as in Fig. 5.46, the incidence would have been at least one per hpf. H & E, × 238

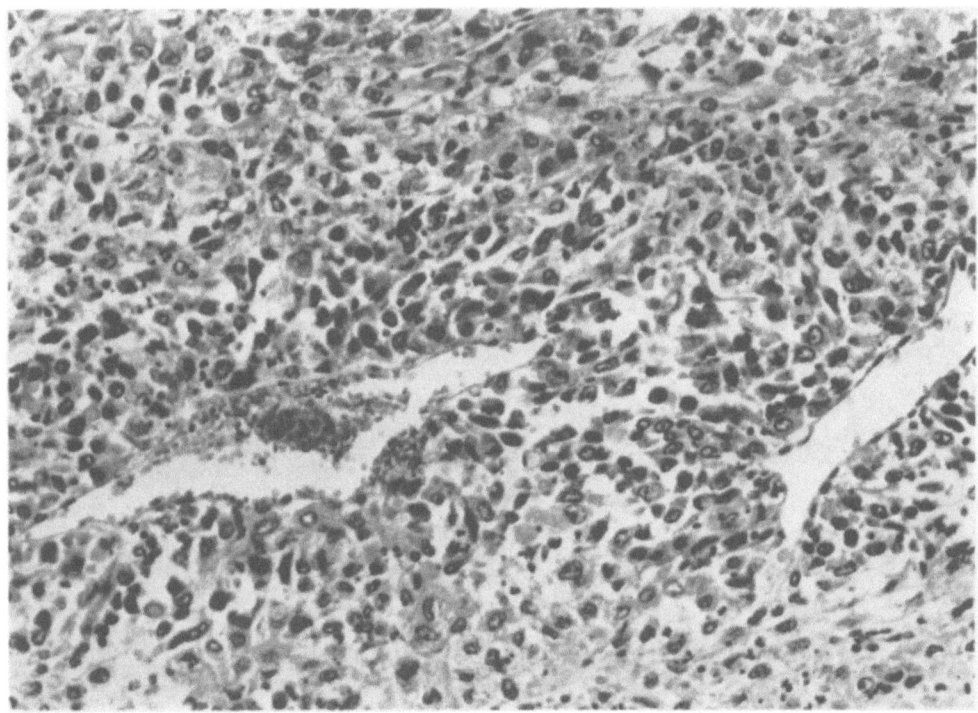

**Fig. 5.46.** The strikingly high and pleomorphic cellularity of the tissue obtained at necropsy. This pattern was as characteristic of the tissue terminally as was that in Fig. 5.43 of it initially. H & E, × 361

cidence could easily have been 1 or more in every hpf. A wider excision and, possibly, irradiation at the time of initial diagnosis might have been better treatment. This advice would certainly be given now (on the assumption, of course, that from this experience such a lesion would not again be under-diagnosed).

### Case 5.29

M (67 years) with mass in right popliteal fossa that had reached a palpable 3 × 2 × 1 cm over the previous 2 years.

Sections from the excised mass (20 × 10 × 5 mm) showed foci of highly cellular tissue in a generally fibroblastic background (Fig. 5.47). The cells were notably uniform, frequently arranged in uninterrupted sheets, and commonly in mitosis (Fig. 5.48). Mitotic figures had an average frequency of 1 per 4 hpf, and certainly aberrant forms were occasionally present. Of possibly equal importance, at least half of the mitoses, though not certainly aberrant, were sufficiently unusual to raise the question whether they were.

The tissue certainly seemed to be neoplastic. The only reason for any reservation at all was an awareness of the misleading appearance of the giant-cell tumour variant of fibrous histiocytoma as exemplified by Case 5.6 in the present series. However, there were no giant cells and no foci of haemosiderin, and, more positively, the cells were much more uniform. Frankly aberrant mitotic figures were no more numerous than in Case 5.6 but the total amount of marginal or borderline abnormality, and the uncertainty it induced, was much greater. In all, the question reached was not 'whether malignant' but what form of malignancy?

There was a main preference for 'synovial sarcoma' (the immediate proximity to the knee may have had some influence in this) but the suggestion was made that the possibility of metastasis from, say, lung or testis should be considered. By the time the patient left hospital, the chest X-ray was known to be clear, and the testes normal on palpation.

No further treatment followed the initial excision, until 2½ years later the swelling reappeared. Microscopy of the now rather larger

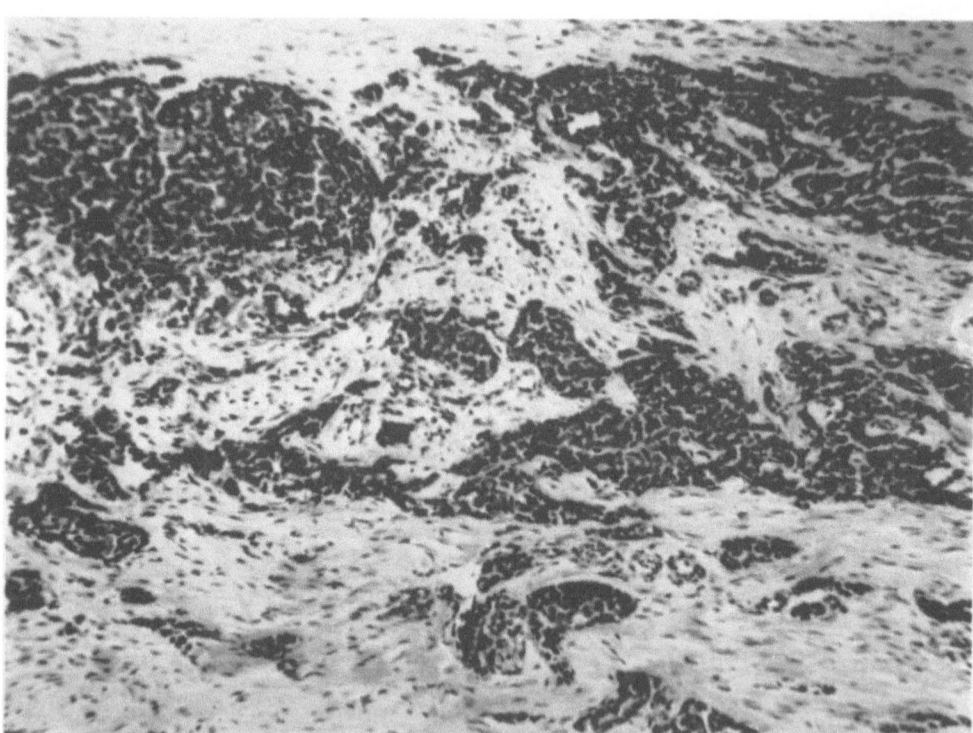

**Fig. 5.47.** Foci of highly cellular tissue disposed in clumps and sheets in a loose fibroblastic stroma. Metastatic carcinoma was considered as possibly its nature though synoviosarcoma was generally favoured. H & E, × 119

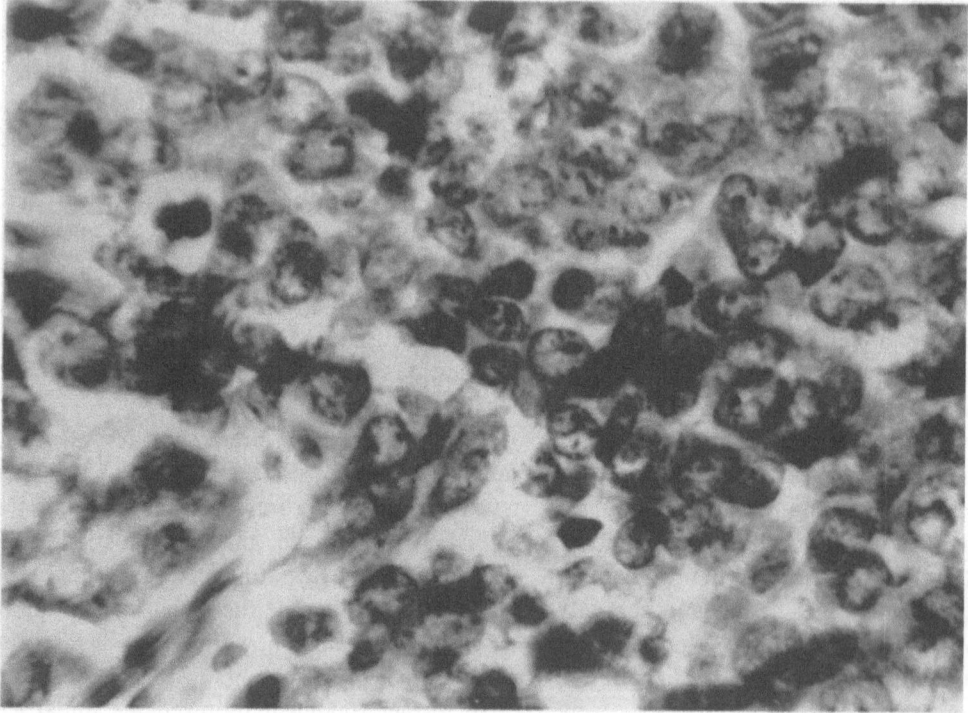

**Fig. 5.48.** The large and variable size of the nuclei, and many mitoses, established the diagnosis as 'malignant' even if the precise type was uncertain. H & E, × 985

mass (8 × 3 × 2 cm) showed a more diffusely than focally cellular lesion with less mitotic activity than originally; it was now, for no understandable reason, widely infiltrated by eosinophil polymorphonuclears. Still some histological doubt persisted that the lesion might be carcinoma rather than sarcoma; however, if this had originally been a metastasis, its recurring before any other metastases had appeared would have been unusual.

Almost exactly one further year later there was again a mass at the same site, by now 8 × 8 × 3 cm. Without further ado, a mid-thigh amputation was performed.

The tissue on this occasion had the appearance shown in Figs. 5.49 and 5.50. The neoplastic foci are now smaller and have adopted a pseudoglandular or pseudo-epithelial character with similar cells forming a quite undifferentiated neoplastic background. This is an expression of the biphasic pattern of many or most synovial sarcomas; it had taken some 3½ years to emerge in full and to confirm the originally preferred diagnosis as *appropriate*.

The patient remains well 9 years after his amputation. In view of the relatively high mortality of this form of sarcoma he has been fortunate to resist the neoplastic cells that must have entered the circulation in plenty, certainly on the occasion of the two episodes of excision, and doubtless from time to time throughout.

### Case 5.30

M (40 years) whose complaint was inability to 'bend his hip', so much so that it seriously interfered with his work as a lorry driver. In fact, he could hardly flex his (right) hip at all, a not surprising consequence of his having what the orthopaedic surgeon described on the initial biopsy request form as '. . . a mass the size of an adult head at the upper end of thigh and encroaching on the groin'. It had first been noticed 3 years earlier. The material first received comprised many fragments of rather soft yellowish-brown tissue resembling skeletal muscle in some places.

Figure 5.51 shows the general texture and largely papillary pattern of the tissue. The darkest areas represent deposits of haemosiderin. There were synovial-type spaces with a pseudo-epithelial lining in many areas (Fig. 5.52).

These are seen also in Fig. 5.53, as is the edge of an area of frondose pattern, but there is, in addition, transition to a much more highly cellular type of tissue. Within this, besides mononuclear siderophages, there were not infrequent multinucleate giant cells (Fig. 5.54) and, with a frequency of approximately 1 per 10 hpf, mitotic figures (Fig. 5.55).

The lesion was diagnosed as an unusually exuberant pigmented 'villo-nodular synovitis'. The high cellularity and mitotic activity were accepted as features of a lesion of this kind rather than an indication of a frank sarcoma although the difficulties of achieving total local excision raised serious doubts whether amputation could be avoided.

Following the biopsy report, an attempt was made to remove the mass as completely as possible and a large amount of tissue was received. Most of the representative sections showed, as expected, the same appearances as before but there were also many areas where the tissue was even more highly cellular, mitotically active and devoid of both giant cells and pigment. Rightly or wrongly this was regarded as now frankly 'synovial sarcoma'. In consequence, any doubt about the advisability of amputation was changed to certainty and the leg was disarticulated.

Dissection of the thigh showed extensive invasion and destruction of all the muscles, anteriorly and posteriorly, around the femur in the upper 18 cm. Local excision, even if technically feasible, would have left an unbridgeable gap and thus a functionless limb. As it was, doubt remained whether all of the abnormal tissue on the pelvic face of the plane of resection had been removed; tissue excised from the area of attachment of the ligamentum teres to the margins of the notch showed it to be of the same highly cellular character and of generally malignant neoplastic appearance.

Despite this, the area healed quickly and the patient is alive and healthy, well adapted to his prosthesis, 11 years later.

In view of the outcome it may be doubted whether this really was synovial sarcoma; it seems unlikely, and to this extent the second report was an *over-diagnosis*. Certainly, because of the extent of muscle destruction, the leg could not have been saved but this in no way minimises the problem; if the mass *had* been technically excisable, would amputation *then*

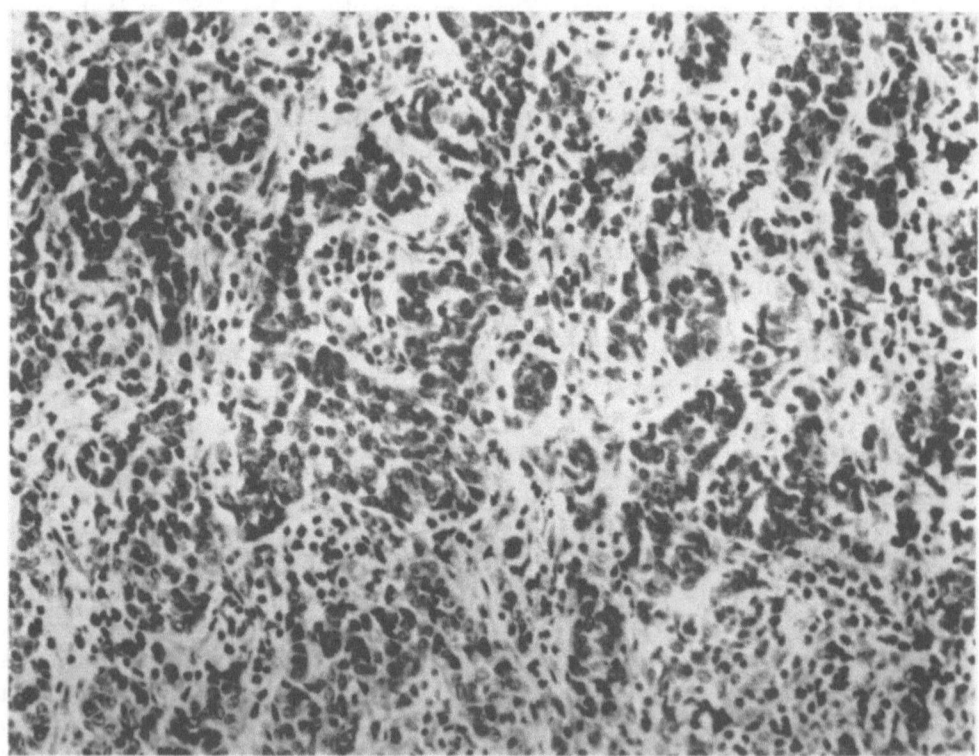

**Fig. 5.49.** From the recurrent growth 3½ years later: the epithelioid foci, some pseudo-glandular, are in a stroma that is now also polymorphic and neoplastic. H & E, × 119

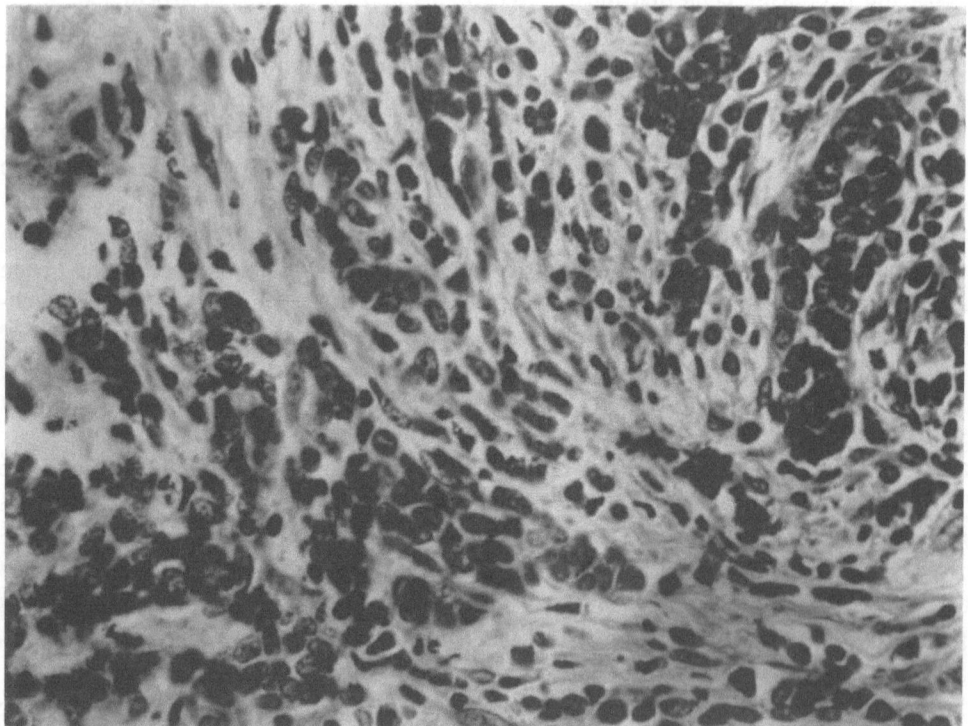

**Fig. 5.50.** The pseudo-glandular character of the hypercellular foci is evident as is the polymorphic cellularity of the stroma. H & E, × 476

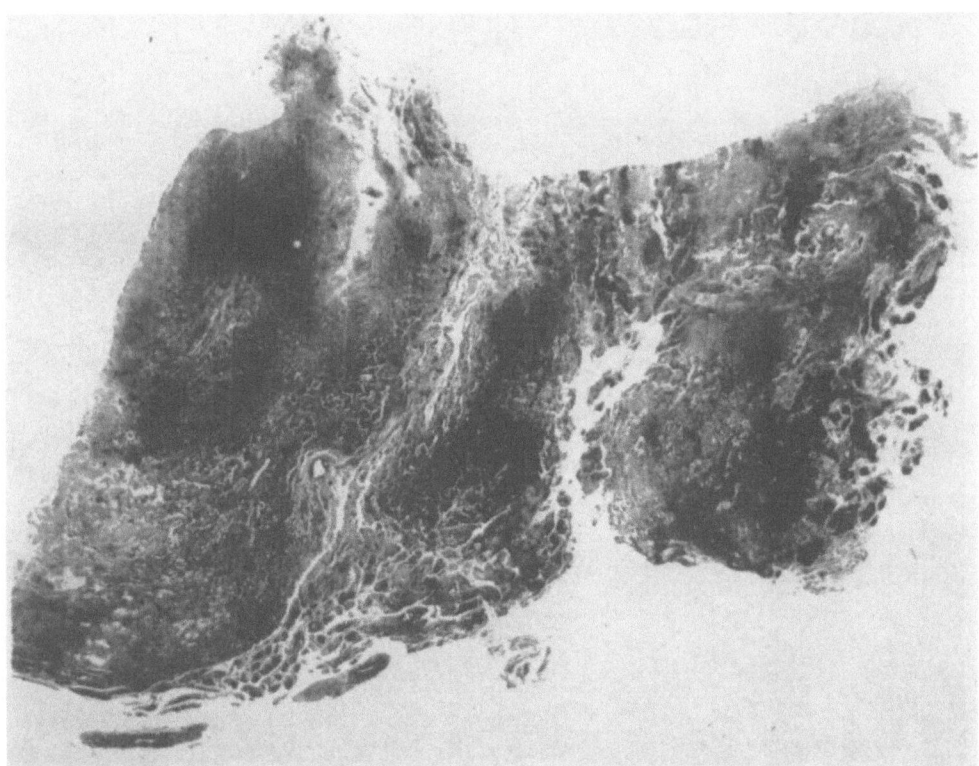

**Fig. 5.51.** Part of the frondose, heavily pigmented mass. H & E, × 5

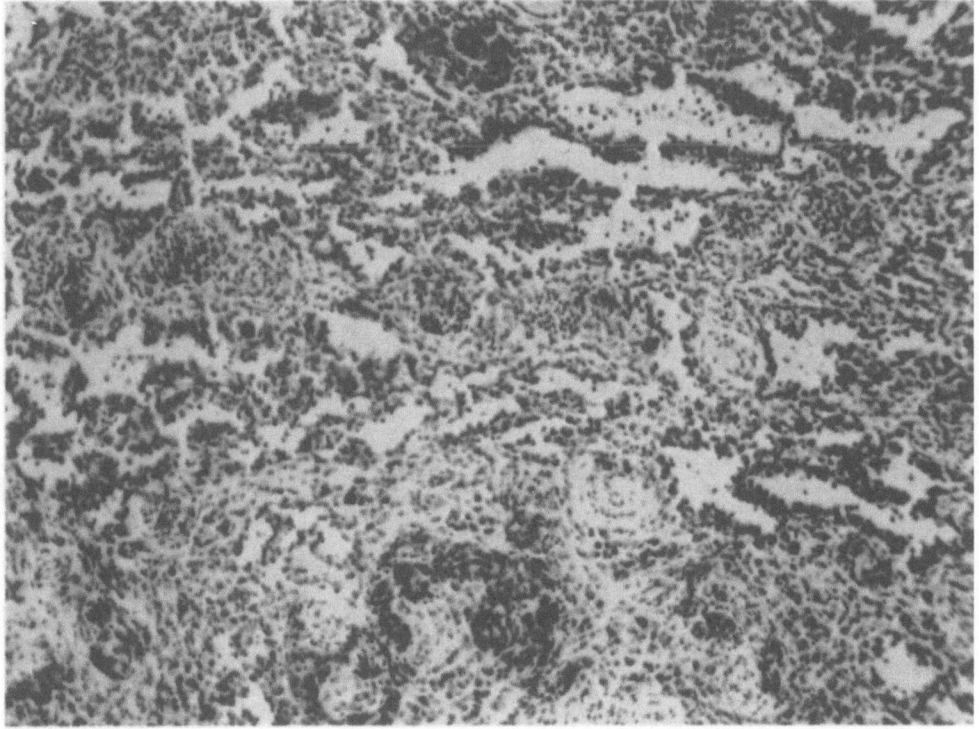

**Fig. 5.52.** The pseudo-epithelial glanduliform structures indicated a basically synovial nature. H & E, × 123

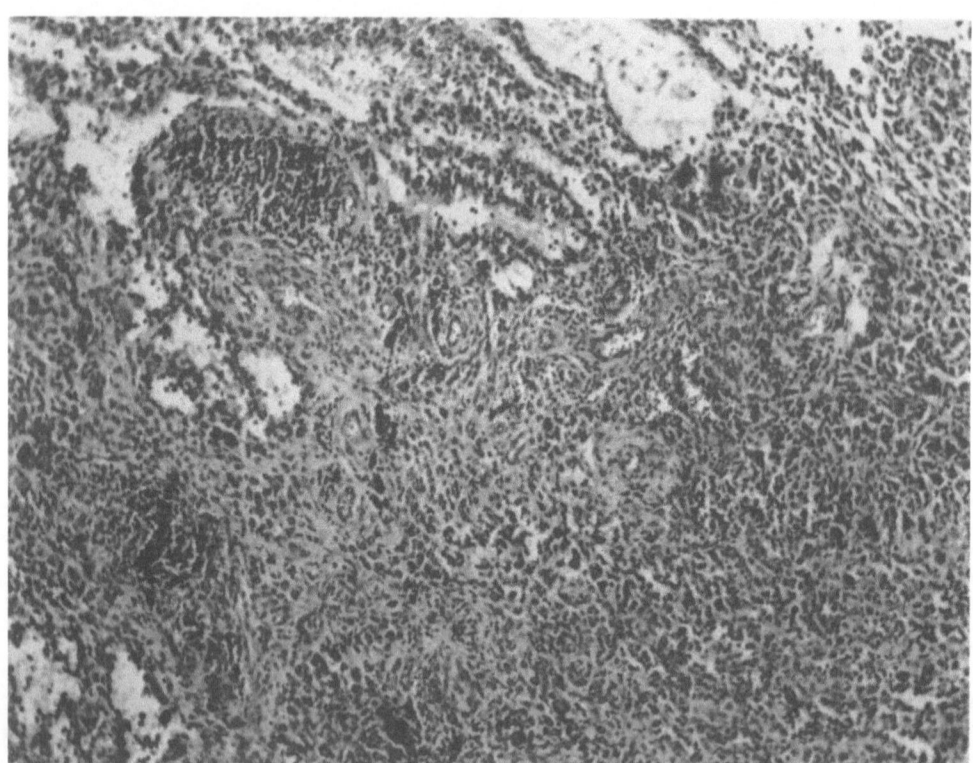

**Fig. 5.53.** The pseudo-glandular frondose pattern merged into one of much denser cellularity. H & E, × 123

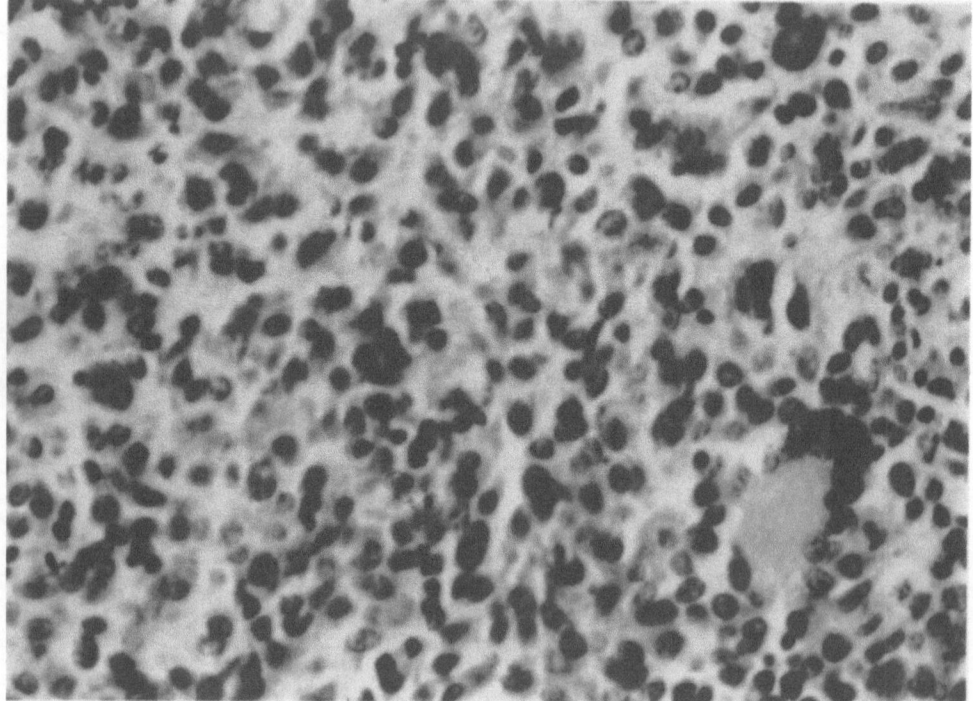

**Fig. 5.54.** Here there is considerable polymorphism and one of the not infrequent multi-nucleate giant cells. H & E, × 476

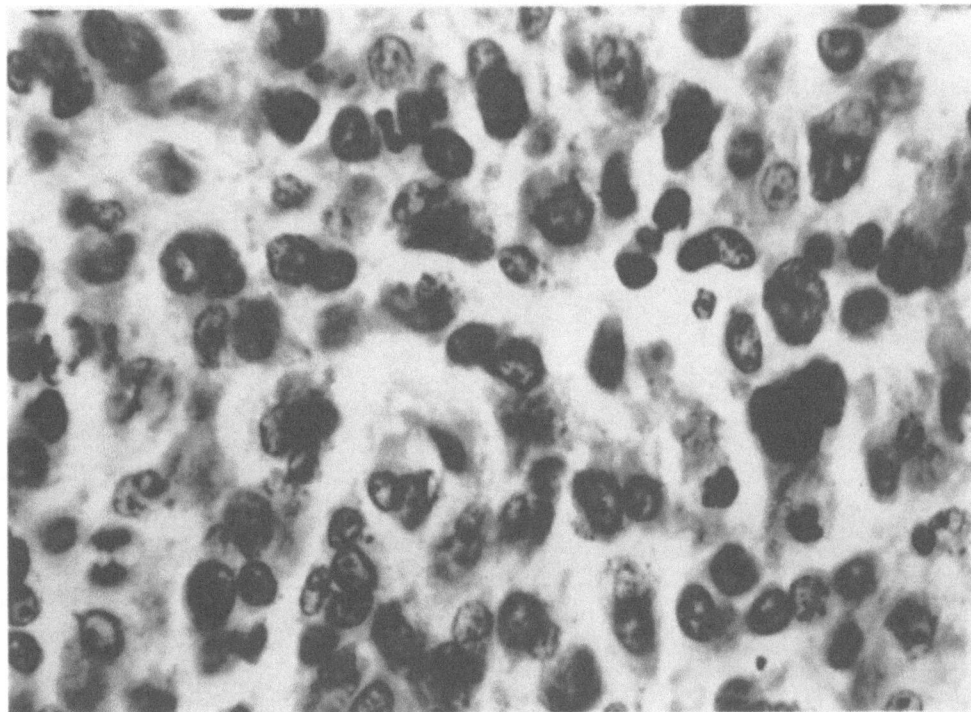

**Fig. 5.55.** The polymorphism is again evident. The pyknotic mass (*lower right*) was a polyploid mitotic figure. H & E, × 985

have been advised? In this respect the problem is the same as that met in Case 5.18.

### Case 5.31

M (26 years) with a small hard painless swelling of 18-months duration on dorsum of right foot.

Biopsy showed highly cellular and what seemed to be obviously malignant neoplastic tissue. Initially, little more could be said than that sarcoma seemed likelier than metastatic carcinoma. Examination of further material, and the occasional presence of small amounts of stromal mucinous substance, led to a marginal preference for 'synovial sarcoma'.

The high cellularity and the generally uniform round or just oval-celled pattern are shown in Figs. 5.56, 5.57 and 5.58. A below-knee amputation was performed within 1 week of the biopsy. Dissection showed the mass to be unexpectedly large though possessing a well-defined, almost rounded edge throughout. It extended between the 2nd and 3rd metatarsal bones to lie just deep to the sole and had an outline measurement of 8 × 5 × 5 cm.

The patient had no further trouble and was well 12 years later. The true nature of the lesion remains debatable but with the benefit of hindsight, it could be seen to have many of the features, including intracellular glycogen, of the extraskeletal lesion described by Angervall and Enzinger (1975) as resembling 'Ewing's sarcoma'. The original diagnosis may nevertheless be regarded as *appropriate*.

### Case 5.32

F (54 years) with complaint of an abdominal swelling. Laparotomy yielded some 3000 g of fibrofatty tissue forming a retroperitoneal mass.

Microscopy showed relatively vascular, widely oedematous but hardly myxoid, fatty tissue with a scanty fibrous stroma. As shown in Figs. 5.59 and 5.60, it contained many large bizarre and frequently multilobular nuclei, and multinuclear masses besides, but few if any mitotic figures (none was seen in three adequately representative sections).

The mass was diagnosed as 'liposarcoma'.

The patient reappeared 20 years later when a further 3700 g of identical tissue was removed from the abdomen; again, after a further 4 years,

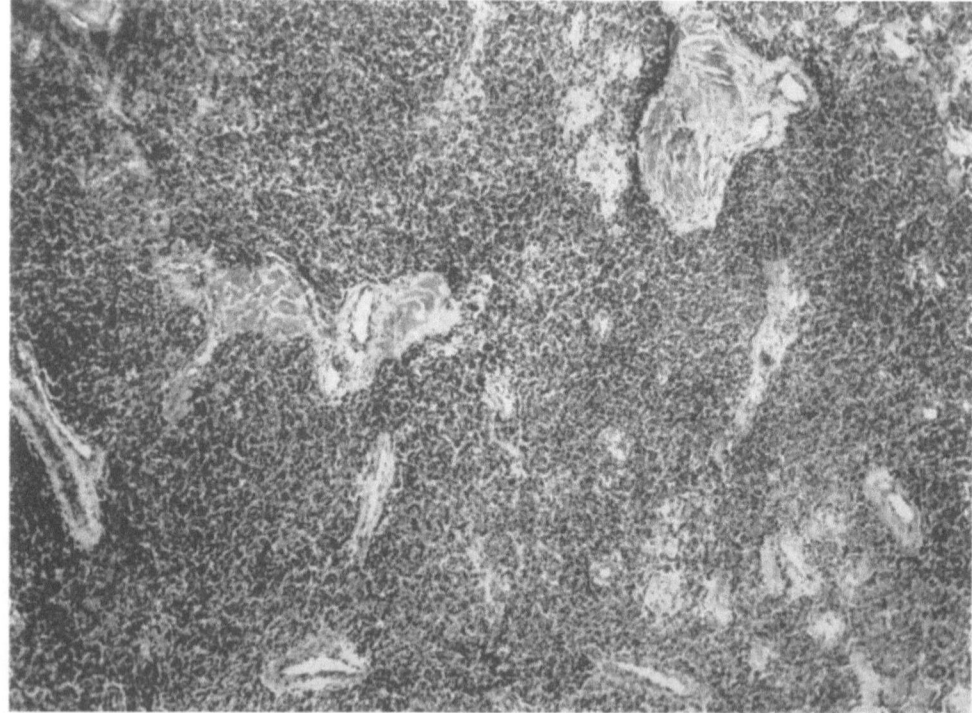

**Fig. 5.56.** The neoplasm was a dense mass of cells infiltrating all tissues forming the substance of the mid-part of the foot, though not eroding the metatarsal bones between which it had grown. H & E, × 60

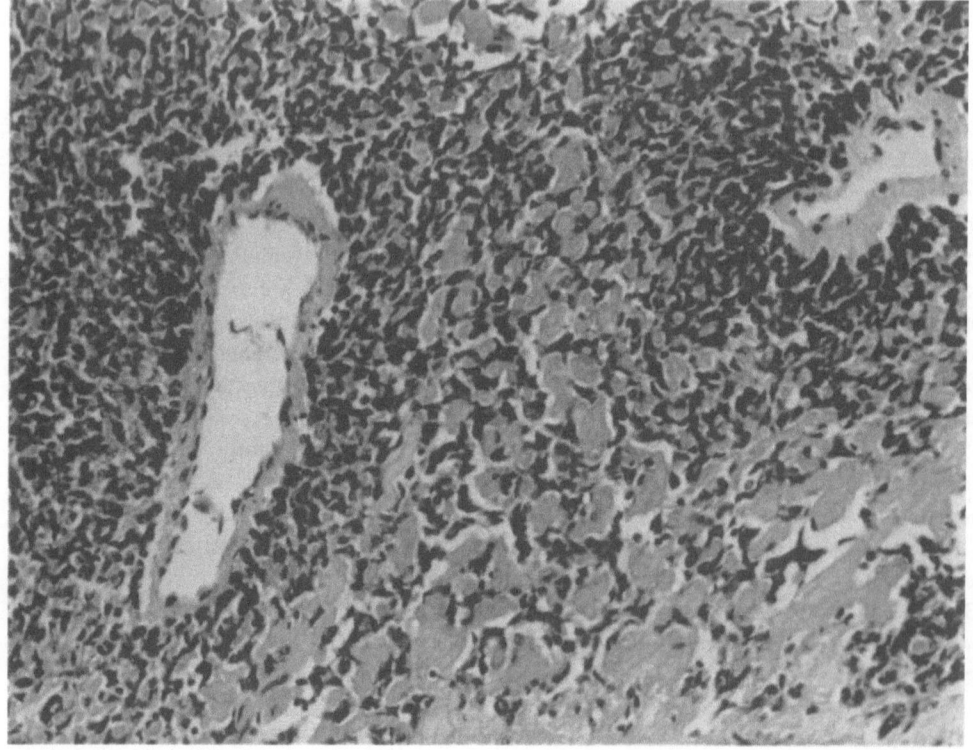

**Fig. 5.57.** Shows permeation of the paucicellular plantar fascia. H & E, × 225

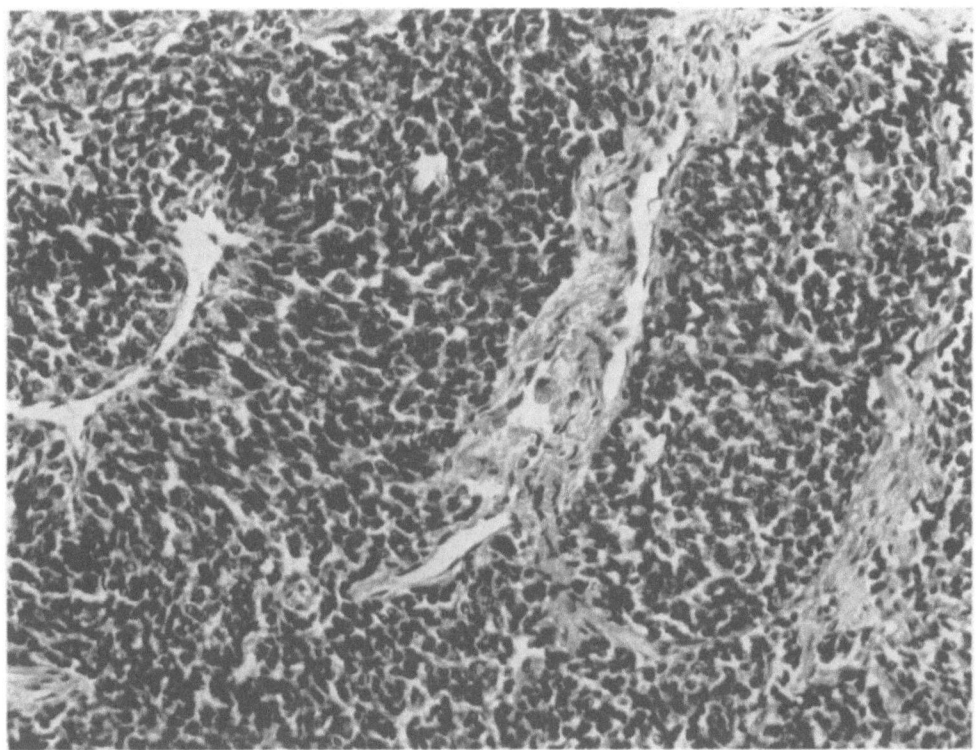

**Fig. 5.58.** The cells are relatively small and round with uniform nuclei. H & E, × 225

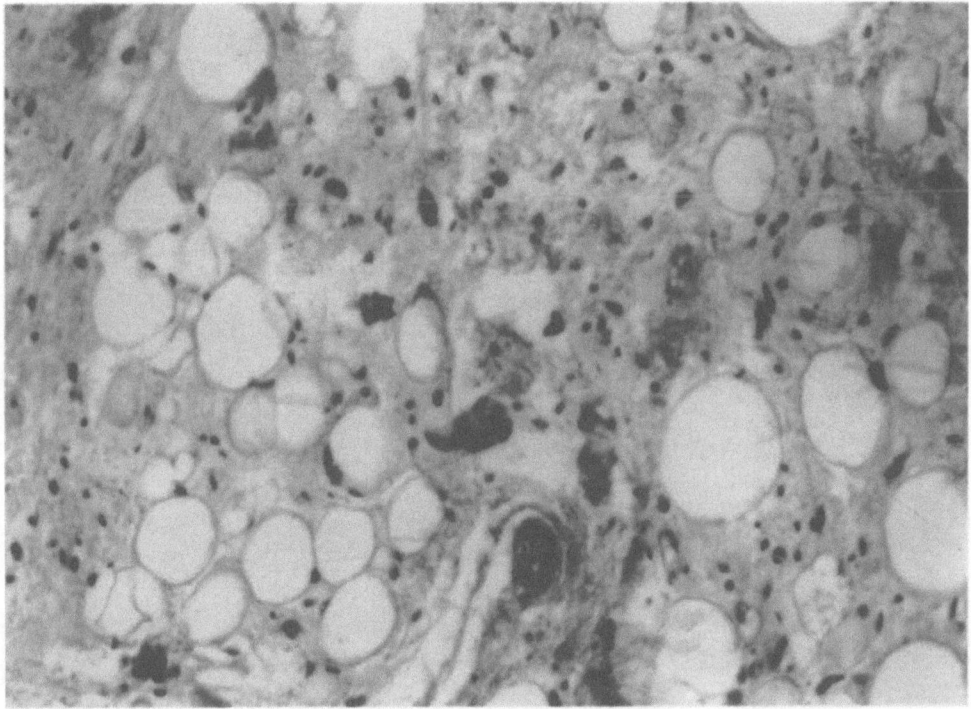

**Fig. 5.59.** Nuclear polymorphism of this degree seems sometimes to be an indication of degenerative rather than aggressively neoplastic change. It may have been so here, but the tissue as a whole continued to recur over many years: liposarcoma, albeit nonmetastasising. H & E, × 952

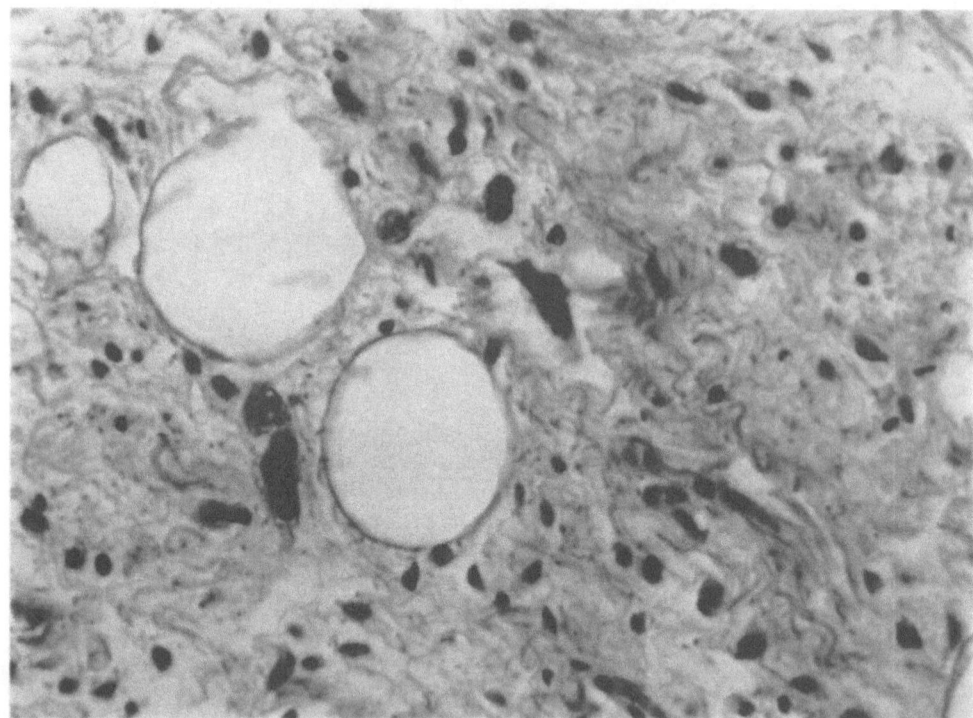

**Fig. 5.60.** Bizarre nuclei similar to those in Fig. 5.59, this time in tissue much more fibro-blastic/myxoid than adipose. H & E, × 952

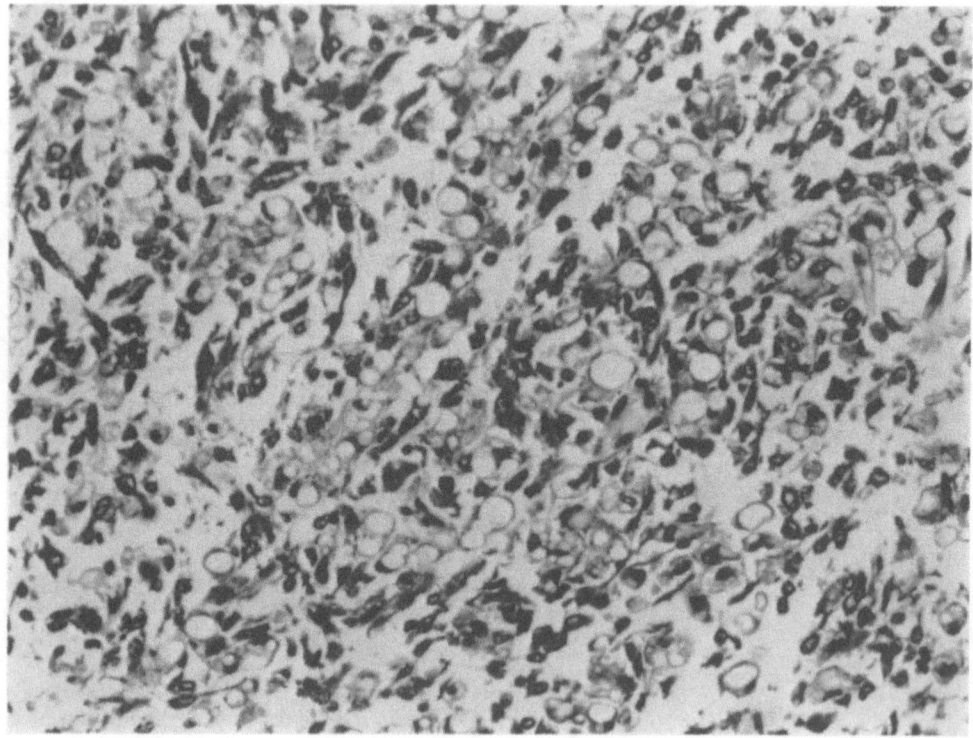

**Fig. 5.61.** Tissue from the last-removed recurrence, now much more highly cellular but still easily recognisable as fatty. H & E, × 374

when the yield was 3000 g; and on three further occasions at intervals of 2 years, 1 year and 9 months. She died 24 years after the initial operation, having sustained and resisted her liposarcoma from age 54 to age 78.

Review of the material in sequence showed a steadily increasing cellularity (Fig. 5.61); bizarre multilobulate and multinuclear forms persisted with approximately the same relative frequency, while, despite the obviously increasing rate of growth, mitotic cells remained extremely few. The diagnosis was *appropriate*.

### Case 5.33

F (63 years) with a 'wart' that had been growing slowly on her chin for the past 12 months.

Examination of the excised nodule, 12 × 10 × 10 mm with an ellipse of overlying skin, showed a typical 'granular cell myoblastoma' with characteristically associated pseudo-epitheliomatous hyperplasia. Excision was incomplete at one edge but the transected area was no more than 1-mm wide in the sections examined. Review in 6 months was advised.

There was no regrowth and consequently no indication for further treatment.. The small remnant of abnormal tissue had presumably regressed. The patient was trouble-free 11 years later. The diagnosis was *appropriate*; only the incompleteness of removal caused concern.

### Case 5.34

F (40 years) with a mass which had been growing slowly in the suprapubic region for 13 years. The excised mass was 13 × 7 × 5 cm, soft and elastic, with a whitish whorled cut surface and, in a few small foci, a myxoid appearance.

The general features are shown in Figs. 5.62 and 5.63. The tissue is of spindle-celled character and has markedly polymorphic nuclei: in different areas it is variably fatty, fibrous, and myxoid. No mitoses were seen; this fact and the extremeness of the nuclear aberrancy together suggested a degenerative rather than a malignant process. It was diagnosed as a degenerative 'fibroma'. However, in view of the capacity of tumours known to be myomas, as for example in the uterus, to show striking nuclear aberrancy, this one was probably a 'myoma'.

No further treatment was given, there was no

recurrence and the patient remains well 12 years later. The diagnosis was *inappropriate* though only technically so.

### Case 5.35

M (56 years) with paraesthesiae over outer aspect of leg in association with a lump over head of fibula. Exploration showed a 7 × 3 × 3 cm mass apparently arising from tibio-fibular joint and firmly adherent to surrounding muscle. It was multilocular with walls up to 8 mm in thickness.

The cysts had a flattened synovial-type lining and walls of simple myxoid connective tissue. It was reported as possibly a bursa or a 'ganglion' or a 'mucinous synovioma', with recurrence quite likely.

Swelling appeared at the site 13 months later. Operation showed a cystic mass, some 14 × 4 × 4 cm, around and possibly arising from the tibio-fibular joint. The tissue was now much more highly cellular, and the cells showed what was considered to be a significant degree of polymorphism and not infrequent mitoses in association with extensive invasion and destruction of muscle (Figs. 5.64, 5.65 and 5.66): the diagnosis given was 'synoviosarcoma', probably incompletely excised. After discussion with the surgeon, the decision was made that further local excision should be used. Total clearance was attempted and included removal of the head of the fibula, tibio-fibular joint capsule, and all surrounding tissue that seemed involved.

Microscopy of this collective specimen suggested that complete clearance had now probably been achieved; the head of the fibula was mildly eroded but not invaded. Opportunity was taken during the operation to remove also a 20-mm nodule on the dorsum of one hand. It also had, basically, the structure of an 'infiltrative' ganglion, excision doubtfully complete.

There has been no further trouble with either leg or hand, and the leg remains fully functional 9 years later. This was a significant *over-diagnosis*, generated by the hypercellularity, mitotic activity and widely destructive invasion of muscle, but at least the leg was not amputated. Review of the sections interpreted as showing synoviosarcoma suggest that such polymorphism as there was had been allowed too much weight. Also, not only were all mitoses wholly normal but a larger

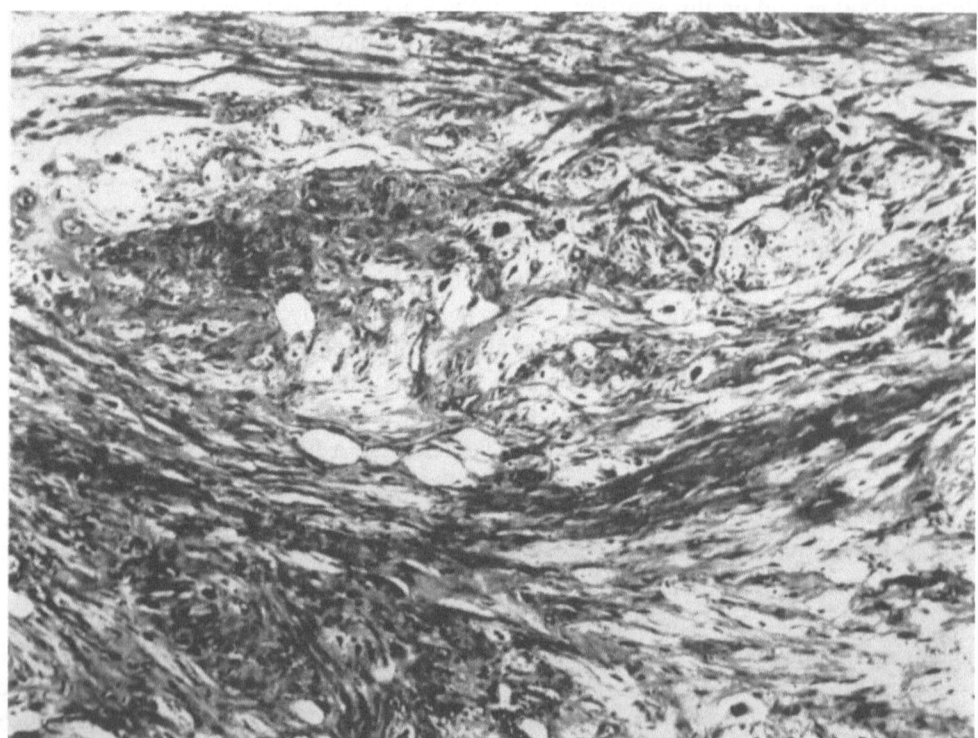

**Fig. 5.62.** General features of case 5.34. See text. H & E, × 62

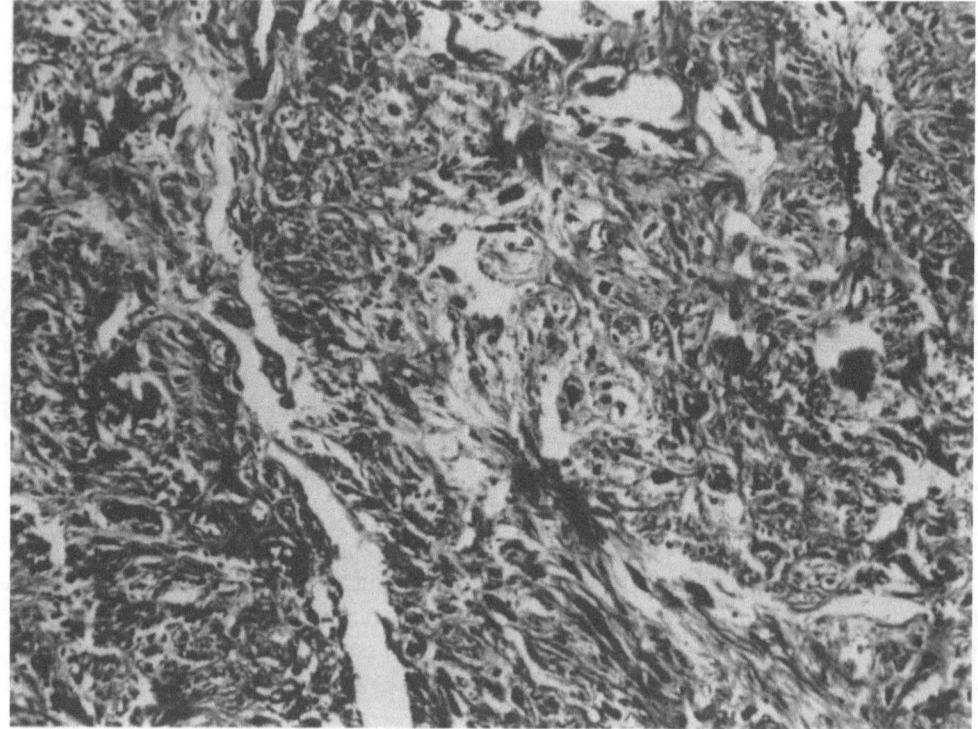

**Fig. 5.63.** General features of case 5.34. See text. H & E, × 123

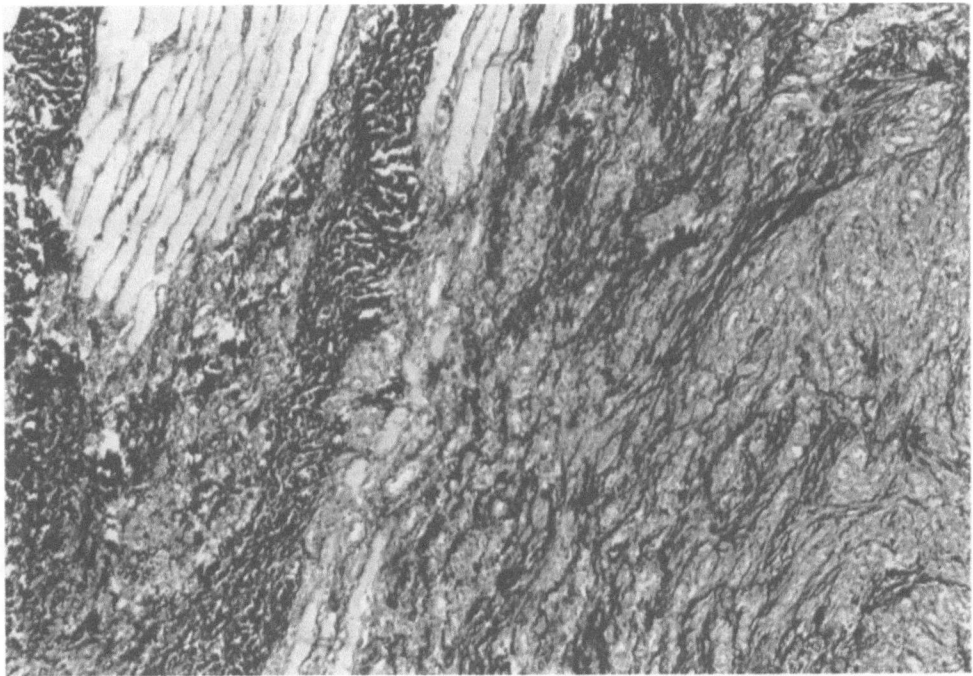

**Fig. 5.64.** The lower end of the mass of skeletal muscle (*upper left*) is being eroded, and the band of muscle running down the centre part of the field totally interrupted by the ingrowth of fairly highly cellular and vascular spindle-form tissue. H & E, × 60

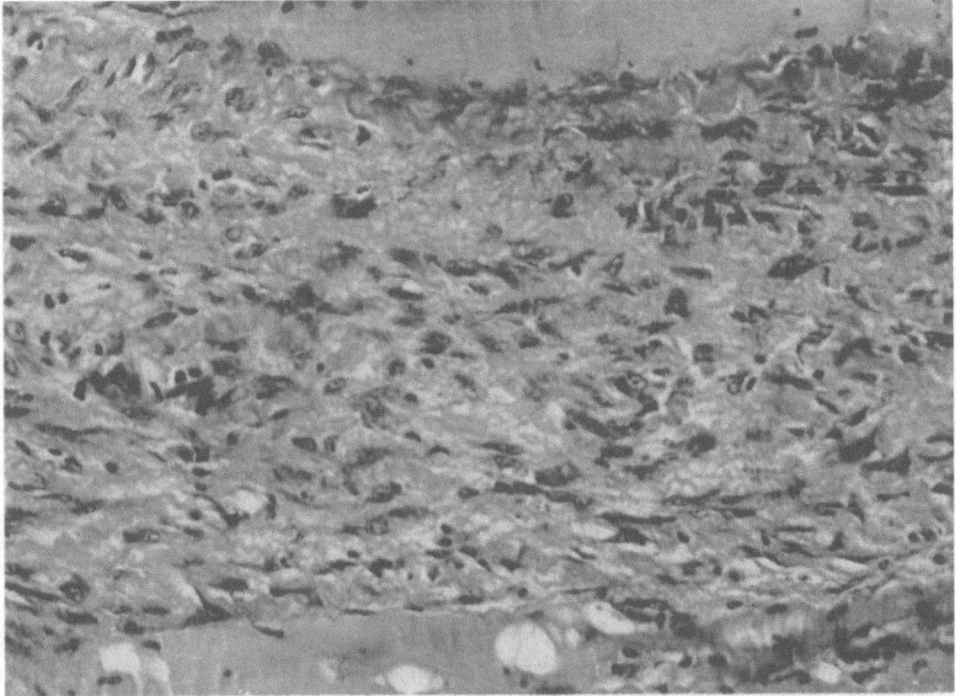

**Fig. 5.65.** Edges of the two adjacent muscle fibres forming upper and lower edges of the field are widely separated by an ingrowth of rather polymorphic tissue. Mitotic figures were present with a maximum frequency in places of one per 10 hpf. H & E, × 320

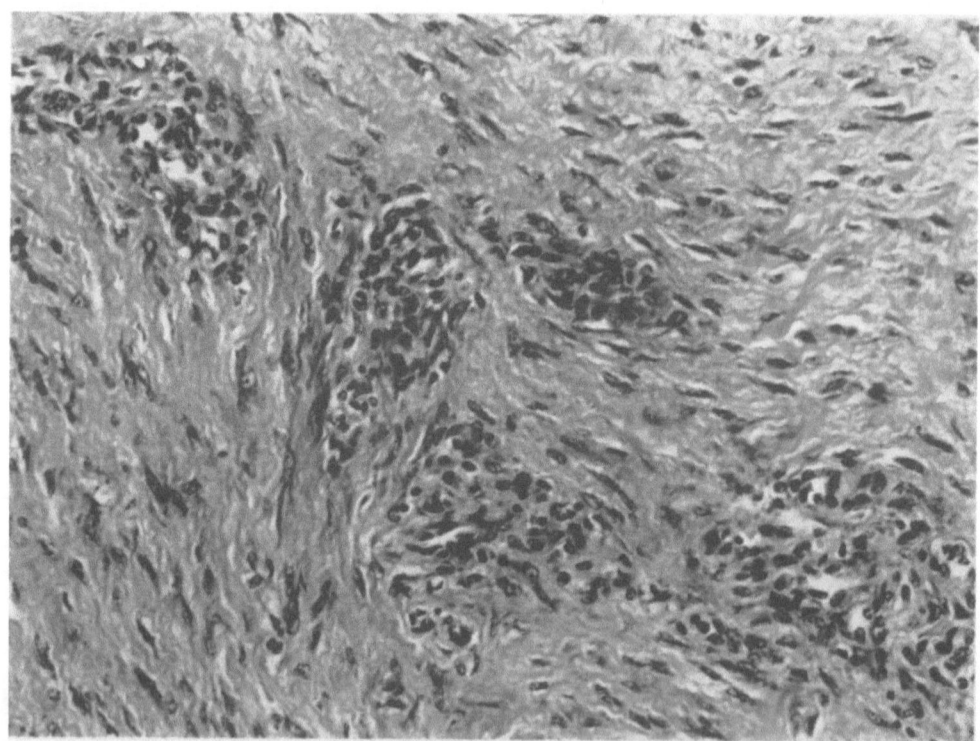

**Fig. 5.66.** Farther from the main area of infiltration of muscle, the tissue was more collagenous but contained small and relatively dense clusters of, again, rather polymorphic cells. Some were surrounding small vessels but most were not: the general impression was that the clusters were not merely overgrowths of vascular endothelium. H & E, × 230

proportion of the cells than was probably believed at the time can now be seen to be endothelial, not fibroblasts or synovially differentiating fibroblasts. The tissue response to what was almost certainly the cause, extruded 'ganglion' content, was nevertheless exuberant and strongly reminiscent of the response that attended the extruded nucleus pulposus in Case 5.25.

*Case 5.36*

M (37 years) with tender lump on palmar aspect of web between thumb and index finger, noticed for 3 weeks, 15 × 10 × 8 mm on excision.

The mass was a solidly cellular, spindle-celled growth of broadly fasciculate pattern, uniform cells and mitotic incidence at 1 per 10 hpf on average: no aberrant mitoses were seen. It contained quite numerous nerve fibrils and was diagnosed as a 'neurofibroma'.

Three years later a mass again grew at the

site, again of approximately the same size when excised.

Histologically the tissue was essentially the same as before with mitoses still numbering on average 1 per 10 hpf. The lesion was regarded as 'not really more malignant' than on the original occasion but further recurrence was considered highly probable.

The expected recurrence appeared 15 months later. It was described by the surgeon as being intimately associated with a nerve, encapsulated, freely mobile, and not infiltrating surrounding tissue.

Histologically, there was a slight but definite increase in both degree of cellularity and mitotic incidence though the cells remained generally uniform and mitotic figures normal. The pattern was now considered to warrant diagnosis as sarcoma. In the absence of any hint of a neurilemmomatous pattern, the diagnosis given was 'fibrosarcoma', of presumably endo- or perineurial origin.

No further recurrence developed during at

least the next 10 years: contact was lost thereafter.

Both the original and final diagnoses seem reasonable and *appropriate*. Also, the policy of strictly local excision, on the last occasion apparently curative, was justified. Any more radical excision would have been difficult without significant mutilation of the hand.

COMMENTARY ON LOCAL SERIES

The seven over-diagnoses per se led to loss of neither life nor limb. Where amputation had been performed, in two patients, the amount of tissue destruction would have necessitated amputation whatever the aetiology. Of the four under-diagnoses, two may have been responsible for death from metastasis; doubt remains. None of the five technically inappropriate diagnoses caused trouble.

As mentioned in the opening chapter, in the series as a whole, only laboratory reports expressing significant diagnostic doubt of some kind were assessed. Diagnoses given forthrightly were assumed to be correct: validation of every one was impracticable. However, with so many overgrowths of soft tissue reputedly mimetic of sarcoma, it seemed essential to try, by reviewing the relevant material, to discover how many patients, if any, had been wrongly diagnosed as having sarcoma: that is, how many lesions appeared on review to be certainly or almost certainly pseudosarcomas. To this end, a list was made of all cases of nonvisceral soft-tissue sarcoma notified to the local Cancer Registry during the years in question. The total, already noted, was 51: the outcome was known in 50. Any patients whose lesions were pseudosarcomas could be expected to figure among those who survived or died, apparently cancer-free, from an unrelated cause. The total of 51 had to be corrected in terms of the over- and under-diagnoses identified on review (Table 5.1); also, for immediate purposes, patients known to have died from an unrelated cause 5 years or longer after diagnosis were regarded as 'survivors'. The corrected figures then became: cases of sarcoma, 48; survivors, 12. The other 36 died of their sarcoma, almost all within 2 years (Case 5.32, the protracted retroperitoneal liposarcoma, was a notable exception). Details of the survivors, amongst whom, to repeat, should appear any patients with lesions considered on review to be pseudo-sarcomas, are contained in Table 5.2.

Review of none of the cases in this table gave any reason for changing the original diagnosis. True, by definition, an element of uncertainty surrounded the seven cases included in the borderline series (the first group in Table 5.2) but only one was a realistically possible candidate qua pseudo-sarcoma; this did not apply to the other six. In all, therefore, pseudo-sarcomatous lesions have not proved a problem over the 25 years. It may be that they have occurred, been not correctly identified, and been given names other than, for example, fasciitis, proliferative myositis, atypical fibroxanthoma, but at least, with the one dubious exception, they have not been diagnosed as sarcomas.

Analysis may be taken further than this, for the matter raises questions of almost philosophical as well as practical significance. An example of a lesion which, because of the outcome, could be regarded as possibly a pseudo-sarcoma, is the last contained in Table 5.2. This satisfied every criterion for high histological malignancy; it also recurred but has not metastasised during the last 12 years. One hesitates with any cancer to make a sharp distinction between 'cure' and 'sustained remission' but, in so far as a distinction can be made, this patient has been cured. However, since some lesions, the atypical fibroxanthoma, for example, may evidently be morphologically indistinguishable from a sarcoma (Gordon, 1964), we should perhaps conclude that this patient's lesion, since it has not metastasised, was not a true sarcoma but a pseudo-sarcoma. Metastasis, therefore, would be the sole criterion for diagnosis as a sarcoma. By this reasoning, then, we are denying the possibility that a potentially metastasising apparent sarcoma can be cured; for if it fails to metastasise it would, *ex hypothesi*, be not a true sarcoma but a pseudo-sarcoma; and this seems unrealistic. A possible explanation of the striking discrepancy between histology and behaviour in pseudo-sarcomas of any kind (assuming adequate sampling) is that, like granulation tissue only more so, these tissue reactions are sarcomas *manqués* or formes frustes. The factor that frustrates is as elusive here as it is with, say, the halo naevus or actinic reticuloid eruption.

The obvious danger of such lesions in practice is false-positive over-diagnosis and the pro-

**Table 5.2.** Details of patients who survived 'sarcoma'.

| Cases | Comment |
|---|---|
| 5.2, 15, 16, 18, 29, 31, 36 | These are already included in Table 5.1. Of these, only Case 5.16 seems a possible candidate *qua* pseudosarcoma, as pseudosarcomatous fasciitis rather than the originally diagnosed neurofibrosarcoma: on review, sarcoma (fibrosarcoma) still seems the likelier diagnosis. |
| M, 69 yr | Mass on back, excised, recurred after 2 yr, re-excised, no radiotherapy. Diagnosis on both occasions *leiomyosarcoma*. Alive to date 10 yr later. |
| F, 34 yr | Mass in thigh, excised, diagnosed *liposarcoma*, no radiotherapy. Alive to date 12 yr later. |
| F, 69 yr | Mass on dorsum of hand, nodular, haemorrhagic, cystic. Microscopy: a mixture of slits and acinar spaces, papillary and solidly cellular pattern (up to 10 mitoses per hpf). Diagnosed *synoviosarcoma*. No further excision or radiotherapy. Alive to date 7 yr later. |
| F, 34 yr | Nodule on scalp, recurred and re-excised after 15 yr. Diagnosed both occasions *fibrosarcoma*. No radiotherapy. Unrelated death 15 yr later. |
| M, 73 yr | Giant-cell tumour of soft tissue of thigh (registered for practical purposes as 'sarcoma'). Excision plus radiotherapy. Recurrence and re-excision after 4 yr. Well to date 6 yr later. |
| F, 18 yr | Mass on buttock, highly cellular, mitotically active (10% of figures aberrant), 'textbook' *fibrosarcoma*. Excision plus radiotherapy. Recurrence, histologically identical, 2 yr later, re-excised. Now trouble-free aged 38 yr. |

nouncement of an over-gloomy prognosis. Further, since a pseudo-sarcoma may evidently be indistinguishable from a true sarcoma, it follows that a deeply gloomy prognosis should never be given for any sarcoma of soft tissue: the patient might be fortunate in having one of the formes frustes. In practice, in the local series, amputation was performed as primary treatment in only 2 of the 36 borderline cases, and then only because total local excision was otherwise impossible. The policy in this region, and it seems to be widely the policy of choice, is virtually always to give local excision every opportunity to cure; and this has been sound. Retrospective analysis of any such series of cases as these would reveal the occasional patient whose life might have been saved by primary amputation; but the cost of this, as routine procedure, to other patients in terms of limbs unnecessarily amputated would be quite unacceptable. For sarcomas of soft tissue, especially in children, it is doubtful whether instant amputation, performed in the hope of forestalling metastasis, is ever justified.

## General Commentary

### PSEUDO-SARCOMATOUS LESIONS

The terms 'pseudo-sarcoma' and its adjective may be used with three quite different connotations:

a) That a lesion is an undoubted 'carcinoma' but has assumed a spindle-celled pattern: the spindle-celled epidermoid carcinoma and (*pace* debate on the precise histogenesis) spindle-celled melanocarcinoma are examples;

b) That a lesion, though arising certainly from mesenchymal tissue, has a close morphological resemblance to, and may even be morphologically indistinguishable from, a sarcoma but in truth is not a sarcoma;

c) That the lesion is a sarcoma but one that rarely metastasises.

In the *first* group, assuming for immediate purposes that the morphological variant has been recognised and the diagnosis correctly made, the malignant nature of the lesion is not in doubt. Examples are considered in other chapters that deal with carcinomas at different sites: implications of the counterpart term 'pseudo-lymphoma' are also considered elsewhere. In the *second* group the malignant nature of the lesion is almost by definition in doubt: or, at the least, no lesion ought to be designated pseudo-sarcoma unless diagnostically and prognostically it is very much of a borderline problem. Used in the *third* sense, the term is merely misleading.

Inevitably, since mesenchymal tissue is ubiquitous and highly versatile, such dangerously misleading tissue patterns may be met virtually anywhere in the body. The remarkable capacity of connective tissue to indulge in exuberant reactive or reparative growth is well recognised and was emphasised by Ewing (1919) long ago, but only relatively recently, as pathologists have followed more closely the after-history of some of their patients, has the frequency of false-positive diagnosis as sarcoma been realised. Such lesions are met mainly in the skin and subcutaneous tissues but examples occur elsewhere as, for example, in the oesophagus (examples of this latter kind are considered in the appropriate anatomical chapters). Some of the main varieties of pseudo-sarcomatous overgrowth are mentioned in the pages that follow.

## Myxoma

'Myxo'- has long been a frequent descriptive insertion in the name of a neoplasm: in these circumstances, descriptive is all it should be. A pure myxoma does exist, as the title of Stout's (1948) definitive paper states, in the form of "the tumor of primitive mesenchyme". Debate

whether mesenchyme can persist into adult life is needless and sterile.

As mentioned later in relation to the fibrous histiocytoma, all mesodermal cells once had the capacity to form mesenchyme, and only de-repression is necessary for the same capacity to be expressed later by some reserve cell somewhere. To merit the term, a lesion should consist of tissue indistinguishable from primitive mesenchyme apart from occasional areas of fibroblastic overgrowth. Such tumours are prone to recur, and may eventually kill by local extension, but, with one partial exception (*see* later), they rarely if ever metastasise. Virtually any other benign or malignant neoplasm of soft tissue, and some that are cartilaginous, may contain areas of myxoid appearance; for example, fibroma, lipoma, mesenchymoma, but, in these circumstances, fibroma, lipoma, and so on is nevertheless what they basically are. Even so, it is proper to ask whether neoplasms of the kinds that do have a myxoid component differ in any clinically significant way from those that do not. The matter has not, so far as I know, been analysed by the morphometric techniques necessary to decide the essential first point, namely, how myxoid a tissue is: we cannot otherwise know how much greater aggressiveness, if indeed any, is to be associated with minimally (say 10%) myxoid versions in comparison with maximally (say 80%) versions.

Such evidence as is available suggests that a neoplasm of whatever type tends to be regarded as 'myxoid' if more than some 50% has that appearance, and that this feature in some examples indicates a lesser tendency to metastasise. The myxoid variety of fibrous histiocytoma will later be cited as an example but even here, of the 80 cases analysed by Weiss and Enzinger (1977), the 32 most 'myxoid' had a rate of metastasis of 16% (and the 19 most 'cellular' a rate of 31%). Other lesions cited by these authors as behaving similarly are the myxoid varieties of chondrosarcoma and liposarcoma. The suggestion advanced by Weiss and Enzinger for the lesser aggressiveness is that the production of myxoid substance rather than of increased numbers of cells may betoken a form of differentiation, the lesser tendency to produce cells denoting a lesser tendency to metastasise: and this is at least plausible. Even so, the experience of our Cases 5.26 and 5.28, in retrospect almost certainly a malignant mesenchymoma and lipo-sarcoma respectively but diagnosed as benign at the outset, has left a lasting mistrust of a myxoid element. In the 144 cases of myxoma surveyed by Stout (1948), most had occurred in subcutaneous tissue (32 cases), bone, mostly jaw (26), genitourinary tract (23) and skin (22): none elsewhere reached double figures. Two series have been published, however, of the lesion's occurring purely in muscle, mostly in thigh or shoulder: 34 examples by Enzinger (1965) and 18 by Kindblom and his colleagues (1974). Despite their infiltrative character, in-tramuscular myxomas seem never to metastasise and scarcely ever to recur even if, as in many of Enzinger's cases, removal is performed by 'enucleation' rather than by radical excision. This calls in question the standing of the lesion qua neoplasm: Enzinger made the reasonable suggestion that it may represent a focus of fibroblasts of arrested development, able to pro-duce much mucopolysaccharide but not mature collagen.

Myxomas are sometimes multiple: when they are, and especially when in muscle, search should be made for a coexistent fibrous dysplasia of bone. This association was first clearly estab-lished by Wirth and his colleagues (1971) and has been re-emphasised since (Editorial, 1974).

The exception to the rule that myxomas do not metastasise is the cardiac myxoma. So ap-parently exceptional is this that either the cardiac form is biologically unique among myxomas or it is not a myxoma. The reaction of Stout was to voice a suspicion that ". . . such lesions are probably not true myxomas but sarcomas of some other types masquerading as myxoma . . ." There is something of a logical fallacy here but it does nevertheless seem likely that a closer examination of some of the metastasising lesions would have shown them to be basically leiomyo-, lipo- or some other type of sarcoma, all of which have been recorded (Burnett, 1975). We our-selves have encountered a metastasising neoplasm which seemed certainly to be an angiosarcoma: it had arisen on the aortic valve, but an identical lesion could presumably arise equally from the wall of the atrium and raise the question of 'myxoma' or 'myxosarcoma'. At least, however, histological niceties have little bearing on the management of an intracardiac mass such as

this. Clinical diagnosis is notoriously difficult (systemic disturbances of various kinds are a curious and frequent accompaniment) but, once diagnosed, only excision carries any hope of saving or prolonging life no matter whether the neoplasm can metastasise or not.

## MESENCHYMOMA, BENIGN AND MALIGNANT

The term 'mesenchymoma', unqualified, may mislead. It was first publicised by Stout (1948a) with its added definition 'the mixed tumor of mesenchymal derivatives'; that is, a neoplasm consisting of two or more types of tissue such as fat, muscle, cartilage. Almost simultaneously, however, the same author (Stout, 1948), in analysing the many myxoid forms of connective tissue overgrowth that there are, invoked mesen-chyme in another context. He concluded that amongst such overgrowths a definable entity could be discerned; this, for him, was the true 'myxoma', defined as 'the primitive tumor of mesenchyme'. We have therefore to distinguish between, on the one hand, benign and malignant neoplasia of mesenchyme, in the myxomas; and, on the other, benign and malignant neoplasia of mesenchymal derivatives, in the mesenchy-momas.

With this practical distinction firmly in mind, we may note and apply as we think fit the recent ultrastructural investigation of a malignant mes-enchymoma by Klima and his colleagues (1975), and their conclusion that such lesions originate in a ". . . precursor primitive mesenchymal cell and that the differentiation of these cells is in-complete, deviated, intermixed, and immature". In addition to these various interpretations, the term, at any rate in the form of 'feminising mesenchymoma', has been used to describe such stromal neoplasms of the ovary as the granulosa cell tumour and thecoma but significant confu-sion is unlikely to arise here. However, it can arise in the context of another group of neo-plasms in the (usually female) genital tract, the so-called mixed mesodermal tumours. These contain two or usually more types of tissue and were acknowledged by Stout as, technically, forms of mesenchymoma. The obvious difference between the two groups is the presence, in the mixed mesodermal tumours, of epithelium; and it is probably this that has frequently served to divorce the two entities in the mind of the pathologist. Logically or histogenetically there is no reason for divorcing the two since the epithelium of the upper 90% or so of the female genital tract is of mesodermal origin; so, by the same token and logic, the endometrial carcinoma and even the fibroid could equally be regarded as mesenchymomas. However, this is little more than a debating-point, summarily dismissed by Nash and Stout (1961) as "prostituting the word 'mesenchymoma' ".

The mixed mesodermal tumour is a structurally well-recognised entity of equally well-recognised behaviour; examples may at times pose something of a borderline problem histologically but for practical purposes all are malignant. The implications of the term 'mesenchymoma' are less widely appreciated, mainly because the term per se conveys no behavioural information. In order to avoid ambiguity, such as may cost the patient (as in our Case 5.27) an avoidable operation, it is essential that the term be qualified as 'benign' or 'malignant' (similarly undesirable ambiguity surrounds the term 'melanoma' unqualified).

*Benign mesenchymomas* are dysontogenetic growths, and as such usually classified as, and submerged in the group of, hamartomas. The terms is thus rarely seen but an exception was the helpful report by Bugg and Mathews (1970) of four examples named as such. These authors stressed the discrepancy there may be between the structural normality of the cells and their infiltrability and gives a warning against over-diagnosis, because of this apparent invasiveness, as sarcoma. The bronchial hamartoma, with its complement of cartilage, fibrous tissue and possibly muscle is, for example, a benign mesenchymoma. The presence of epithelium in most, though not all, seems sometimes no more than a simple anatomical infolding or accident but, even when epithelium is apparently inherent, the mesodermal component would still qualify as mesenchymomatous.

Similarly hamartomatous mesodermal masses may occur in uterus, skin, nerve, muscle and bone, and especially in the kidney where they comprise a quite consistently definable entity, the angiomyolipoma. This has a curious and still unexplained association with tuberous sclerosis but may also occur sporadically. Any seemingly sporadic case clearly calls for investigation concerning tuberous sclerosis and also for assess-

ment of the state of the other kidney. The lesion may reveal itself by producing symptoms such as pain, haematuria and renal colic, and a series of 30 such examples was described by Price and Mostofi (1965). Malignancy has been recorded but is rare. None of the lesions in that series of 30 had metastasised but in as many as 13 cases the tumour had been diagnosed as malignant, as some form of sarcoma. The risk of over-diagnosis as malignant is therefore high, and it is due in particular to the polymorphism, giant-cell formation, mitotic activity and apparent invasion of vessels that the smooth-muscle component may show. The only safeguard against such over-diagnosis is recognition of the lesion, with its tripartite tissue make-up, for what it is, and familiarity with the fact that the histological features just mentioned, however suggestive, may appear in lesions wholly benign.

*Malignant mesenchymomas* according to Stout (1948a) are the "potentially or actually malignant neoplasms composed of two or more cellular types any one of which, if taken by itself, might be considered a primary malignant neoplasm". The word 'potential' here can have relevance only in retrospect, and in prospect the phrase 'might be' is of no value to the pathologist. A more practical version of the definition would be 'a neoplasm composed of two or more cellular types, any one of which would, if taken by itself, be considered a primary malignant neoplasm'. There are two further points, one important, one less important. First, fibrosarcoma is so commonly a component in these lesions that diagnosis of one as malignant mesenchymoma is more certain if based on histological malignancy in, say, a cartilaginous or muscular component (otherwise a fibrosarcoma amongst normal adipose tissue might be wrongly diagnosed as a malignant mesenchymoma); second, lesions already well-known as composite, for example the osteosarcoma and malignant osteoclastoma, though literally admissible, should not be included in the category of malignant mesenchymoma.

The myxoma, by Stout's definition, is an essentially monoclonal overgrowth. The mesenchymoma is a polyclonal overgrowth; that is, it includes at least two, and perhaps five or more, of the types of tissue into which the primitive mesenchymal cell may differentiate such as fibrous tissue, smooth muscle, striped muscle, cartilage, bone and haemopoietic tissue. In Stout's original series (1948a), eight cases included amongst them 11 different forms of differentiated malignant tissue such as chondrosarcoma and liposarcoma (one form was 'reticulum cell sarcoma': the others were more immediately recognisable as pertaining to the musculo-skeletal connective tissues).

Points to note in practice are two. First, the presence of more than two types of tissue may be overlooked, or, if recognised, the significance of the mixture may not be fully appreciated. Second, if only one of the component tissues is cytologically aberrant, and especially if the other tissues have been overlooked, the problem becomes that of the borderline fibrosarcoma or liposarcoma or some other sarcoma. It is here that recognition of the composite nature of the lesion is important, for its recognition would help to remove the '?' from the ? fibrosarcoma, or ? liposarcoma, or ? other sarcoma. No matter whether, say, the fibrous element or the cartilaginous element appears wholly benign, the appearance of a frankly sarcomatous other element would establish the lesion as a malignant mesenchymoma, and, as such, a lesion demanding the widest excision possible, for they have a formidable capacity for both local recurrence and metastasis. In the 201 cases referred to by Stout and Lattes (1967), the mortality in adults had been 60% and in children 43%. Even so, surprisingly gratifying results are sometimes achieved, to the point where Nash and Stout (1961) comment that the behaviour of the lesion in children is "unpredictable to a remarkable degree". Prognostic assessment on biopsy is clearly equally difficult but, of the various expressions of the neoplasm, the rhabdomyosarcomatous has proved the most consistently ominous. The not infrequently pseudo-sarcomatous appearance of myositis ossificans will shortly be mentioned. Reciprocal misdiagnosis with malignant mesenchymoma is an obviously possible danger.

NEOPLASMS OF FAT

The liposarcoma, in the words of Reszel and associates (1966) is a "deceptive and dangerous tumor". The possibilities of both over-diagnosis and under-diagnosis, and the obviously associated dangers, are correspondingly high. Lesions that may be misinterpreted histologically as liposarcoma fall broadly into two groups: (a) truly fatty lesions that either infiltrate, or show some minor structural change from normal adipose tissue, or both; (b) others of an essentially different kind, such as pseudo-sarcomatous fasciitis, that may be over-diagnosed as liposarcoma and must figure in the differential diagnosis; they are considered presently. Clinically, it would be well if pathologists constantly broadcast to surgeons that no mass, however like a lipoma, and however seemingly simple, should ever be discarded. I can recall two instances where a fungating mass had developed at the site of an earlier excision: in each case the lesion was a liposarcoma, and in each the original lesion had been considered a simple lipoma, too inconsequential to be worth sending to the laboratory.

*Lipoma and Angiolipoma*

The infiltrating lipomas and angiolipomas are intrinsically harmless but the degree of infiltration of surrounding tissue may be difficult to judge and completeness of excision therefore difficult to attain. Complete removal is essential, for, as with the fibromatoses, continued infiltration will interfere with blood supplies and destroy tissue. In one of the cases described by Dionne and Seemayer (1974) a lesion of this kind was intentionally over-diagnosed as liposarcoma ". . . to indicate the invasive and destructive growth qualities of the tumour, despite the benign histologic qualities", an illustrative and not indefensible use of the pathologist's prerogative. The lesion may be purely intramuscular, as were the 46 examples (3 were hibernomas) reported by Kindblom and his colleagues (1974), but even one of these cases had extended beyond muscle into fascia and tendon. A distinction was made by both Dionne and Seemayer (1974) and Lin and Lin (1974) between lipoma and angiolipoma; this difference in structure, however, implies no significant difference in behaviour. Both these groups of observers comment on the absence from the lipoma and angiolipoma of such features as high cellularity, myxoid areas, pleomorphism and mitotic activity. Since these features, if present, would presumably shift the diagnosis to liposarcoma, they could hardly be other than absent from the lesions judged benign.

*Liposarcoma*

Found by Enzinger and Winslow (1962) to be the commonest malignant mesenchymal tumour of adults coded at the AFIP, liposarcoma is as malignant a lesion as any of the soft tissue sarcomas. Of the 222 patients with liposarcoma of the limbs and limb-girdles in the series of Reszel and associates (1966), 94 were known to have died of the lesion within 10 years; only 38 were alive longer than this, and some 70% had suffered recurrence of the lesion after attempted local excision. Those in the series of Enzinger and Winslow (1962) with retroperitoneal lesions had a 5-year survival of less than 40%. This location was found prognostically ominous also by Spittle and his colleagues (1970), as was the appearance of a liposarcoma during pregnancy.

The structural range of liposarcoma is wide, and examples are customarily and conveniently subdivided, as, for example, by Enzinger and Winslow and others into myxoid, round-celled, well-differentiated and pleomorphic forms, or, as by Reszel and colleagues, into myxoid, lipogenic and pleomorphic. The myxoid form is the least aggressive, the pleomorphic form the most aggressive. In this last group the degree of polymorphism attained, with cells sometimes 300 μm in diameter (Enzinger and Winslow), is probably as great as occurs anywhere in malignant neoplasms. Mitotic activity, however, is a variably reliable index. In the myxoid forms, even those that eventually prove fatal (as in our own Case No. 5.32 admittedly only after 24 years) mitoses may be extremely few or even apparently absent, and even far from abundant in the polymorphic form. This, at any rate, was the experience of Enzinger and Winslow. In the survey of Enterline and colleagues (1960), on the other hand, ". . . the frequency of mitotic figures was roughly proportional to the ultimate death rate": lesions with more than 5 mitoses per 100 hpf were associated with a 5-year mortality of 90%, those with no mitoses per 100 hpf with a 5-year mortality of 22%. Almost certainly, in our Case 5.28, had the scanty cellularity of the tissue, with its 'diluting' effect on the apparent mitotic incidence, been given its proper significance, the lesion would not have been under-diagnosed.

Prognostic uncertainty lies not, as it were, at the top of the range but, as almost always, at the bottom, namely, whether a particular lesion merits diagnosis as a sarcoma at all. The essence of the difficulty is exemplified in the statement of Stout (1944) apropos the well-differentiated forms that, "It is questionable whether such tumors ever metastasise while they remain in this state of good differentiation". Lesions of this kind, as already noted, would probably be diagnosed and classified by others as infiltrative lipomas. Similarly, the advice was given long ago by Seids and McGinnis (1927) that the presence of mucoid tissue in a lipomatous growth should arouse suspicion of 'malignancy': how much mucoid tissue should engender how much suspicion is obviously a wholly subjective decision (however, accurate volumetric measurement could well provide the surgeon with an approximate but valuable percentage probability of 'malignancy', in effect, metastasis). A possibly helpful diagnostic clue seen by Spittle and his colleagues (1970) in 10% of their cases of liposarcoma is pyrexia. The significance or existence of this is probably more likely to be uncovered by a pathologist's specific enquiry than by clinical suspicion of the nature of a fatty mass.

The difficulties of designation, the likelihood of overdiagnosis and uncertainties of statistics have been illustrated by Evans and his colleagues (1979) whose 30 cases, originally diagnosed as well differentiated liposarcoma, were rediagnosed on review as: atypical lipoma, 9: atypical intramuscular lipoma, 13: and the remaining 8, all in the same region, well differentiated retroperitoneal liposarcoma. We may note that, in conflict with the advice of Seids and McGinnis just cited, most of the lesions in the Evans series contained at least some myxoid tissue.

Besides the predominantly fatty borderline tumours there are lesions of other kinds that may be misdiagnosed as liposarcoma. The acknowledged significance of mucoid or myxoid areas in a lipoma brings into this group the simple 'ganglion', myxoma and neurofibroma with myxoid stroma mentioned by Tremblay and Bonenfant (1969). Also, the next-mentioned pseudo-sarcomatous fasciitis, must, qua *pseudosarcoma*, be identified and excluded. This lesion was included in the list by Enterline and his co-workers (1960) as were fat necrosis (including sclerema neonatorum) and xanthogranuloma, both of which may may contain areas of misleadingly high cellularity, and the malignant fibroxanthoma. By comparison with the misdiagnosis of, say, a fasciitis as liposarcoma, the misinterpretation as liposarcoma of a malignant fibroxanthoma or one of the 'other mucoid sarcomas' mentioned by Enterline and his colleagues, however regrettable academically, would be of little consequence in practice.

### Fasciitis (Pseudo-sarcomatous, Nodular)

In 1955 an account was published by Konwaler and his colleagues of eight patients with what they termed *subcutaneous pseudo-sarcomatous fibromatosis (fasciitis)*. A few years later the recommendation was made by Stout (1961), from his study of 123 cases, that the term 'subcutaneous' be dropped since the lesions may occur elsewhere as, for example, in skeletal muscle, breast and trachea. He commended and recommended the term *pseudo-sarcomatous fasciitis*, first introduced by Culberson and Enterline (1960). Almost simultaneously there appeared the papers by Price and his associates (1961) designating the entity *nodular fasciitis*, Soule (1962) using *proliferative (nodular) fasciitis* and Hutter and colleagues (1962) simply *fasciitis*, all giving useful descriptions of the lesions in a total of, together, 191 cases. Further series since then have been presented by Kleinstiver and Rodriguez (1968) and Dahl and co-workers (1972). The total number of cases covered by the articles so far cited is 397.

The composite clinical picture that emerges is that of a 2–3 cm nodule (rarely multiple) generally subcutaneous, frequently in the upper extremity, and sometimes of rapid growth (in four of the patients seen by Kleinstiver and Rodriguez (1968) for example, the 2-cm diameter was attained within 2 weeks). The original statement by Konwaler and his colleagues that a frequent initial clinical impression was subcutaneous abscess emphasises both the rapid growth and the not uncommon further features of tenderness and hyperaemia.

Pathologically, the lesion is highly cellular and vascular with a variably muco-oedematous stroma, several authors likening the pattern to that of large hyperchromatic spindle-shaped cells growing in all directions as in a tissue culture.

Sometimes it may show focal calcification or osteoid formation. Inflammatory cell infiltration is often minimal or absent, though Stout described the presence of lymphocytes and histiocytes in many. Mitotic figures may be numerous but all reports have stressed their normality: unlike some other pseudo-sarcomatous lesions, shortly to be mentioned, fasciitis does not show aberrant mitoses. A tendency to invade surrounding tissue is usual, and with adipose tissue so commonly nearby there is some risk that the lesion will be misdiagnosed as liposarcoma. In spite of this infiltrative character, and the fact even that in one of Stout's cases a lymph node had been invaded (whether directly or by vascular spread was uncertain), none of the nearly 400 patients in these series had suffered significant harm, at any rate from the lesion itself: the greatest risk lies in wrong diagnosis and inevitable over-treatment, as in the case of two patients (Hutter et al., 1962) who suffered mastectomy for a 'mammary sarcoma'. Nowadays, almost the only neoplastic lesion for which amputation of a limb is performed is the osteosarcoma (other neoplasms may lead to this but usually only after one or more episodes of recurrence or if adequate local excision would entail a useless limb). Over-diagnosis of fasciitis as a sarcoma, therefore, should not cost a limb. However, a comparable danger exists elsewhere. Fasciitis has been reported in the oral cavity (Rakower, 1971); the consequences of excision as for a sarcoma here need no emphasis.

Recurrence sometimes occurs, almost certainly due to incomplete excision, though in some cases inadequately excised remnants have apparently regressed. In short, despite the exuberant histological appearance, local excision is curative.

Lesions to be considered by the pathologist in the differential diagnosis include desmoid, simple fibromatosis, the juvenile aponeurotic fibroma, and the group of connective tissue overgrowths covered by the increasingly accepted terms *fibrous histiocytoma* and *fibrous xanthoma*, terms which include the lesions better known so far as histiocytoma, sclerosing angioma and dermatofibrosarcoma protuberans (DFSP). In some countries, Kaposi's sarcoma should be added to the list.

The 'histiocytoma' family merits particular mention and will be considered now.

## HISTIOCYTOMA

Some uncertainty still surrounds this term and its close relatives 'fibrous histiocytoma' and 'fibrous xanthoma', mainly because the term includes within a single histogenetic group many forms of abnormal tissue pattern hitherto regarded as representing individually distinct entities. This unifying concept owes much to the late Dr A. P. Stout whose basic tenet it was that the histiocyte could function at times as a fibroblast: overgrowths of histiocytes, whether inflammatory, neoplastic or dubiously neoplastic, could thus appear under the microscope as more or less fibroblastic, or more or less phagocytic, or in some degree as a mixture of the two. The concept was based largely on the mergence or sharing of morphological pattern by so many growths of spindle-celled type but partly also, as shown by Ozzello and his colleagues (1963), on the sharing of certain characteristics in tissue-culture by histiocytomas and 'xanthomas'. A recent histological, ultrastructural and tissue-cultural study of histiocytomas by Fu and his colleagues (1975) has extended and largely vindicated this concept. However, even with the help of the many articles by Dr Stout, often with co-workers, and repeated statements of his belief in the histiocyte as a 'facultative fibroblast', it has not been easy to gain from current texts, or even from the AFIP fascicle on *Tumors of Soft Tissues*, of which Dr Stout was co-author (Stout and Lattes, 1967), a clear synoptic view of the histiocytoma family.

The list that follows as Table 5.3 includes probably most of the lesions considered by various workers to have the facultative histiocyte/fibroblast as the parent cell. Some of the lesions present particularly difficult prognostic problems for the pathologist and will be briefly examined later for this reason. For the same reason it is hardly possible to make a sharp distinction between 'benign' and 'malignant' but the three groups do so approximately. Terms in the first column that appear to be largely synonyms have been bracketed but even these bracketed groups are not sharply separable one from another.

In view of this array, it is natural to ask more about the status of the 'facultative' histiocyte/fibroblast. This presumably has itself a precursor

**Table 5.3.** Lesions believed to arise from the histiocyte/fibroblast, and all, to that extent, 'histiocytomas'.

| Histiocytoma | 'Atypical' Histiocytoma | Malignant Histiocytoma |
|---|---|---|
| { Naevoid histiocytoma<br>{ Juvenile xanthogranuloma | Atypical fibroxanthoma<br>Atypical fibrous histiocytoma | Fibroxanthosarcoma<br>Malignant fibroxanthoma |
| { Histiocytoma<br>{ Sclerosing angioma<br>{ Angioendothelioma<br>{ Subepidermal nodular fibrosis | Pseudo-sarcomatous reticulo-<br>    histiocytoma<br>Pseudo-sarcomatous dermato-<br>    fibroma<br>Paradoxical fibrosarcoma<br>Pseudo-sarcoma | Malignant fibrous histiocytoma<br>Malignant histiocytoma<br>Malignant giant-cell tumour of soft<br>    tissue<br>Reticulum-cell sarcoma of soft tissue<br>Epithelioid sarcoma |
| { Xanthoma<br>{ Fibrous xanthoma<br>{ Xanthogranuloma<br>{ Xanthofibroma<br>{ Reticulohistiocytoma<br>{ Reticulohistiocytic granuloma | | |
| { Fibrous histiocytoma<br>{ Dermatofibroma<br>{ Dermatofibrosarcoma<br>{     protuberans (DFSP)<br>{ Storiform neurofibroma | | |
| { Giant-cell tumour of tendon sheath<br>{ Nodular synovitis | | |
| Villo-nodular synovitis | | |

or parent cell, a matter given close attention by Fu and his colleagues (1975) in the paper already cited. They offer three possible candidates as the parent cell; the fibroblast, the histiocyte, and a postulated stem cell that may beget either or both of these. Further, they doubt whether morphological evidence alone is enough to allow a firm choice of any one of the three. There, meantime, the matter rests; and perhaps that is where it will continue to rest, at least histogenetically, for the following reason. When an ancestral 'stem cell' is invoked in such circumstances we are within sight of the embryonic mesenchyme, which is multipotent, almost within sight of the inner cell mass or the morula, and not far from the ultimate stem cell itself, the zygote, which is omnipotent. *All* cells, au fond, have the same ancestor.

The practical problem for the pathologist is how to deal with the array of terms and entities in Table 5.3, and it presents a classical example of the choice, Shall we be 'lumpers' or 'splitters'? Conceptually, with its scientific backing, 'lumping' has the greater appeal; that is, we report the lesion to the surgeon as a 'histiocytoma (sclerosing angioma variety)' or 'histiocytoma (fibroxanthoma variety)', and similarly for the others. Alternatively, we may report or designate the lesions the other way round, as it were, thus appearing to underwrite their separable identity, for example, 'dermatofibrosarcoma protuberans (a form of histiocytoma)' or 'villo-nodular synovitis (a form of histiocytoma)'. The choice is for the individual pathologist to make, and no doubt he will compromise. Many of the terms in Table 5.3 are well established and well known to the surgeon, and probably already too mature to be uprooted or significantly modified with impunity. Others are less familiar, for example, 'atypical fibroxanthoma' and 'fibroxanthosarcoma', and put the pathologist under some obligation to explain, no matter whether he be a 'lumper' or a 'splitter'. For this reason, I believe that further comment on some of these lesions, and on others of the soft tissues that can cause problems, is in order.

### Dermatofibrosarcoma Protuberans (DFSP)

The term DFSP, at least, has long been familiar. To what extent the lesion it denotes is a true entity is debatable, essentially for the following

reason. The characteristic by which DFSP is usually defined is a particular kind of plexiform tissue pattern; descriptive terms include whirligig, cartwheel, spiral nebular, storiform (mat-like), but this pattern is not specific. It may be seen in lesions elsewhere than in skin, and sometimes, as in the case described and illustrated by McPeak and his associates (1967), in circumstances where the histogenesis is not in doubt: in this case the lesion was one among many in a patient with von Recklinghausen's disease. The pattern was seen also by Taylor and Helwig (1962) in two deep subcutaneous 'differentiated fibrosarcomas', while O'Brien and Stout (1964) indicate that it is also found in some of the other types of histiocytic/fibroblastic overgrowth, already mentioned, to which they gave the generic name 'fibrous xanthoma'. It seems better, therefore, to define the lesion primarily according to its clinical behaviour, that is, relatively bulky and commonly nodular subcutaneous growth with a frequent tendency to recur after excision; and to expect most to show the whirligig pattern on sectioning (ingenious three-dimensional reconstructions of the fascinating pattern have been illustrated by Meister and his colleagues, 1979).

The behaviour of this type of histiocytoma (or fibrous xanthoma) is generally familiar. It is notoriously prone to recur and may, rarely, metastasise. In the series analysed by McPeak and his colleagues, 21 patients had a collective total of 75 recurrences, due almost certainly to incomplete excision. This may be of relatively little consequence when re-excision is technically feasible, but in two cases the inherent invasiveness of the lesion had led to death from intracranial extension of lesions in the scalp. Initial excision seems commonly to underestimate the extent of the growth to the point where in the average case there is a 50% chance of recurrence. It therefore seems wise for the surgeon, should there be doubt about adequacy of excision, at any rate to consider a further excision at once. Occurrence in the retroperitoneal region has been reported by O'Brien and Stout (2 cases), and by Rosas-Uribe and his colleagues (1970). Metastasis and death occurred in all three. Occurrence on the face is surprisingly rare (Sauter and De Feo, 1971).

Frank metastasis has thus been recorded but the true frequency is difficult to estimate, partly on account of the problems created by differences in nomenclature and classification. Thus, Brenner and his co-workers (1975) describe the case of a DFSP that metastasised from the dorsum of the foot to the inguinal nodes 5 years later as the "24th instance of metastasis and the 7th case of lymphatic metastasis" of a DFSP recorded in the world literature. In fact, several other instances had already been reported though by another name; for example, as 'fibrous xanthoma' by Kauffman and Stout (1961) and by O'Brien and Stout in the series just mentioned; as 'malignant fibrous histiocytoma' by Wasserman and Stuard (1974); and as 'fibroxanthosarcoma' (*see* later) by Kempson and Kyriakos (1972). The development in two patients with DFSP of apparent metastases virtually identical with Hodgkin's disease (cervical node) and reticulum cell sarcoma (lytic lesion in ilium) was reported by Fisher and Hellstrom (1966). These authors were inclined to favour, as the explanation, aberrant differentiation by the DFSP in the light of "inter-relationship between primitive recticular, histiocytic and fibrocytic elements" but themselves acknowledged the difficulty of excluding the possibility that each of the patients did in fact have two independent neoplasms.

There is general agreement that the microscopic appearances are an uncertain guide to probability of metastasis, though the general working principle applies that high cellularity and a high mitotic rate (in the experience of McPeak and his colleagues, more than 8 mitoses per 10 hpf) is ominous but that a low mitotic rate (less than 2 per hpf) in no way precludes metastasis. It has been almost unknown hitherto for metastasis to occur with a lesion that has not recurred locally one or more times. However, in the light of what has been said about 'fibroxanthoma' and 'fibroxanthosarcoma' this assessment requires to be reconsidered. Along with other aspects it will now be reconsidered as part of the general problem of the relation of 'fibrous xanthoma' to the 'atypical fibrous xanthoma'.

### Atypical Fibroxanthoma

This term, growing in acceptance, applies to lesions with components essentially the same as those of the fibroxanthoma described above but arranged in a histological pattern so aberrant or 'atypical' as closely, sometimes indistinguish-

ably, to mimic a sarcoma. Since the lesion is almost always harmless, its correct recognition is obviously important.

The term was first used by Helwig (1963), who, with a colleague (Fretzin and Helwig, 1973), later published a valuable review of 140 cases in which the lesion was described as a ". . . mesenchymal proliferation of the dermis characterized by a bizarre and pleomorphic sarcoma-like histologic appearance but with a disposition to benign biologic behavior" arising in response to ". . . a variety of cutaneous insults".

Besides the series of Fretzin and Helwig, there have been published not only those by Kempson and McGavran (1964), Kroe and Pitcock (1969), Hudson and Winkelmann (1972) and Soule and Enriquez (1972) but also other smaller series and single case reports by others of what seem fairly certainly to be examples of the same lesion though given some other name. These include the 44 'reticulohistiocytomas' of Purvis and Helwig (1954); the 5 'sarcoma-like tumors of the skin' that followed irradiation described by Rachmaninoff and his colleagues (1961); 13 examples of 'paradoxical fibro-sarcoma' or 'pseudo-sarcoma' of the skin reported by Bourne (1963); the 4 cases of 'pseudo-sarcomatous reticulo-histiocytoma' of Gordon (1964); and the 53 'possible potential malignant tumors' selected from their 979 fibrous xanthomas and cases of DFSP by O'Brien and Stout (1964).

Details of age-incidence, sites of predilection, histogenesis, clinical behaviour, histology and differential diagnosis are well presented in these publications and will not be re-written in précis here. Certain general characteristics can, however, be discerned amongst these data that could be diagnostically and therefore prognostically useful. It may be helpful to anticipate here a later comment by stating that in this lesion, as would be suspected from the types and variety of designation used, correlation between histology and later clinical behaviour is low.

*Age and Site.* The condition may occur in children but is one predominantly of adults, and of the skin of head and neck in particular: elsewhere, especially on the trunk and limbs, the lesion is more likely to be seen in younger adults and children. In the series of Fretzin and

Helwig, it was in the head/neck region in 109/140 patients, the general circumstances being summed up by these observers thus: "Atypical fibroxanthoma is usually recognized clinically as a solitary, firm nodule on the sun-exposed skin of the head and neck of elderly Caucasian men". This is a useful vignette but the qualification 'usually' should not be overlooked.

*Clinical Behaviour.* With adequate excision of the lesion, which seems almost always possible, probably because the mass is usually well demarcated, the patient is cured. In some 10% of cases it will recur (for example, 9/101 in the Fretzin/Helwig series), perhaps by continued growth of remnants, perhaps, as always in these circumstances, as a fresh clonal response to the same persisting stimulus. On the other hand, despite the pleomorphic histology and even the aberrant mitoses, it seems virtually never to metastasise. The tantalising, indeed frustrating, character of the situation was well expressed by O'Brien and Stout who, despite an earlier statement by Ozzello and associates that "The mitotic activity of fibrous xanthoma is of great importance", said ". . . there are fibrous xanthomas that behave in a malignant fashion. It is gratifying to find that only approximately 1% of fibrous xanthomas prove themselves malignant but alarming to find that there are no reliable criteria that will enable one to recognize the malignancy from histological features".

*Histology and Pseudo-malignant Mimicry.* In none of the series cited above, other than that of O'Brien and Stout (to be discussed further presently), was the lesion described as in any degree microscopically storiform; that is, as resembling the DFSP (or fibrous xanthoma). Any resemblance is either positively denied by the authors or, if not, cannot be construed by the reader from either text or illustration. To this extent, atypical fibroxanthoma cannot be regarded as an aberrant member of the DFSP subgroup.

The components of the lesion are, intimately intermingled, fibroblasts, histiocytes of varying lipid content, and multinucleated giant cells (that is, in line with Stout's concept, the essential component is a histiocyte with a varying capacity to form fibroblasts, to ingest lipid, and to form multinucleated cells). These features do, of course, characterise many a granuloma. What distinguishes them here is their bizarrerie; many of the cells may show not only polymorphism and nuclear variability but also mitotic activity and, to be emphasised, mitotic aberrancy.

With this histological character, the lesions may closely or exactly mimic not only certain benign lesions but also, especially, sarcomas; yet, with the rarest exceptions, they do not behave as sarcomas (and when they do, the question naturally arises of a false-negative diagnosis). To give but two illustrations: the size of the problem may be judged, *first*, by noting some of the lesions included in the differential diagnosis by workers mentioned above, thus:

| | |
|---|---|
| myoblastoma | anaplastic carcinoma |
| fibrosarcoma | spindle-cell carcinoma |
| 'primitive' sarcoma | melanocarcinoma |
| rhabdomyosarcoma | reticulum-cell sarcoma |
| liposarcoma | |

and, *second*, by quoting the experience of Gordon with his Case 4: "Case 4 was recently presented at a seminar attended by over 35 pathologists. All . . . (but one) . . . made a diagnosis of some form of malignant neoplasm . . ."

These circumstances emphasise how frail our histoclinical correlations may be. We may note, as a further reminder of this, the way in which Hudson and Winkelmann obtained their series of 19 cases. They were analysing, retrospectively, lesions originally diagnosed as cutaneous spindle-cell carcinoma in 25 patients. On review, six were re-diagnosed; two as melanocarcinoma, and one each as fibrous histiocytoma, morpheiform basal-cell carcinoma, blue naevus and metastasising fibrosarcoma. The remainder formed their series of 19 cases of atypical fibroxanthoma. Thus, in not a single case was the original diagnosis confirmed. It is not surprising that almost all who have published series of cases of atypical xanthoma have stressed, positively, the difficulty of predicting the future behaviour of the lesion from the histology, and, negatively, the unreliability of the aberrant mitotic figure as a guide to prognosis.

The inclusion of forms of carcinoma in the above list of conditions figuring in the differential diagnosis is given added point by the report of Hood and co-workers (1973) who saw 13 examples of carcinoma of breast metastatic to the eyelid. The resulting lesion was highly mimetic of a histiocytoma. In four of the cases the lesion had, however, been correctly identified as metastatic carcinoma: in six, the initial diagnosis had been histiocytoma or a xanthomatous lesion of some other kind or a chronic inflammatory reaction. Similarly, histiocytoma-like appearances were seen with carcinoma metastatic to axillary nodes and closely resembling 'sinus histiocytosis'; the commonest form of mammary carcinoma to do this was lobular carcinoma.

*Differential Diagnosis.* To those confronted by the problems of differential diagnosis within this group as a whole, some useful advice has been given by Hudson and Winkelmann. They wrote that *atypical fibroxanthoma* is a polymorphic, exophytic, dermal and superficially ulcerative growth, while *fibrosarcoma* tends to be monomorphic and deeply infiltrative, and that degree of mitotic activity and cellularity are of little help in distinguishing the two. Further, as points of difference from *spindle-cell carcinoma*, the atypical fibroxanthoma shows no squamous differentiation and no close relation to the epidermis, and is not accompanied by epidermal dysplasia or carcinoma in situ. Even so, the distinction may be far from easy. We have recently had experience of an ulcerative lesion beside the ear in a woman of 72, highly cellular, aberrant, mitotically active, and not recognisably associated with the epidermis except insofar as it had ulcerated. With the possibility of fibroxanthoma in mind, the parallel possibility of a relatively good prognosis was given. Within a year, however, the lesion had recurred and metastasised to a retroauricular lymph node. With little doubt it was a spindle-cell carcinoma. Review of the sections showed probably too few multinucleated giant-cells to match the above descriptions completely; their scarcity should have been allowed more weight in the assessment.

There remain to be mentioned the 12 (possibly 14) cases of fatally metastasising 'malignant fibrous xanthoma' of O'Brien and Stout, exceptions apparently to the general rule that these lesions do not metastasise. It will be recalled that these workers, besides including DFSP with its storiform pattern in the broad group of fibrous xanthoma, remarked that this pattern ". . . is also found in many other fibro-xanthomas"; and indeed they recognised, as well as a 'giant-cell' subgroup, another characterised by a storiform pattern and multinucleated giant-cells together. The lesions that metastasised came from these two storiform subgroups exclusively, with the important implication that the presence or persistence of the storiform pattern indicates a metastasising potential largely or completely lacking in the fibroxanthomas without it. This deduction seems all the more valid in view of the studies of Kempson and Kyriakos (1972) into the entity they designate 'fibroxanthosarcoma', the subject of the next section.

*Fibroxanthosarcoma*

In view of the comments above, that atypical or 'malignant' fibroxanthoma sometimes recurs and occasionally metastasises in a quite unpredictable manner, it may be wondered whether there is any need for a category of fibroxanthosarcoma. Can it do anything but aggravate an already confusing situation?

The term was introduced in the particularly well-illustrated article by Kempson and Kyriakos (1972), and its mode of introduction and definition has merit. Its merit lies in the way the lesion was defined. These observers examined all cases in their file of 'soft tissue tumors' and excluded all those of generally agreed and well-recognised character. They were then left with a ". . . heterogeneous group of tumors, some of which were markedly pleomorphic". Within this group there were ". . . 30 tumors composed of varying mixtures of fibroblasts, histiocytes, xanthoma cells, and giant cells. At least focally, a storiform fibroblastic pattern was present in every tumor, and many cells were pleomorphic". Normal and abnormal mitoses were frequent, as was marked polymorphism, and, as they said, the overall pattern was that of a highly pleomorphic sarcoma. These lesions, *without knowledge of the clinical findings or course*, the authors designated fibroxanthosarcoma. This is histopathological assessment with validity. By contrast, O'Brien and Stout selected their examples of 'malignant xanthofibroma', not only prospectively on histological assessment, but also retrospectively by including amongst their material sections of lesions *already known* to have recurred or metastasised. By contaminating their series in this way they robbed themselves of the opportunity of objective assessment and were therefore not surprisingly unable to frame any closer an estimate of prognosis than that ". . . only approximately 1% of fibrous xanthomas prove themselves malignant . . ." The much closer assessment of probability of recurrence and/or metastasis attained by Kempson and Kyriakos, about to be noted, is a good example of the value of initially analysing sections 'blind'. This is not, as has been censoriously said, the pathologist 'playing games', but the pathologist making a valid attempt to extract from the available evidence the most helpful information possible for his clinical colleague. That the pathologist *afterwards* appraises his histological conclusions in the context of the clinical circumstances before issuing his report needs hardly to be repeated.

The most pleomorphic of the lesions described by Kempson and Kyriakos were, as we have seen, all characterised by a storiform pattern in some degree. In 9 of 30 patients the lesion recurred; in 3 of 30 it metastasised (one after, two without, local recurrence). This grouping therefore allowed a prediction of *metastasis* with a 10% probability, and of *local recurrence* with a 30% probability. This may still not be very high but it at least represents a greater prognostic precision than that attained by O'Brien and Stout. In fact, Kempson and Kyriakos state that ". . . fibroxanthosarcoma is a malignant variant of storiform fibrous xanthoma . . ." In other words, by the old terminology, it is recognisably the most aggressive form of DFSP. Substantially similar observations were made by Soule and Enriquez (1972), who subdivided their 65 cases of lesions in the general 'histiocytoma' group into sub-groups of increasing clinical malignancy, and by Fu and his colleagues (1975) in the article already cited. More recently, Weiss and Enzinger (1977) have drawn attention to the myxoid element that characterises some malignant fibrous xanthomas, and, along with other histological features, assessed its significance in 80 cases all in some degree myxoid (some had been diagnosed originally as myxofibrosarcoma). In general, the more myxoid the lesion, the less the likelihood of metastasis: the larger the lesion, above 5 cm, and the deeper the invasion into fascia or muscle the greater the likelihood of metastasis: mitotic activity was

of little predictive value. The occurrence of the lesion in bone is described in Chap. 6.

The practical conclusion to be drawn is that the storiform pattern must be accorded respect, and increasingly so in parallel with its cellular aberrancy. Of all the lesions currently diagnosed as fibroxanthoma, the storiform type is the most likely to recur, and, when markedly pleomorphic, to metastasise. When relatively uniform and monomorphic it may rarely metastasise but is most unlikely to do so without recurring locally at least once: when pleomorphic, and mitotically active and aberrant, it may metastasise without any early warning local recurrence. This, then, is the reconsideration that must be given to the earlier belief that DFSP virtually never metastasises without earlier local recurrence. In its most aberrant form, as fibroxanthosarcoma, it may.

JUVENILE FIBROMATOSES

Lesions of this type may occur almost anywhere in soft tissue but are seen most commonly in the form of palmar and plantar, and sternomastoid, fibromatosis. When the lesion is generalised, as rarely it may be, the explanation is more probably multifocal development than metastasis (Stout, 1954). In some series, the more highly cellular forms are designated as differentiated fibrosarcomas. The desmoid tumour and DFSP are rare in children but the juvenile aponeurotic fibroma and the recurrent digital fibroma are relatively well-defined entities. Points to note regarding the juvenile aponeurotic fibroma are that it may be partly chondroid, and thus mimic a chondroma, and that all such lesions at age 5 years or less, so far reported, have recurred (Allen and Enzinger, 1970). The recurrent digital fibroma is a lesion obviously worrying to parent, patient and surgeon alike: it is not formally a cancer but for a child it is almost worse. In our own case (Case No. 5.19), as mentioned earlier, there was at any rate suggestive evidence that the child had sustained significant psychological trauma as it grew (the emotional strains engendered by childhood cancer have been sympathetically described by Murphy [1968]).

The curious eosinophilic inclusions, first described by Reye (1965), that commonly characterise the cells of the digital fibroma (in 14 of the 15 cases of Allen, 1972), raise the possibility of a viral aetiology but despite a recent ultra-microscopic study of the condition by Battifora and Hines (1971), who suggest aggregates of fibrillary proteins or of products of cells as other possibilities, this remains unconfirmed.

In a mainly surgical account of 44 'hand tumors' in children (18 were forms of angioma, and 17 neoplastic), Woods and co-workers (1970) described one fatal case, an apparently orthodox fasciitis in a girl of 9 years that nevertheless recurred, then metastasised to axillary nodes after 2 years and caused death with pulmonary metastasis 18 months later. This, however, is a quite exceptional experience.

## DESMOID TUMOUR

Sometimes termed musculo-aponeurotic fibromatosis, this lesion appears to behave in the same familiar way whether characteristically in the anterior abdominal wall or elsewhere. The 30 cases located around the shoulder-girdle, described by Enzinger and Shiraki (1967), showed the same tendency to repeated recurrence and progression, and the same lack of prognostically helpful histological criteria. One of the rare instances of metastasis (as a fibrosarcoma) was reported by Soule and Scanlon (1962); in this patient, however, the desmoid had been energetically treated by radiotherapy 7 years earlier. There are those, like Willis (1960), who hold that these lesions, despite their relentless recurrence and invasive behaviour are 'not malignant'. They may not ordinarily metastasise but a lesion that can by its relentless invasive progression lead directly to death, as in our own Case 5.21, merits the term 'malignant' at least as much as the basal-cell carcinoma. Amply wide excision still seems to carry the only realistic hope of cure. At times, this will certainly be difficult but, with the patient almost always an adult, the hope can usually be greater than with, say, the recurrent digital fibroma in a baby. Some further hope resides in the experience of McDougall and McGarrity (1979): the lesion in two of their three patients with an extra-abdominal desmoid of long standing underwent regression after the menopause.

Fibromatosis may occur as so-called *idiopathic retroperitoneal fibrosis*. This should be a diag-nosis of last resort, for sometimes the condition is only apparently idiopathic. Cases are on record in which the fibrosis has been an unduly collagenous stromal response to some infiltrating neoplasm, for example, carcinoma of prostate (Piper, 1969), carcinomas of breast, cervix and unknown origin, and Hodgkin's disease (Nitz et al., 1970).

## FIBROSARCOMA

From the uncommon simple fibroma, through the increasingly cellular and recurrent fibromatoses, to highly cellular and rapidly metastasising fibrosarcoma is a classically smooth histopathological progression. How far along this path a fibroblastic overgrowth has to go before the pathologist decides 'fibrosarcoma' is a largely subjective decision. Mitotic incidence may be of only limited value as a prognostic indicator but it is the best we have: reticulin pattern and proportion of collagen, for example, give little help. In an analysis of 139 cases of fibrosarcoma, Werf-Messing and Unnik (1965) compared mitotic frequency with the frequency of spread by the blood. With an incidence of mitoses (per 10 hpf) of 0, 1–6, 7–11 and 12 and over, the incidence of blood-borne metastasis was respectively 24%, 37%, 69% and 100% (whether the incidence was an average figure or the incidence in only the most highly cellular and active areas is not stated: it is probably best, as with degree of anaplasia, always to work by the areas of greatest activity). A similarly useful correlation between 'grade' and prognosis was found in their series of 199 fibrosarcomas of the trunk and limbs in adults by Pritchard and co-workers (1974), who concluded that "No other soft-tissue sarcoma except liposarcoma would seem to lend itself to useful histologic grading". Interestingly, however, they preferred a subjective assessment of degree of differentiation by wide sampling of the tissue to the actual counting of mitoses.

### Fibrosarcoma in Youth

The above correlation is valuable, but it seems not to hold with fibrosarcoma in the young. Thus, Stout (1962), in his assessment of the lesion in infants and children, found mitotic incidence of no value. Of the 23 children in his personal series, 3 were known to have died, 2 of them with metastatic spread; the mitotic incidence in them (per *50* hpf) was 0, 1 and 5; in others, still alive at up to 5½ years, the incidence had reached a maximum of 19 per 50 hpf. Similar conclusions had been reached by Chung and Enzinger (1976) who found no useful correlation between degree of cellularity or mitotic incidence or amount of necrosis and clinical outcome, and by Soule and Pritchard (1977) who were ". . . unable to detect any microscopic factors that would allow (them) to predict the clinical course of a given tumor with regard to local recurrence or metastatic spread". The death rates in the series of these authors, 8.3% and 7.3% respectively, stand in marked contrast to the 41% 5-year and 29% 10-year survival rates found in the series of adult patients of Pritchard and his colleagues (1974); and this confirms the general belief that fibrosarcoma threatens life much more seriously in the adult than in the infant and child.

However, even 10 years of freedom from trouble is no guarantee of security. A patient described by Hitchens and Platt (1972) developed a 'fibromyxosarcoma' at age 18 years, had some 20 local excisions thereafter and died from intra-abdominal metastasis and intestinal obstruction at the age of 71. Two children, aged 5 and 9 at the time of initial diagnosis, were described by Horne and his colleagues (1968) as developing pulmonary metastases from fibrosarcoma 13 and 15 years later respectively (the original lesion in the first case showed no mitoses and was diagnosed as a simple fibroma; the lesion in the second case, highly cellular but with mitoses no more frequent than 1 figure per 100 hpf, was diagnosed as a 'spindle-cell sarcoma'). By contrast and emphasising the unpredictability of the neoplasm, Dobson and Dickey (1956) describe the case of a fibrosarcoma diagnosed in the upper thigh and abdominal wall of a baby of 5 months. At 18 months after the biopsy the mass was no longer palpable, and the child was well at the age of 13. In all, it appears that the usual criteria, degree of differentiation and mitotic frequency, are of some predictive value after puberty but not before, and perhaps no patient should ever be regarded as entirely immune from reappearance of the lesion. Cancer makes many claims to be a systemic disease.

*Post-irradiation Fibrosarcoma*

Post-irradiation fibrosis is common. In contrast, post-irradiation fibrosarcoma is rare but, in view of the explanation offered by Pettit and his colleagues (1954), perhaps not surprisingly rare. These authors suggest that it is most likely to follow what they term excessive and poorly conceived or 'pugilistic' irradiation: its rarity may therefore be a tribute to the skills of radiotherapists. As would be expected, distinction between radiation fibrosis and fibrosarcoma may be as difficult microscopically as it is between the spontaneous fibromatoses and fibrosarcoma. The most dependable criterion found by Pettit and his colleagues was the presence of aberrant mitoses. Cellular pleomorphism, well known as a frequent consequence of irradiation, was an unreliable index. A further finding by these workers was that such sarcomas tend much more to infiltrate than to metastasise.

GRANULATION TISSUE SARCOMA: HAEMATOMA-SARCOMA

Years ago, Ewing (1919) stated that "Many clinical observations point to the development of sarcoma from granulation tissue . . ." but cited no examples in support. That this sequence occurs is undoubted (*see*, for example, the reports by Dawson and McIntosh, 1971, and Johnston and Miles, 1973) but it is rare; indeed, in view of the universally vast amount of granulation tissue, freakishly rare, for every reparative reaction is a sarcoma *manqué*.

In the report by Dawson and McIntosh, the lesion was an angiosarcoma that developed at the site of a 20-year varicose ulceration and killed by metastasis 21 months after mid-thigh amputation of the leg. The two patients reported by Johnston and Miles developed lesions in osteomyelitic sinuses, one a probable angiosarcoma, the other, probably, a rhabdomyosarcoma, both of which killed by metastasis. Further examples of similar developments are cited by both pairs of authors but the total number remains remarkably small.

The more usual cancer arising in association with long-standing ulcers and scars is, of course, carcinoma, and the associated borderline problem the familiar pseudo-epitheliomatous hyperplasia of which exuberant granulation tissue is the mesodermal analogue. The continuation of the above-quoted sentence of Ewing is, ". . . and the histological study of granulation tissue and of organizing blood-clots occasionally reveals pictures which closely approach the structure of sarcoma". Both these situations were fully exemplified by our Cases 5.18 and 5.19. In Case 5.18, as already described, the hypercellular reaction was regarded by all who saw it as certainly fibrosarcoma. For anatomical reasons the leg could not be saved but the nonappearance of metastases during the next 20 years (to date) suggests, as the first practical point, that local excision should be the treatment of first choice in such cases whenever technically possible. It was partly the experience of this case that counselled conservatism in Case 5.19 but partly also the fact that the histological pattern here was not that of a 'textbook' sarcoma. Not even local excision was suggested, and with little more than symptomatic treatment the exuberant tissue response subsided. A rather similar problem was posed by our Case 11.9 where the lesion, a 'papilloma' arising beneath a toe, had been diagnosed histologically, evidently correctly, as a granuloma pyogenicum: when shown 'blind' to a visiting colleague from tropical Africa it produced the response, "Had I been at home, I should probably have called this Kaposi sarcoma". From these last two cases emerges the second practical point that, with the histological pattern of granulation tissue so hypercellular, polymorphic and mitotically active as strongly to suggest sarcoma, a delay long enough at least to allow the hoped-for regression to occur is fully justified. An unusual example of exuberant tissue response of this kind was seen by Scully and his colleagues (1977) in the organising interstitial exudate of a 'shock' lung. The fibroblasts were described as ". . . spectacular . . . with large hyperchromatic nuclei . . .", and, while mitoses were few, ". . . descriptively the degree of nuclear pleomorphism could be termed 'pseudosarcomatous'."

The types of wound-associated or repair-associated sarcoma so far mentioned are angio-, fibro- and suggestively rhabdomyosarcoma. A rather more academic consideration has emerged with the report by Ryan and his co-workers (1974) that apparent fibroblasts in granulation tissue have many of the features of smooth muscle cells, hence their designation as 'myo-

fibroblasts'. Ultrastructural observation in the future will no doubt tell us whether a lesion such as that in our own haematoma-sarcoma should be diagnosed as myofibrosarcoma rather than simply fibrosarcoma. The myofibroblast, if generally confirmed and shown to be present in such a lesion, may be the factor to be correlated with the essentially local rather than metastatic aggressiveness that seems to obtain: should this be so, the ultramicroscopy of a lesion like this might go far to determine decision whether a limb is to be amputated or not. It may be well to note, however, that some doubt has recently been voiced (Watts, 1979) whether the myofibroblast really is a distinctively individual type of cell.

## GRANULAR CELL MYOBLASTOMA

Increasingly, examples are being reported of multiple granular cell myoblastomas, as for example by Moscovic and Azar (1967). In these circumstances the question arises whether the lesions represent metastases from a primary source or a multifocal development. The further question naturally follows whether, if multiple lesions really are metastases, the likelihood of their development can be predicted from an individual example.

The conclusion reached by Moscovic and Azar, from an analysis of 36 reported instances of multiple lesions, was that, with one possible exception, the phenomenon is one of independent multicentric development within tissue of mesenchymal origin, and that ". . . this behavior is suggestive of a selective implantation or action at a distance of a specific provoking agent, released from the tumor, which could be metabolic or infectious". This, if true, could solve the paradox, reported of some earlier examples, of the primary tumour's being 'clinically malignant but histologically benign'.

The possible exception was an example reported by Švejda and Horn (1958) as a 'disseminated granular cell pseudo-tumour': even here, however, the authors had considered the lesion as a possible form of 'storage reticulosis' and as a ". . . generalised degeneration of the mesenchyme of unknown aetiology and of pseudo-tumorous appearance". The histology had been 'benign' throughout.

There is no intention to examine here the still

controversial nature of the cells comprising this familiar lesion beyond noting the recent report of Shousha and Lyssiotis (1979) that the cells can be shown (by an immunoperoxidase technique) to contain carcinoembryonic antigen. To the extent that cells from Schwannomas, neurofibromas, dermatofibromas and leiomyomas were shown to contain no CEA, the procedure could be of considerable diagnostic, and therefore prognostic, value. Its relevance to the histogenesis of the lesion is evident.

## PROLIFERATIVE MYOSITIS

This lesion, first described and named by Kern (1960), appears usually as a rapidly growing nodule in skeletal muscle. It has a mottled, finely septate appearance and produces what Enzinger and Dulcey (1967) describe and illustrate as a 'vague checkerboard effect', on gross or microscopic section. Histologically, it is characterised in particular by fields of giant-cells, often with two but sometimes more nuclei, and an associated fibroblastic overgrowth but little leucocytic infiltration. The amount of damage to muscle varies: it was described by Kern in his five cases as 'prominent' but found by Enzinger and Dulcey in their 33 cases to be minimal. The giant-cells, fibroblastic proliferation, general polymorphism and mitotic activity in both giant-cells and fibroblasts comprise the suggestively sarcomatous picture. A diagnosis had been made of rhabdomyosarcoma in 8, and of sarcoma of some other kind in a further 6, of the above-mentioned 33 cases; yet none had metastasised, and none even recurred. The nature of the giant-cells remains in debate. Some have favoured an origin in muscle (Kern), some an origin in fibroblasts (Enzinger and Dulcey). More recent ultramicroscopic evidence has suggested an origin in histiocytes (Stiller and Katenkamp, 1975) or, less precisely, cells of 'mesenchymal' origin (Gokel et al., 1975): none of the electron microscopy has supported an origin in muscle. An earlier ultrastructural investigation by Rose (1974) had proved inconclusive.

Our own Case 5.23 was judged to be an example of the condition but differed in that, of the giant-cells present, some were certainly simple 'muscle' giant-cells, that is, damaged skeletal muscle 'rounding-up' to form multi-nucleated symplastic masses of the kind so

familiar in many destructive lesions of skeletal muscle. It is puzzling that such cells have not figured conspicuously in published accounts of the entity, for it seems hardly possible for a destructive process in skeletal muscle *not* to produce such cells. If our own case, otherwise so typical, is not an example of proliferative myositis, any other diagnosis is difficult to suggest. This case recalled a report by Cappell and Johnstone (1958) of two highly cellular, polymorphic and mitotically aberrant lesions in thigh diagnosed as unequivocally sarcoma and probably rhabdomyosarcoma (no striations were demonstrable): yet, after local excision only, both patients were well 9 and 12 years later. There must be some possibility that these were instances of proliferative myositis in an unusually florid form. The clinical features were wholly in keeping with this suggestion.

The account by Enzinger and Dulcey supplies an interesting commentary on currently conservative trends in treatment. The 14 of their patients diagnosed initially as having sarcoma were probably not the same 14 as those whose lesions were in a limb but, in however many the 'sarcoma' *was* in a limb, none had been amputated.

## MYOSITIS OSSIFICANS

Proliferative myositis may occasionally contain minute foci of osteoid tissue, and this, in turn, may raise the question of its being myositis ossificans. However, there seems to be general agreement now that the osteoid tissue in these circumstances reflects no more than metaplasia, and that proliferative myositis is not myositis ossificans at an early stage (Stiller and Katenkamp, 1975). The hypercellularity and mitotic activity of myositis ossificans are sometimes conspicuous, to the point where, in the opinion of Ackerman (1958), there may be "a central undifferentiated zone impossible to distinguish from sarcoma". A feature that is diagnostically important and may be crucial—since upon its recognition may depend distinction from a true sarcoma, almost always osteosarcoma—is that, with diminishing cellularity, this central zone merges around the edge into osteoid tissue and then into well-differentiated bone. With a fully excised mass this distinction should always be possible but the dangers of a limited biopsy are evident. The closest cooperation should be maintained with the surgeon so that the pathologist knows exactly the disposition of the mass and the site of biopsy; perhaps best of all, as with any biopsy of bone, the pathologist should attend the operating table. Even after that, the pathologist should at some stage show the sections to a colleague 'blind'; only in this way can every bit of information be gained from the biopsy, and every lesson learned that it teaches.

Accounts appear from time to time of a so-called *pseudo-malignant osseous tumour of soft tissue*, particularly in journals of mainly orthopaedic interest; for example, those of Angervall and associates (1969), Valentin, also with associates (1969), and Chaplin and Harrison (1972). In each instance the lesion is mentioned as requiring to be distinguished from myositis ossificans but the points of distinction described by these various authors are not entirely convincing. In the opinion of Angervall and his colleagues, the five cases described by Ackerman (1958) as myositis ossificans were "apparently the same lesion", that is, pseudo-malignant tumour of soft tissue; yet few now would doubt that Ackerman's diagnosis was appropriate and correct. The main reason for Angervall's rejection of the lesion as myositis ossificans appears to be objection to the term 'myositis' on the grounds that in some instances muscle was minimally involved. With its implication of inflammation, the term 'myositis' is certainly inappropriate (as it is equally in proliferative myositis) but that is not a sufficient reason for regarding myositis ossificans and the pseudo-malignant lesion as different entities.

The lesion was first given its name by Fine and Stout (1956) who stated quite clearly that they regarded it as an atypical or pseudo-malignant form of myositis ossificans; it is just unfortunate that their other name for it gained the popularity it has, so much so that, as just described, attempts are made to distinguish it separately from myositis ossificans. The appearance of 'zoning', so important diagnostically and emphasised by Ackerman, is not stressed to the same degree by Fine and Stout but the description is there, with its mention of circumscribed periphery yet central zone so cellular and mitotically active as to mimic osteosarcoma. Paradoxically, were an example to be over-diagnosed as osteosarcoma, the natural absence of (visible) pulmonary metastases during the succeeding months would virtually assure amputation.

## BONY NEOPLASMS OF SOFT TISSUE

Lesions of these types comprise three groups:

a) Those analogous to the skeletal osteoclastoma;

b) Those analogous to the skeletal malignant osteoclastoma;

c) Those analogous to the skeletal osteo-(genic) sarcoma or chondrosarcoma;

and confident allocation of an appropriate case to one of these groups rather than the others is not always possible. Distinction should, however, be attempted since the prognosis in the first group is so notably better than in the others.

A series of ten *cases analogous to the skeletal osteoclastoma* was described by Salm and Sissons (1972). Little more need be said of the histology than that these authors of great experience found it indistinguishable from that of the giant-celled tumour of bone. Prognostically also the similarity held: of the eight patients traced, seven were known to be alive and well at 1–6 years later, one died from an unrelated cause, without recurrence, 6 years after excision. Since the publication of that report, one patient suffered recurrence 4 years after the initial excision (sections from the lesion were originally referred from Dundee Royal Infirmary to Dr Sissons who included the data as Case No. 7 in the series of Salm and Sissons); he remains well 6 years after the re-excision, and is now aged 82. Histologically and prognostically, then, there is much resemblance to the lesion as it occurs in bone. With age-incidence, however, the similarity ends. Of the 10 patients, 6 were aged 50 or more; the others were 1, 15, 18 and 23 years old. Thus, only three of the ten were within the 'usual' ages for skeletal osteoclastoma of 15–30 years.

Every skeletal osteoclastoma confronts the pathologist with the problem whether its histology warrants the term 'malignant' or not; the same holds for the extraskeletal version. The after-history of their patients indicates that Salm and Sissons had read the position correctly throughout. Included also in that series were patients with lesions of rather similar appearance that therefore figured in the differential diagnosis. Two were notably vascular and cystic; they were possibly related to the aneurysmal bone cyst. One other was believed to be a fibrosarcoma with a prominent and coincidental osteoclastic component; whether this should be regarded as a 'one-sided' or clonal fibroblastic development within the same osteoclastoma-like lesion is speculative, as indeed is the pathogenesis of the group as a whole. Prognostic guides are the usual two, cellular polymorphism and mitotic activity in both giant-cells and stromal cells, and with this lesion, unlike most of the pseudo-sarcomas, they appear to be reasonably dependable.

The *other forms* of extraskeletal giant-celled tumours, those analogous to the malignant osteoclastoma and the osteosarcoma of bone, are also not always sharply distinguishable. Thus, Guccion and Enzinger (1972) include among their 32 cases of malignant giant-cell tumour, 2 that were originally reported by Fine and Stout (1956) as osteogenic sarcoma of soft tissue, while, despite the frequently close similarity, Allan and Soule (1971), in describing 26 cases of the soft-tissue osteogenic sarcoma make no mention of the giant-celled tumour in the differential diagnosis. Much clearly depends on the assessment of such osteoid and/or bony tissue as may be present, and this commonly occurs in both types of lesion.

As with the benign form of extraskeletal giant-cell tumour, both the malignant form and the osteosarcoma of soft tissue occur predominantly at ages outwith the usual range, in this instance 15 to 25 years. In the 32 cases of Guccion and Enzinger, only one was within this range; of the others, 27 were over 40 years of age. Of the 26 cases described by Allan and Soule, 3 were within the range 15–25 years, 17 were over 40. The fact that the prognosis is equally bad with both types of lesion again raises the question whether we really are dealing with only one entity, admittedly histologically variable, not two; or, if not that, with remarkably near neighbours in the same histological street. The mortality in the Guccion/Enzinger series was 18/32, in the Allan/Soule series 21/26. The mortality in the original series of Fine and Stout, 10/12, strongly suggests that here too the lesion was the same entity.

A useful prognostic distinction was made by Guccion and Enzinger between lesions that were 'superficial', those involving superficial fascia

and subcutaneous tissue, and those that were 'deep', involving deep fascia, muscle and tendon. In the superficial group, 2/12 died, in the others, 16/20. The components of the lesions were essentially the same, namely, multinucleated giant-cells and stromal cells of mononuclear histiocytic and fibroblastic appearance with frequent transformation in places to a fibrosarcomatous pattern; foci of osteoid differentiation were present in almost half the cases. In general, however, the prognostic distinction between the two groups was paralleled by cellular polymorphism and increasing mitotic activity. The mitotic incidence ranged from 1 to 11 figures per 10 hpf in the superficial growths to 11 to 22 per 10 hpf in not only the deep lesions but also in the two superficial lesions that metastasised. A feature that, according to Guccion and Enzinger, may be unique among neoplastic cells is the occasional presence within the giant cells of asteroid bodies, ordinarily seen only in the giant cells of granulomatous lesions. At times the histology may closely simulate that of a malignant fibroxanthoma. However, the scarcity or absence of both xanthoma cells and a storiform pattern serve to distinguish the two conditions.

The problem facing the pathologist is that which faces him with osteoclastoma in bone: can the likelihood of metastasis be predicted? In bone, as noted later, this can be achieved to an approximate but nevertheless useful extent. Grading depends on the already mentioned degree of anaplasia and mitotic activity, and use of these criteria in conjunction with an assessment of location, 'superficial' or 'deep', should enable the pathologist to give the surgeon at least some guidance. As a group these lesions appear to be much more aggressive than the osteoclastoma in bone. They have the guise of a skeletal osteoclastoma but the habit rather of a skeletal osteosarcoma.

Extraskeletal osteogenic sarcoma may be a rare sequel to irradiation therapy. Two examples were reported by Boyer and Navin (1965), while a malignant neoplasm of essentially the same appearance in the soft tissue of the neck has been reported by Hasson and his colleagues (1975) as a sequel to the intracarotid injection of thorotrast. It was diagnosed initially as an atypical fibroxanthoma, perhaps understandably in view of the similarity mentioned above, but as osteogenic sarcoma on its recurrence. The lesion appeared 30 years after the injection of thorotrast, and the patient died 3 years later.

A series of 34 cases of extraskeletal myxoid chondrosarcoma has been described by Enzinger and Shiraki (1972). The lesion is less aggressive than chondrosarcoma of bone but is nevertheless serious. Thus, of the 31 patients traced by these authors, 4 had died with metastasis, while 7 were still alive with recurrence and/or metastasis; remarkably, the 3 patients still alive with metastasis (two had also recurrence) had their original operation 10, 20 and 20 years earlier.

## Synovial Overgrowths

Diagnostic and prognostic difficulties may arise with the nodular tenosynovitis, long familiar as the giant-cell tumour of tendon sheath, and with the probable or possible synoviosarcoma.

### Nodular Tenosynovitis

The nodular tenosynovitis is still to some extent aetiologically debatable as to whether it is basically inflammatory and a form of fibrous histiocytoma or truly neoplastic (Lichtenstein, 1972). It may mimic a sarcoma, at times it may *be* a sarcoma, and at times it may simulate the osteoclastoma. A fair assessment of the evidence might be that it is an essentially granulomatous lesion that may nevertheless on rare occasions behave as a sarcoma. A series of 118 examples (91 on the fingers) was described by Jones and his associates (1969) in which 17% recurred at least once but none metastasised; all had been treated by local excision. In contrast, an account was given by Bliss and Reed (1968) of four examples of the malignant form; of these, three metastasised, two ultimately causing death.

Distinction between the benign and malignant forms may be far from easy. In the experience of Bliss and Reed, features characterising the malignant lesion were greater polymorphism amongst cells, mainly polygonal, a relative lack of giant cells and more frequent mitoses (there was no resemblance to the 'usual' synoviosarcoma with its biphasic pattern). However, these features may be found also in lesions that do not recur and metastasise. In our own Case 5.6, not only were there abundant cellularity and mitotic activity, there was aberrant mitotic ac-

tivity; and mitotic activity was not inconspicuous in several of the others in the series. The problem in practice appears closely similar to that holding for fibrosarcoma. The obvious tendency to recurrence after local excision, perhaps 10% (though none of our local patients experienced this), will be countered so far as possible by local measures; only recurrent growth to the point where a digit is made useless will demand amputation, and then only of the digit. It is doubtful whether even 'alarming' histology in an otherwise typical nodular tenosynovitis in an extremity would justify amputation of a whole limb.

### Synovial Sarcoma

The synovial sarcoma is a treacherous neoplasm of quite another order. Beyond a general tissue kinship it has little clinically significant relation to the nodular tenosynovitis. Even if the nodular lesion in its rarely malignant expression emerges as a synoviosarcoma, synoviosarcomas in general start de novo. The biphasic histological pattern, so mimetic of a carcinosarcoma (and I have known it misdiagnosed as such) is generally familiar and has been the subject of ultramicroscopic study by Gabbiani and colleagues (1971). The differences between the epithelial-like and the stromal cells, so obvious under the light microscope, were not only confirmed in detail but both types of cell were shown to carry desmosomes. Possession of desmosomes or maculae adherentes is widely accepted as a feature characterising only epithelial tissues, thus allowing a distinction in undifferentiated neoplasms between the carcinoma and the sarcoma or lymphoma. Here at least is an exception. Our own Case 5.27 was educative in that the biphasic pattern did not emerge for 3½ years (inadequate sampling of the original lesion was almost certainly not the explanation). This behaviour has possible implications vis-à-vis the lesion described by Enzinger (1970) as 'epithelioid sarcoma' and considered at the end of this section.

The bad prognosis with synoviosarcoma has been repeatedly confirmed, as, for example, in the series of Cadman and his co-workers (1965), Cameron and Kostuik (1974) and Gerner and Moore (1975). Points gleaned from these accounts are that there is little relation between the duration of symptoms or the histology and the outcome; that even 10 years' 'cure' must be viewed with reservation; and that without question the optimum treatment is amputation; in the first series mentioned the rate of recurrence after simple excision was 77%. In view of this virtually mandatory amputation it is imperative that the diagnosis be unequivocal, and here an important practical point emerges; any biopsy must be adequately representative. The tissue pattern in a synoviosarcoma may vary greatly from place to place, and biopsy of a small single area might well lead to the erroneous diagnosis of fibrosarcoma for which, as already noted, amputation would very possibly *not* be the treatment of choice. This point has been emphasised and well illustrated by Lichtenstein (1972) in his fig. B7, which shows three quite different patterns from within the same synoviosarcoma. The 5-year survival rate found by Cameron and Kostuik (1974) was 45% but they, too, stress the insecurity of even a 10-year survival.

The outlook seems no less gloomy in children, indeed, of the 43 patients described by Crocker and Stout (1959), 22 had died. Even so, from comparison of the survivors and nonsurvivors, these workers believe that complete local excision can achieve as good a long-term result as amputation. Their rather frustrating conclusion on the value of histology was that ". . . one can feel no assurance that tumors with a comparable histological structure will behave in the same way in children as they do in adults".

EPITHELIOID SARCOMA

The epithelioid sarcoma of Enzinger (1970) is a curious lesion of still uncertain histogenesis. It has a characteristically multinodular disposition and appears mostly in the soft tissues of the hand, forearm and pretibial region at age 30 years or less. It is relentlessly recurrent and may eventually metastasise if not completely extirpated in its early stages. Despite its close similarity to nodular tenosynovitis, and even though commonly desmoplastic, it does not show the sharpness of biphasic pattern of a synoviosarcoma; and this raises doubts about its being a form of this entity. However, as happened in our Case 5.29, the biphasic pattern may take years to emerge, and in some cases possibly never does. Therefore, the mainly monophasic epithe-

lioid pattern of the epithelioid sarcoma may be no more than an atypical feature of a basically synovially derived neoplasm.

The differences in mucin-staining from the synoviosarcoma, noted by Enzinger, may also be just another atypical feature. The cells are notably eosinophilic, epithelioid (and much prone to necrosis in the centre of the nodular foci) to the point where a granulomatous inflammation of some kind has been the usually favoured diagnosis in early cases. Pleomorphism is not marked, but mitotic activity is common, sometimes with an incidence of 2 to 6 figures/10 hpf. The dangerous deceptiveness of the lesion, and the great likelihood of under-diagnosis, is emphasised by the fact that, in the 62 cases comprising Enzinger's series, 11 different 'benign' diagnoses had been made at the outset. Also, when larger or recurrent and recognisably aggressive, 20 different 'malignant' diagnoses had been made (synoviosarcoma in 15 cases, some other sarcoma in 22, carcinoma in 8, malignant melanoma in 4). Of the 54 patients traced, 13 were alive with recurrence, 4 were alive with metastasis, and 11 dead with metastasis. Clearly, for a lesion as aggressive as this, correct diagnosis and early thorough excision are crucial. Even so, and understandably, probably few patients will lose a forearm or a leg as first treatment. Recurrence, however, will make this almost mandatory.

'STAGING' OF SOFT TISSUE SARCOMAS

The most fitting final note to this fragmented survey of tumourous growths of soft tissues must be a reference to the enormous volume of work undertaken by Russell and his many colleagues (1977), the 'Task Force for Soft Tissue Sarcomas', to devise a system of clinical and pathological staging for these cancers. The TNM + G (grading) scheme evolved was based on the data from 1215 cases of soft tissue sarcomas that had been histologically confirmed and that had adequate follow-up.

The 1215 had been culled from 13 institutions. The preliminary screening and histological confirmation had presumably been dealt with at source, and with care, for all 1215 were acceptable to the Task Force. Not all of the sections were reviewed by this group but the probable correctness of diagnosis on the nonreviewed sections was neatly validated by demonstration that the survival curves for patients with a non-reviewed lesion were not significantly different from those for patients whose lesion had been reviewed. In the present context it is natural to wonder how many cases had been proffered originally as sarcomas but were rejected; that is, in how many the original diagnosis was a false-positive, and just how big the borderline problem had been. The desirability of a scheme of grading is not in doubt, and this one may have come in time to prevent the chemotherapeutic chaos already here in the case of some cancers. However, the allocation of a grade to a unanimously agreed sarcoma is not, for the pathologist, a 'front-line' action: *his* front-line action is to decide whether the lesion is a sarcoma or not. How hard-fought this action was in the 13 institutions we do not know but, in the light of much of the substance of this chapter, it cannot have been easy. In its own way, the population of cases rejected would make a subject for study as valuable as the system of grading itself.

## Conclusions

1) Lesions that may closely simulate a sarcoma of soft tissue form two groups:
   a) Where the difference from sarcoma is essentially quantitative: these have long been familiar:
   Desmoid tumour
   Fibromatosis (e.g. juvenile digital: plantar/palmar)
   Post-irradiation fibrosis
   Infiltrating lipoma;
   b) Where the difference from sarcoma is essentially qualitative: some of these entities are less familiar as significant simulators:
   Nodular fasciitis
   Atypical fibroxanthoma (histiocytoma)
   Proliferative myositis
   Reparative reactions (including that to fat necrosis)
   Myositis ossificans
   Extraskeletal giant-cell tumour.
2) The term 'histiocytoma' embraces lesions of many types, as diverse as DFSP, nodular synovitis and sclerosing angioma. If it is used in pathological reports, its relation to lesions of these kinds, long familiar under the older names, should be made clear.

The atypical fibroxanthoma is especially mimetic of sarcoma.

3) The juvenile digital fibroma and juvenile aponeurotic fibroma are notoriously recurrent.

4) Apparently idiopathic retroperitoneal fibrosis may be the scirrhous reaction to metastatic carcinoma.

5) Fibrosarcoma is intrinsically less malignant in children than in adults. In children, however, mitotic incidence is prognostically less helpful.

6) Myxomas when multiple (and especially in muscle) frequently co-exist with fibrous dysplasia of bone.

7) The angiomyolipoma of kidney (a benign mesenchymoma or hamartoma) has a significant association with tuberous sclerosis. It may also mimic a liposarcoma.

8) Malignant mesenchymoma has a high mortality. Diagnosis is best based on sarcomatous change in a component other than the fibroblastic. A rhabdomyosarcomatous component is prognostically the worst.

9) All seemingly simple lipomas should be examined microscopically. Liposarcoma is a dangerous lesion, made more so by pregnancy. It may be simulated by fasciitis, fat necrosis (including sclerema neonatorum) and xanthogranuloma.

10) Nodular synovitis may show areas of notably high cellularity and mitotic activity yet be curable by local excision. Amputation of a digit is rarely required. Sarcomatous forms are few.

11) An 'epithelioid sarcoma' has been described; it could be the malignant form of nodular tenosynovitis. It is liable to be under-diagnosed as benign yet may metastasise in some 30% of cases.

12) Synoviosarcoma, after attempted local excision, has a rate of recurrence close on 80% and a high mortality. In children, local excision may achieve results no worse than amputation. The patchy and varied pattern demands adequately representative biopsy, preferably from more than one area.

13) Myositis ossificans carries an especial risk of overdiagnosis as sarcoma. Only an ade-

quate biopsy will show the correctly indicative 'zonal' architecture.

14) The giant-cell tumour of soft tissue is morphologically identical with the giant-cell tumour (osteoclastoma) of bone but has a rather better prognosis. It occurs as often outwith the 15–30 year age-group as within.

15) The extraskeletal malignant osteoclastoma and osteosarcoma equally have a high mortality: they may be morphological variants of the same entity. Both are commoner outwith the 15–25 year age-group. Prognostic assessment histologically should be as for the skeletal equivalents.

16) Granulation tissue may be suggestively sarcomatous but granulation tissue sarcoma is extremely rare. Extruded material of synovial origin may provoke a particularly active cellular response.

17) Variations in tissue texture and cellularity make assessment of mitotic incidence more accurate and informative in terms of number per 100s or 1000s of cells than of number per 10s or 100s of hpfs.

18) A TNM + G (grading) system of staging for sarcomas of soft tissue has recently been proposed.

# References

Ackerman LV (1958) Extra-osseous localized non-neoplastic bone and cartilage formation (so-called myositis ossificans): Clinical and pathological confusion with malignant neoplasms. J Bone Joint Surg [Am] 40: 279–298

Allan CJ, Soule EH (1971) Osteogenic sarcoma of the somatic soft tissues. Clinicopathologic study of 26 cases and review of literature. Cancer 27: 1121–1133

Allen PW (1972) Recurring digital fibrous tumours of childhood. Pathology 4: 215–223

Allen PW, Enzinger FM (1970) Juvenile aponeurotic fibroma. Cancer 26: 857–867

Angervall L, Enzinger FM (1975) Extraskeletal neoplasm resembling Ewing's sarcoma. Cancer 26: 240–251

Angervall L, Stener B, Stener I, Ahren C (1969) Pseudomalignant osseous tumour of soft tissue. A clinical, radiological and pathological study of five cases. J Bone Joint Surg [Br] 51: 654–663

Battifora H, Hines JR (1971) Recurrent digital fibromas of childhood. An electron microscope study. Cancer 27: 1530–1536

Bliss BO, Reed RJ (1968) Large cell sarcomas of

tendon sheath: Malignant giant cell tumors of tendon sheath. Am J Clin Pathol 49: 776–781

Bourne RG (1963) Paradoxical fibrosarcoma of skin (pseudo-sarcoma): A review of 13 cases. Med J Aust 1: 504–510

Boyer CW, Navin JJ (1965) Extraskeletal osteogenic sarcoma. A late complication of radiation therapy. Cancer 18: 628–633

Brenner W, Schaefler K, Chhabra H, Postel A (1975) Dermatofibrosarcoma protuberans metastatic to a regional lymph node. Report of a case and review. Cancer 36: 1897–1902

Bugg EI, Mathews RS (1970) Benign mesenchymoma. South Med J 63: 268–273

Burnett RA (1975) Primary cardiac leiomyosarcoma with pulmonary metastases: A diagnostic problem. Scott Med J 20: 125–128

Cadman NL, Soule EH, Kelly PJ (1965) Synovial sarcoma: An analysis of 134 tumors. Cancer 18: 613–627

Cameron HU, Kostuik JP (1974) A long-term follow-up of synovial sarcoma. J Bone Joint Surg [Br] 56: 613–617

Cappell DF, Johnstone JM (1958) Pleomorphic sarcoma of thigh with long survival. J Clin Pathol 11: 139–141

Chaplin DM, Harrison MHM (1972) Pseudomalignant osseous tumour of soft tissue. Report of two cases. J Bone Joint Surg [Br] 54: 334–340

Chung EB, Enzinger FM (1976) Infantile fibrosarcoma. Cancer 38: 729–739

Crocker DW, Stout AP (1959) Synovial sarcoma in children. Cancer 12: 1123–1133

Culberson JD, Enterline HT (1960) Pseudo-sarcomatous fasciitis: A distinctive clinical-pathologic entity; report of five cases. Ann Surg 151: 235–240

Dahl I (1976) Atypical fibroxanthoma of the skin. A clinicopathological study of 57 cases. Acta Pathol Microbiol Scand [A] 84: 183–197

Dahl I, Angervall L, Magnusson S, Stener B (1972) Classical and cystic nodular fasciitis. Pathol Eur 7: 211–221

Dawson EK, McIntosh D (1971) Granulation tissue sarcoma following long-standing varicose ulceration. J R Coll Surg Edinb 16: 88–95

Dionne GP, Seemayer TA (1974) Infiltrating lipomas and angiolipomas revisited. Cancer 33: 732–738

Dobson L, Dickey LB (1956) Spontaneous regression of malignant tumors: Report of a twelve-year spontaneous complete regression of an extensive fibrosarcoma with speculations about regression and dormancy. Am J Surg 92: 162–171

Editorial (1974) Myxoma of soft tissues. Br Med J 1: 170

Enterline HT, Culberson JD, Rochlin DB, Brady LW (1960) Liposarcoma: A clinical and pathological study of 53 cases. Cancer 13: 932–950

Enzinger FM (1965) Intramuscular myxoma. A

review and follow-up study of 34 cases. Am J Clin Pathol 43: 104–113

Enzinger FM (1970) Epithelioid sarcoma. A sarcoma simulating a granuloma or a carcinoma. Cancer 26: 1029–1041

Enzinger FM, Dulcey F (1967) Proliferative myositis. Report of thirty-three cases. Cancer 20: 2213–2223

Enzinger FM, Shiraki M (1967) Musculo-aponeurotic fibromatosis of the shoulder girdle (extra-abdominal desmoid). Analysis of thirty cases followed up for ten or more years. Cancer 20: 1131–1140

Enzinger FM, Shiraki M (1972) Extraskeletal myxoid chondrosarcoma. An analysis of 34 cases. Hum Pathol 3: 421–435

Enzinger FM, Winslow DJ (1962) Liprosarcoma: A study of 103 cases. Virchows Arch [Pathol Anat] 335: 367–388

Evans HL, Soule EH, Winkelmann RK (1979) Atypical lipoma, atypical intramuscular lipoma, and well differentiated retroperitoneal liposarcoma. A reappraisal of 30 cases formerly classified as well differentiated liposarcoma. Cancer 43: 574–584

Ewing J (1919) Neoplastic Diseases. A textbook on tumors. Saunders, Philadelphia

Fine G, Stout AP (1956) Osteogenic sarcoma of the extraskeletal soft tissues. Cancer 9: 1027–1043

Fisher ER, Hellstrom HR (1966) Dermatofibrosarcoma with metastases simulating Hodgkin's disease and reticulum cell sarcoma. Cancer 19: 1165–1171

Fretzin DF, Helwig EB (1973) Atypical fibroxanthoma of the skin. A clinicopathologic study of 140 cases. Cancer 31: 1541–1552

Fu Y-S, Gabbiani G, Kaye GI, Lattes R (1975) Malignant soft tissue tumors of probable histiocytic origin (malignant fibrous histiocytomas): General considerations and electron microscopic and tissue culture studies. Cancer 35: 176–198

Gabbiani G, Kaye GI, Lattes R, Majno G (1971) Synovial sarcoma: Electron microscopic study of a typical case. Cancer 28: 1031–1039

Gerner RE, Moore GE (1975) Synovial sarcoma. Ann Surg 181: 22–25

Gokel JM, Meister P, Hübner G (1975) Proliferative myositis. A case report with fine structural analysis. Virchows Arch [Pathol Anat] 367: 345–352

Gordon HW (1964) Pseudosarcomatous reticulohistiocytome: A report of four cases. Arch Dermatol 90: 319–325

Guccion JE, Enzinger FM (1972) Malignant giant cell tumor of soft parts. An analysis of 32 cases. Cancer 29: 1518–1529

Hasson J, Hartman KS, Milikow E, Mittelman JA (1975) Thorotrast-induced extraskeletal osteosarcoma of the cervical region. Report of a case. Cancer 36: 1827–1833

Helwig EB (1963) Atypical fibroxanthoma. Tex J Med 59: 664–667

Hitchens EM, Platt DS (1972) Fibrosarcoma. Cancer 29: 1369–1375

Hood CI, Font RL, Zimmerman LE (1973) Metastatic mammary carcinoma in the eyelid with histiocytoid appearance. Cancer 31: 793–800

Horne CHW, Slavin G, McDonald AM (1968) Late recurrence of juvenile fibrosarcoma. Br J Surg 55: 102–103

Hudson AW, Winkelmann RK (1972) Atypical fibroxanthoma of the skin: A reappraisal of 19 cases in which the original diagnosis was spindle-cell squamous carcinoma. Cancer 29: 413–422

Hutter RVP, Stewart FW, Foote FW (1962) Fasciitis. A report of 70 cases with follow-up proving the benignity of the lesion. Cancer 15: 992–1003

Johnston RM, Miles JS (1973) Sarcomas arising from chronic osteomyelitic sinuses. A report of two cases. J Bone Joint Surg [Am] 55: 162–168

Jones FE, Soule EH, Coventry MB (1969) Fibrous xanthoma of synovium (giant-cell tumor of tendon sheath, pigmented nodular synovitis). A study of one hundred and eighteen cases. J Bone Joint Surg [Am] 51: 76–86

Kahn LB, Wood FW, Ackerman LV (1969) Fracture callus associated with benign and malignant bone lesions and mimicking osteosarcoma. Am J Clin Pathol 52: 14–24

Kauffman SL, Stout AP (1961) Histiocytic tumors (fibrous xanthoma and histiocytoma) in children. Cancer 14: 469–482

Kempson RL, Kyriakos M (1972) Fibroxanthosarcoma of the soft tissues. A type of malignant fibrous histiocytoma. Cancer 29: 961–976

Kempson RL, McGavran MH (1964) Atypical fibroxanthomas of the skin. Cancer 17: 1463–1471

Kern WH (1960) Proliferative myositis: A pseudosarcomatous reaction to injury. A report of seven cases. Arch Pathol 69: 209–216

Kindblom L-G, Stener B, Angervall L (1974) Intramuscular myxoma. Cancer 34: 1737–1744

Kleinstiver BJ, Rodriguez HA (1968) Nodular fasciitis. A study of forty-five cases and review of the literature. J Bone Joint Surg [Am] 50: 1204–1212

Klima M, Smith M, Spjut HJ, Root EN (1975) Malignant mesenchymoma: Case report with electron microscopic study. Cancer 36: 1086–1094

Konwaler BE, Keasbey L, Kaplan L (1955) Subcutaneous pseudosarcomatous fibromatosis (fasciitis). Report of 8 cases. Am J Clin Pathol 25: 241–252

Kroe DJ, Pitcock JA (1969) Atypical fibroxanthoma of the skin. Report of ten cases. Am J Clin Pathol 51: 487–492

Lendrum AC (1948) The surgical significance of some so-called simple tumours. Ann R Coll Surg Engl 3: 32–43

Lichtenstein L (1972) Bone tumors, 4th edn. Mosby, St. Louis

Lin JJ, Lin F (1974) Two entities in angiolipoma. A study of 459 cases of lipoma with review of literature on infiltrating angiolipoma. Cancer 34: 720–727

McDougall A, McGarrity G (1979) Extra-abdominal desmoid tumours. J Bone Joint Surg (Br) 61: 373–377

McKenna RJ, Schwinn CP, Soong KY, Higinbotham NL (1966) Sarcomata of the osteogenic series (osteosarcoma, fibrosarcoma, chondrosarcoma, parosteal osteogenic sarcoma, and sarcomata arising in abnormal bone). An analysis of 552 cases. J Bone Joint Surg [Am] 48: 1–26

McPeak CJ, Cruz T, Nicastri AD (1967) Dermatofibrosarcoma protuberans. An analysis of 86 cases—five with metastasis. Ann Surg 166: 803–816

Meister P, Höhne N, Konrad E, Eder M (1979) Fibrous histiocytoma. An analysis of the storiform pattern. Virchows Arch A. Path Anat 383: 31–41

Moscovic EA, Azar HA (1967) Multiple granular cell tumors ("myoblastomas"). Case report with electron microscopic observations and review of the literature. Cancer 20: 2032–2047

Murphy ML (1968) Curability of cancer in children. Cancer 22: 779–784

Nash A, Stout AP (1961) Malignant mesenchymomas in children. Cancer 14: 524–533

Nitz GL, Hewitt CB, Straffon RA, Kiser WS, Stewart BH (1970) Retroperitoneal malignancy masquerading as benign retroperitoneal fibrosis. J Urol 103: 46–49

O'Brien JE, Stout AP (1964) Malignant fibrous xanthomas. Cancer 17: 1445–1455

Ozzello L, Stout AP, Murray MR (1963) Cultural characteristics of malignant histiocytomas and fibrous xanthomas. Cancer 16: 331–344

Pettit VD, Chamness JT, Ackerman LV (1954) Fibromatosis and fibrosarcoma following irradiation therapy. Cancer 7: 149–158

Piper JV (1969) Malignant retroperitoneal fibrosis presenting as a vascular emergency. Br J Clin Pract 23: 390–391

Price EB, Mostofi FK (1965) Symptomatic angiomyolipoma of the kidney. Cancer 18: 761–774

Price EB, Silliphant WM, Shuman R (1961) Nodular fasciitis: A clinicopathologic analysis of 65 cases. Am J Clin Pathol 35: 122–136

Pritchard DJ, Soule EH, Taylor WF, Ivins JC (1974) Fibrosarcoma—a clinicopathologic and statistical study of 199 tumors of the soft tissues of the extremities and trunk. Cancer 33: 888–897

Purvis WE, Helwig EB (1954) Reticulohistiocytic granuloma ("reticulohistiocytoma") of the skin. Am J Clin Pathol 24: 1005–1015

Rachmaninoff N, McDonald JR, Cook JC (1961) Sarcoma-like tumors of the skin following irradiation. Am J Clin Pathol 36: 427–437

Rakower W (1971) Fasciitis, an unusual diagnosis, and the clinician's dilemma: Report of case. J Oral Surg 29: 503–506

Registrar-General (1973) Statistical review of England and Wales for the year 1973. Part I (B) tables, medical. HMSO, London

Reszel PA, Soule EH, Coventry MB (1966) Liposarcoma of the extremities and limb-girdles. A study of two hundred twenty-two cases. J Bone Joint Surg [Am] 48: 229–244

Reye RDK (1965) Recurring digital fibrous tumors of childhood. Arch Pathol 80: 228–231

Rosas-Uribe A, Ring AM, Rappaport H (1970) Metastasizing retroperitoneal fibroxanthoma (malignant fibroxanthoma). Cancer 26: 827–831

Rose AG (1974) An electron microscopic study of the giant cells in proliferative myositis. Cancer 33: 1543–1547

Russell WO, Cohen J, Enzinger F, Hajdu SI, Heise H, Martin RG, Meissner W, Miller WT, Schmitz RL, Suit HD (1977) A clinical and pathological staging system for soft tissue sarcomas. Cancer 40: 1562–1570

Ryan GB, Cliff WJ, Gabbiani G, Irlé C, Montandon D, Statkov PR, Majno G (1974) Myofibroblasts in human granulation tissue. Hum Pathol 5: 55–67

Salm R, Sissons HA (1972) Giant-cell tumours of soft tissues. J Pathol 107: 27–39

Sauter LS, Feo CP de (1971) Dermatofibrosarcoma protuberans of the face. Arch Dermatol 104: 671–673

Schoenfeld RJ (1964) Epidermal proliferations overlying histiocytomas. Arch Dermatol 90: 266–270

Scully RE, Galdabini JJ, McNeely BU (1977) Weekly clinicopathological exercises. Case 22-1977. N Engl J Med 296: 1279–1287

Seids JV, McGinnis RS (1927) Malignant tumors of fatty tissues. Surg Gynecol Obstet 44: 232–243

Shousha S, Lyssiotis T (1979) Granular cell myoblastoma: Positive staining for carcinoembryonic antigen. J Clin Pathol 32: 219–224

Soule EH (1962) Proliferative (nodular) fasciitis. Arch Pathol 73: 437–444

Soule EH, Enriquez P (1972) Atypical fibrous histiocytoma, malignant fibrous histiocytoma, malignant histiocytoma and epithelioid sarcoma. A comparative study of 65 tumors. Cancer 30: 128–143

Soule EH, Pritchard DJ (1977) Fibrosarcoma in infants and children. A review of 110 cases. Cancer 40: 1711–1721

Soule EH, Scanlon PW (1962) Fibrosarcoma arising in an extra-abdominal desmoid tumor: Report of case. Proc Mayo Clin 37: 443–451

Spittle MF, Newton KA, Mackenzie DH (1970) Liposarcoma: A review of 60 cases. Br J Cancer 24: 696–704

Stiller D, Katenkamp D (1975) The subcutaneous fascial analogue of myositis proliferans. Electron microscopic examination of two cases and comparison with myositis ossificans localisata. Virchows Arch [Pathol Anat] 368: 361–371

Stout AP (1944) Liposarcoma—the malignant tumor of lipoblasts. Ann Surg 119: 86–107

Stout AP (1948) Myxoma, the tumor of primitive mesenchyme. Ann Surg 127: 706–719

Stout AP (1948a) Mesenchymoma, the mixed tumor of mesenchymal derivatives. Ann Surg 127: 278–290

Stout AP (1954) Juvenile fibromatoses. Cancer 7: 953–978

Stout AP (1961) Pseudosarcomatous fasciitis in children. Cancer 14: 1216–1222

Stout AP (1962) Fibrosarcoma in infants and children. Cancer 15: 1028–1040

Stout AP, Lattes R (1967) Atlas of tumor pathology, 2nd ser, fasc 1: Tumors of the soft tissues. Armed Forces Institute of Pathology, Washington, D.C.

Švejda J, Horn V (1958) A disseminated granular-cell pseudotumour: So-called metastasising granular-cell myoblastoma. J Pathol Bacteriol 76: 343–348

Taylor HB, Helwig EB (1962) Dermatofibrosarcoma protuberans. A study of 115 cases. Cancer 15: 717–725

Tremblay M, Bonenfant J-L (1969) Embryonal liposarcoma (myxoid liposarcoma): A study of six cases. Can Med Assoc J 100: 281–285

Valentin P, Godenèche JL, Piollet J, Laguillaumie B de (1969) Tumeur osseuse des parties molles dite 'pseudo-maligne'. Rev Chir Orthop 55: 351–357

Wasserman TH, Stuard ID (1974) Malignant fibrous histiocytoma with widespread metastases. Autopsy study. Cancer 33: 141–146

Watts GT (1979) Myofibroblasts. Lancet I: 335

Weiss SW, Enzinger FM (1977) Myxoid variant of malignant fibrous histiocytoma. Cancer 39: 1672–1685

Werf-Messing B van der, Unnik JAM van (1965) Fibrosarcoma of the soft tissues: A clinicopathologic study. Cancer 18: 1113–1123

Willis RA (1960) Pathology of tumours, 3rd edn. Butterworth, London

Wirth WA, Leavitt D, Enzinger FM (1971) Multiple intramuscular myxomas. Another extraskeletal manifestation of fibrous dysplasia. Cancer 27: 1167–1173

Woods JE, Murray JE, Vawter GF (1970) Hand tumors in children. Plast Reconstr Surg 46: 130–139

# 6　Lesions of Bone and Cartilage

As with malignant neoplasms of the soft tissues, the incidence of malignant neoplasms of bone and cartilage in comparison with those of any other anatomical system of similar size is low. The number of deaths from malignant neoplasms of the digestive system in England and Wales for 1973, 39,300, was cited in the previous chapter. The equivalent figure for deaths from malignant neoplasms of bone was 518: deaths from multiple myeloma were 1,155. However, in the local series, and again as with lesions of soft tissue, the proportion of borderline lesions to forthright diagnoses is high.

## Local Series

During the 25 years covered by the local series, the number of lesions diagnosed as primary malignant neoplasms of the skeletal system was 43: osteosarcoma, 13; osteoclastoma, 7; chondrosarcoma, 8; Ewing's tumour or ? neuroblastoma, 6; myeloma or myelomatosis, 9. The number of lesions causing significant diagnostic difficulty was 15.

### SUMMARISED TOTALS

#### Inflammatory or Reparative Lesions

Each of three cases raised a different problem: (a) whether prominent areas of cartilage around a focus of undoubted inflammation in a pelvic bone were neoplastic; (b) whether, at the site of a known fracture, highly cellular and proliferative osteoid/fibroblastic tissue was callus or osteosarcoma; and (c) whether quite numerous plasma cells in company with other leucocytes indicated myeloma rather than non-specific osteo-

myelitis. In only the last of these instances did a significantly expressed suspicion of myeloma amount in some degree to an over-diagnosis.

#### Predominantly Fibrous Lesions

In three of four cases the problem had been that of deciding whether a predominantly fibroblastic overgrowth accompanied by not infrequent multinucleated giant cells could represent an osteoclastoma. The fourth lesion was also basically fibrous but showed a prominently myxoid change and no giant cells. All four lesions were evidently cured by curettage.

#### Cartilaginous or Chondroid Lesions

Four cases each presented a different facet of the unpredictability of cartilaginous overgrowths. One was a well-differentiated chondroma in the pubic ramus (it necessitated caesarean section) which called for cautious prognosis more on account of the site than the histology: it recurred after 11 years but has not reappeared during the 7 years since then. The chondromyxoid fibroma in the series showed some possibly significant differences from an earlier typical example. It was more chondroid and more pervasive of surrounding bone but was eradicated nevertheless by en bloc removal. A highly cellular and notably chondroid exostosis recurred once but was then adequately removed, while the pleomorphism that may seemingly characterise the normal laryngeal cartilages led to some concern about an apparently enlarged cricoid cartilage.

#### Osteoclastoma or Osteosarcoma?

Of two cases, one, diagnosed initially as osteoclastoma, showed histological appearances demanding a more cautious prognosis than was given at the time; it became, or perhaps from

**Table 6.1.** Fifteen cases of equivocal lesions of the skeletal system.

| Case No. | Diagnosis on review | Treatment | Outcome |
|---|---|---|---|
| *1 case under-diagnosed* | | | |
| 6.13 | Osteosarcoma > osteoclastoma | Curettage × 3 + amputation | Death @ 6 yr |
| *2 cases over-diagnosed* | | | |
| 6.3 | ? osteomyelitis > ? plasmacytoma | Curettage | Alive @ 12 yr |
| 6.9 | Probably normal cartilage > chondrodysplasia | Excision | Alive @ 7 yr |
| *12 cases appropriately diagnosed* | | | |
| 6.1 | Osteomyelitis | Chemotherapy | Alive @ 14 yr |
| 6.2 | Callus | Reduction | Unrelated death @ 2 yr |
| 6.4 | Non-osteogenic fibroma > 'fibroma' | Curettage | Alive @ 3 yr |
| 6.5 | Non-osteogenic fibroma | Curettage | Alive @ 8 yr |
| 6.6 | Fibrous dysplasia | Curettage | Alive @ 11 yr |
| 6.7 | Periosteal myxofibroma | Curettage | Alive @ 11 yr |
| 6.8 | Chondroma | Excision × 2 | Alive @ 7 yr since recurrence |
| 6.10 | Chondromyxoid fibroma | Excision | Alive @ 9 yr |
| 6.11 | Exostosis | Excision × 2 | Alive @ 3 yr since recurrence |
| 6.12 | Osteoclastoma | Excision × 4 | Recurrence × 3 then amputation |
| 6.14 | Probable myeloma | Excision + radiotherapy | Alive @ 10 (possibly 20) yr |
| 6.15 | Myeloma | Radiotherapy | Death @ 6 yr |

the outset was, an osteosarcoma. The second lesion was, and behaved characteristically as, an osteoclastoma. However, tissue removed at one of the three operations for recurrence, would of itself have warranted diagnosis as the fibrosarcomatous expression of an osteosarcoma.

### 'Small Round Cell' Lesions

Two lytic lesions in bone consisted of cells of this type. On later evidence, one was shown certainly to be, and the other almost certainly to be, a plasma-cell myeloma. The diagnostic uncertainty would have been greatly reduced, if not abolished, by the use of cytological techniques on the occasion of first biopsy.

*Review has yielded:*
  Under-diagnoses, 1
  Over-diagnoses, 2
  Appropriate diagnoses, 12
These 15 cases comprise Table 6.1

### Case Data

*Case 6.1*

F (12 years) with pain in the hip, radiating to the knee, present for 5 weeks and ascribed to a local injury 2 months earlier (followed by a vague febrile illness for 2 weeks). Radiology showed a localised lesion in left inferior pubic ramus, nature uncertain but possibly neoplastic. At operation, partly bony, partly fibrous material was removed from an area of poorly defined erosion in the substance of the bone.

Near-purulent exudate and spicules of necrotic bone indicated a subacute or chronic 'osteomyelitis'. Relatively large areas of cartilage did raise the question of a chondroma but their generally regular architecture and cytology suggested that they were part of the normal pelvic structure and not neoplastic.

A coagulase-positive staphylococcus was isolated from the lesion and all subsided satisfactorily with chemotherapy. The history of injury and febrile illness possibly was of aetiological significance.

The patient fully recovered, had a normal pregnancy 7 years later, and after a further 7 years remains well. The histological diagnosis was relatively straightforward and *appropriate*.

I can recall at any rate four other instances where, in children, clinical findings and radiological appearances have been regarded as virtually diagnostic of a neoplasm in bone, all, it so happens, in the lower limb (head of femur, lower end of femur ($\times$ 2), upper end of tibia), all shown histologically to be due to osteomyelitis. The X-ray appearances can thus be indistinguishable, but I recollect no instance where radical treatment was carried out on the basis of radiology alone.

## Case 6.2

F (87 years) fell heavily on hip. No fracture-line was visible on X-ray and conservative treatment was advised. Pain and disability persisted until, 20 days later, the patient "turned over in bed and heard a loud crack from the hip". X-ray now showed a subtrochanteric fracture of femur. At open reduction, "suspicious-looking tissue" was seen partly surrounding the site of fracture; pieces were taken for histology.

The material consisted essentially of a mixture of damaged skeletal muscle, granulation tissue and areas of highly cellular tissue not only mingled with the granulation tissue but so abundantly proliferative elsewhere as to form wide sheets of cells quite unlike any 'ordinary' granulation tissue. Part of one of these areas is shown in Fig. 6.1 where highly cellular and not notably vascular tissue is permeating fat; it was infiltrating nearby skeletal muscle also. It is seen in more detail in Fig. 6.2. The cells are relatively large, often with ample cytoplasm, and their nuclei are also large, generally hyperchromatic and mildly polymorphic. Amongst these cells, mitoses were frequent, sometimes as many as 5 per hpf; in this illustration there are three. Numerous multinucleated muscle giant-cells added to the widely varying picture of the reaction but were generally easily recognised as such.

There was no serious suggestion radiologically that this was a neoplasm of bone, either primary or secondary, but independently of this information and despite the exuberance and mitotic

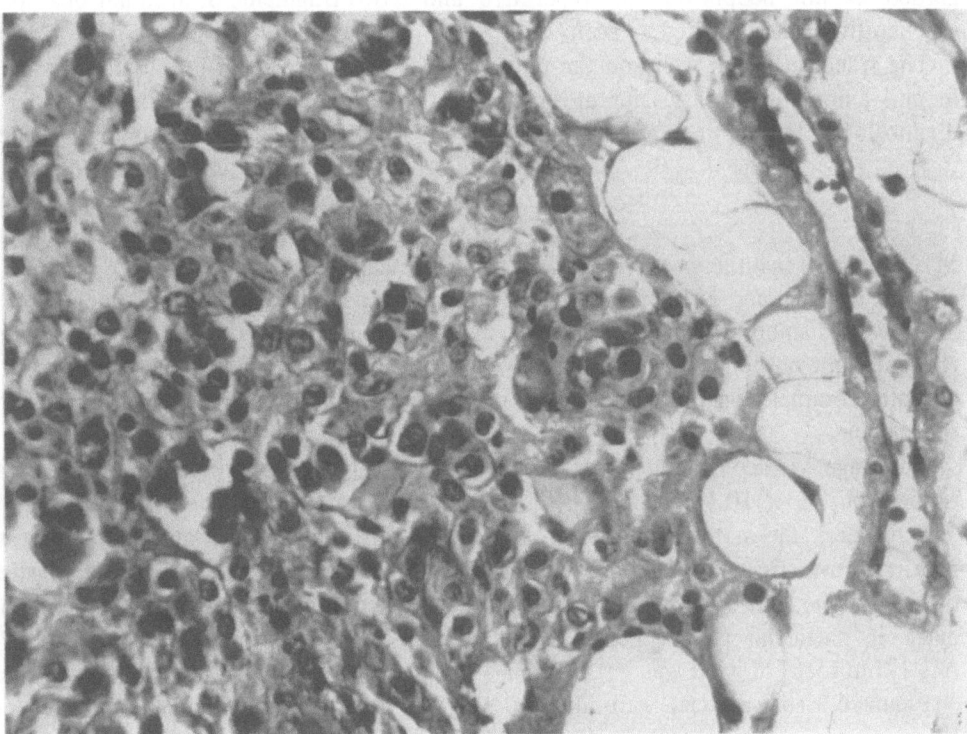

**Fig. 6.1.** Highly cellular tissue extending into adjacent fat. H & E, $\times$ 493

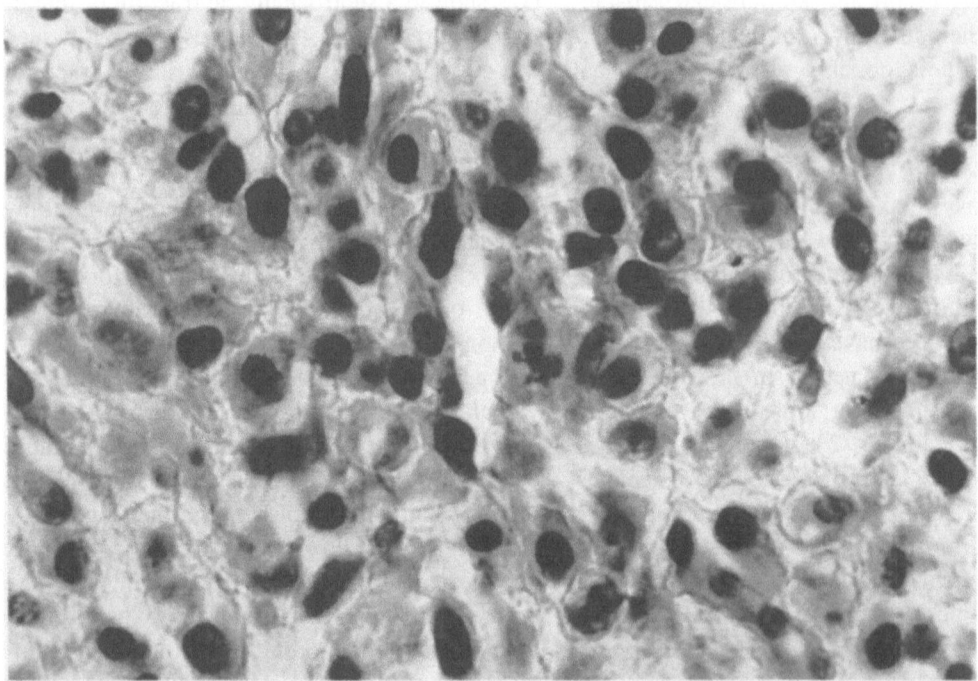

**Fig. 6.2.** There is some polymorphism of the nuclei, also mitotic activity. One mitotic figure lies at right edge of the lumen in centre, another below this and slightly to right, near lower edge of the figure; a third (less obvious) is opposite left of lumen, half-way towards edge of field. H & E, × 952

activity of the tissue the reaction was finally regarded as not neoplastic but 'reparative and regenerative', and reported as such.

The fracture healed well and the patient was fit and ambulant 6 years later at age 93. The diagnosis had been *appropriate*.

### Case 6.3

M (56 years) with 4-week history of painless swelling over inner end of left clavicle. The swelling was smooth, oval, 4 × 3 × 2 cm and reddened but not tender. Radiology showed apparently complete disappearance of the head of the clavicle.

Curettage yielded fragments of soft whitish tissue up to 15 × 10 × 5 mm.

In general, the material consisted of variably mature fibrous tissue containing scattered flecks of dead bone and widely infiltrated by leucocytes, in particular plasma cells, but including one 1-mm focus of what was virtually pus.

Figure 6.3 shows (left) well-differentiated fibrous tissue and (centre) a large, densely-populated focus of leucocytes amongst which are two fragments of acellular dead bone.

Figure 6.4 shows, in the lower left half, moderately vascular granulation tissue and maturing fibrous tissue; and, in the upper right half, a uniformly dense infiltration by leucocytes.

Figure 6.5 was selected to show the considerable polymorphism of the plasma cells in many places; all the larger, darker cells here are plasma cells, the smaller, darker cells are lymphocytes, the relatively large pale nuclei are those of either monocyte/endothelial or young fibroblastic type. Here, as almost everywhere except for the focus of pus already mentioned, polymorphonuclears are not present.

The problem was, plasmactyoma or not, and, if not, what? The final opinion, purely on the histology, was that the lesion was almost certainly inflammatory, not neoplastic, but that no aetiological clues such as tubercle bacilli or fungi had been seen. A parallel search for clues with serological, biochemical and further radiological investigation yielded nothing of positive value. The final comment was made, however, that the

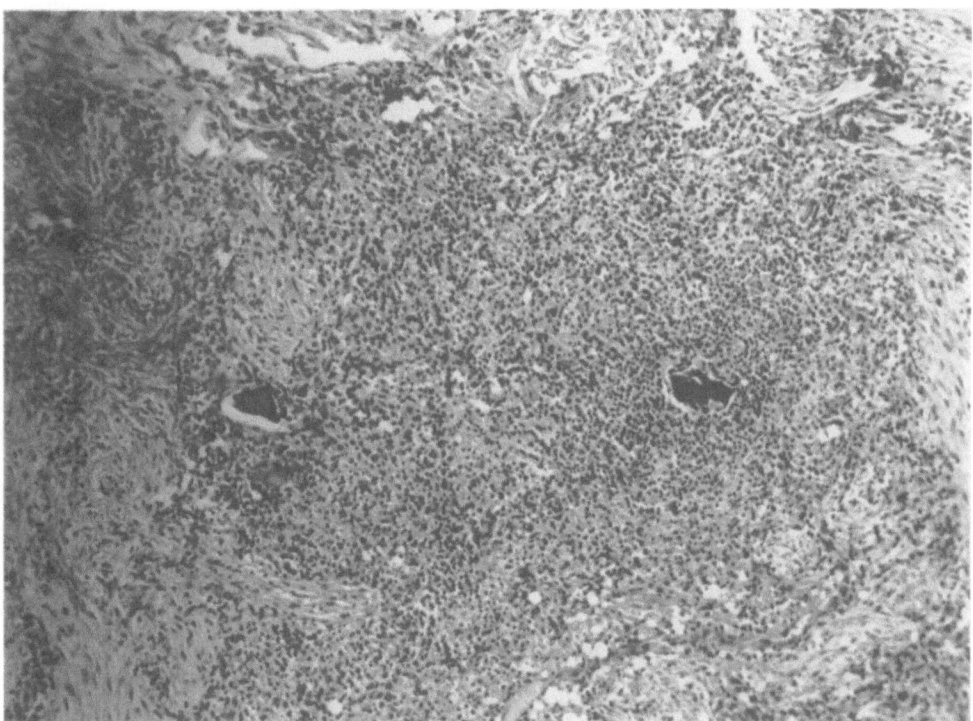

**Fig. 6.3.** The central mass is virtually pus, with two flakes of bone, surrounded by moderately highly cellular fibrous tissue. H & E, × 123

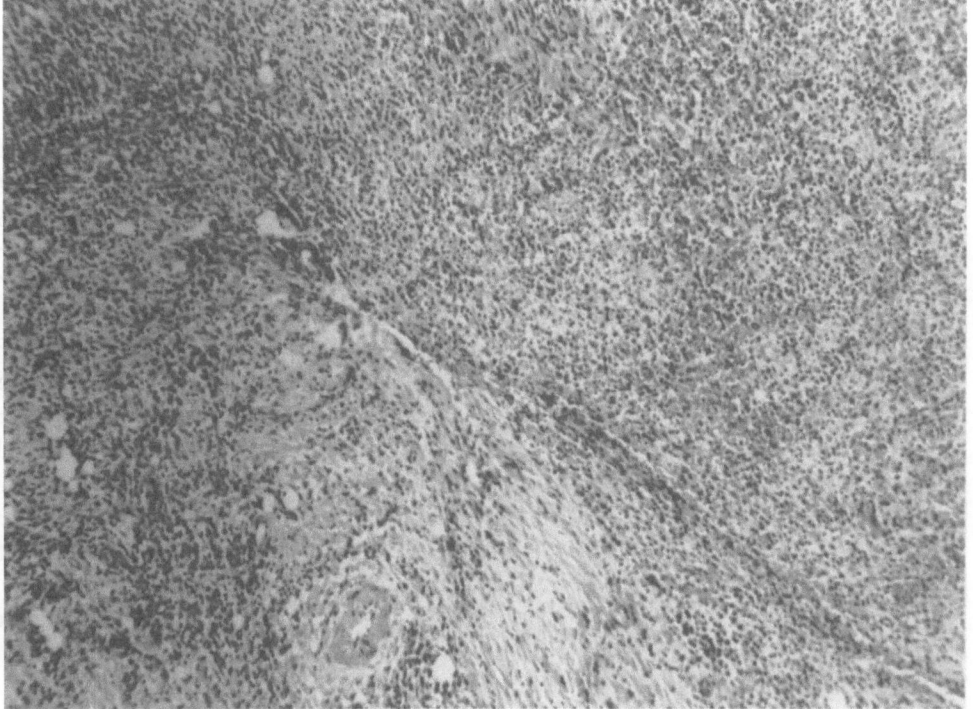

**Fig. 6.4.** Much of the material consists of a mixture of granulation tissue, young fibrous tissue and abundant leucocytes. H & E, × 123

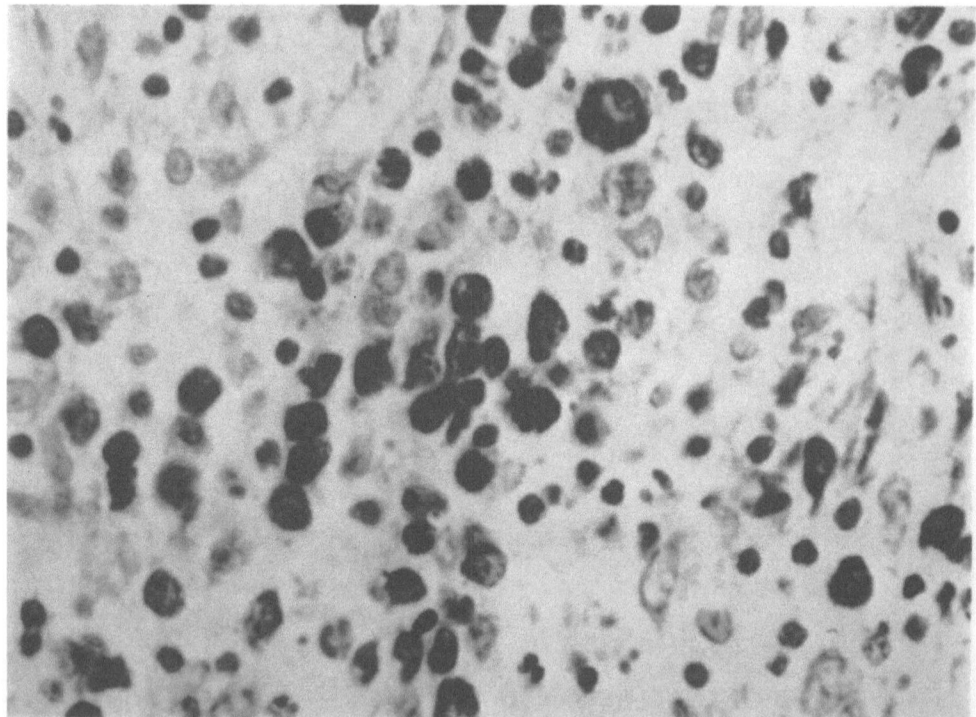

**Fig. 6.5.** Amongst the leucocytes, plasma cells such as these were not only numerous but notably polymorphic. This had raised the possibility of plasmacytoma. H & E, × 985

possibility of this lesion's being the first expression of a 'myelomatosis' could not be entirely excluded.

Shortly after this the possibility was raised that this might be an example of 'disappearing bone disease' or 'massive osteolysis' (Jones et al., 1958). However, within 18 months of the curettage, the area had fully recalcified and regained a completely normal radiological appearance. The patient has had no further trouble during the 12 years since then. The suggestion of myelomatosis was at any rate a partial *over-diagnosis*.

### Case 6.4

F (12 years). Complained of pain in the ankle of 6-weeks duration. Radiology showed an oval area of rarefaction in the lower third of tibia; its distal margin was level with the upper edge of the malleoli.

Exploration showed the lesion to be a defect, 4 × 3 × 2 cm, expanding the marrow cavity and largely replacing the anterior cortical bone. It contained soft brownish, partly fatty tissue. Despite the virtually indistinguishable similarity

between the X-ray pattern of this lesion and of chondromyxoid fibroma (CMF), the brownish fatty content of the cavity was entirely different from the homogeneous pure white material that characterises the CMF.

The difference from CMF was as striking microscopically as macroscopically. This was a moderately highly vascular, spindle-celled growth of seemingly fibroblastic character. The pattern varied little throughout and had the generally swirling appearance illustrated in Fig. 6.6 which shows also that multinucleated giant cells are relatively frequent. Two other examples of such cells are seen in Fig. 6.7, which illustrates also, approximately, the extremes of the range of cellularity of the abnormal tissue. The general nuclear disposition and mild polymorphism are shown in Fig. 6.8. The pyknotic mass at the lower right-hand edge was one of the rather scanty mitotic figures that were present. As expected from the gross appearance, haemosiderin was abundant: no foam cells were seen.

The lesion was diagnosed as a 'fibroma' though only after much consideration of both low-grade fibrosarcoma and osteoclastoma.

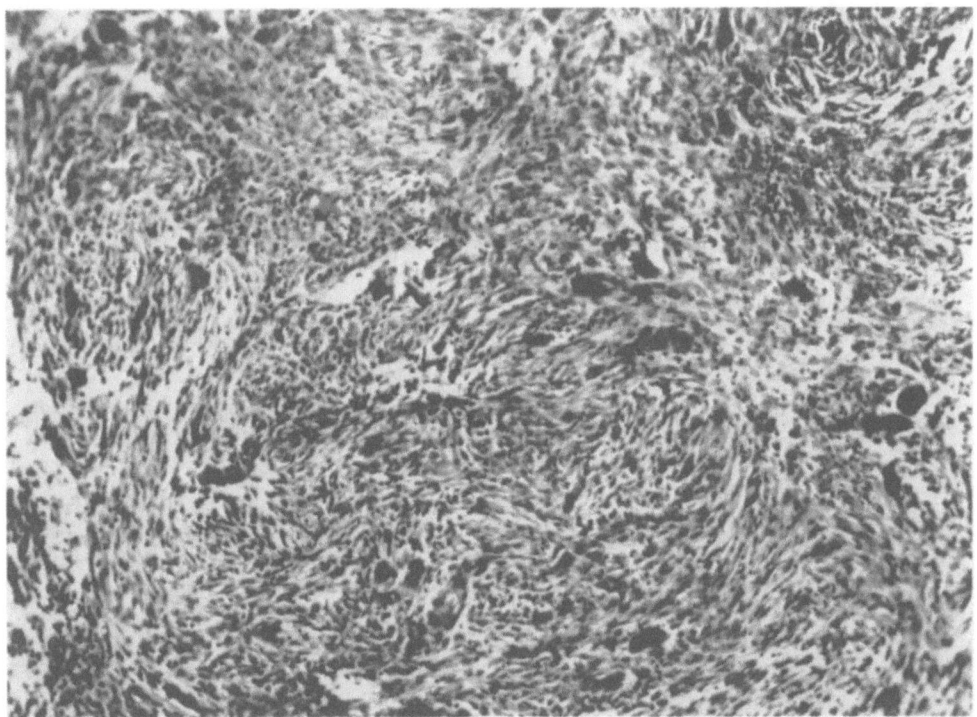

**Fig. 6.6.** The stroma was formed of mingling swathes of rather polymorphic spindle-type cells interpreted as fibroblastic. Multinucleated giant-cells are prominent. H & E, × 123

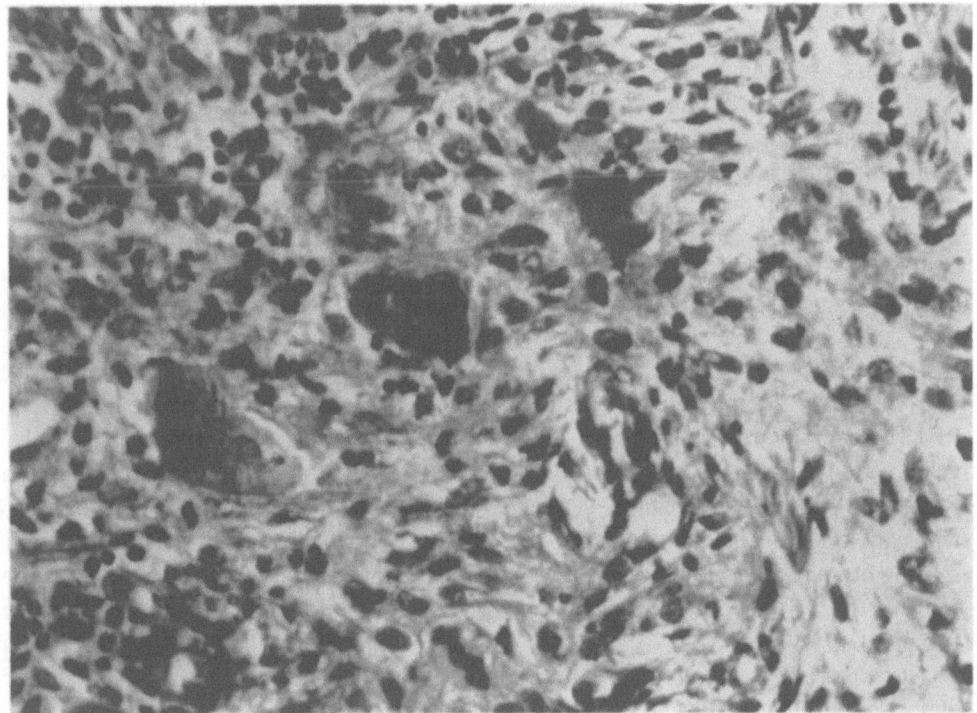

**Fig. 6.7.** Shows the variable degree of cellularity of the tissue: to right it is loosened by apparent oedema. The giant-cells rarely contain as many or as uniform nuclei as those usually characterising an osteoclastoma. H & E, × 493

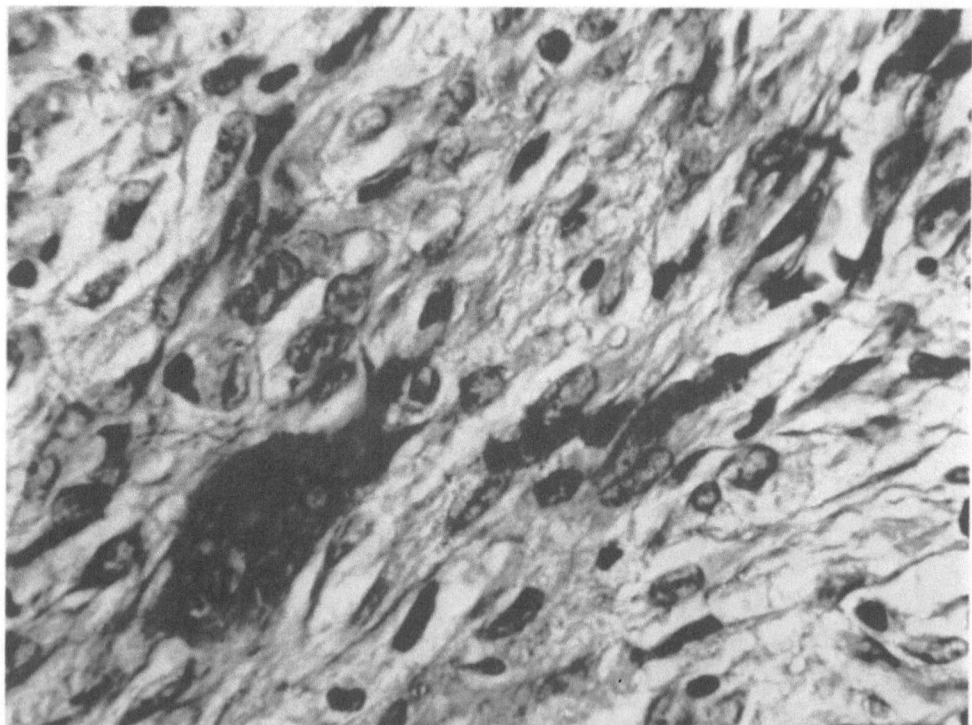

**Fig. 6.8.** The nuclei in the giant-cell vary in size as do those of the stroma in general. H & E, × 985

The lesion healed well after curettage and the patient was known to be trouble-free three years later. She was not traced thereafter but at least no enquiry has been received on her behalf during the 15 years since then.

This was almost certainly a 'non-ossifying fibroma' (fibrous cortical defect) in the differential diagnosis of which Lichtenstein (1972) particularly mentions low-grade fibrosarcoma and osteoclastoma as strong contenders. The original diagnosis was wholly *appropriate*.

### Case 6.5

M (31 years) with pain in the right heel for 7 years, and recently becoming more disabling. Radiology showed replacement of virtually the whole of the calcaneus by material resembling a mass of small soap-bubbles. Biopsy and later full curettage with bone-chip packing were performed.

The material, as shown in Fig. 6.9, consisted of moderately highly fibrous tissue amid which were scattered spicules of bone. The bone was still live bone but there was no osteoblastic activity such as would suggest active osteogenesis.

There were also areas containing multinucleated giant-cells, sometimes but not always associated with foci of haemosiderin and siderophages: they appeared to be of nonspecific RE type rather than osteoclasts. Figure 6.10 shows them in an area of tissue of higher cell-density than that characterising the lesion as a whole. Areas of this kind, however, were the main reason for concern for they showed an appreciable degree of mitotic activity at about one mitotic figure per 10 hpf; no aberrant forms, however, were seen.

The lesion was diagnosed as a 'non-ossifying fibroma' with a warning that, even with thorough curettage, recurrence was possible.

The curettage and packing proved curative, and the patient remained fully fit 8 years later.

Comparison of the first (biopsy) sections with those from the tissue obtained at definitive curettage 5 weeks later showed this later tissue to be marginally the more highly cellular and mitotically active, suggesting that a degree of reparative reaction had been induced by the biopsy procedure. If this can happen, there is clearly some risk that a tissue obtained later may be wrongly 'overestimated' and lead to unnecessarily radical

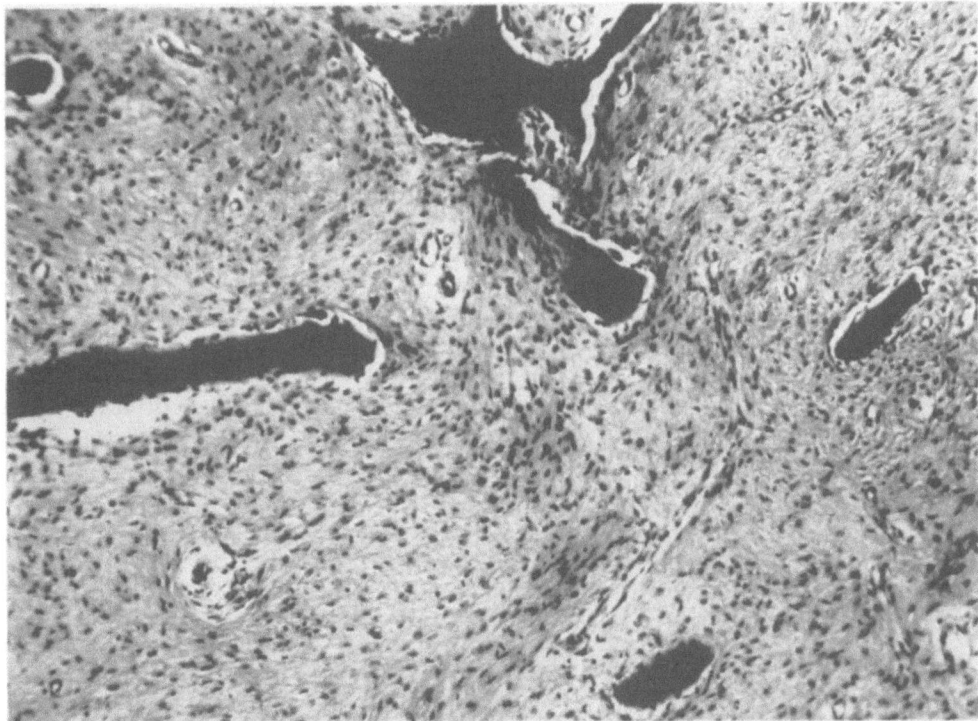

**Fig. 6.9.** Material of this mixed bony and fibroblastic character replaced almost the whole of the cavity of the calcaneus. H & E, × 123

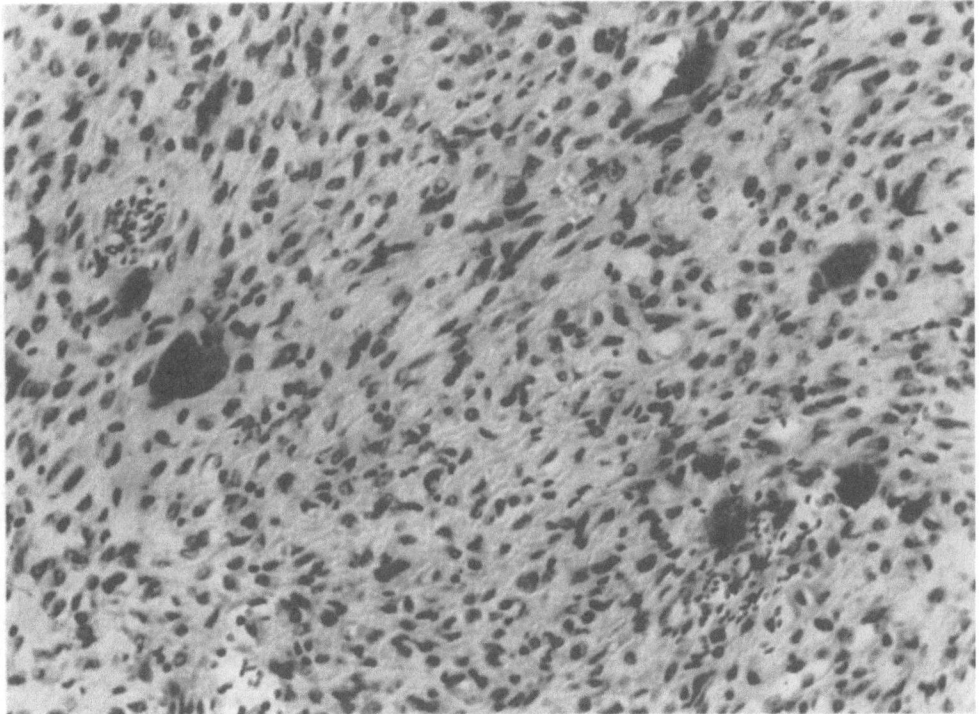

**Fig. 6.10.** An area of the mildly polymorphic stroma that includes multinucleated giant-cells considered not to be osteoclasts. Mitotic figures were moderately numerous. H & E, × 246

treatment. However, despite the histology, it would probably have been right to take into account the fact that the lesion had been present, at any rate according to the clinical history, for 7 years. The outcome confirmed the diagnosis as *appropriate*.

### Case 6.6

F (13 years). Referred for treatment by a dental surgeon. Complaint was swelling of right lower jaw. Radiology showed a 25 × 20 mm polycystic rarefaction 20 mm anterior to the angle of the jaw. The cavity was found to be filled with brownish, occasionally finely gritty, fibrotic tissue. There was resorption of tooth roots with loosening.

The material was composed essentially of quite highly cellular fibrous tissue containing a scattering of haemosiderin, occasional clusters of multi-nucleated giant cells and foci of what could reasonably be described as bony 'pellets'. These objects were round or oval and sharply circumscribed, some 150 μm in diameter on average, recognisably bony or osteoid, or sometimes simply acellular and marginally calcific. They had some resemblance to so-called 'cementicles' but were insufficient by themselves to identify the lesion as a cementifying fibroma. Instead, the mass was considered to be a 'focal fibrous dysplasia'. The fibrous tissue, though quite highly cellular was neither unduly polymorphic nor mitotically active.

There were no skeletal abnormalities elsewhere and blood chemistry was normal. The main concern was possible liability to recurrence. However, the curettage proved adequate treatment and the patient was trouble-free at least 11 years later. The diagnosis had been *appropriate*.

### Case 6.7

M (48 years). Complained of pain in the shoulder for three months since receiving a 'knock'. Radiology showed a subperiosteal cystic area, 3 × 2 cm, just below the lateral aspect of the head of the humerus. Exploration showed the cyst to be partly filled with glairy fluid but mostly with myxoid tissue.

The soft tissue consisted of poorly cellular material with abundant mucoid or myxoid matrix. The cells, presumably fibroblasts, were stel-

late, or compressed into other shapes, and only occasionally in mitosis. The lesion was diagnosed as a 'periosteal myxofibroma' pending later examination of bony tissue from the margins of the defect. This material, when decalcified, showed an appreciable amount of young cartilage and newly-formed trabeculae of bone. This was regarded as reactive or reparative and not as evidence that the lesion was a 'juxta-cortical chondroma' (Jaffé). Some possibility of recurrence was mentioned.

No further treatment was given after evacuation and curettage of the cyst, and the area healed satisfactorily. All was known to be well 11 years later. The diagnosis, even if little more than descriptive, was *appropriate*.

### Case 6.8

F (18 years). Required caesarean section because of a hard mass on the upper medial border of the descending ramus of the pubis. When removed, it was hemispherical and 5 × 5 × 5 cm.

The pattern was that of a moderately highly cellular 'chondroma', a little unusual in having many bands of fibrous tissue coursing through it. It was insufficiently aberrant or mitotically active to warrant diagnosis as chondrosarcoma but, quite apart from the doubtful adequacy of excision, a warning was given about high probability of recurrence, and, possibly, even conversion to chondrosarcoma.

Eleven years later the patient was seen at an antenatal clinic when a nodule, 'the size of a grape', was discovered at the site of the original chondroma. Despite the difficulties there would be, it was decided that excision was the proper course. This was performed and yielded tissue virtually identical with that seen originally. Clearance on this occasion did seem to be adequate.

The defect left by the excision healed well and the patient remains fully fit 7 years later. During this interval she had a further successful caesarean section.

This case exemplifies well the insidious character of cartilaginous growth in the pelvic bones. Even the most benign-looking chondroma at this site represents some risk of recurrence. Also, despite the seeming adequacy of the last excision, there can be no guarantee that this patient will not have further trouble. With its warning of likely recurrence, the original diagnosis was wholly *appropriate*.

## Case 6.9

M (37 years) with complaint of pain and swelling over region of cricoid cartilage. Exposure showed some irregularity of the surface with mild enlargement of the anterior half of the cartilage. Biopsy was performed.

The biopsy had the appearance seen in Fig. 6.11, and caused concern because of, as shown in both this figure and in Fig. 6.12, the wide variation both in nuclear size and the number of cells per cluster of chondrocytes. Mitotic figures were not seen: mainly for this reason, the lesion was designated 'dysplastic' rather than neoplastic though with a recommendation that any further tissue of similar macroscopic appearance should be removed. This was done, the further fragments showing essentially the same histology.

No further treatment was given, and the patient has had no further trouble during the 7 years to date. The possibility that the lesion was a chondrosarcoma was seriously considered: had that diagnosis been given, laryngectomy would have been performed. In the event, as already said, local removal was evidently curative though there is even yet no clear explanation for the 'pain and swelling'.

The cytology here was so disturbing, and the clinical consequences of any histological overresponse to it so grave, that further cricoid cartilages were later examined for comparison (the range of histological variability amongst cricoid cartilages is perhaps not immediately familiar to all). Figures 6.13 and 6.14, from one such 'control' cartilage, show that a comparable degree of polymorphism is entirely within physiological limits. This, therefore, had been something of an *over-diagnosis*.

## Case 6.10

F (8 years) with pain and swelling in right knee. Examination showed an area of rarefaction, 20 × 15 × 10 mm, in the upper posterior part of the tibia almost abutting on the epiphyseal plate. The cavity was curetted and packed with bone chips. The material obtained was almost pure white, rather translucent, firm and resilient, similar to the flesh of a green coconut.

Microscopically, the material was a mixture of 10% chondroid and 90% myxomatous or myxomatoid tissue: adjacent areas of both are shown in Fig. 6.15. The most likely diagnosis was chondromyxoid fibroma. Many of the features, both clinical and histological, were characteristic of this condition, others were not.

We had previously had experience with a typical chondromyxoid fibroma (Hutchison and Park, 1960). In that case the lesion was also abutting on the upper tibial epiphyseal plate but was treated by curettage alone. It recurred after 2½ years but was completely eradicated by a block removal that included a shell of surrounding bone (this was then possible thanks to bone growth's having moved the epiphyseal plate well away from the recurrent focus).

Histologically, the present lesion differed from the first in showing a rather greater amount of chondroid differentiation and in containing many more multinucleated giant-cells. Figure 6.16 shows one of the quite numerous clusters of these; in all, they were far from abundant but relative to the incidence in the first case they were numerous. A further point of difference, at first sight possibly significant prognostically, was a plentiful permeation or invasion by the abnormal tissue amongst well-formed bony trabeculae (Fig. 6.17). In fact, this seemed largely a matter of sampling. With the first case in mind, the surgeon this time removed more of the bony surroundings of the cavity.

Despite the differences from our earlier case, the lesion was diagnosed also as 'chondromyxoid fibroma' (CMF).

There was no recurrence, and all was well 9 years later. The diagnosis had been *appropriate*.

The myxoid type of tissue shown in part of Fig. 6.15 (and illustrated more fully by Hutchison and Park on the earlier occasion) does appear to be reasonably distinctive and diagnostic. CMF seems quite frequently to produce areas of chondroid differentiation but a chondroma rarely contains areas of this type of myxoid differentiation. Remnant tissue almost certainly can regress, as Jaffé and Lichenstein (1948) believed, for, although the abnormal tissue surrounded by bone in this case was adequately removed, hardly every cell can have been scraped from the epiphyseal plate.

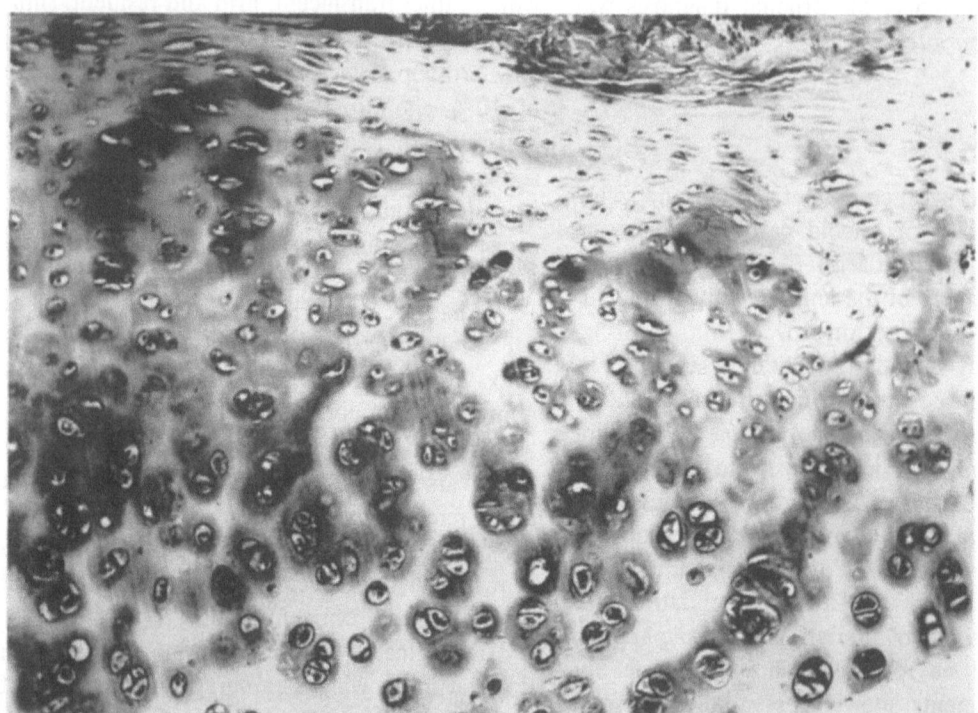

**Fig. 6.11.** *See text.* This degree of architectural variability was considered aberrant and probably at least dysplastic. H & E, × 123

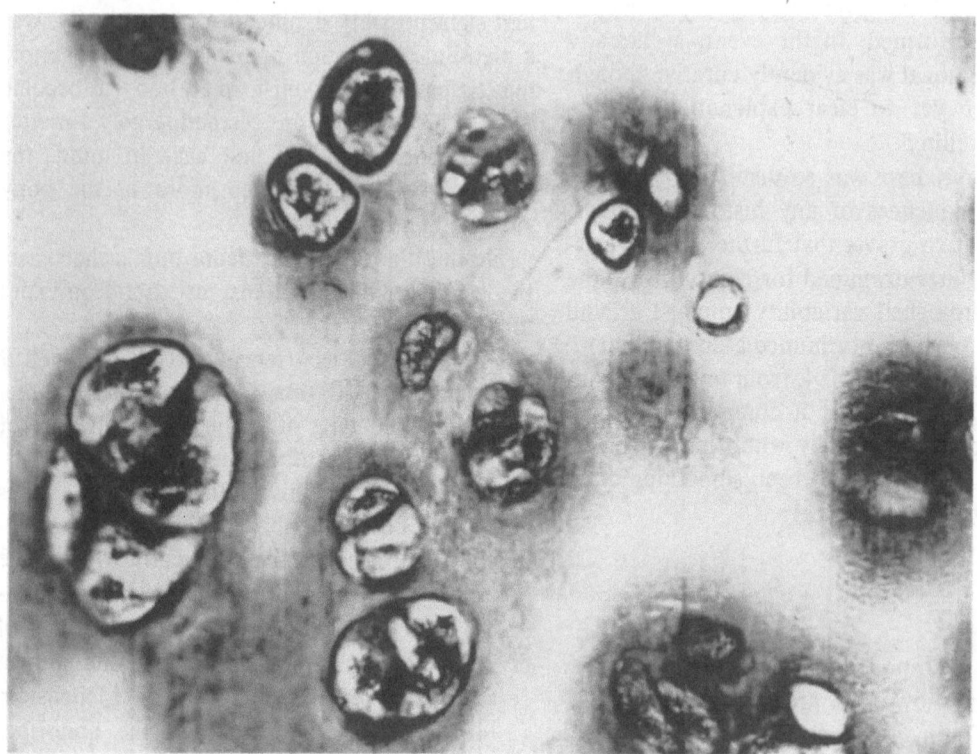

**Fig. 6.12.** The variability in nuclear size and number per cluster is great. H & E, × 493

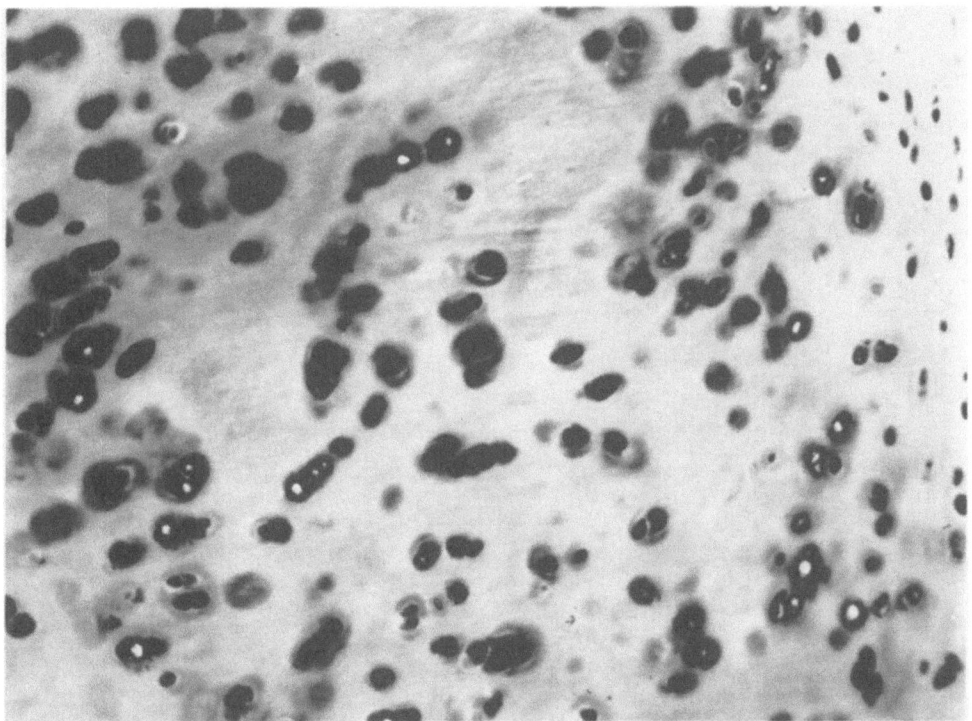

**Fig. 6.13.** This 'control' cricoid cartilage shows little, if any, less structural variability than that in the suspect cartilage. H & E, × 123

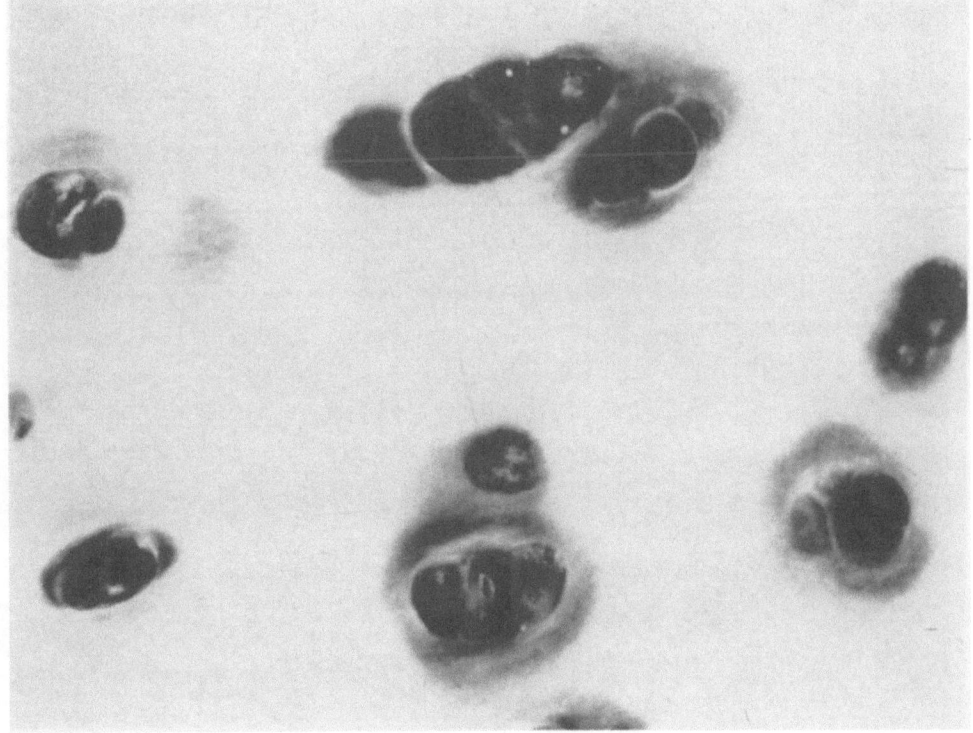

**Fig. 6.14.** Comparable variability is again present in the 'control' cartilage. H & E, × 493

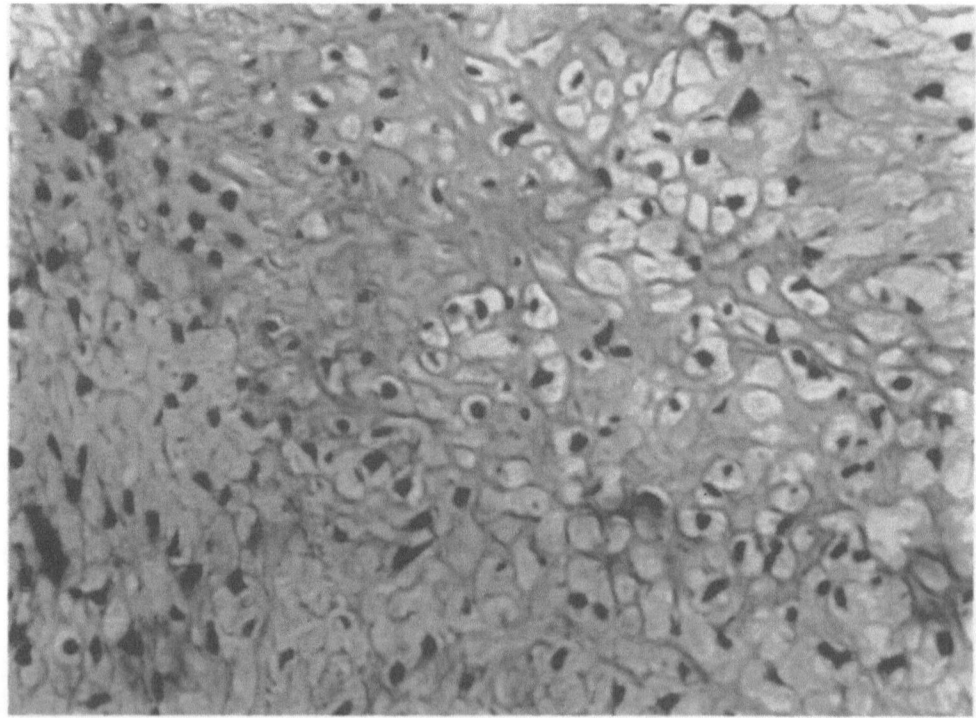

**Fig. 6.15.** The quite characteristic conjunction of myxoid and chondroid tissue. H & E, × 246

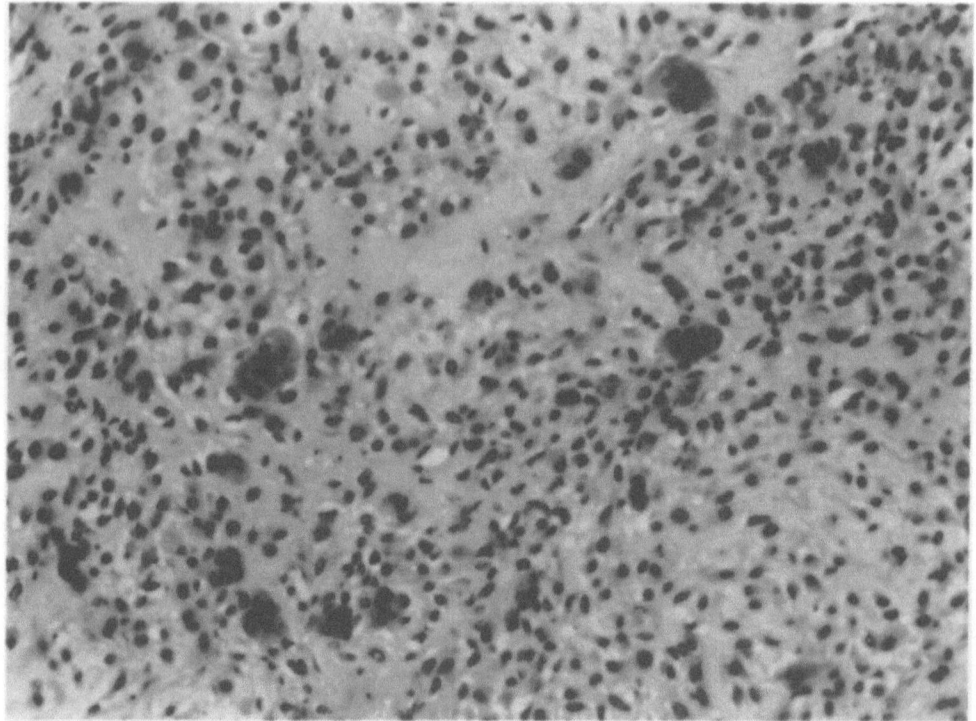

**Fig. 6.16.** Scattered multinucleated giant-cells, similar in appearance to those seen in an earlier typical chondromyxoid fibroma. H & E, × 246

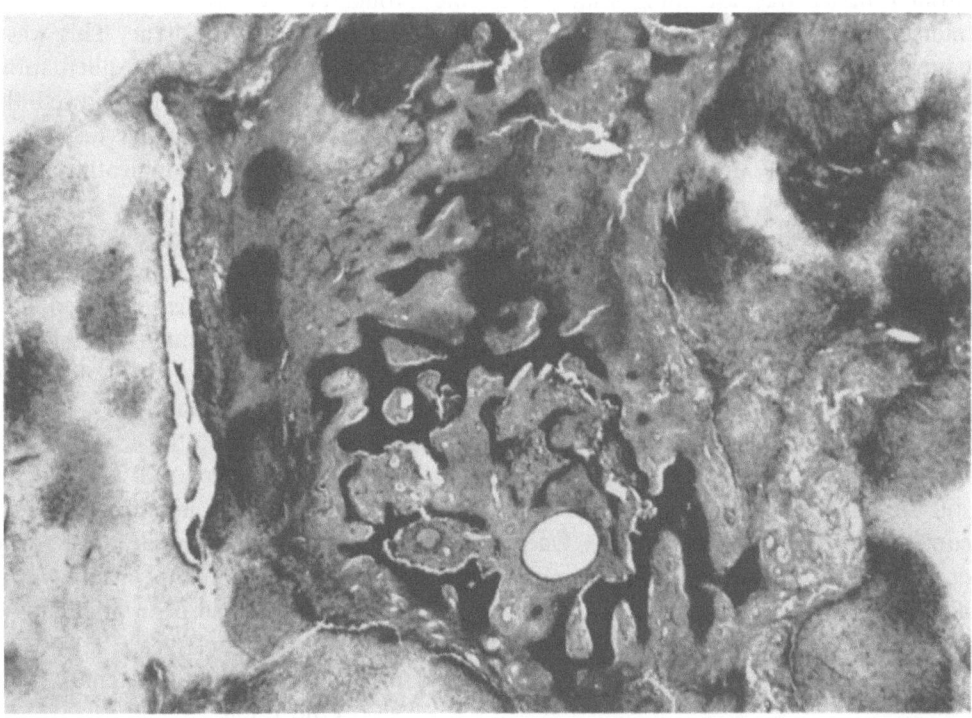

**Fig. 6.17.** The chondromyxoid tissue is seen in relatively solid sheets to right and left. In the centre it is totally permeating what appeared certainly to be pre-existing normal bone. H & E, × 17

*Case 6.11*

F (20 years) with pain in right hallux for several months. The lesion was a subungual exostosis: it was excised.

The cartilage was rather highly cellular and merged into undifferentiated fibrous tissue also of rather high cellularity. There was no undue polymorphism in either component but occasional mitotic figures were present in both. Further excision of the base and margins of the mass, diagnosed as a 'highly cellular exostosis', was recommended but nothing further was done.

The lesion recurred, recognised at first radiologically then visibly. It was removed again 11 months after the original excision, and this time the excision included the distal half of the phalangeal bone from which it arose, but, for whatever reason, this further specimen was not submitted for histology. However, the removal proved curative to the extent that the patient was free from trouble when last traced 3 years later. The diagnosis and advice, even if too lightly regarded, had been *appropriate*.

Solitary exostoses, which Willis (1960) believes for this reason are better designated 'oste-omas' or 'osteochondromas', do not always stop growing when skeletal maturation is attained. An amply thorough removal at the beginning would probably spare a patient what happened here, a second operation.

*Case 6.12*

F (27 years) with complaint of pain in the knee for 10 months. A destructive lesion, 4 × 4 × 3 cm, in the head of the tibia was shown on biopsy to be an osteoclastoma. The mass was then removed by curettage and the cavity packed with bone chips.

The pattern was typically that of an 'osteoclastoma'. The giant-cells were abundant and morphologically characteristic. The stroma was highly cellular with areas showing up to three mitoses per hpf but was reported nevertheless as "not frankly sarcomatous".

The area healed well but regrowth occurred 2 years later, with an area of destruction rather larger than originally. The tissue now showed some difference: giant-cells were relatively few and the stromal tissue even more highly cellular, polymorphic and mitotically active. Further, this stromal tissue was extending widely into the interstices of the otherwise healthy surrounding bone: wide areas could reasonably be diagnosed of themselves as fibrosarcoma. On this occasion the aggressiveness of the lesion was emphasised, as was the difficulty in assessing adequacy of excision: the possible need for amputation should the neoplasm appear yet again was very much in mind.

After a further 5 years it did reappear, and a block of bone, 6 × 3 × 1 cm, including the affected area was removed. Regrowth, with tissue now even more fibrosarcomatous, led to amputation 5 years later still (at the time of writing), that is, 12 years since the first operation, and still the outlook is uncertain. The diagnosis was correct and of course *appropriate*. On a future occasion, with tissue as cellular and actively dividing as this, a more thorough first extirpation, if technically feasible, would be recommended.

### Case 6.13

M (44 years) with pain in hip for 'a few months'. Radiology showed obvious abnormality in region of greater trochanter. Exploration revealed a rough-lined cavity, 25 × 20 × 20 mm, containing soft but gritty tissue. This was removed by curettage and the cavity filled with bone chips.

The abnormal tissue showed the dimorphic appearance seen in Fig. 6.18: in part it was wholly acceptable as indicating an osteoclastoma; elsewhere it was totally lacking in giant cells, purely stromal, and quite highly cellular. In some areas (Fig. 6.19) active osteogenesis was evident. The diagnosis preferred and given was 'osteoclastoma' though the alternative suggestion was made that the lesion might represent "an osteoclastic reaction to a bony lesion of some other kind".

The lesion recurred after 12 months, and again 12 months after that. On each occasion treatment was again curettage and packing, and on each occasion the histology was essentially the same as it had been originally.

After a further 3 years, now 5 years since the original treatment, the femur fractured at the site of the lesion.

On submitting tissue from the area of fracture, the surgeon specifically enquired whether the character of the lesion had changed—for one thing, it felt much less gritty—and indeed it had;

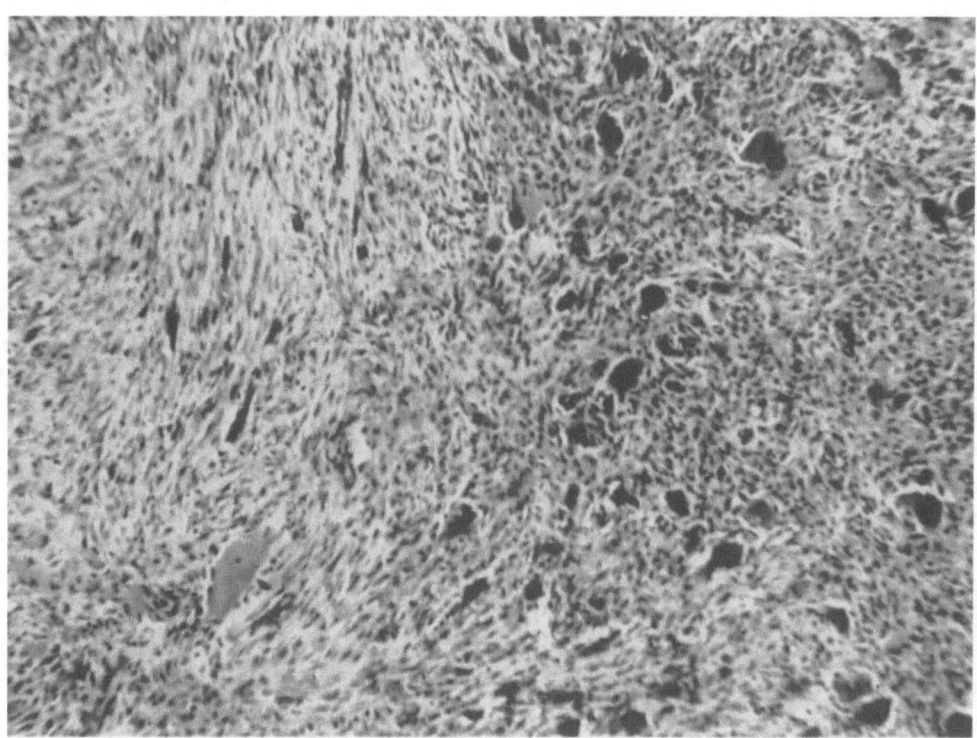

**Fig. 6.18.** To left is tissue representing ? highly cellular fibroma, ? fibrosarcoma. To right is what could be osteoclastoma. H & E, × 123

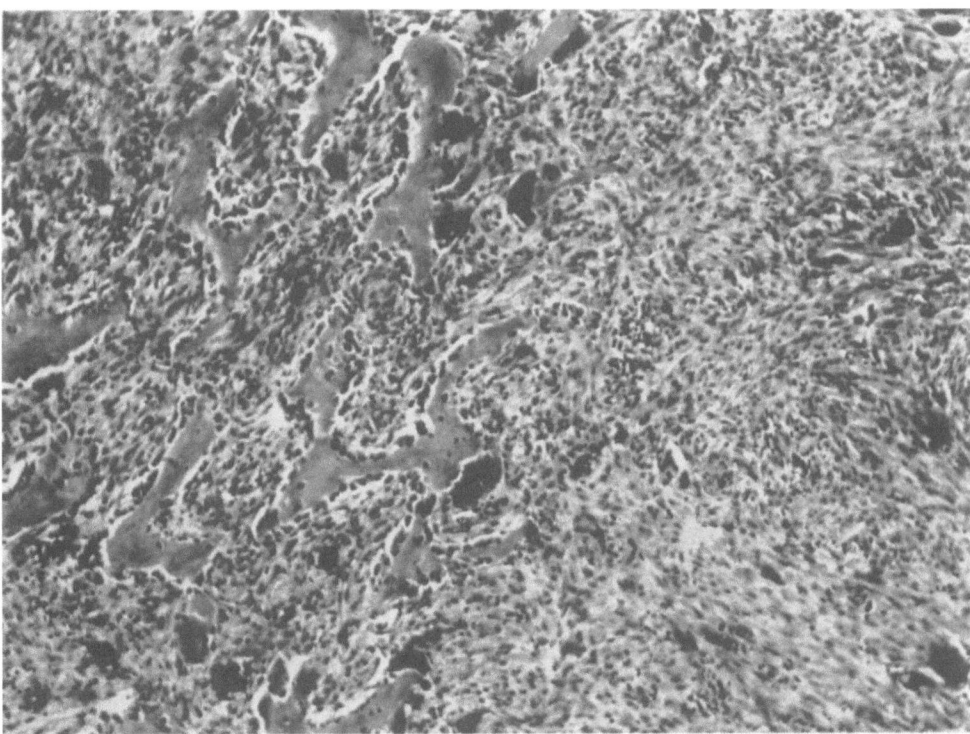

**Fig. 6.19.** Well-established osteogenesis was prominent in some places. These trabeculae were almost all amply surrounded by osteoblasts. H & E, × 123

it was now frankly a 'fibrosarcoma'. As seen in Fig. 6.20, it consisted purely of bands and swathes of closely packed spindle-shaped cells, not strikingly polymorphic but frequently in mitosis (Fig. 6.21). On this diagnosis, disarticulation was performed and the patient adapted well to his prosthesis during the next 6 months. However, he developed pelvic and pulmonary metastases and died 10 months after this procedure—that is, 6 years after the onset of trouble. There was no necropsy.

The amount of material sectioned on this last occasion was relatively large, and reasonably acceptable as representative. It seemed therefore that the giant-cell component had completely disappeared. So, what was the true nature of the neoplasm, and had it originally been 'culpably' underestimated (for it obviously had been so biologically)? Osteosarcomas may sometimes contain areas identical with fibrosarcoma; they may also contain foci of giant-cells. On balance, therefore, this seems likelier to have been an 'osteosarcoma' than an osteoclastoma from which such a purely stromal emergence is less common. On review of the original sections it is still hardly

possible to dogmatise on the *type* of the lesion. In terms of likely *behaviour*, however, more concern should have been expressed than was. Indeed, with its suggestion of a possible 'reactive' abnormality, the report was giving a hint away from metastasising malignancy. As seen in Fig. 6.22 the stromal cells (in both components) were appreciably polymorphic and quite frequently in mitosis (1 per 6 hpf) though none was certainly aberrant. Even so, on this evidence, the original report has to be regarded as an *under-diagnosis*. Whether, however, on the rather equivocal evidence, the formidable advice to disarticulate the limb should have been, or on a similar occasion now would be, given remains highly debatable.

### Case 6.14

M (52 years) with complaint of back-ache of 3 months' duration. Radiology showed collapse of 6th thoracic vertebra: all other investigations negative: clinical diagnosis made of 'eosinophil granuloma'. Radiotherapy produced some symptomatic relief: patient reasonably well until 10

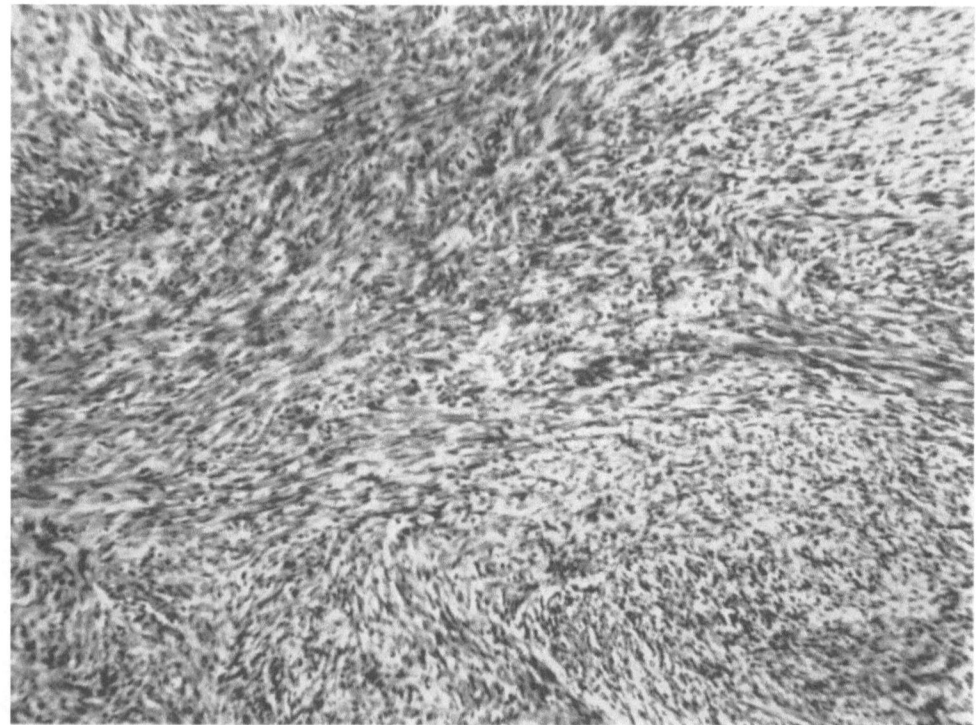

**Fig. 6.20.** Tissue from the late recurrence: it appeared to be unequivocally fibrosarcoma, and there was no neoplastic tissue of any other type. H & E, × 123

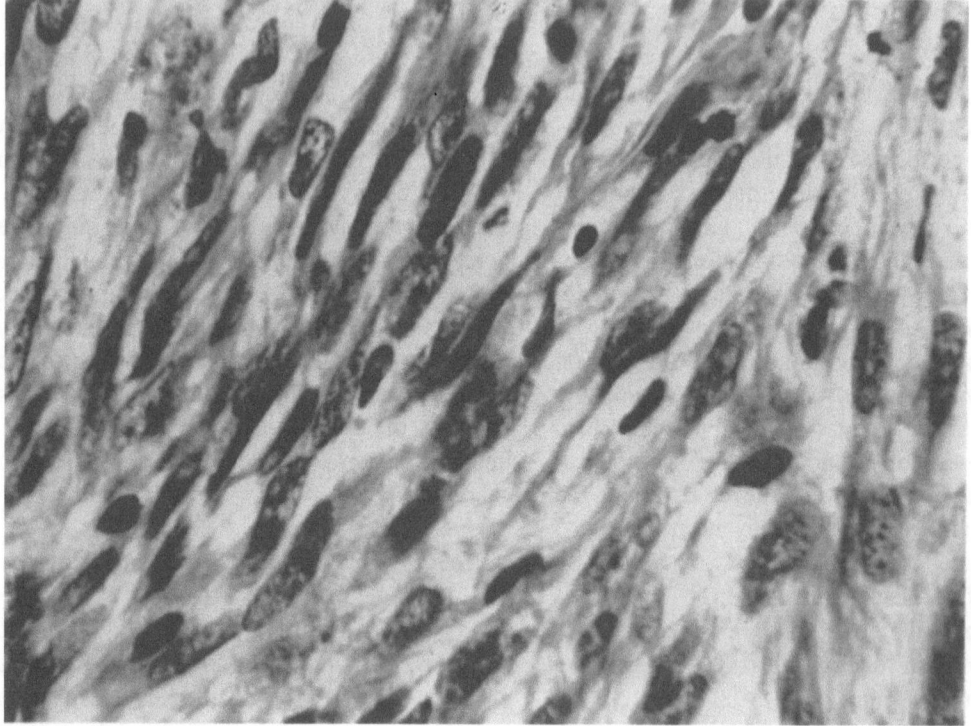

**Fig. 6.21.** The typically spindle-cell character of the finally recurrent growth. It is mildly polymorphic and mitotically active (one figure towards top right corner). H & E, × 985

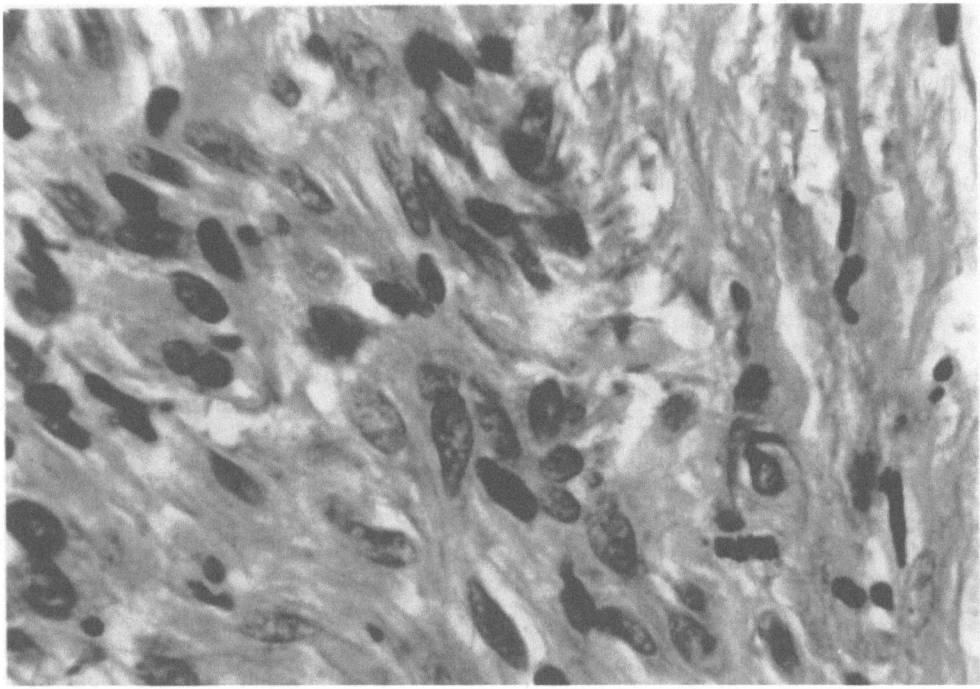

**Fig. 6.22.** Stromal tissue from the original biopsy, less highly cellular than the finally recurrent tissue but at least as polymorphic and with not infrequent mitoses (one lies towards lower right corner). H & E, × 985

years later when signs of cord compression developed. Exploration showed neoplastic tissue largely replacing collapsed body of T6, destroying adjacent ends of ribs and invading soft tissue.

Diagnosis was first requested by frozen section during the operation: the most that could be said was that the tissue was neoplastic, possibly lymphosarcoma, possibly metastatic carcinoma (the story of the events 10 years earlier had not then been conveyed). Paraffin sections showed solidly cellular sheets of tissue devoid of structural differentiation. Nuclei were remarkably uniform, rarely in mitosis (not more than 1 per 50 hpf), rather larger than those of normal lymphocytes and now with more punctate chromatin than was evident on FS. Cell outlines were rarely definable, the cytoplasm almost universally 'melting' and merging to form a finely but variably vacuolated and almost symplastic background. However, in a few places around the edge of the sheets, where cell density was less, outlines were better preserved and sufficient to show that many cells had a suggestively plasma-cell-like structure. Scattered clusters of cells were strongly pyroninophilic, not a diagnostic feature but one again hinting at myeloma. None of the cells contained glycogen. Later experience with Case 6.15 made it seem likely that a film preparation of the cells would have revealed at any rate some as being certainly of the plasma cell series, but the opportunity had not been offered. On the evidence available at the time, the diagnosis could not be taken further than (and remained at) 'probably myeloma': as such, it was *appropriate*.

Further radiotherapy was given, again with symptomatic relief, and the patient remains alive 8 years later, i.e. 10 years since the laminectomy and 20 years since discovery of his collapsed vertebra. The blood picture remains normal, and there is still no abnormality of an immunoglobulin pattern. Despite this, the likeliest diagnosis is still myeloma or 'solitary myeloma of bone (SMB)', of the behavioural type that Azar and his colleagues (1972) designate 'non-secretory'. This patient's long survival recalls the case reported by Willis (1941) of a patient whose solitary myeloma (of C2 vertebra) was also almost certainly present for 20 years before causing collapse of the vertebra and death from compression of the cord.

*Case 6.15*

M (49 years) with unsteadiness of gait over 3 months. Positive findings were bilateral weakness of distal leg muscles; a 15-mm osteolytic lesion in anterior end left 7 rib; cystic areas in body of T4 vertebra. Immunoelectrophoresis showed 'an abnormal group in IgG'. The lesion in the rib was biopsied.

The tissue was virtually identical with that seen in the preceding Case 6.14: sheets of uniform cells with 'melting' cytoplasm, which were occasionally pyroninophilic, glycogen-free and rarely in mitosis but none of them with sufficiently well-defined cytoplasmic outline or character to make myeloma histologically the most favoured diagnosis. Taking all the evidence into account, however, the final diagnosis at this time was 'probable myeloma'.

The spinal lesion was irradiated. The clinical picture was that of a peripheral neuropathy. It slowly progressed until, 5 years later, the arms became involved. There were now lytic lesions in the 2nd sacral vertebra and a further three ribs, with moderate enlargement of liver and spleen. The Ig pattern was essentially unchanged. Laparotomy, with biopsies, showed no significant abnormalities of liver, spleen, and mesenteric nodes. However, on this occasion an imprint preparation was made from one of the lytic lesions in a rib: some 70% of the cells were unquestionably of plasma cell type. Correlation with the Ig abnormality was thus attained and the diagnosis of myelomatosis fully established. The doubt that surrounded this case for 5 years was technical or academic only. Had specific treatment been available, or amputation been in question, the diagnosis from the outset would have been 'for practical purposes, myeloma'. The originally suggested diagnosis, though less than firm, was reasonably *appropriate*.

The patient developed increasing congestive cardiac failure and died within a few months of the laparotomy. There was no necropsy. The spreading neuropathy remained unexplained but was no different in this respect from the neuro- or myo-pathy seen sometimes in association with, say, a carcinoma of bronchus.

COMMENTARY ON LOCAL SERIES

None of the diagnostic/prognostic uncertainty had led to unnecessarily radical treatment or to delay in treatment. In the two instances of over-diagnosis, the over-diagnosis was one of degree, not one of complete error. In the first, some preference was expressed for myeloma rather than osteomyelitis. In the second, the architectural variability in a cricoid cartilage was regarded over-gloomily as a dysplasia. Neither limb nor larynx was lost: both patients made a full recovery and remain well. Whether the one patient whose lesion was initially under-diagnosed as osteoclastoma instead of osteosarcoma would have been saved by correct diagnosis, then irradiation and hind-quarter amputation, remains doubtful.

To the above extent, the position has been generally satisfactory. At the same time, however, as with the neoplasms of soft tissue, it seemed proper, with manageably small numbers, to examine, over the years, the outcome in the case of patients firmly diagnosed locally as having a malignant lesion of bone or cartilage, and then to review the material from such survivors as there were. Of the 36 'other-than-osteoclastoma' patients there were (and are) but 4 survivors: osteosarcoma 1/13: chondrosarcoma, 1/8: Ewing's tumour or ? neuroblastoma, 0/6: myeloma, 2/9. Review of the histology from these few surviving patients still finds the diagnosis wholly appropriate. In this small group, therefore, survivorship has probably not been a spurious survivorship due to over-diagnosis.

General Commentary

There are few texts that do not stress how important, indeed mandatory, it is for the pathologist to take into account the clinical and radiological evidence when he is assessing the histology of a lesion in bone. Thus, to quote as just one instance the statement by Spjut and his colleagues (1971, p. 16) in the current AFIP Fascicle on Tumors of Bone and Cartilage, "To merely 'read slides' without full comprehension of the clinical setting (age of patient, bone involved, location in bone) and the radiologic clues of the biologic behavior of the tumor can easily lead to an erroneous diagnosis". This is, of course, true but the way in which 'comprehension of the clinical setting' is used is crucial. As illustrated by the following examples, it is not always used in the same way: at times its uncritical use may be actively misleading.

Again to cite Spjut and his colleagues (1971), they illustrate in their fig. 2 an area of callus from the surface of a humerus in a patient of 29 years with the subscription "Without clinical data and knowledge of radiologic findings, this frightening histologic picture could be mistaken for osteosarcoma". What, then, of a lesion occurring in just the same clinical circumstances that was indeed osteosarcoma, for osteosarcoma does occur at both this age and site? In these circumstances, the pathologist, equally conditioned by the same clinical data and radiological findings, would presumably be as likely again to diagnose the lesion as not osteosarcoma: that is, the lesion would be under-diagnosed. The radiological appearances of an osteosarcoma are not always diagnostic: as we were reminded by Mirra and his co-workers (1976), "The benign-appearing radiographic features an osteosarcoma may assume are rarely reported". The best hope of avoiding under-diagnosis, and thus loss of potentially valuable time, lies with the pathologist who assesses the histology quite objectively. If, to him, the histology indicates osteosarcoma, he should say so, but he will, we hope, recognise the diagnostic hazard and frame his report along such lines as, 'Though virtually diagnostic of osteosarcoma, this appearance may be produced by exuberant callus: could the lesion be a simple fracture?' The parenthetical thought occurs that normal callus cannot often be the object of biopsy. Ordinarily, one would think, if callus is biopsied, it must be in some way unusual. In our own Case 6.2, the circumstances were fortuitous, namely, operation for fixation of a fracture that became distracted 3 weeks after initial impaction.

One of the few contributions to analyse the histological difficulties that callus may cause is that by Kahn and his associates (1969). In this, these authors describe (Case 2) a femoral lesion diagnosed histologically as a 'sarcoma', treated by curettage only (disarticulation was refused), and apparently fully healed 6 years later. The diagnosis was later revised to one of aneurysmal bone cyst, "only because the histologic sections were studied together with the roentgenograms". In the same article, however, in connection with their Case 3, also an aneurysmal bone cyst but in the humerus, they state that the radiological

opinion suggested osteosarcoma: that "The pathologist in turn was influenced by this radiologic. opinion . . .": and that the humerus was excised. Also, in relation to their Case 4 (a femoral lesion, found later to be metastatic bronchial carcinoma, diagnosed on biopsy as osteosarcoma), the authors comment, "This case illustrates most dramatically how readily the pathologist may err, when confronted with pieces of callus, especially when presented with a roentgenogram which he is led to believe shows a primary osteosarcoma". In saying this, the authors seem to have undermined, if not largely demolished, their own thesis; on these two occasions, foreknowledge of clinical circumstances was the very factor that induced the pathologist to err.

A final example, less intrinsically contradictory than that just cited, is seen in the contribution by Unni and his associates (1977) on intra-osseous osteosarcoma. In line with the general approach, they state that, "As in all bone lesions, there should be a close correlation between the roentgenographic and the histologic appearance before the diagnosis of central low-grade osteosarcoma can be made", yet shortly thereafter we read that "no pattern emerged to allow a definite diagnosis to be made roentgenographically". In the light of this, we may wonder whether, at any rate with intraosseous osteosarcoma, and with probably many other lesions, the radiographic evidence should ever take precedence over the histological. On many occasions there is a quantum of histological evidence, a quantum of radiological evidence, and a quantum of more purely clinical (including biochemical) evidence; and only joint consultation will determine the weighting to be given to each. Where events finally prove that radiological appearances or biochemical findings had established the diagnosis correctly, while the histology had not, the pathologist will come to appreciate, not so much the superiority of other techniques as the shortcomings (and perhaps remediable shortcomings) of his own.

This short section concludes, as it began, with a further quotation in similar vein from Spjut and his colleagues (1971, p. 161), "It is essential with any doubtful lesion for the pathologist to review all clinical data and radiographs to assist in determining the true nature of the lesion". This is absolutely correct. However (and the reader by now will know what is coming), the time for review is after the histological survey, pure and unbiased, not before.

Unlike the borderline problems in many systems, those met with lesions of bone and cartilage appear to take relatively well-defined though certainly many forms, some of greater practical or clinical significance than others. The various categories to be examined in turn, are those shown in Table 6.2.

## CLINICAL EVIDENCE VS HISTOLOGICAL EVIDENCE

Circumstances must be rare when a radiologically suspicious lesion in the skeletal system, as elsewhere in the body, cannot be investigated by biopsy. The limitations of radiological techniques and interpretation are recognised and acknowledged by radiologists, and need neither description nor emphasis. Nevertheless, even if radiological appearances are sometimes misleading, a biopsy-based opinion that fails to confirm the diagnosis favoured by the radiologist should be reviewed and if necessary followed by further biopsy. As stressed already, the biopsy should be adequately representative, for tissue changes may be patchy. Though sometimes expensive of time, attendance by the pathologist at the orthopaedic theatre has probably more to contribute to the selection of suitable tissue for biopsy than attendance at any other theatre: overall, it may well on occasions save time. In my own limited experience, the lesion producing the widest discrepancy between radiological and histological findings has been also the commonest to do so, namely, osteomyelitis.

**Table 6.2.** Borderline problems with lesions of bone and cartilage

---

A. Clinical/radiological evidence vs histological evidence
B. Equivocal histology
  I   Inflammatory patterns vs neoplastic patterns (osteomyelitis vs myeloma vs Ewing's tumour vs lymphoma)
  II  Chondroma vs chondrosarcoma
  III Callus vs osteosarcoma vs chondrosarcoma
  IV  Predominantly fibroblastic lesions containing giant cells

---

## INFLAMMATORY PATTERNS VS NEOPLASTIC PATTERNS

This problem may present itself in different ways: (a) whether the number of plasma cells in a particular lesion is sufficient to warrant a diagnosis of myeloma; (b) whether 'small round cells' are normal or neoplastic plasma cells, or lymphocytes, or the cells of a Ewing's tumour, or metastatic neuroblastoma, or even carcinoma. There are useful guides to the solution of these versions of the basic problem, and they will be mentioned presently, but the pathologist may be asked to provide a solution by means of frozen section when the surgeon first explores the lesion; and the difficulty then may be great. My own approach is broadly similar to that adopted in similar circumstances when confronted with tissue from a lymph node, thyroid gland, or melanotic lesion: either the tissue is blatantly 'malignant', even if the exact type of neoplasm cannot be decided, or the decision must await paraffin sections.

However, paraffin sections, no matter how perfect, offer no guarantee that the pathologist can give a firm answer to either of the questions, whether neoplastic, and, if so, what kind of neoplasm. Distinction between myeloma and osteomyelitis may be a matter of degree involving both numbers and types of cells. Few if any myelomas consist of a 100% population of morphologically obvious plasma cells. At one end of the scale, therefore, we may visualise a destructive lesion consisting of relatively uniform cells of which some 50% are obvious plasma cells, almost certainly a myeloma. At the other end of the scale is a lesion that includes, besides plasma cells, leucocytes of other kinds as well as proliferating vessels and fibroblasts, almost certainly inflammatory. The morphology of the cells that are or may be plasma cells is not valueless but it has limitations. Bi- and trinucleate forms may be as frequent in inflammatory aggregates as in myelomas; on the other hand, mitotic activity amongst cells that probably are plasma cells is rare in purely inflammatory lesions but relatively common in myelomas.

The opinion of the pathologist may or may not be available earlier than that of the biochemist but there is no certainty that confirmatory abnormalities of immunoglobulin pattern, whether in blood or in urine, would be detectable at that stage: the lesion might be what Azar and his colleagues (1972) call a 'non-secretory' plasma cell myeloma (or which they had five examples in their series of 123 cases). In one of the local cases, Case 6.14, even yet, after the presence of a destructive plasma cell lesion in the vertebral column for 10 (and possibly 20) years there is no demonstrable disturbance of immunoglobulin pattern but myeloma still seems the most appropriate diagnosis. The protracted course of this lesion stands in interesting contrast to the experience of Azar and his colleagues that 'non-secretory' myelomas are prognostically worse than the others. They were inclined to regard the phenomenon as an expression of poor differentiation, and as such, reasonably to be correlated with a greater aggressiveness. However, they still regard 'non-secretion' as a 'complex and obscure phenomenon'.

A second case in the local series, Case 6.15, was also relevant to the problem of the 'round cell tumour' in bone, though in a different way. For 5 years the paradox remained that the patient had an abnormal pattern of immunoglobulins yet the cells of the lesion, also in the vertebral column, were not diagnostically plasma cells. However, on this occasion a cell-imprint showed that they were, after all, plasma cells. Whether an imprint from the original lesion would also have revealed their identity we cannot know but the suspicion remains that it would. Be that as it may, the experience was enough to act as a reminder that there is nothing to be lost, and perhaps much to be gained, by having imprint preparations made from any lesion that gives a radiological hint that it might be a myeloma; if open biopsy is for any reason impracticable, this provides one of the few indications for needle biopsy with aspiration and cytological study thereafter. The basic technique was well described by Erf and Herbut (1946) many years ago (it may be used with advantage in other circumstances also, as, for example, and as illustrated by Garfinkel and Bennett [1969], with dubious lesions of lymph nodes).

The relation of the solitary myeloma of bone (SMB) to extramedullary plasmacytoma (EMP) and myelomatosis has been analysed by Wiltshaw (1976). In his opinion, SMB is "but one mode of presentation of myelomatosis rather than a separate entity" while EMP, though also characterised by disseminated lesions in bone, has a pattern of distribution within bone (random, rather than within the axial skeleton) and a response to treatment (much more favourable) identifying it as a disturbance of a different order. A consideration of these features in a patient from whom a 'myeloma' biopsy had been obtained might thus allow a better assessment of prognosis than study of the biopsy in isolation. Of the patients with EMP in Wiltshaw's series, 50% were alive 10 years after diagnosis, while, with a relatively low dosage of radiotherapy, 15 year survival was not uncommon. By contrast, mortality amongst patients with SMB was high, most dying with widely disseminated disease. Substantially similar findings have been published by Corwin and Lindberg (1979) in the case of 24 patients studied over 20 years: of 12 with SMB, six developed myelomatosis: of 12 with EMP, two developed myelomatosis.

By now, the time has passed when the diagnosis of myeloma is likely to depend solely on histology, whether supplemented by cytology or not. Techniques of histochemistry, immunoelectrophoresis and ultramicroscopy have all a significant contribution to make, and it may well be that with their widening use there will come a reduction in the number of lesions of bone hitherto diagnosed with varying degrees of assurance as malignant lymphoma (usually RCS), Ewing's tumour and metastatic neuroblastoma or carcinoma. The correct identification of these, and distinction of one from the others, is of less immediate practical importance than the already mentioned distinction of any one of them 'from osteomyelitis; here we are deciding, not whether the patient has a neoplasm or not, but which neoplasm he has of several highly dangerous forms.

The discovery by Schajowicz (1959) that the cells of a Ewing's tumour contain glycogen went far to reduce the differential diagnostic problem, and it has largely stood the test of time. As noted in chap. 5 the same PAS positivity has been the essential basis of recognition of morphologically similar lesions in soft tissue, as also Ewing's tumour. With knowledge of this, and the diagnostic resources available anent myeloma, and also the features that broadly characterise the other neoplasms in question, it is possible to construct an outline guide to diagnosis of the familiar dichotomous type as shown in Table 6.3.

There are, of course, factors other than those

**Table 6.3.** 'Small round cell' neoplasms in bone[a].

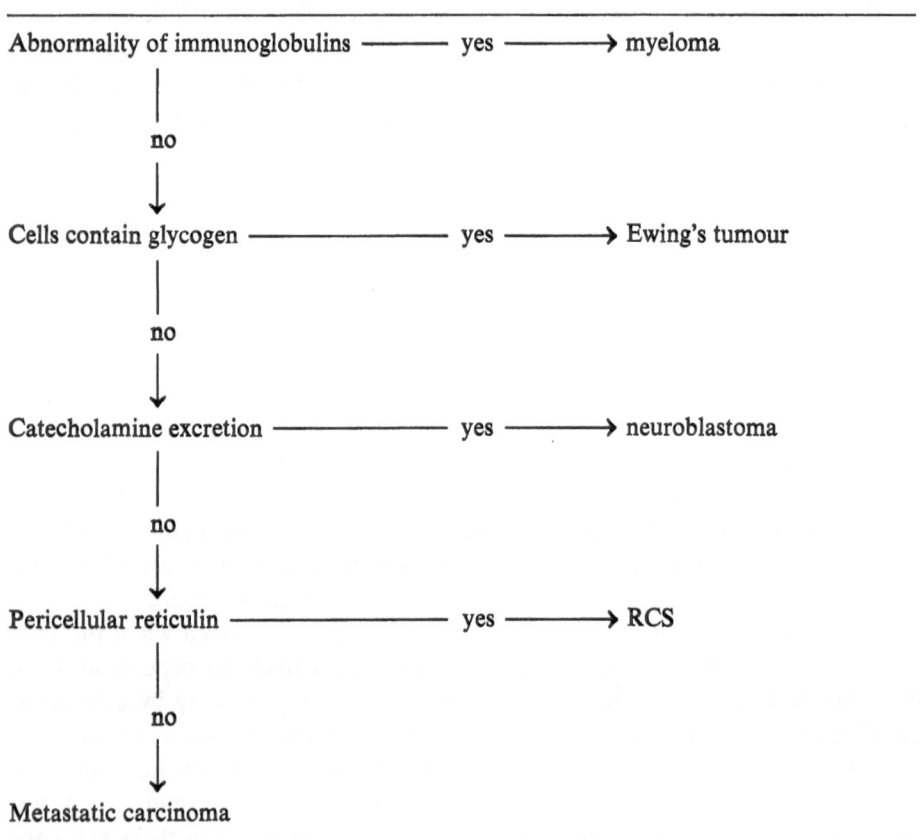

| | |
|---|---|
| Abnormality of immunoglobulins ——— yes ———→ | myeloma |
| │ | |
| no | |
| ↓ | |
| Cells contain glycogen ——————— yes ———→ | Ewing's tumour |
| │ | |
| no | |
| ↓ | |
| Catecholamine excretion ————— yes ———→ | neuroblastoma |
| │ | |
| no | |
| ↓ | |
| Pericellular reticulin ——————— yes ———→ | RCS |
| │ | |
| no | |
| ↓ | |
| Metastatic carcinoma | |

[a] An outline scheme of analysis to be supplemented by other observations as mentioned in the text.

shown in this most elementary outline to be taken into account but it is a framework on which to build a more detailed scheme of analysis. One such factor is age (of which more anon): others are the possible presence and type of tumour metabolites: the sometime presence of rosettes in neuroblastoma: the tendency for RCS to show a greater degree of polymorphism than the other lesions: and the ultramicroscopic characteristics.

A valuable survey of 229 examples of Ewing's tumour has been published by Pritchard and his colleagues (1975) with particular reference to the clinical and pathological features of the lesions in the 37 patients in the series who survived for five years or longer. Only two factors appeared to be usefully correlated with such survival, namely, location of the lesion in an extremity and "inclusion of surgery as part of the initial treatment". Of patients with a primary lesion in a limb, 21.8% survived 5 years: for those with the lesion elsewhere, the correspond-

ing figure was only 8.3%. Neither radiological nor histological appearances were useful guides to prognosis: indeed, in the authors' words, "Histological study of the lesions of the survivors revealed that no pathological features relative to an improved prognosis could be identified. The histological features of the lesions of the survivors were not different from those of the non-survivors".

Age as a factor to be considered in assessment of round or oval cell lesions merits further comment. Knowledge of the age of the patient may have an insidious influence on diagnosis here as elsewhere. The usual age-incidence of the lesions in question is well known: neuroblastoma in infancy: Ewing's tumour, 10–30 years: RCS, over 30 years: carcinoma, over 50 years. With totally equivocal histology and no supplementary evidence, the likeliest diagnosis among these naturally lies directly in line with the age of the patient. However, the danger here is that age may be allowed an overriding importance. If a lesion in a patient of 40, for example, is less than totally equivocal, giving perhaps just a hint of neuroblastoma, any pathologist dominated by considerations of the age incidence might reason that such a lesion at age 40 would be so far outside the usual age range as to make this diagnosis highly unlikely and indeed unacceptable: that is, the factual histological evidence is being dismissed on grounds that have nothing to do with morphology: and this is illogical. Neuroblastoma does occur in the adult (*see*, for example, the report of nine cases by Mackay and his colleagues [1976] where the diagnosis was established on firm ultramicroscopical evidence): therefore, there is every reason here, and in other comparable circumstances, for the pathologist to abide by his histological impressions and relegate considerations of age to second place.

A further danger in allowing age incidence to dominate as a factor in diagnosis is that, if an age range is virtually built into the definition of a neoplasm, that neoplasm will 'never' be found in any patient outside the prescribed age-range. Occurrence of what appears to be a neoplasm $X$ outside the 'usual' age-range will certainly lessen the probability that the diagnosis in indeed $X$ but it cannot reduce the probability to nil; it cannot alter morphological fact. Fortunately for diagnostic accuracy, newer techniques and their revelation of more nearly incontrovertible evidence, as in the case of the adult neuroblastomas just mentioned, are gradually downgrading age as a factor in diagnosis and further upgrading the roles of morphology and biochemistry.

An analysis of the 'malignant round-cell tumour' of bone was carried out by Sissons (1975) and four other pathologists to obtain information (a) on whether, after a 'careful attempt' to exclude myeloma, lymphoma, carcinoma and metastatic neuroblastoma, distinction between a primary and a secondary round-cell neoplasm was possible, and (b) on the degree of concordance between observers on the assessment of tissue patterns. The first matter is clearly not relevant to borderline decisions (the investigation left the problem largely unresolved). The second matter is relevant to the extent that it bears on the interpretation of tissue patterns in general. In the event, a significant variation in the opinion of the observers was revealed, of a degree leading Sissons to conclude that ". . . the examination of a section, on one occasion, by

one pathologist, was not a reliable way to answer the particular questions in which we were interested".

## CHONDROMA VS CHONDROSARCOMA

The essential problems posed by cartilaginous overgrowths are: first, when should a borderline chondroma be regarded as a chondrosarcoma; second, for manifest chondrosarcoma, how radical should treatment be? In practice, the second question is the more important. The more radical the treatment, certainly, the better the outlook (at least so far as concerns eradication of the neoplasm) but equally clearly, every effort will be made to avoid unnecessarily radical treatment. The first question, considered in more detail later, is self-answering to the extent that any chondrosarcoma initially under-diagnosed as a chondroma will reveal its true identity sooner or later. A series of 27 cases of chondrosarcoma of bones of the limbs, illustrative in this general context, was described by Méary and Roger (1972). In this series, 3 lesions treated by wide excision all recurred, 2 fatally metastasising: of 16 treated by resection, 8 recurred, one fatally metastasising: of 8 treated by primary amputation, 7 were probably cured. Perhaps, if primary amputation had been used in all 27 patients, some 90% would have been cured but at the cost of how many limbs 'needlessly' amputated? This is the surgeon's dilemma; and very largely the pathologist is called upon to resolve it.

As would be expected, there is, with chondrosarcomas, a broad correlation between degree of histological aberrancy and clinical behaviour. Its level has not often been expressed mathematically but this has been done in a helpful analysis of 71 cases by Evans and his associates (1977). Sections from the 71 cases, of which almost one-third were in the pelvis, were examined 'blind' with mitotic incidence the main criterion of grade, namely, number of mitoses per 10 hpf in the most highly cellular areas (usually at the periphery of the mass and often in areas where the pattern approached that of a spindle-celled sarcoma with minimal chondroid or myxoid matrix). Grades I, II and III had, respectively, a mitotic incidence of nil, less than 2, 2 or more per 10 hpf. The 10-year survival rates were, again respectively, 83%, 64% and 29%, and the frequency of metastasis 0%, 10% and 71%.

Likelihood of local recurrence bore little relation to histological grade but, as in the series of Méary and Roger (1972), was notably correlated with the form of treatment used: recurrence appeared in 46% of the patients treated by local excision but in only 9.5% of those treated by 'amputation or resection of all or part of the involved bone'.

Figures such as these are of the greatest value. The remark was made earlier that assessment of probability in percentage terms is the most helpful advice the pathologist can give. The assessing of probability is what biopsy reporting is. Its expression in mathematical terms, especially when based on objectively 'blind' histology, is not purported or spurious accuracy; it is an opinion as close to accuracy as the facts and techniques allow. What use thereafter the surgeon makes of the percentage probability, what weighting he gives it, is his concern.

Further figures of value were provided by Dahlin and Beabout (1971) from their analysis of 370 examples of well-differentiated or low-grade chondrosarcoma. Observant sampling of the lesions had led to the recognition of 33 cases containing foci of pure fibrosarcoma or of osteosarcoma, a combination described by the authors as a "bimorphic combination of almost benign and highly malignant tumor". Such lesions are highly malignant: 30 of the patients had died. It is therefore prognostically important that sarcomatous islands like these be identified and sectioned, and Dahlin and Beabout maintain that this can be done; the foci of de-differentiated tissue were relatively well demarcated and distinguishable by their pink or greyish-white and opaque appearance. Failure by pathologists in the past to sample such areas may well account in part for the notoriously evident unpredictability of chondromas and chondrosarcomas. A subsidiary point of biological interest is that foci of this kind were found in the 26 neoplasms obtained by primary removal as well as in the 7 that were recurrent. The appearance of focal de-differentiation was thus not a regrowth 'reactive' to earlier removal but a feature present probably from the start. The relation of lesions of this kind to osteosarcoma is considered presently.

The anatomical location of a chondroma matters greatly to prognosis. Thus, in a review of 110 cases of chondroma in bones of the hand treated mostly by curettage and autologous cancellous bone grafting, Takigawa (1971) reported 'excellent' results in 87. The follow-up period was relatively short, rarely more than 2 years, but even so results of this kind are inconceivable with chondromas of the axial skeleton or proximal bones of the limbs. In the local series, Case 6.8, a chondroma in the pubic ramus seemed histologically wholly benign, yet it recurred after 12 years; and none can be sure this will not happen again. The anatomical location takes precedence even over histology. Thus, as mentioned by Spjut and his co-authors (1971), aberrant nuclear forms that would cause concern in other circumstances may be accepted with equanimity in enchondromas, periosteal chondromas, and synovial chondromatosis. The ribs, though small bones relative to the femur, humerus and those of the pelvis, are dangerous sites for cartilaginous overgrowths. From their experience with 35 cases in ribs, Marcove and Huvos (1971) regard all masses more than 4 cm in diameter, however benign the histology, as 'borderline chondrosarcomas', and for all these adequate local excision is essential; local excision in their view implies the excision of adjacent uninvolved ribs and pleura en bloc. Despite this, of 28 patients with lesions of this kind, 17 died.

Electron microscope studies of chondrosarcomas such as those by Erlandson and Huvos (1974) and Fu and Kay (1974) have shown ultramicroscopic abnormalities increasing approximately in parallel with the abnormalities visible by light microscopy. They have taken us little nearer to answering the basic question, When is a chondroma a chondrosarcoma? This is a subjective decision; each pathologist will, from his experience, have laid his own diagnostic threshold in terms of nuclear and cellular aberrancy. However, he will recall the significance of the site and size of the mass, and also recall, as illustrated in Figs. 6.13 and 6.14, that normal cartilage may show a wide range of patterns, including anisocytosis, binucleate cells and more than 1 cell per lacuna.

The fact may be highly frustrating but we have to conclude that correlation between histology and prognosis at the 'lower end' or in the borderline zone is particularly low. We just have to accept our impotence which not even the electron microscope has helped; as Erlandson and Huvos (1974) resignedly said, "one would be hard pressed to point out differences between 'normal' chondrocytes and neoplastic cartilage cells present in low-grade chondrosarcomas".

Fortunately, our incapacity matters little in practice. The governing principle has emerged that, apart from chondromas of the hands and feet, en bloc resection must be the aim, and at times the only way to achieve this will be amputation, perhaps at forequarter or hindquarter level. In extreme circumstances, as with extensive pelvic involvement, the question of translumbar resection or hemisomatectomy ('hemicorporectomy' to some) will arise. This is a formidable procedure with implications far beyond those of surgical technique alone. In the case described by Thomine (1972), the operation was successful but the patient "could not sustain his infirmity and in the end . . . became quite mad".

Two lesions, with little doubt once over-diagnosed as chondrosarcoma but probably no longer so, are the chondromyxoid fibroma and benign chondroblastoma.

### Chondromyxoid Fibroma

A valuable review of 76 cases of CMF has been published by Rahimi and his associates (1972), who note the possibly misleading feature that its cells may have disturbingly large nuclei. Further aids, proposed by these observers, to the distinction of the lesion from chondrosarcoma are the more distinct resemblance in places to hyaline cartilage, the characteristic admixture of fibrous elements (which in local Case 6.10 amounted virtually to fibrocartilage), and the often relatively sharp margination of the neoplastic tissue.

The basic architecture of the lesion is illustrated by the recommendation of Schajowicz and Gallardo (1971) that it should rather be designated 'fibromyxoid chondroma'. These authors and others suggest that, where feasible, treatment should be by en bloc resection rather than by curettage. The notorious tendency to recurrence was unusually demonstrated by reappearance of a focus of the neoplasm in the soft tissues of the incision 19 years after removal of a CMF (Mikulowski and Östberg, 1971).

### Chondroblastoma

The chondroblastoma, like CMF, is prone to recurrence and is also basically benign. The histo-

logical pattern is, however, much more distinctively chondroid and has been aptly described by Huvos and his associates (1972a) as consisting of "Close-packed polyhedral cells, separated by scant interstitial occasionally chondroid matrix". Despite the general uniformity of pattern (sometimes rather reminiscent of frog spawn) there may be enough polymorphism sometimes to suggest chondrosarcoma, as had happened, with resultant amputation, in one of the cases in the series of Huvos and his colleagues.

### CALLUS VS OSTEOSARCOMA VS CHONDROSARCOMA

To some extent the problems arising here blend with those considered below apropos the mainly fibrous overgrowths: however, some points merit separate mention. Almost always when tissue is submitted as '? callus', the clinical circumstances will be appropriate; there will have been a known fracture. Some examples of tissue from such a biopsy may show such a mixture of tissue, bony and cartilaginous, osteoid and chondroid, as raises the triple problem 'callus or osteo- or chondro-sarcoma' but more usually the problem is double, either 'callus or osteosarcoma' or 'osteosarcoma or chondrosarcoma'. Chondrosarcoma, because of its generally less gloomy prognosis, should be distinguished whenever possible from osteosarcoma but the more important distinction to be made in practice is that between callus and osteosarcoma. Some of the attendant difficulties were considered earlier in this chapter but then mainly to illustrate the interrelationships between clinical, radiological, and histological data in the diagnosis of skeletal lesions. There are further aspects more directly relevant to the histology.

By definition, callus follows a fracture. Conceivably, a fracture could be subclinical, fail to heal, produce a mass of callus and instigate biopsy but histological recognition of the tissue as callus, and enquiry of the patient, is unlikely to fail to uncover an appropriate history of trauma. As exemplified by our Case 6.2, and as agreed in many texts (for example Kahn et al., 1969), young active callus may histologically be indistinguishable in places from osteosarcoma. The *ingredients* of the problem are: highly cellular tissue, possibly or probably callus, and an appropriate history. The *nature* of the problem is:

has the fracture been a pathological fracture superimposed upon an osteosarcoma? (and the telangiectatic osteosarcoma that may be confused with an aneurysmal bone cyst must especially be remembered here.)

The contribution of the pathologist in these circumstances may be crucial. The histological evidence and the radiological evidence may concur or conflict. Even if the radiological evidence is virtually diagnostic of osteosarcoma, any reservations by the pathologist demand discussion and review. On occasion, the histological evidence may be unarguable and directly contradict the radiological, as, for example, when the lesion is manifestly metastatic carcinoma, or, in the opposite direction, when the lesion is wholly benign, as with the enchondroma illustrated by Spjut and his colleagues (1971, fig. 166) that was suspected radiologically to be osteosarcoma. The position is then straightforward. When the histology is arguable, on the other hand, further biopsy may or may not be indicated, and again it is the pathologist in essence who will decide. If the radiologist, for example, says 'virtually certainly lesion *X*', the pathologist need say no more than that the histology is 'compatible with lesion *X*' for the diagnosis to be substantiated in full. However, in circumstances such as these, where the histology is equivocal, 'lesion *X*' will almost certainly not be the only lesion with which the histology is compatible, and responsibility then lies with the pathologist to put before the surgeon for evaluation his list of diagnostic possibilities and their respective probabilities.

The problems involved when fracture + callus is superimposed upon some underlying lesion have been clearly stated by Kahn and his co-workers (1969). These authors offer as advice that, while distinction from osteosarcoma may on occasion be extremely difficult, uncomplicated callus does not show the 'obvious anaplasia' of an osteosarcoma, and that, from about the 3rd week, 'the osteoid and bony trabeculae are regularly arranged and are usually rimmed by a single layer of osteoblasts'. Perhaps, in our Case 6.2, if the callus had been aged 4 weeks instead of 3 weeks the morphology would no longer have been so highly mimetic of osteosarcoma: as it was, the callus, with its exuberant cellularity, polymorphism and mitotic activity, was diagnosed on a later occasion as osteosarcoma when examined 'blind' by several in a group of pathol-

ogists (though it was correctly identified on the original occasion). As mentioned earlier, callus is unlikely to be the object of biopsy unless circumstances are unusual and probably suspicious. It seems wise, therefore, to take the biopsy request per se as a warning: every biopsy of callus should be searched for evidence of some underlying and possibly causative lesion—inflammatory, degenerative, dysplastic or neoplastic. Finally, and especially since trauma will equally figure in the patient's history, myositis ossificans should always remain in mind in this general context as a lesion to be positively identified or excluded.

Distinction between chondrosarcoma and osteosarcoma is important in view of the likely difference in treatment. In chondrosarcoma, local en bloc excision will be attempted wherever possible; in osteosarcoma, amputation is still the likeliest outcome (*pace* such chemotherapeutic advances as may emerge). The distinction may be objectively-based and well-defined, or subjectively-based and ill defined: it depends on the answer to the question, How much, if any, osteoid tissue is acceptable wtihin the diagnosis 'chondrosarcoma'? If the answer is 'none', the position is clear: otherwise, as just said, the matter is vague, depending on the amount of osteoid tissue allowed.

Reference has been made to the description of areas of dedifferentiation in low-grade chondrosarcoma by Dahlin and Beabout (1971). In 11 of their 33 cases, "malignant cells produced osteoid . . . making the complicating tumors in these osteogenic sarcomas". Since, in 26 of these cases, areas of either fibrosarcoma or osteosarcoma were present on first biopsy, tissue of this kind could not have been a new development or 'reaction' stimulated by an earlier incomplete removal. It could equally be held, therefore, that the lesions containing foci of osteosarcoma were indeed osteosarcomas, characterised, as is not rare, by wide areas of chondroid differentiation. Of 28 patients in this series treated before a certain date, 23 were dead, mostly with known metastatic spread: this is more comfortably acceptable as the behaviour of osteosarcoma than of low-grade chondrosarcoma with focally atypical histology.

The distinction between chondro- and osteosarcoma had to be made by Evans and his associates (1977). Their policy, in their own words, was, "In some neoplasms otherwise resembling high-grade chondrosarcoma, there are foci in which neoplastic osteoid arises directly from a sarcomatous stroma. This feature is considered indicative of osteosarcoma . . .". On the whole, this policy seems best, for it is simple: the presence of any osteoid tissue in an otherwise apparent chondrosarcoma warrants classification as osteosarcoma. By this, an occasional patient may or might be over-treated but many fewer will or would be under-treated.

### Osteosarcoma

Osteosarcoma may have to be distinguished from many lesions other than chondrosarcoma and simple callus; and, of these others, the aneurysmal bone cyst (ABC) takes a foremost place. Osteosarcoma and ABC may be mistaken histologically (and, equally, radiologically) for each other. In two of the cases described by Kahn and his colleagues (1969), an ABC was wrongly over-diagnosed as osteosarcoma. In contrast, 9 of the 25 examples of telangiectatic osteosarcoma described by Matsuno and coworkers (1976) were initially diagnosed as benign; 3 of them as ABC, 3 as haemangioendothelioma, 2 as benign giant-cell tumour and 1 as blood clot. Similarly, in a series of 80 cases of juxtacortical osteosarcoma described by Heul and others (1967), 16 had been initially diagnosed histologically as a 'benign lesion'. The possibilities of reciprocal misdiagnosis for either lesion in either direction are thus considerable. A valuable working principle lies in the writings of Lichtenstein (1972, p. 391), ". . . however extensive or otherwise impressive the tendency to new bone formation may be, an essential prerequisite for the diagnosis of osteogenic sarcoma is the presence of a connective tissue stroma that is frankly sarcomatous".

There is no completely satisfactory classification of osteosarcoma, partly because anatomical location may be a better prognostic guide than the histology. The kinds of groupings that have been used, a mixture of the anatomical and the histological, are approximately as follows:

*General anatomical:*
  a) Lesions around the jaw
  b) Lesions in soft tissue (analysed earlier)
  c) The remainder

*Local anatomical:*
  a) Juxtacortical or parosteal
  b) Periosteal (distinguished from parosteal by Unni et al., 1976a, 1976b)
  c) Intraosseous (Unni et al., 1977)
  d) Other or 'orthodox', i.e. most osteosarcomas

*Functional:*
Osteosarcoma in association with Paget's disease

*Histological:*
  a) Osteoblastic
  b) Chondroblastic
  c) Fibroblastic
  d) Sclerosing
  e) Telangiectatic

Osteosarcomas around the jaw, and the juxtacortical, are in general less aggressive than those occurring elsewhere; also, of histological types, the telangiectatic are seemingly the most aggressive (whether site or type would take precedence in, say, a telangiectatic osteosarcoma of mandible is difficult to discover: in the series of telangiectatic lesions of Matsuno and his colleagues [1976] all but one, in the ribs, were in the limbs). Beyond this, there is much to be said for the synoptic view of Willis (1960) that all are but structural variants of the one entity. Accepting this, it is natural to look in more detail at the histology and cytology to see whether prognostically useful information can be gained from 'grading', and here again opinions differ.

From statistical analysis of mitotic incidence in a series of 88 patients, Price (1961) concluded that a prognostically helpful level of grading could be found. On the other hand, this has not emerged from some later series. Studies of long-term survivors were made by both O'Hara and his associates (1968) and Gravanis and Whitesides (1970), and in neither series were any features found that could be consistently correlated with the outcome. In a 20-year review of 54 cases, Scranton and his colleagues (1975) found a modest correlation between the general cytological pattern (degree of cellularity, pleomorphism and vascularity) and the outcome, but not so with either mitotic frequency or amount of lymphocytic infiltration. Of 16 patients in this series with a raised serum alkaline phosphatase, 11 had died, while of 22 patients with a single normal reading, 10 had died. In contrast, O'Hara and his group had found phosphatase levels valueless; however, none of their patients had shown any 'marked elevation'. The experience of Unni and others (1977) was similar to the extent that, in their analysis of 27 cases subgrouped as 'intraosseous' osteosarcoma, they also found mitotic incidence of little value but the cytological pattern otherwise of some value.

In all, therefore, the attempted grading of unequivocal osteosarcoma appears to have little to offer; and all the time the nagging suspicion will remain around the long-term survivors that perhaps the lesion was not an osteosarcoma but one of its many imitators (to the ranks of which 'malignant fibrous histiocytoma' of bone, considered later, is a recent recruit). In a case described by Mirra and colleagues (1976), a lesion that appeared histologically to be certainly an osteosarcoma (of fibula at age 17 years) had been radiologically static for at least 15 months before treatment: only curettage was used, and all was well 4½ years later. The authors believed a more likely explanation to be that the lesion was a 'pseudo-malignant osteoblastoma' rather than an arrested osteosarcoma. They also appropriately cite (though with an incorrect reference) the description by Levin (1957) of an apparently spontaneous cure of what again appeared to many who saw the sections to be an osteosarcoma (it was a histologically unequivocally malignant neoplasm of the upper humerus); without treatment, the widely destructive lesion was fully recalcified 4 years later. The same context recalls the case reported by Francis and his colleagues (1962) where radiologically demonstrable pulmonary metastases from an osteosarcoma twice disappeared (at an interval of 14 months) after only palliative radiotherapy; the patient was well 5 years after last treatment, aged 8 years at the time of reporting.

Evidence has been given by Broström and his associates (1979) on a matter sometimes referred to the pathologist for advice, the question whether biopsy per se carries any threat of provoking metastasis. A comparison by these observers of two closely comparable groups of patients with osteosarcoma showed that ". . . the performance of a biopsy, with or without a delay of not more than thirty days between the biopsy and the definitive operation, had no adverse effect on survival".

## Osteoblastoma

The osteoblastoma, just mentioned, may simulate a well-differentiated osteosarcoma to the extent that it contains anastomosing trabeculae of osteoid tissue. It may also contain vascular spaces so prominent as to suggest an aneurysmal bone cyst. It shares these features with the osteoid osteoma, and is indeed sometimes designated 'giant osteoid osteoma'. Distinction between the two, for example, is based by McLeod and his colleagues (1976) on a diameter of 1 cm: those at or below 1 cm are osteoid osteomas, those above are osteoblastomas. The lesion is intrinsically innocuous. Thus, in two of the cases of McLeod and his colleagues, the lesion subsided after biopsy only.

There are other lesions, less closely mimetic of osteosarcoma, or less certainly osteosarcomas of curious behaviour, than these but deserving a comment nevertheless as offering troublesome borderline patterns and problems: they comprise those where the lesion, though in bone, has a predominantly fibroblastic background.

### PREDOMINANTLY FIBROBLASTIC LESIONS CONTAINING GIANT-CELLS

The lesions most commonly causing diagnostic difficulty within this general grouping include osteoclastoma, aneurysmal bone cyst, fibrous dysplasia and its allies, and some others later mentioned. Each in its typical form may be diagnosed without difficulty but each has its atypical forms, hence the many problems.

An impression of the extent of the diagnostic difficulty can be gained from two lists of diagnoses-on-review given to lesions originally diagnosed as giant-cell tumour (osteoclastoma) but reassessed by experts in bone pathology. A series of 218 cases of giant-cell tumour was analysed by Goldenberg and colleagues (1970). The number of cases before review was 299; after review the pattern was as shown in Fig. 6.23.

Thus, in the series as a whole, 44 lesions that were benign had been diagnosed originally as giant-cell tumour: that is, a minimum false-positive rate of 44/299 or approximately 15%.

Comparable analysis of the other series, that of Larsson and his associates (1975), gives the pattern displayed in Fig. 6.24, the rate of false-positive diagnosis of which was thus 18/73 or some 25%.

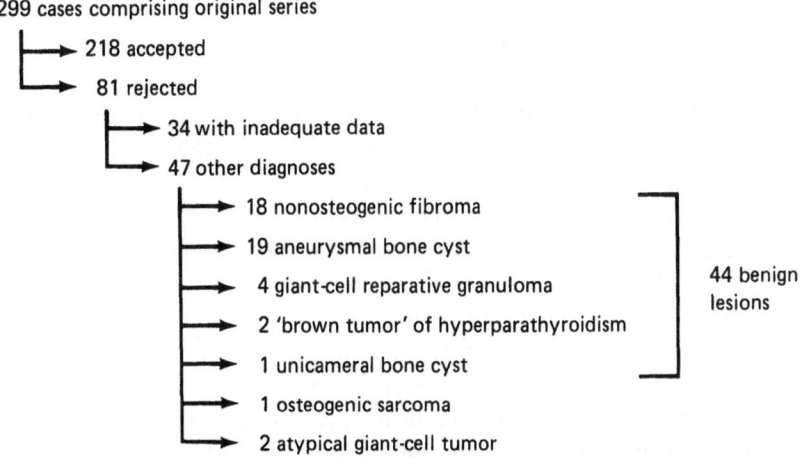

**Fig. 6.23.** An analysis of the diagnoses on review of 299 lesions originally diagnosed as 'giant-cell tumor' (Goldenberg et al., 1970).

If, to the lesions named in these two analyses, we add fibrous dysplasia, we have before us a list that impressively illustrates the problem for the general pathologist who is confronted by the histological syndrome 'fibroblastic stroma + giant-cells': and, indeed, not much more need be said, for, often enough, all that is required to 'make' a diagnosis is that the existence of a particular entity be remembered. Were a pathologist, examining sections of a lesion of the kind in question, to ask himself whether they could represent an example of each of these entities in turn, he would at least greatly lessen, perhaps altogether remove, the likelihood of over-diagnosing one of the many benign lesions as a giant-cell tumour. However, in these and some other texts there are useful guides to diagnosis and prognosis.

## Osteoclastoma

Increasingly, the unequivocal osteoclastoma is being recognised as, to use Lichtenstein's (1972) apt term, a 'formidable neoplasm'. The same author has succinctly summarised the prognosis: at least one-half are likely to have a favourable outcome: one-third or more are likely to recur: and the remaining 10%–15% are frankly malignant and liable to metastasise, especially to lung. The experience of others has been broadly similar. In the two series just cited, the rates of recurrence and directly tumour-associated mortality were, respectively, 35% and 7% (Goldenberg et al., 1970) and 42% and 13% (Larsson et al., 1975): also, in other series, 45% and 6% (Dahlin et al., 1970) and 33% and 10% (McGrath, 1972). As always, when some pa-

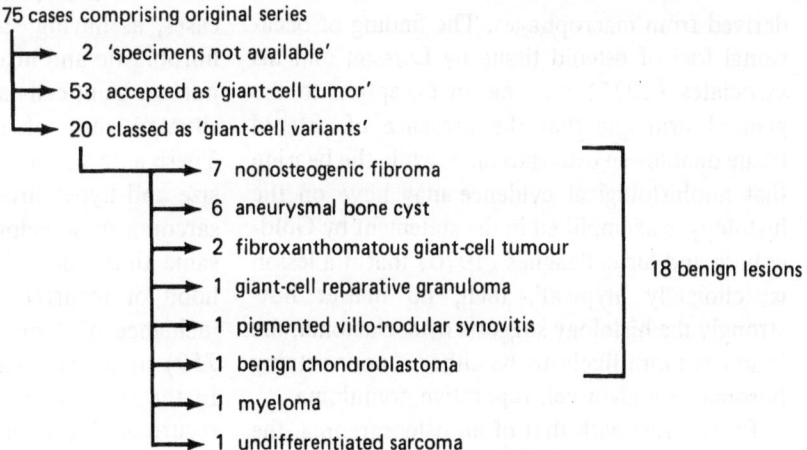

**Fig. 6.24.** An analysis of the diagnoses on review of 75 lesions originally diagnosed as 'giant-cell tumor' (Larsson et al., 1975).

tients are still alive but with metastases, these figures express a minimum mortality.

Attempts at the histological grading of osteoclastomas have generally tended to be abandoned: the histoclinical correlation is worthlessly low. A striking example of this occurred in the case of one patient included in the series of Dahlin and his colleagues (1970): a distal radial lesion (M, 61 years) of seemingly quite benign appearance recurred after 18 months, and then emerged as a solitary pulmonary metastasis 4½ years after that; tantalisingly, because perhaps not unconnected with the benign histology, after removal of the metastasis by lobectomy, the patient was still well 11 years later. These authors advise that, if, in a highly cellular lesion, the nuclei of the mononuclear stromal cells are similar to those of seemingly benign giant-cells, the lesion is almost certainly not a sarcoma: if, on the other hand, the stromal cells appear malignant throughout, then, no matter how many or seemingly benign the giant-cells, the lesion is almost certainly an osteosarcoma or a fibrosarcoma. This advice, to concentrate attention on the mononuclear stromal cells, accords well with recent observations, largely confirmatory of earlier but less firmly based impressions, that the stromal cell is the essentially neoplastic element. Ultrastructurally, the multinucleated giant cells (indistinguishable from osteoclasts) appear to be formed by the mergence of stromal cells which, in one investigation, were the only cells to show proliferative activity (Hanaoka et al., 1970). Further, though less direct, confirmation lies in the demonstration by Wood and his colleagues (1978) on immunological evidence that the multinucleated giant cells are at any rate not derived from macrophages. The finding of occasional foci of osteoid tissue by Larsson and his associates (1975) may be an exception to the general principle that the presence of osteoid tissue denotes an osteosarcoma, while the bearing that nonhistological evidence may have on the histology is exemplified in the statement by Goldenberg and his colleagues (1970) that if a lesion is 'clinically atypical', then, no matter how strongly the histology suggests osteoclastoma, the lesion is more likely to be either a nonossifying fibroma or a giant-cell reparative granuloma.

By contrast with that of an osteosarcoma, the occurrence of an osteoclastoma in association with Paget's disease is rare. The example in mandible reported by Brooke (1970) brought the number of recorded cases to 30. Most examples occur in the skull and jaws, and here the possibility of confusion with the giant-cell reparative granuloma is particularly high. In Brooke's case the diagnosis was amply established: the patient had Paget's disease in femora, tibia and pelvis as well as in the skull, and the lesion recurred after 15 months. The example reported by Schajowicz and Slullitel (1966) was in the tibia and was at that time only the third such lesion recorded in a long bone. The extreme difference in prognosis between the osteoclastoma and the much commoner osteosarcoma associated with Paget's disease makes accurate distinction between them imperative.

### Aneurysmal Bone Cyst

Neither radiological nor clinical impressions can be relied upon to distinguish this benign lesion from others that are malignant. No matter how persuasive the clinical evidence, dismissal of, or failure to seek, histological evidence may lead to needless amputation as in the two cases described by Hadders and Oterdoom (1956). This is not to say that the histology is always diagnostic, for it is not, but at least it offers the best chance of avoiding unfortunate error. Confusion with an unusually vascular or 'telangiectatic' osteosarcoma, even histologically, is the greatest danger: though mentioned already, the point is reemphasised that each of these lesions may be mistaken for the other.

Close attention needs to be given to the lining of the cysts and septa, described by Ruiter and his co-workers (1977), with their series of 105 cases, as having "a superficial layer of cellular fibroblastic and histiocytic tissue in which multinuclear giant cells are present, covering a deeper situated zone of less cellular fibrous tissue". These authors have described the greater nuclear size and hyperchromatism of the cells in osteosarcoma as a helpful discriminator but, at the same time, the guide they found best to likelihood of recurrence was mitotic incidence; an incidence of 7 or more figures per 50 hpf ($\times$ 750) indicated a significantly greater likelihood. In the series as a whole, 30.5% of the lesions recurred, due mainly, in their view, to incomplete excision.

The aetiology of the lesion, whether primarily

maldevelopmental, either essentially dysplastic or associated with skeletal haemangiomatosis, or secondary and a 'reaction' that develops for no known reason to the presence of some other lesion such as chondromyxoid fibroma or benign osteoblastoma, remains uncertain and is not a matter of main concern here. Some points, however, are relevant to diagnostic practice.

First, both a haemangioma in a phase of active growth, and a fibrovascular or more purely fibrous secondary reaction could equally produce highly cellular, mitotically active tissue entirely analogous to examples of granulation tissue that may at times be so exuberant as to mimic a fibro- or angiosarcoma; and the ABC may indeed mimic these. The addition of multinucleated giant-cells is the further complicating factor that brings the giant-cell tumour into the list of diagnostic contenders. Second, the tendency of the lesion to local recurrence (the younger the patient, the likelier this is) and its apparent capacity to spread from one bone to another, perhaps exclusively in vertebrae and adjacent ribs, together give at least a hint of neoplastic behaviour. Available evidence, however, leaves little doubt that the lesion is not a neoplasm. The tendency to involve adjacent bones was described thus by Tillman and his colleagues (1968), "Extension from one bone to another proved to be a useful roentgenographic sign because it is almost non-existent in other benign processes and is rare even with malignant ones". A reasonably plausible explanation for the phenomenon would be a simultaneous accession of growth in haemangiomas in adjacent vertebrae, rather than 'spread' of some unspecified form; for angiomas in the vertebral column are not uncommon (refs. in Hadders and Oterdoom, 1956) though admittedly often small and likely to be overlooked unless specially sought. Finally, the occasional coexistence of the ABC with other bony lesions is acknowledged (*see*, for example, Spjut et al., 1971, pp. 361-2) even though rare; no such coexistence was seen, for example, by Tillman and his colleagues in their 95 cases. However, when it is present, it could cause some diagnostic confusion.

*Fibrous Dysplasia and Allied Lesions*

A note on the terminology of disorders of this type may be in order, for there are difficulties, mostly concerned with the term 'ossifying'. Ossifying means 'bone-making', and bone-making implies activity by osteoblasts. However, bone may be seen in lesions that lack osteoblasts but are nevertheless described as 'ossifying'. The problem can perhaps best be analysed by examining various published statements. All the following have been taken from the AFIP Fascicle on Tumors of Bone and Cartilage (Spjut et al., 1971), not because the statements appear only in that publication but because it is a widely consulted text on the subject, and one where various opinions are conveniently gathered together.

1) A diagnostic feature of *fibrous dysplasia*, with only an occasional exception, is ". . . the lack of osteoblastic rimming of the bony trabeculae." (p. 276).

2) Synonyms for fibrous dysplasia that have been used but are 'not recommended' by these authors are ossifying fibroma and fibrous osteoma (p. 270).

3) 'Ossifying fibroma' differs from fibrous dysplasia histologically: in it are found ". . . randomly distributed bone spicules . . . in a fibrous stroma . . . rimmed with osteoblasts" (p. 261).

4) Nonossifying fibroma is substantially synonymous with *fibrous cortical defect*: the cortical lesion has enlarged to reach the medullary cavity. In both, "Evidence of new bone formation is not observed in the uncomplicated lesion" (p. 257).

5) Observations by Reed (1963) have been rendered (p. 277) as, "if one concedes that fibrous dysplasia in part represents a defect (in the maturation of bone) . . . confusion of this lesion with ossifying fibroma, fibrous osteoma . . . (etc.) . . . will not occur". The implication here is that these two terms indicate separate entities, and that fibrous dysplasia makes a third; yet, as noted in (2) above, both terms have been used at times as synonyms for fibrous dysplasia and were 'not recommended'.

From the above, three broad conclusions may be drawn concerning the osseous component, and to these may be added two concerning the fibroblastic and giant-celled components:

1) Bony elements of which few, if any, bear osteoblasts indicate *fibrous dysplasia*.

2) Bony elements of which most, if not all, bear osteoblasts indicate *ossifying fibroma*.

3) Absence or near-absence of bony elements

indicates *fibrous cortical defect* (non-ossifying fibroma).

4) Cytological features will determine the significance of the fibroblastic tissue; that is, whether fibrosarcoma seems possible.

5) The number of giant-cells will vary from almost none to so many as to raise the question of osteoclastoma.

*Fibrous dysplasia* is characterised by a content of bone almost wholly of woven type; lamellar bone is rarely seen in the trabeculae. This is largely the basis of the view that the lesion is essentially a defect in maturation of bone (Harris et al., 1962; Reed, 1963). The defect may be a permanent maturation arrest since, as reported by Reed, repeated biopsies in three patients over 3, 8 and 10 years respectively showed no change in bone structure. Therefore, predominance of woven bone in a biopsy does not indicate that the lesion is either young or recent. Two further points made by Reed are that the histology may be exactly simulated by a unicameral bone cyst, distinction depending upon whether the lesion was found at operation to be actually cystic or not; and that occasional trabeculae may show a mosaic of cement lines quite similar to that seen in Paget's disease.

In describing their series of 50 cases (37 polyostotic, 13 monostotic), Harris and his colleagues (1962) remarked on the presence of foci of cartilage in seven cases; this in their opinion was not an integral part of the lesion but represented the remains of callus from some earlier fracture. Their comment that chondrosarcoma had never been recorded as a complication has since been overtaken by several reports of this, including that of Huvos and co-workers (1972) who reported 12 cases in which sarcomas had developed (eight osteo-, two chondro-, two spindle-celled sarcoma); in five of these cases the pre-existence of fibrous dysplasia was known, in the other seven it was discovered simultaneously with the sarcoma.

The difficulty in diagnosing fibrous dysplasia is emphasised by the observation of Harris and his colleagues (1962) that in 28% of their cases the lesion was diagnosed initially not as fibrous dysplasia but as, for example, unicameral bone cyst or aneurysmal bone cyst: other lesions may be simulated, fibrosarcoma by those of high fibroblastic cellularity, and giant-cell tumour by those containing many multinucleated giant-cells. The clinical course varies greatly but, as might be expected, the younger the patient and the more widespread the lesion, the likelier the condition is to advance, with increasing bone damage, liability to fracture and likelihood of sarcoma. In patients treated by radiotherapy, the usual long-term risk of sarcoma exists. In their account of fibrosarcoma of bone, Dahlin and Ivins (1969) reported that 20% of their cases had followed the treatment of some lesion by irradiation (this form of therapy is doubtless the best available sometimes but so relatively frequently is sarcoma reported as a sequel to the irradiation of benign lesions of bone that it must surely be the treatment of last resort?). In all, these authors found that in nearly a third of their cases the fibrosarcoma had been a complication of a primary lesion or other disturbance of some kind. This was the experience also of Eyre-Brooke and Price (1969): in their 50 cases, 11 had arisen in association with Paget's disease.

A hereditary form of fibrous dysplasia restricted to the jaws, so-called *cherubism*, has been comprehensively described from both the genetic and pathological standpoints by Anderson and his collaborators (Anderson et al., 1962; McClendon et al., 1962) and from the therapeutic by Hamner and Ketcham (1969). The strong hereditary element is suggestive of an association with the Albright syndrome.

*Ossifying fibroma*, characterised by bands and islands of bone wherein both osteoblasts and an admixture of lamellar bone may be seen, occurs mainly in the jaws. When it arises in a long bone, as may rarely happen, it is likely to be much more aggressive than fibrous dysplasia (Kempson, 1966). Histological distinction from fibrous dysplasia is therefore of some therapeutic importance: curettage may prove curative in fibrous dysplasia but en bloc resection is more likely to be required for the ossifying fibroma.

*Fibrous cortical defect* has a nearly certain diagnostic appearance on X-ray and is characterised histologically by highly cellular fibrous tissue, often with a whorled pattern, multinucleated giant-cells and foam cells (recalling in some degree the fibrous histiocytoma), and an absence of bone. Spontaneous regression occurs often enough for this to be optimistically awaited.

Should this fail to happen, especially when fracture seems a significant risk, active treatment is indicated (Bollman, 1969).

The whorled or storiform pattern is seen also in the entity now identified as *malignant fibrous histiocytoma* (MFH) of bone. The diagnostic features are the storiform pattern, aberrancy of the constituent cells including polymorphism and (often atypical) mitotic activity, a variable content of intracellular lipid and, in most cases, areas of tissue indistinguishable from osteoclastoma. The lesion is highly aggressive. In a series of seven cases described by Kahn and his colleagues (1978), three of the patients had developed metastases within two years of amputation, while, of a total of 71 examples comprising four earlier series of other workers and cited by Kahn, 42 had died: that is, since many of the patients had been followed for only a short time, a minimum mortality rate of some 60%. In a comparable series of 35 cases (average age 34 years) reported by McCarthy and co-workers (1979), of 21 patients followed for up to 3 years, ten had died and two were alive with apparently solitary metastases. Among lesions considered in the differential diagnosis of the neoplasm, which these authors regard as ". . . an important complication of bone infarction", were, besides the malignant osteoclastoma, osteosarcoma, malignant lymphoma and metastatic carcinoma. The treatment recommended by these authors is amputation.

The lesson to be learned here is that any apparent osteoclastoma should be thoroughly searched for areas of cytologically aberrant stromal tissue of storiform pattern: for the presence of this, qua MFH, promotes the degree of malignancy to one of a predictably higher order than that of the osteoclastoma. As earlier mentioned, the 'grading' of pure or straightforward osteoclastoma is widely regarded as worthless.

Additional points of prognostic importance are that, as noted by two groups of workers (Spanier et al., 1975; Dahlin et al., 1977), the least fibrogenic, most histiocytic, forms merge with the histiocytic lymphomas (RCS). Further, unlike the fibrosarcoma and osteosarcoma, the MFH may metastasise to lymph nodes, and, in the words of Dahlin and his colleagues, ". . . the lesions are likely to occur at ages and locations that would be unusual for the accepted entity they mimic most often, nonosteogenic fibroma (metaphyseal fibrous defect)". It is instructive to recall that, on an earlier occasion apropos the occasional osteosarcoma that metastasises in the form of a pure fibrosarcoma, Dahlin (1975) had remarked that ". . . some such metastases have the aura of malignant fibrous histiocytoma".

## Conclusions

1) The histology of a lesion of bone or cartilage should first be assessed independently of all other evidence: preconditioning by knowledge of radiological appearances may mislead. Lack of concordance between radiological/histological/clinical opinion demands joint review.

2) Plasma cells may appear in chronic osteomyelitis. Only mitotic activity in such a population suggests myeloma (but evidence of other kinds may be more nearly diagnostic).

3) Distinction between chondroma and chondrosarcoma is a largely subjective decision but degree of mitotic activity may be prognostically helpful. The anatomical site also is important: cartilaginous tumours of hands and feet are relatively nonaggressive.

4) Osteoid tissue in an otherwise typical chondrosarcoma is widely regarded as an index of osteosarcoma.

5) Callus, in its first three weeks, may be histologically indistinguishable from osteosarcoma (myositis ossificans may be equally mimetic).

6) Stromal tissue in part frankly sarcomatous is a requisite for the diagnosis of osteosarcoma. An apparent osteoclastoma with sarcomatous stroma is likely to be an osteosarcoma.

7) Histological grading of osteosarcoma for prognostic purposes is unreliable. The lesion is prone to over-diagnosis.

8) Osteoclastoma has a 30% to 40% likelihood of recurrence, and a 10% to 15% likelihood of metastasis; it also is prone to over-diagnosis, and cannot be usefully graded.

9) The aneurysmal bone cyst may closely mimic both osteosarcoma and osteoclastoma.

10) Fibrous dysplasia may be mistaken for aneurysmal bone cyst, fibrosarcoma or osteoclastoma.

# References

Anderson DE, McClendon JL, Cornelius EA (1962) Cherubism—hereditary fibrous dysplasia of the jaws. I. Genetic considerations. Oral Surg 15: Suppl 2, 5–16

Azar HA, Zaino EC, Pham TD, Yannopoulos K (1972) "Non-secretory" plasma cell myeloma: Observations on seven cases with electron microscopic studies. Am J Clin Pathol 58: 618–629

Bollmann L (1969) Zur Klinik und Pathologie des nichtossifizierenden Knochenfibroms Jaffé Lichtenstein. Dtsch Med Wochenschr 94: 221–224

Brooke RI (1970) Giant-cell tumor in patients with Paget's disease. Oral Surg 30: 230–241

Broström L-A, Harris MA, Simon MA, Cooperman DR, Nilsonne U (1979) The effect of biopsy on survival of patients with osteosarcoma. J Bone Joint Surg (Br) 61: 209–212

Corwin J, Lindberg RD (1979) Solitary plasmacytoma of bone vs. extramedullary plasmacytoma and their relationship to multiple myeloma. Cancer 43: 1007–1013

Dahlin DC (1975) Pathology of osteosarcoma. Clin Orthop 111: 23–32

Dahlin DC, Beabout JW (1971) Dedifferentiation of low-grade chondrosarcomas. Cancer 28: 461–466

Dahlin DC, Ivins JC (1969) Fibrosarcoma of bone. A study of 114 cases. Cancer 23: 35–41

Dahlin DC, Cupps RE, Johnson EW (1970) Giant cell tumor: A study of 195 cases. Cancer 25: 1061–1070

Dahlin DC, Unni KK, Matsuno T (1977) Malignant (fibrous) histiocytoma of bone—fact or fancy ? Cancer 39: 1508–1516

Erf LA, Herbut PA (1946) Comparative cytology of Wright's stained smears and histologic sections in multiple myeloma. Am J Clin Pathol 16: 1–12

Erlandson RA, Huvos AG (1974) Chondrosarcoma: A light and electron microscopic study. Cancer 34: 1642–1652

Evans HL, Ayala AG, Romsdahl MM (1977) Prognostic factors in chondrosarcoma of bone. A clinicopathologic analysis with emphasis on histologic grading. Cancer 40: 818–831

Eyre-Brooke AL, Price CHG (1969) Fibrosarcoma of bone. Review of fifty consecutive cases from the Bristol Bone Tumour Registry. J Bone Joint Surg [Br] 51: 20–37

Francis KC, Hutter RVP, Phillips RK, Eyerly RC, Schechter L (1962) Osteogenic sarcoma. Sustained disappearance of pulmonary metastases after only palliative irradiation. N Engl J Med 266: 694–699

Fu Y-S, Kay S (1974) A comparative ultrastructural study of mesenchymal chondrosarcoma and myxoid chondrosarcoma. Cancer 33: 1531–1542

Garfinkel LS, Bennett DE (1969) Extramedullary myeloblastic transformation in chronic myelocytic leukemia simulating a coexistent malignant lymphoma. Am J Clin Pathol 51: 638–645

Goldenberg RR, Campbell CJ, Bonfiglio M (1970) Giant-cell tumor of bone: An analysis of two hundred and eighteen cases. J Bone Joint Surg [Am] 52: 619–663

Gravanis MB, Whitesides TE (1970) The unreliability of prognostic criteria in osteosarcoma. Am J Clin Pathol 53: 15–20

Hadders HN, Oterdoom HJ (1956) The identification of aneurysmal bone cyst with haemangioma of the skeleton. J Pathol Bacteriol 71: 193–200

Hamner JE, Ketcham AS (1969) Cherubism: An analysis of treatment. Cancer 23: 1133–1143

Hanaoka H, Friedman B, Mack RP (1970) Ultrastructure and histogenesis of giant-cell tumor of bone. Cancer 25: 1408–1423

Harris WH, Dudley HR, Barry RJ (1962) The natural history of fibrous dysplasia. An orthopaedic, pathological and roentgenographic study. J Bone Joint Surg [Am] 44: 207–233

Heul RO van der, Ronnen JR von (1967) Juxtacortical osteosarcoma: Diagnosis, differential diagnosis, treatment, and an analysis of eighty cases. J Bone Joint Surg [Am] 49: 415–439

Hutchison J, Park WW (1960) Chondromyxoid fibroma of bone: Report of a case. J Bone Joint Surg [Br] 42: 542–548

Huvos AG, Higinbotham NL, Miller TR (1972) Bone sarcomas arising in fibrous dysplasia. J Bone Joint Surg [Am] 54: 1047–1056

Huvos AG, Marcove RC, Erlandson RA, Miké V (1972a) Chondroblastoma of bone. A clinicopathologic and electron microscopic study. Cancer 29: 760–771

Jaffé HL, Lichtenstein L (1948) Chondromyxoid fibroma of bone: A distinctive benign tumor likely to be mistaken especially for chondrosarcoma. Arch Pathol 45: 541–551

Jones GB, Midgley RL, Smith GS (1958) Massive osteolysis—disappearing bones. J Bone Joint Surg (Br) 40: 494–501

Kahn LB, Wood FW, Ackerman LV (1969) Fracture callus associated with benign and malignant bone lesions and mimicking osteosarcoma. Am J Clin Pathol 52: 14–24

Kahn LB, Webber B, Mills E, Anstey L, Heselson NG (1978) Malignant fibrous histiocytoma (malignant fibrous xanthoma: Xanthosarcoma) of bone. Cancer 42: 640–651

Kempson RL (1966) Ossifying fibroma of the long bones. A light and electron microscopic study. Arch Pathol 82: 218–233

Larsson S-E, Lorentzon R, Boquist L (1975) Giant-cell tumor of bone. A demographic, clinical and histopathological study of all cases recorded in the Swedish Cancer Registry for the years 1958 through 1968. J Bone Joint Surg [Am] 57: 167–173

Levin EJ (1957) Spontaneous regression (cure ?) of a malignant tumor of bone. Cancer 10: 377–381

Lichtenstein L (1972) Bone tumors, 4th edn. Mosby, St. Louis

McCarthy EF, Matsuno T, Dorfman HD (1979) Malignant fibrous histiocytoma of bone: A study of 35 cases. Hum Pathol 10: 57–70

McClendon JL, Anderson DE, Cornelius EA (1962) Cherubism—hereditary fibrous dysplasia of the jows. II. Pathologic considerations. Oral Surg 15: Suppl 2, 17–42

McGrath PJ (1972) Giant-cell tumour of bone: An analysis of fifty-two cases. J Bone Joint Surg [Br] 54: 216–229

Mackay B, Luna MA, Butler JJ (1976) Adult neuroblastoma. Electron microscopic observations in nine cases. Cancer 37: 1334–1351

McLeod RA, Dahlin DC, Beabout JW (1976) The spectrum of osteoblastoma. Am J Roentgenol 126: 321–335

Marcove RC, Huvos AG (1971) Cartilaginous tumors of the ribs. Cancer 27: 794–801

Matsuno T, Unni KK, McLeod RA, Dahlin DC (1976) Telangiectatic osteogenic sarcoma. Cancer 38: 2538–2547

Méary R, Roger A (1972) Chondrosarcoma of the long bones of the extremities. In: Price CHG, Ross FGM (eds) 'Bone—certain aspects of neoplasia'. Colston papers, 24th Symposium, Univ. Bristol. Butterworth, London, pp 471–474

Mikulowski P, Östberg G (1971) Recurrent chondromyxoid fibroma. Acta Orthop Scand 42: 385–390

Mirra JM, Kendrick RA, Kendrick RE (1976) Pseudomalignant osteoblastoma versus arrested osteosarcoma. A case report. Cancer 37: 2005–2014

O'Hara JM, Hutter RVP, Foote FW, Miller T, Woodard HQ (1968) An analysis of thirty patients surviving longer than ten years after treatment for osteogenic sarcoma. J Bone Joint Surg [Am] 50: 335–354

Price CHG (1961) Osteogenic sarcoma. An analysis of survival and its relationship to histological grading and structure. J Bone Joint Surg [Br] 43: 300–313

Pritchard DJ, Dahlin DC, Dauphine RT, Taylor WF, Beabout JW (1975) Ewing's sarcoma. A clinicopathological and statistical analysis of patients surviving five years or longer. J Bone Joint Surg [Am] 57: 10–16

Rahimi A, Beabout JW, Ivins JC, Dahlin DC (1972) Chondromyxoid fibroma: A clinicopathologic study of 76 cases. Cancer 30: 726–736

Reed RJ (1963) Fibrous dysplasia of bone. A review of 25 cases. Arch Pathol 75: 480–495

Ruiter DJ, Rijssel TG van, Velde EA van der (1977) Aneurysmal bone cysts. A clinicopathological study of 105 cases. Cancer 39: 2231–2239

Schajowicz F (1959) Ewing's sarcoma and reticulum-cell sarcoma of bone, with special reference to the histochemical demonstration of glycogen as an aid to differential diagnosis. J Bone Joint Surg [Am] 41: 349–356

Schajowicz F, Gallardo H (1971) Chondromyxoid fibroma (fibromyxoid chondroma) of bone. A clinicopathological study of thirty-two cases. J Bone Joint Surg [Br] 53: 198–216

Schajowicz F, Slullitel I (1966) Giant-cell tumor associated with Paget's disease of bone. A case report. J Bone Joint Surg [Am] 48: 1340–1349

Scranton PE, Cicco FA de, Totten RS, Yunis EJ (1975) Prognostic factors in osteosarcoma. A review of 20 years' experience at the University of Pittsburgh Health Center Hospitals. Cancer 36: 2179–2191.

Sissons HA (1975) Agreement and disagreement between pathologists in histological diagnosis. Postgrad Med J 51: 685–689

Spanier SS, Enneking WF, Enriquez P (1975) Primary malignant fibrous histiocytoma of bone. Cancer 36: 2084–2098

Spjut HJ, Dorfman HD, Fechner RE, Ackerman LV (1971) Atlas of tumor pathology, 2nd ser, fasc 5. Tumors of bone and cartilage. Armed Forces Institute of Pathology, Washington, D.C.

Takigawa K (1971) Chondroma of the bones of the hand. A review of 110 cases. J Bone Joint Surg [Am] 53: 1591–1600

Thomine JM (1972) Cartilaginous tumours of the pelvic girdle. In: Price CHG, Ross FGM (eds) 'Bone—certain aspects of neoplasia'. Colston papers, 24th Symposium, Univ. Bristol. Butterworth, London, pp 451–459, 461

Tillman BP, Dahlin DC, Lipscomb PR Stewart JR (1968) Aneurysmal bone cyst: An analysis of ninety-five cases. Mayo Clin Proc 43: 478–495

Unni KK, Dahlin DC, Beabout JW (1976a) Periosteal osteogenic sarcoma. Cancer 37: 2476–2485

Unni KK, Dahlin DC, Beabout JW, Ivins JC (1976b) Parosteal osteogenic sarcoma. Cancer 37: 2466–2475

Unni KK, Dahlin DC, McLeod RA, Pritchard DJ (1977) Intraosseous well-differentiated osteosarcoma. Cancer 40: 1337–1347

Willis RA (1941) Solitary plasmocytoma of bone. J Pathol Bacteriol 53: 77–85

Willis RA (1960) Pathology of tumours, 3rd edn. Butterworth, London

Wiltshaw E (1976) The natural history of extramedullary plasmacytoma and its relation to solitary myeloma of bone and myelomatosis. Medicine (Baltimore) 55: 217–238

Wood GW, Neff JR, Gollahon KA, Gourley WK (1978) Macrophages in giant cell tumours of bone. J Pathol 125: 53–58

# 7  Lesions of the Skin

The skin, with its epidermis, adnexa, pigment cells, corium and immediately related subcutaneous tissue, provides histologically borderline problems in plenty. Those posed by the stratified squamous epithelium of the epidermis are supplemented by the many others, essentially identical in such areas as larynx and cervix uteri, to the point where stratified squamous epithelium in general has fair claim to be regarded as the provider of more 'benign or malignant?' problems than any other tissue. The subjective element in histopathological diagnosis is nowhere seen more sharply than in the hyperplasia/ dysplasia/carcinoma sequence of stratified squamous epithelium, and the decision reached can have consequences far more significant than in the case of, say, the lesion that may or may not be a melanocarcinoma: nowadays, it is almost unknown for a diagnosis of, 'for practical purposes, melanocarcinoma' to be followed by amputation of a limb but 'for practical purposes, squamous cell carcinoma' may mean the loss of a larynx or oesophagus.

Adnexal problems are rarely so prognostically grave; mostly they involve the decision 'adenoma or carcinoma', and few such lesions are more aggressive than the usual basal cell carcinoma (BCC). Problems posed by the aberrant melanocyte are not infrequent, and they are worrying, but at least, as already mentioned, the pathologist is safe in the knowledge that, whatever his diagnosis, the patient will not suffer a major amputation (some would say undeservedly safe, for the changed situation has not been of the pathologist's making; it has come about in essence from the observation of many surgeons over many years that amputation of a limb, even as soon as the diagnosis of melanocarcinoma was received, was all too rarely life-saving; all it meant for so many was a brief interval to death mutilated rather than intact). Whether, however, a diagnosis of 'for practical purposes, melanocarcinoma' will again in the future expose the patient to the risks of newer techniques of regional perfusion or the dangers, known and unknown, of immunotherapy, remains to be seen.

The borderline melanocytic lesions will be considered separately as will mycosis fungoides (MF). Both conditions will be given what may be considered undue attention but there seems ample reason for doing so. In comparison with, say, BCC, the number of patients reported on biopsy over the years as certainly having melanocarcinoma or MF is quite small. However, the amount of diagnostic difficulty and uncertainty they have caused is quite disproportionately great. Worry naturally attaches to a lesion that may be a melanocarcinoma or MF in a way that does not apply to the BCC or even the SCC (squamous cell carcinoma), and recurrent imprecision on the diagnosis of either is disquieting to pathologist and clinician alike.

Overgrowths of the mesodermal cells of corium and subcutaneous tissue such as the dermatofibrosarcoma protuberans and xanthofibroma were examined in Chapter 5 along with other mesodermal lesions. The problems of aberrant stratified squamous epithelium elsewhere than in skin are considered also in other chapters: those of the skin itself are considered now.

# Part A   Epithelial Lesions Other than Melanocarcinoma

## Overgrowths of Stratified Squamous Epithelium

### LOCAL SERIES

The problems caused by overgrowths of the epidermis are of a mainly standard type. Most involve an assessment of 'invasion', sometimes by cells almost morphologically normal; others, when the lesion is judged to be not invasive, involve the assessment of individual cells. At some sites, to be sure, assessment of invasion is straightforward; eyelid, lip and tongue have immediately subjacent muscle, the extremities have subjacent bone, and only scarring is likely to cause confusion. Elsewhere the assessment is wholly subjective: one man's severe dysplasia or solar keratosis is another's 'for practical purposes, carcinoma', while, as mentioned in chap. 1, apparent transgression of the basement membrane as a criterion of invasion is for various reasons valueless. It is scarcely too much to say that a borderline lesion is invasive when a pathologist of experience says it is.

This uncertainty has made it difficult to decide from the local files just which of the lesions reported should be included in this section: how much of a hint of possible recurrence should 'count'? The cases eventually chosen were those where the lesion appeared certainly to have been incompletely excised; where treatment as for a SCC seemed the only safe course for the patient; where the later history had been instructive; or where the original diagnosis was, in retrospect, wrong. Those selected comprise Table 7.1. The clinical data are so relatively similar and the histological problem so standard that only the briefest details of some of the cases are included (the data of patients with certain or possible MF have been treated in the same way). For essentially the same reason there seemed little need to add photomicrographs to this section; the basic morphology of the problem at least is familiar to all.

Assessment of the quality or validity of diagnosis was similarly difficult. In six cases (see Table 7.1) lesions were certainly over-diagnosed

as SCC. In four others the lesion seemed with little doubt to have been a keratoacanthoma (KA) but the clinical data contributed more to this verdict than re-examination of the sections: if, as mentioned later, KA and SCC are in truth histologically indistinguishable though biologically different, clinical behaviour is inevitably the final arbiter. None of the 37 cases was under-diagnosed, to the extent that at least none recurred without some warning of the possibility in an earlier report.

Probably all papillomas when apparently incompletely excised are reported as such to the surgeon (or dermatologist) but the risk of recurrence seems small. Each of the two recurrent papillomas in the local series appeared to have been completely excised yet each had a successor; one, in the external auditory meatus, within 2 years; the other, in eyelid, after 11 years. Timing suggests true regrowth in the case of the ear, the development of a second independent lesion in the case of the eye. Lesions in the external auditory meatus should not be underestimated, essentially because of the anatomical danger that SCC represents in this area. The only fatal lesion in Table 7.1 was a carcinoma at this site.

Carcinoma in situ in the skin rarely progresses to frankly invasive carcinoma. Our experience confirms this. Over a period of 20 years, in only the three cases included in the table did a warning of possible invasion seem warranted, and in only one did it develop. However, the just-mentioned fatal case in the series began in part in this way. Of the two initial biopsies, one, from the external auditory meatus, showed carcinoma in situ: the other, 'granulations from middle ear', contained a flake of bone partly permeated by epithelium that was only mildly aberrant yet nevertheless, from its location, demanding diagnosis as carcinoma. The lesion recurred after 13 months, now a frankly polymorphic carcinoma that caused death with metastasis 15 months later.

Seborrhoeic keratosis is familiar as a lesion sometimes over-diagnosed as SCC, usually in inverse proportion to the experience of the

**Table 7.1.** Borderline squamous cell overgrowths in the local series.

---

*Recurrent squamous cell papilloma* (F. 17 yr, ext. auditory meatus)

Completeness of excision doubtful; recurrence 2 yr later; further excision curative.

*Recurrent conjunctival papilloma* (M. 40 yr)

First excision apparently complete; further papilloma at same site 11 yr later; trouble-free 5 yr later.

*Bowen's disease* (3 cases with ? invasion)

1 recurred after 16 yr, again as Bowen's disease but now with SCC; trouble-free till unrelated death 5 yr later.

*Borderline SCC or SCC incompletely excised* (32 cases)

10  retrospective diagnoses other than SCC (6, ?10, over-diagnoses)

    1  chondrodermatitis nodularis helicis
    1  hypertrophic lichen planus
    2  florid venereal warts
    2  seborrhoeic keratosis
    4  keratoacanthoma

 4  SCC incompletely excised

    3 'orthodox' SCC    }   3 had subsequent radiotherapy:
    1 spindle cell SCC }   none of the 4 recurred.

17  diagnosed 'for practical purposes' SCC

    12  received radiotherapy    }  all trouble-free or
    5  thought adequately excised, }  died from unrelated
    not further treated      }  cause 2 to 18 yr later.

 1  (M, 68 yr; 'granulations' ext. auditory meatus and middle ear) died from metastatic SCC, the only patient from the 37 to die from carcinomatosis.

---

SCC, squamous cell carcinoma

---

pathologist. Hypertrophic lichen planus is an uncommon lesion that just has to be remembered as a producer of exuberant and mildly aberrant epidermal overgrowth. The diagnosis is not always clinically obvious, and the possibility may not be offered by the dermatologist in his request to the laboratory; the suggestion may come first from the pathologist[1].

---

[1] All too often outside specialist hospitals the routine histological report of a biopsy of skin is cast in the pattern ". . . (one or two morphologically descriptive sentences) . . . appearances conformable with . . . (lichen planus, erythema multiforme or whatever the clinically suggested diagnosis may be)'. In fact, many more lesions of skin have distinctive or even virtually diagnostic histological features than is realised by many non-dermatological pathologists, The most reliable way to teach oneself is, again, to cultivate the 'blind' approach.

## GENERAL COMMENTARY

### *'Leukoplakia'*

The term 'leukoplakia' has long been the source of prognostic uncertainty, largely sustained, it has to be admitted, by persistent use of the term by many pathologists. Leukoplakia is a descriptive clinical term and should be used in that sense only. Its associations with subsequent carcinoma have been recognised from the earliest days but 'it' is no more than an area or areas of shiny whitish discolouration of varied aetiology of epidermal or other stratified squamous epithelium (the lesion could be discussed as well in connection with the mouth or genitalia as here). What matters to the pathologist is not the colour of the lesion, whether red, pink or white, or the degree of induration, whether mild, moderate or marked, all of which depend on varying degrees of keratosis, leucocytic infiltration and oedema, but the architecture and cytology of the stratified squamous epithelium; and this will be variably atrophic, hypertrophic or dysplastic in the one patient or in a group of patients.

Sometimes the dysplasia will be extreme, and understandably, as with KA, attempts have been made to find forms of tissue pattern or association of tissue patterns that could be significantly correlated with the subsequent development of carcinoma. One such was made by Kint (1963) in a histophotometric investigation of nuclear DNA in normal and abnormal epidermis including such lesions as seborrhoeic keratosis, keratosis senilis, SCC and BCC. There was some parallelism between increasing DNA content and biological aggressiveness but not enough to provide prognostically useful information. Another attempt was that of Kramer and co-workers (1970, 1970a) who carried out a relatively complex discriminant analysis of 39 histological features in 235 cases of oral lesions comprising keratosis (127), leukoplakia (60) and lichen planus (48). There emerged from the cases of leukoplakia and keratosis a cluster of 11 placed by the computer in the category 'carcinoma', and 4 (36%) of these did subsequently develop a frankly malignant lesion. This is still a long way from totally accurate prediction but the technique indicates the lines along which greater accuracy might be achieved. A 36% probability of subsequent cancer would be held in most circumstances as quite high enough to warrant the most radical procedure possible.

Clinicians and pathologists equally know, without microscopy, that a 'leukoplakic' epidermis is an unstable epidermis in which carcinoma is prone to develop though the degree of risk involved is difficult to define. Some indication of the risk was provided by Einhorn and Wersäll (1967) in relation to oral lesions (defined in essence as a white patch that could not be attributed to any other defined disease such as stomatitis, lichen planus or carcinoma) in 782 patients. Carcinoma developed in 2.4% in 10 years, and in 4.0% in 20 years. Surprisingly, there were fewer cases of carcinoma amongst smokers with leukoplakia than amongst non-smokers with leukoplakia, a finding that prompted the comment, "The leukoplakia in tobacco users seems not to be of great precancerous significance". Until discriminant analysis of the kind just mentioned yields clearer guidance, the best course open to the pathologist is to assess the epidermal pattern in the presence of reported whiteness or leukosis just as he would in the absence of leukosis. He is likely at times to use, or wish to use, the valuable designation 'squamous carcinoma, Grade ½' though, if he does, he is under obligation to the surgeon to make his meaning clear.

In some circumstances, governed by anatomy, the position is straightforward. The report on a localised epidermal lesion of this pattern in, say, lip or pinna could be qualified by some such phrase as 'adequate excision, which this lesion appears to have had, should make the risk of recurrence minimal'. When a precisely similar pattern is seen in one of several biopsies from vulva/perineum such advice is obviously inappropriate; only joint consultation and the experience of the surgeon can properly assess the circumstances there.

### Keratoacanthoma

Attempts to distinguish the KA from SCC continue but still with little success. Thus, a recent close investigation of 108 KAs and 14 SCCs by both light and electron microscopy (Fisher et al., 1972) ". . . failed to reveal any consistent, single feature allowing for their distinction". As these authors say, the growth rates of KA and SCC may both vary considerably. Crateriform lesions with marked epithelial overgrowth and frequently 'elephant bell' downgrowths of qualitatively normal epidermis at the edge, that is, seeming KAs, do in general have a history of 10–20 weeks duration. On the other hand, lesions less distinctive macroscopically and without such downgrowths, the seeming carcinomas, rarely have histories of only 10–20 weeks. Thus, the probability is high that a histologically equivocal lesion with the above features and a short history is a KA and thus almost always innocuous.

This statistical fact, however, is of little comfort to the 1 in 100 or so patients whose rapidly growing crateriform lesion is an invasive and metastasising SCC. Four such cases, two of them fatal, were described by Jackson (1969) whose account suggests that in some of the cases at any rate the initial histological diagnosis of KA had been wrong, an error due entirely to the inevitably biasing foreknowledge of the clinical features, including short history, of the lesions. In saying the following, ". . . examination of histological sections . . . should not be influenced by clinical history and preliminary diagnosis" Jackson allied himself with the growing number of pathologists who appreciate just what the proper relation of clinical data is to histological interpretation. In contrast, in the immediate context of KA, are those such as Ghadially and his colleagues (1963) who write, "It would appear that correct diagnoses are more likely to be made by a careful analysis of clinical data in combination with microscopic study of the lesions than by histological examination alone", and Emerson and his associates (1971), similarly, "In all cases, the correlation of the history and gross and microscopic appearance is necessary to make the diagnosis". A similar opinion has been advanced by Davies (1969) who, nevertheless, offered the useful advice that a histological diagnosis of KA in the nasal vestibule should be viewed with suspicion.

Assessments of this kind, I believe, are largely if not wholly responsible for mistaken diagnoses and therefore unfortunate prognoses of the kind applied to the patients in Jackson's series. If the sections are examined without foreknowledge, either the diagnosis is certainly carcinoma or certainly KA or the appearances are equivocal and the matter insoluble. Stratified squamous epithelium that is structurally equivocal is not made unequivocal by knowledge of clinical data. In describing two cases of unusually aggressive KA in patients with Hodgkin's disease, Lowry and his associates (1972) made the reasonable suggestion that, ". . . perhaps keratoacanthoma and squamous-cell carcinoma are the same disease, in a different host", a brisk or defective immune response leading to rejection, on the one hand, or aggressive malignancy, on the other. If true, this would provide an acceptably plausible explanation for the histologist's difficulty; the solution lies rather in assessment of the patient's immunocompetence than in the histology.

## Pseudo-epitheliomatous Hyperplasia

This form of reactive overgrowth is so familiar as scarcely to merit a mention. The diagnostic difficulty remains, nevertheless, and certain distinction from carcinoma may at times be impossible. The hyperplasia may arise eventually in association with any ulcerative lesion, of whatever aetiology, and the causes of these are many. Difficulty will be greatest when no underlying cause can be demonstrated but every effort should be made to do so (fungal infection, perhaps exotic, may remain undetected for long; bromoderma is probably now of historical interest only). The occurrence of the phenomenon in company with 'granular cell myoblastoma' is well known: epithelial hyperplasia in the tongue, in particular, should prompt instant search for a myoblastoma.

## Pseudo-sarcoma

The possible implications of this term were outlined earlier in the context of borderline lesions of the soft tissues. Briefly to recall, the term may mean a sarcoma that rarely metastasises; a spindle-celled lesion that is truly a carcinoma; and an overgrowth that seems to be sarcoma but proves to be not even a neoplasm. Lesions of this last kind have been reported by Finlay-Jones and his colleagues (1971): they occurred almost exclusively on the face and ears of elderly persons and were characterised histologically by, "Abundant mitotic figures, multinucleated and bizarre cellular forms, together with lack of circumscription . . ." yet were virtually always curable by surgical excision. The problems of diagnosis are obviously great, in particular from fibrosarcoma but also from other conditions mentioned by these authors, including spindle-celled amelanotic melanocarcinoma and leiomyosarcoma. There is a strong possibility that the lesion is a variant of the atypical fibroxanthoma, already considered as one of the histologically misleading lesions of soft tissue.

Yet other pseudo-malignant patterns, those that simulate a malignant lymphoma, may be produced by infiltration of the skin by normal and abnormal leucocytes. They are considered presently in the general context of MF.

*Verrucous Carcinoma*

The massively exophytic epidermal lesion now often designated verrucous carcinoma (Ackerman, 1948) has been described in a helpful study of 105 cases (oral cavity, larynx and genitalia) by Kraus and Perez-Mesa (1966). In this lesion, the essential abnormality is a voluminous hyperplasia of the epithelium in the form of what these authors call 'bulbous masses' in which, in distinction to the condyloma acuminatum, there is no connective tissue core. The neoplastic epithelium may be destructive of surrounding tissue, even of bone, while still retaining a notably well-differentiated and cyto-logically benign character. This discrepancy be-tween histology and clinical behaviour can lead to a situation well described by these authors as ". . . a sort of impasse during which the clinician, sure of his ground, doggedly performs biopsy after biopsy which the pathologist doggedly refuses to recognize as carcinoma"[2] (this is substantially what happened with the local Case 8.2 where the lesion was in the oral cavity). The lesion is locally destructive but intrinsically non-metastasising. In the 77 oral cases described by Kraus and Perez-Mesa, nodal metastasis oc-curred in four; all had been treated by irradia-tion. In the opinion of these authors, irradiation may well be a factor provoking the lesion to metastasise. Irradiation had been used in 17 cases and failed to control the disease in every one; the results of excision in the other 88, on the other hand, were excellent.

Though metastasisingly malignant only when, apparently, provoked by radiotherapy there seems no more clinical reason to withhold the designation 'carcinoma' from this lesion than from the rodent ulcer. Statistics, however, are at some risk when verrucous carcinoma is held to be synonymous with the 'giant condyloma' or 'papillary tumour' of others. The statement by Newbold (1972) that ". . . florid papillomatosis, giant condyloma and also epidermodysplasia verruciformis are all caused by the wart virus and all of these conditions are premalignant" succinctly summarises the position and, in so far as all these lesions might in some clinics be diagnosed as carcinoma, simultaneously exposes the vulnerability of figures of incidence (and therefore curability) of cutaneous or mucosal SCC. Two reported cases are relevant here. Malignant transformation of an anal condyloma acuminatum was reported by Siegel (1962), who also gives a timely warning of the pseudo-carcinomatous appearance that may be produced in such warty lesions by podophyllin; while co-existing carcinoma in situ was seen, also in an anal lesion, by Oriel and Whimster (1971); this lesion had added interest and significance in containing virus particles demonstrable by electron microscopy.

*Metastasis from SCC*

In comparison with carcinomas of internal stratified squamous epithelia, metastasis from SCC is a relatively slight risk. A survey of 577 SCCs of skin (excluding the vermilion border of the lip) by Katz and his associates (1957) showed metastasis from 15 (2.6%) while an even larger series of 46,000 biopsies analysed by Lund (1965) included 3,700 squamous cell neoplasms of which 780 were aggressive car-cinomas; of these, only 4 had metastasised. The long-term risk with lesions of skin is therefore small, some 1% or less, scarcely enough to warrant ultraradical treatment with node dissec-tion in all, especially when we have no means of knowing that even ultraradical treatment would have saved the few who did develop metastases. In contrast is the analysis published by O'Brien and colleagues (1971) of lesions at internal sites. They describe the patterns of spread in patients with SCC of the head and neck including buccal cavity, tongue, pharynx, hypopharynx and larynx. From their own ob-servations and those of others they reported a frequency of metastasis from cancers at these sites of 10%–57%.

---

[2] And even when, as these authors further remark, the pathologist is invited to see the patient and discovers ". . . that the lesion he regards as benign half fills the mouth, has destroyed the mandible or perhaps has obliterated the glans penis" (or, as I have seen it, virtually fill the larynx), he will still be right in 'dog-gedly refusing' to diagnose carcinoma, at any rate histologically. For practical purposes, certainly, and perhaps to avoid seeming to his clinical colleagues absurd, he will agree that 'carcinoma' is an appropriate term; but no amount of tissue destruction changes be-nign histology into malignant.

# Basal Cell Carcinoma

The name basal cell carcinoma may not be appropriate in terms of either histogenesis or behaviour (to meet this objection some have proposed other terms; for example, Pinkus and Mehregan, 1969, prefer 'basaloma') but its implications are generally understood and unambiguous. The problems posed to the pathologist by the neoplasm are mainly three: (a) distinction between adnexal adenoma and carcinoma, (b) the implications of partial squamous cell differentiation in an otherwise typical BCC (the baso-squamous lesion) and, (c) associated with this, the frequency with which BCC may metastasise.

## Adnexal Adenoma and Carcinoma

The epithelium of sweat glands, both eccrine and apocrine, and their ducts; sebaceous glands and their ducts; and the hair follicle, provides a wide range of structural variants when neoplastic. The terminology of the resulting growths is correspondingly wide and varied. Most such lesions show well differentiated glanduliform spaces or sheets of cells, as in the eccrine poroma, and their cells are orderly; they are usually well circumscribed and thus equally often completely excised. Problems of prognosis arise only when completeness of excision is in doubt, and the usual warning about possible recurrence is then in order. The problem becomes more insistent when structural and cellular uniformity is lost since the occasional carcinoma of adnexal structure can infiltrate, metastasise and kill (*see*, for example, Berg and McDivitt, 1968). Therefore, even though Willis (1960) has advised of sweat gland tumours, that "A disorderly structure does not necessarily denote malignancy", structural and cellular aberrancy in these growths should not be underestimated; any doubt about completeness of excision should warrant a strong recommendation of further treatment. The rare but dangerous malignant eccrine poroma is mentioned later as a lesion that may simulate melanocarcinoma.

The so-called epithelioma adenoides cysticum (trichoepithelioma or Brooke's tumour) should not be confused with the adenoid cystic carcinoma of salivary glands. The epidermal lesion is usually wholly benign and only rarely behaves as a BCC; the salivary lesion is relentlessly recurrent, perhaps over many years, rarely cured and frequently fatal.

## Baso-squamous Carcinoma

Some belief persists that areas of squamous differentiation within an otherwise typical BCC imply a proportional capacity for metastasis. This is rarely fulfilled in practice. An example of one such lesion that spread widely by blood and, curiously, not at all to lymph nodes, was described by Hunt (1940). However, the squamous differentiation appears to represent no more than a focal expression by basal cells of the inherent capacity they have to form squamous cells; and many observers including, for example, Allen (1967) and Lever (1975) have found no evidence that the baso-squamous carcinoma is any more prone to metastasise than the BCC that is wholly undifferentiated.

## Metastasising Basal Cell Carcinoma

Such lesions are rare; the total so far recorded does not exceed 100. They show no morphologically identifiable difference from the common BCC but they have generally been larger and deeper at the time of first excision, a point noted particularly by both Wermuth and Fajardo (1970) and Cranmer and his colleagues (1970) who reviewed cases recorded in the literature up to that time. From these analyses, metastasis was found to occur, as expected, particularly to regional nodes (70%), but also to internal viscera such as lungs, liver and bone (30%), and after an interval of 7–40 (average 11) years. The metastasis in many cases followed a local recurrence. The recurrent BCC has been studied particularly by Menn and his associates (1971). They analysed the outcome of 100 lesions treated initially and at the time of recurrence by standard forms of therapy, and found that no fewer than 47 recurred a second time. Their reasonable recommendation is therefore that treatment of a recurrent lesion should be rather more 'aggressive' than that of an initial lesion.

The suggestion has been made by Sloane (1977) that morphological subdivision of BCC can be helpful in assessing probability of recurrence. Lesions classified as nodular, nodular with infiltrative margin, multifocal, and infiltrative had rates of recurrence after surgical excision of 6%, 12%, 20% and 24% respectively. No other feature, including type of differentiation, mitotic frequency, amount of leucocytic infiltration and ulceration, possessed predictive value.

Two further practical points are that a metastatic lesion may have a close histological resemblance to a carcinoid tumour (Wermuth and Fajardo, 1970); and that, while BCC and SCC sometimes co-exist, BCC may also be accompanied by an epidermal overgrowth that is not SCC but pseudo-epitheliomatous hyperplasia.

## Extramammary Paget's Disease (EMPD)

EMPD, in keeping with the normal distribution of apocrine sweat glands, occurs predominantly in the perineal and axillary areas though occasional examples have been described in the eyelid and external auditory meatus (Fligiel and Kaneko, 1975). The importance of the lesion in the present context is twofold: (a) it may closely simulate both Bowen's disease and the superficial spreading melanocarcinoma; and (b) to the extent that this form of melanocarcinoma may be difficult to distinguish from a junctional naevus, EMPD may create the same problem. The dangers of misdiagnosis are evident in the statement of Allen and Spitz (1953) that, "... radical mastectomies are known to have been done under the impression that a junctional nevus of the nipple was Paget's disease"; and, no doubt, what can happen with the misdiagnosis of Paget's disease when its site is usual, the nipple, can happen also with Paget's disease when its site is unusual. The danger is not particularly that EMPD and Bowen's disease may be mistaken for each other, since each is usually amenable to local excision (though not, of course, with anogenital Paget's disease accompanying a carcinoma of rectum), but that EMPD, a junctional naevus and melanocarcinoma may be confused. The likelihood of the error has been reduced by the wider use of histochemical staining procedures; for example, the Gomori aldehyde-fuchsin stain will usually allow a clear distinction between EMPD (+ve) and both Bowen's disease

and melanocarcinoma (−ve). Details of these and other techniques are given by Helwig and Graham (1963) and by Lever (1975).

## Conclusions

1) Squamous cell overgrowths in the external auditory meatus are potentially dangerous and should not be underestimated.

2) Leukoplakia is a clinically descriptive term, not one for the pathologist. Usefully accurate calculation of the risk of later carcinoma implied by the lesion is not yet possible.

3) KA may be histologically indistinguishable from, and may be a forme fruste of, SCC. Metastasis from seemingly typical examples has been reported.

4) The verrucous carcinoma has a deceptively bland appearance microscopically but is notoriously destructive (treatment should be surgical: irradiation has been reported as dangerously provocative of anaplastic transformation).

5) Squamous differentiation in a BCC carries no implication of metastasis.

6) BCCs that metastasise are usually of long standing, extensive and previously recurrent but show no distinctive histological difference from those that do not.

7) EMPD may have to be distinguished in particular from Bowen's disease and superficial spreading melanocarcinoma.

8) The risk of metastasis from cutaneous SCC is less than 1%.

## References

Ackerman LV (1948) Verrucous carcinoma of the oral cavity. Surgery 23: 670–678

Allen AC (1967) The skin. A clinicopathological treatise, 2nd edn. Heinemann, London

Allen AC, Spitz S (1953) Malignant melanoma. A clinicopathological analysis of the criteria for diagnosis and prognosis. Cancer 6: 1–45

Berg JW, McDivitt RW (1968) Pathology of sweat gland carcinoma. Pathol Annu 3: 123–144

Cranmer L, Reingold IM, Wilson JW (1970) Basal cell carcinoma of skin metastatic to bone. Arch Dermatol 102: 337–339

Davies DG (1969) Kerato-acanthoma or squamous carcinoma ? J Laryngol Otol 83: 333–347

Einhorn J, Wersäll J (1967) Incidence of oral carcinoma in patients with leukoplakia of the oral mucosa. Cancer 20: 2189–2193

Emerson CW, Hillman JW, McSwain B, Wood F (1971) Keratoacanthoma vs. squamous-cell carcinoma. A critical differentiation. J Bone Joint Surg [Am] 53: 143–146

Finlay-Jones LR, Nicoll P, Ten Seldam REJ (1971) Pseudosarcoma of the skin. Pathology 3: 215–222

Fisher ER, McCoy MM, Wechsler HL (1972) Analysis of histopathologic and electron microscopic determinants of keratoacanthoma and squamous cell carcinoma. Cancer 29: 1387–1397

Fligiel Z, Kaneko M (1975) Extramammary Paget's disease of the external ear canal in association with ceruminous gland carcinoma. A case report. Cancer 36: 1072–1076

Ghadially FN, Barton BW, Kerridge DF (1963) The etiology of keratoacanthoma. Cancer 16: 603–611

Helwig EB, Graham JH (1963) Anogenital (extramammary) Paget's disease. A clinicopathological study. Cancer 16: 387–403

Hunt AH (1940) Terebrant rodent ulcer with widespread blood-borne metastases. Br J Surg 40: 151–153

Jackson IT (1969) Diagnostic problem of keratoacanthoma. Lancet I: 490–492

Katz AD, Urbach F, Lilienfeld AM (1957) The frequency and risk of metastases in squamous-cell carcinoma of the skin. Cancer 10: 1162–1166

Kint A (1963) Histophotometric investigation of the nuclear DNA-content in normal epidermis, seborrheic keratosis, keratosis senilis, squamous-cell carcinoma and basal cell carcinoma. J Invest Dermatol 40: 95–100

Kramer IRH, Lucas RB, El-Labban N, Lister L (1970) A computer aided study on the tissue changes in oral keratoses and lichen planus, and an analysis of case groupings by subjective and objective criteria. Br J Cancer 24: 407–426

Kramer IRH, Lucas RB, El-Labban N, Lister L (1970a) The use of discriminant analysis for examining the histological features of oral keratoses and lichen planus. Br J Cancer 24: 673–686

Kraus FT, Perez-Mesa C (1966) Verrucous carcinoma: Clinical and pathologic study of 105 cases involving oral cavity, larynx and genitalia. Cancer 19: 26–38

Lever WF (1975) Histopathology of the skin, 5th edn. Lippincott, London

Lowry WS, Clark DA, Hannemann JH (1972) Skin cancer and immunosuppression. Lancet I: 1290–1291

Lund HZ (1965) How often does squamous cell carcinoma of the skin metastasize? Arch Dermatol 92: 635–637

Menn H, Robins P, Kopf AW, Bart RS (1971) The recurrent basal cell epithelioma. A study of 100 cases of recurrent, re-treated basal cell epitheliomas. Arch Dermatol 103: 628–631

Newbold PCH (1972) Pre-cancer and the skin. Brit J Dermatol 86: 417–434

O'Brien PH, Carlson R, Steubner EA, Staley CT (1971) Distant metastases in epidermoid carcinoma of the head and neck. Cancer 27: 304–307

Oriel JD, Whimster IW (1971) Carcinoma in situ associated with virus-containing anal warts. Br J Dermatol 84: 71–73

Pinkus H, Mehregan AH (1969) A guide to dermatohistopathology. Appleton - Century - Crofts, New York

Siegel A (1962) Malignant transformation of condyloma acuminatum: Review of the literature and report of a case. Am J Surg 103: 613–617

Sloane JP (1977) The value of typing basal cell carcinoma in predicting recurrence after surgical excision. Br J Dermatol 96: 127–132

Wermuth BM, Fajardo LF (1970) Metastatic basal cell carcinoma. A review. Arch Pathol 90: 458–462

Willis RA (1960) Pathology of tumours, 3rd edn. Butterworth, London

# Part B    The Problem of Mycosis Fungoides and Comparable Conditions

During the years under review, the question of a premycotic eruption, MF or some other form of malignant lymphoma/leukaemia, or a benign lymphocytic lesion of skin, was represented by biopsies from 53 patients. The diagnoses suggested histologically, and the outcome where known, are shown in Table 7.2.

## Local Series

Review of the series has shown that, for the diagnosis of MF, maximum reliance had been placed on the presence of the Pautrier microabscess. Where MF had been diagnosed with certainty or near-certainty, this feature had been

**Table 7.2.** Fifty-three cases in which MF was considered by clinician or pathologist: histological diagnosis suggested and outcome.

---

*Mycosis fungoides* (13 cases)

   6 died of MF at 1, 1, 3, 5, 8, 10 yr
   2 reticulum cell sarcoma on review, died at 1 yr, 3 yr
   1 lymphosarcoma at death at 7 yr
   1 death from bronchial ca. at 4 yr: eruption more probably tumour-associated parapsoriasis
   1 lesion subsided: unrelated death at 6 yr
   2 outcome unknown (no further biopsies)

*Suggestive of MF or premycotic* (22 cases)

   1 chronic lymphatic leukaemia, death at 7 yr
   1 nodular vasculitis on later biopsy
   1 syphilitic eruption
   3 condition unchanged till unrelated death at 2, 4, 7 yr
 10 subsided
   6 outcome unknown (no further biopsies)

*Spiegler-Fendt sarcoid* (5 cases)

   1 later diagnosed CDLE
   4 subsided

*Lymphocytoma cutis* (3 cases)

   All subsided, no sequelae

*'? reticulosis'* (8 cases)

   6 subsided
   1 persisting at 7 yr, possibly Spiegler-Fendt sarcoid
   1 outcome unknown (no further biopsies)

*Leukaemic infiltrate* (2 cases)

   Both died of leukaemia

---

present; in its absence, with an infiltrate regarded as histologically ominous, the diagnoses suggested had been either malignant lymphoma (ML) of some other kind or a (relatively easily assessed) leukaemia; or, with a less ominous infiltrate, a premycotic or possibly mycotic or benign lymphocytic lesion.

The data, as shown in Table 7.2, indicate the nature and to some extent the accuracy of the histological diagnoses. As with the squamous overgrowths of skin, accuracy is difficult to assess. At the least, there was no significant degree of under-diagnosis (in the patient who died 7 years postbiopsy of lymphosarcoma, the initial lesion was not malignant and had been reasonably diagnosed as parapsoriasis). In 13 cases MF was considered the correct diagnosis, and review confirms that this was appropriate in at least nine even if three now seem more probably examples of ML of another type. The outright over-diagnoses are thus possibly three

(though no further biopsies were received from two), and to these have to be added most of the 30 cases where the lesion had been regarded as premycotic or a '? reticulosis' but proved not to be so. To this total extent, then, there was over-diagnosis. At any time the line is difficult to draw between over-diagnosis that is alarmist and over-diagnosis that is prudent; opinion will consequently differ whether the amount of over-diagnosis in this series is excessive or in keeping with general, nonspecialist experience. Thoughts of a possibly conditioning factor are inevitable. Over-diagnosis of a lesion of skin as malignant will not cost a patient a viscus. Whether and to what extent this knowledge lowers the diagnostic threshold of a pathologist is also a matter of opinion.

Three main points have emerged from the local study, two instructive, one incidental; (a) impressive mitotic frequency was seen in two wholly benign lesions (one in retrospect, a hypercellular granuloma pyogenicum [M, 12 years]; the other a still unexplained monocytoid infiltration accompanying haemorrhagic blisters on palms [F, 68 years]—the eruptions in both subsided on antibiotic therapy); (b) over-emphasis has been placed on the polytypia[3] of an infiltrate as an ominous appearance; (c) in many of the lesions, both benign and malignant, the epidermis has been notably psoriasiform, sometimes even with parakeratosis.

A somewhat comparable though much larger series of cases has been described by Epstein and colleagues (1972) as ". . . 144 patients in whom the diagnosis of mycosis fungoides was at one time accepted both clinically and pathologically . . . No patient was excluded because later clinical course suggested either a more benign disease such as eczema or a more common lymphoma such as Hodgkin's disease". Patients were finally accepted as having died of MF only on the evidence of necropsy or convincing documentary data; they numbered 75; the rest died either from another disease or from a cause unknown. The rate of over-diagnosis was thus possibly 69/144 and therefore somewhat similar to the possibly 30/53 in the local series. However, comparability between the two series is less than total if only because most of the local over-diagnosis is represented by over-diagnosis not as MF but as premycosis. These same authors

[3] Confusion may be caused by the terms 'polymorphism' and 'monomorphism'. Both terms are sometimes applied to describe the character of a population of cells, whether composed of many different types of cell, polymorphism, or of one type of cell, monomorphism. However, both terms are sometimes applied also to describe the character of a population of cells all of the one histogenetic type: the cells comprising a lymphosarcoma are monomorphic in the sense that all are of lymphoblastic type but they have a variability in size, shape and staining intensity that does not occur in a population of normal lymphocytes; that is, relative to the normal cells they are polymorphic. It would be less confusing if such terms as monotypic and polytypic (with monotypia or-ism, and polytypia or-ism) were used to refer to cell *type*, and monomorphic and polymorphic to cell *structure* or *form*. This terminology is unlikely to be adopted now but, since assessment of malignancy may depend on judgement of both the histogenetic type and the morphology of a cell, it is important to realise that the possibility of confusion does exist. The ambiguities have been acknowledged by the emergence of the term 'mixed cellularity' in the context at least of Hodgkin's disease.

offered the useful prognostic information that MF is less aggressive in patients under 50 years of age than over 60 (even when the age-difference per se is taken into account), and that tumour formation, ulceration and palpable lymph node enlargement are prognostically bad signs.

## General Commentary

Rarely in histopathology is the need greater for the 'blind' approach to biopsy than with specimens from an eruption of skin thought possibly to be premycotic. Should the pathologist read the request '? premycotic eruption' before he examines the sections, he is abnormally on the alert for every mitotic figure, every cell and nucleus marginally larger than the rest and marginally larger than what he had arbitrarily set as his norm hitherto for nonspecific inflammatory infiltrates. The confusion and uncertainty that still prevails would surely have been less, and might never have started, had pathologists from decades ago initially scrutinised their sections with an open mind.

That lymphomatous plaques and lumps in the skin of a patient who dies of unequivocal mycosis fungoides (MF) may be preceded, perhaps for years, by an eruption of some kind is well known. To that extent, in retrospect, these eruptions are 'premycotic'. To diagnose such eruptions in prospect as 'premycotic' is another matter: in the opinion of many, it cannot be done. Most of the eruptions seen in retrospect to have been premycotic are of nonspecific type, commonly those of a simple chronic dermatitis. Certainly, occasional patients with poikiloderma atrophicans (atrophic parapsoriasis; prereticulotic poikiloderma) will progress to develop MF or some other form of ML (Samman, 1972) but even here prediction in the individual case is uncertain.

It is doubtful whether even near-certainty in diagnosis can be reached until the arrival in the infiltrate of the so-called mycosis cell (a debatable entity still) or the appearance of the Pautrier micro-abscess, or preferably both; and, with that, the diagnosis has been made of MF itself. The mycosis cell and other features often regarded as strongly suggestive of the diagnosis will be further examined presently. Meantime, a short examination is in order of the status of

MF as an entity, for recent reports offer some hope of more accurate diagnosis.

For long, two main views have been held on the nature of MF. One, it is a specific entity, a particular form of ML, particular in beginning in and being for long confined to the skin; the other, it is not an entity at all but a syndrome produced by any of the MLs that happen by chance to affect primarily and predominantly the skin. Until recently, the second view was the more widely supported, examplified for example by the comment that ". . . most authorities now accept a fairly wide concept of this disease and include any malignant reticulosis (lymphoma) which originates in the skin" (Editorial, 1972). The suggestion had even been made (Reed and Cummings, 1966) that the term MF be discarded altogether because of its lack of specificity. The same suggestion has been made again, 10 years later (Schein et al., 1976) but, as mentioned later, for quite the opposite reason.

Two detailed and well-illustrated analyses of findings at necropsy in 15 and in 45 patients, with what was regarded as certainly MF, have been given by Long and Mihm (1974) and Rappaport and Thomas (1974) respectively. In general, both pairs of authors agree that the behaviour, distribution, morbid anatomy and histopathology of the lesions are distinctive and virtually always clearly separable from those of other MLs. Rarely, a cell may be seen that is indistinguishable from a Reed-Sternberg cell, but significant difficulty in distinguishing MF from HD is exceptional. However, even though a disease may be sharply separable at necropsy from one-time diagnostic rivals, the findings at necropsy are often of only limited help towards separation in the diagnostically important early stages. A structure virtually always present at necropsy both in skin and internal organs is the already-mentioned 'mycosis cell'. This cell, the Pautrier micro-abscess and a polytypic or mixed cell infiltrate are frequently held to be strong diagnostic indicators in the early stages: all three features merit comment for this reason.

The mycosis cell is described as having a hyperchromatic nucleus that is relatively large and convoluted, deeply indented, or cerebriform. It is regarded by Rappaport and Thomas (1974) as ". . . usually essential for the differentiation of the cellular proliferation of M. F. from those of other malignant lympho-

mas". The concept was broadened by Long and Mihm (1974) to include a range of abnormal lymphoid cells in which "Mycosis cells appeared to vary in size from the small 10–15 $\mu$ in diameter cell, to the large 10–30 $\mu$ in diameter cell, with many intermediate sized variants". On the other hand, the specificity (though not the existence) of such cells has been questioned by Flaxman and his associates (1971) and completely rejected by Brehmer-Andersson (1976), who says that "A cell which is specific for mycosis fungoides, i.e. a 'mycosis cell', does not exist". The opinion of Rosas-Uribe and his colleagues (1974), based on ultrastructural observations, is that cells with a notably indented or cerebriform nucleus are characteristically present in MF but of diagnostic value only when present in clusters. These authors, like Long and Mihm, also believe that the cells are of lymphoid origin.

The typical Pautrier micro-abscess, when present, is probably a more dependable indicator of MF than the postulated 'mycosis cell' but has not enjoyed the same reputation, partly because it is only an epiphenomenon, and partly because it is not invariably present in otherwise undoubted MF (it was present in 29 of the 44 available cases of Rappaport and Thomas, 1974). It may be simulated in the misleadingly pseudomalignant picture of 'actinic reticuloid' (see later) but is usually of great diagnostic help.

The third feature frequently cited as strongly suggestive of MF is the already mentioned polytypia of the inflammatory cell infiltrate. The fact that the scatter of cells may represent a reaction to the neoplastic process rather than be part of the process itself (Clendenning et al., 1964; Rappaport and Thomas, 1974), and gradually disappear as the disease advances, need not detract from its possible value as another indicator. However, polytypia of this kind has been reported many times as commoner in benign lesions than in malignant, as, for example, by Reed and Cummings (1966) and Caro and Helwig (1969).

These various morphological features now seem likely to be overtaken if not replaced as diagnostic pointers by the pattern of cell surface receptors. There is strong evidence that MF is a separately definable form of malignant lymphoma, a neoplastic expression of T-cells. In the opinion of Lutzner and his colleagues

(1973), MF, Sézary's syndrome and (though still a debatable lesion) lymphomatoid papulosis are interrelated and to be grouped as 'cutaneous T-cell lymphomas'; Sézary's syndrome, they believe, is a leukaemic variant of MF. Later individual case reports give added support, namely: an example of MF terminating as an immunoblastic sarcoma with leukaemic blood picture (Schwarze and Ude, 1975); an example of diffuse poorly differentiated lymphoma terminating with leukaemic blood picture and subcutaneous neoplastic plaques (Greenberg et al., 1976); and one of MF terminating with leukaemia (Harrington and Slater, 1978), with good evidence in each case that the neoplastic cells mainly concerned were T-cells. Added support for the concept of the cutaneous T-cell lymphoma has been given by Schein and his associates (1976) from their study of 12 cases; and it is these authors who repeat the advice that the terms MF and, for its leukaemic form, Sézary's syndrome, should be discarded, on this occasion, however, because of the very specificity of the lesion as a T-cell lymphoma.

The evidence, in sum, indicates that the terms 'premycosis' and 'premycotic' are appropriate clinically but not pathologically. To the histologist, MF is characterised by an infiltration of the dermis, and (as the Pautrier micro-abscess) the epidermis by abnormal cells. The build-up of this pattern to a diagnostic level is gradual, and the threshold for *diagnosis* will continue to vary from pathologist to pathologist. However, the threshold for *suspicion* is lower: assessment of this is increasingly likely to lead to investigation of the T-cell status of the lesion, and it is on this rather than the histology that the diagnosis of MF in the early stages is increasingly likely to depend.

## Lymphocytic Infiltrations of the Skin

The presence of crowded lymphocytes or more formally follicle-bearing lymphoid tissue in the skin is always disquieting but these changes are usually benign. In the opinion of Mach and Wilgram (1966), ". . . the cause of cutaneous lymphoplasia is a special tendency of some individuals to react with hyperplasia of pre-existent lymphoreticular tissue to such etiologic stimuli as infection, trauma, and insect

bites", and for this reason they prefer to designate the condition lymphoplasia rather than lymphocytoma.

The significance of 'cutaneous lymphoid hyperplasia' has been well reviewed by Caro and Helwig (1969) who, in analysing 225 lesions in 193 patients, found 138 benign and 87 malignant. The malignant lesions comprised lymphosarcoma, reticulum cell sarcoma, and 'malignant lymphoma not otherwise classified' (HD was specifically excluded as was MF). The benign lesions included lymphocytoma cutis, lymphocytic infiltration of the skin (Jessner), Spiegler-Fendt sarcoid and arthropod bite granuloma. These authors say that there is no single histological criterion that can be used to differentiate cutaneous lymphoid hyperplasia from cutaneous ML (and special stains were of no help) but that certain features are helpful. A monomorphous infiltrate was seen mainly in malignant lesions ("The hallmark of the benign lesion was a polymorphous infiltrate . . ."). Pseudo-epitheliomatous hyperplasia of the epidermis was seen mainly in benign lesions. Mitotic figures and atypical cells were much commoner, but well formed lymphoid follicles much rarer, in the malignant lesions: well formed follicles are particularly a feature of the Spiegler-Fendt form of lymphocytic infiltration.

Broadly similar conclusions were reached by Clark and his colleagues (1974) who stated that, "The vast majority of lymphocytic infiltrates, regardless of how disturbing they may be histologically, are not due to leukemia or malignant lymphoma . . ." and that ". . . as a general rule, the diagnosis of malignant lymphoma or leukemia should not be made on the basis of a skin biopsy alone". This last point is forcibly emphasised by the experience of Ackerman and Tanski (1977) with a lump in the skin confidently diagnosed on biopsy in several clinics as a malignant lymphomatous lesion: it proved on further sections to be the polymorphous inflammatory accompaniment to molluscum contagiosum, and was designated by these authors 'pseudoleukemia cutis'.

## Other Pseudo-malignant Lesions

Some other types of cutaneous lesion closely simulate cancer but are not cancer. What remains are lesions characterised by infiltration of the dermis by cells abnormal in type and/or in number, to the point where a distinction from cancer may be extremely difficult or virtually impossible: if the pathologist is unfamiliar with the lesions, a diagnosis of cancer, perhaps ML or metastatic carcinoma, will be made outright.

*Actinic reticuloid* is possibly the commonest lesion of this kind. First identified by Ive and his colleagues (1969), the condition is a form of photodermatosis in which the skin, clinically thickened and ridged, is heavily infiltrated by mononuclear cells, many of which are likely to be abnormally large, dark and polymorphic, and occasionally in mitosis. As such they closely resemble the infiltrating cells of an early ML though they do not attain the size or the lobulate features of a characteristic R-S cell; also, they may appear in clusters within the epidermis to suggest Pautrier micro-abscesses.

*Pityriasis lichenoides* (Mucha-Habermann disease) is a rarer condition surrounded, like MF, by nosological uncertainty; some authors, for example, regard it as an acute form of parapsoriasis. However, the important point in biopsy practice is that in one of its expressions it may be virtually indistinguishable from a ML. This variant has been separately named by some as 'lymphomatoid papulosis' (Macaulay, 1968; Borrie, 1969) though others regard this as unwarranted (Muller and Schulze, 1971); the compromise term 'lymphomatoid pityriasis lichenoides' has been offered by Black and Jones (1972). The prominent features of this variant are a necrotising vasculitis and a highly cellular infiltrate of which many of the cells are large, polymorphic and hyperchromatic, variously described as ". . . at least twice the size of a small lymphocyte . . . (with) . . . a large hyperchromatic nucleus", the largest "similar in size to Sternberg-Reed cells of Hodgkin's disease but . . . (with) . . . nuclei more hyperchromatic, cytoplasm . . . less prominent . . and lacking the large eosinophilic nucleolus characteristic of Hodgkin's cells" (Black and Jones); ". . . large reticular cells" (Muller and Schulze, whose first case was initially diagnosed as reticulum cell sarcoma); and, most tellingly, ". . . an alarming infiltrate of large pleomorphic hyperchromatic cells which expert histopathologists and hematologists have variously classified as highest grade malignant lymphoma (a majority opinion),

malignant reticulosis, metastatic carcinoma, malignant melanoma, undifferentiated malignant tumor" (Macaulay, 1968). This last author added that mitotic figures were relatively scarce, a point of discrepancy possibly useful in reminding the pathologist of the existence of this non-malignant mimic. While the disease is evidently self-limiting and quite benign, and the true nature of the bizarre cells unknown, the whole matter clearly demands reassessment in view of the already-mentioned claim that 'lymphomatoid papulosis' is a cutaneous T-cell lymphoma.

*Lymphomatoid granulomatosis* is "an angiocentric and distinctive lymphoreticular proliferation and granulomatous disease" (Kay et al., 1974) first described by Liebow and his colleagues (1972) in 40 cases as a condition affecting primarily the lungs but also, in nearly half the cases, the skin; and the lesion in skin may be the first manifestation of the disease (lymph node, spleen and bone marrow are, unexpectedly and unusually, not affected). The infiltrating cells, though predominantly histiocytic, present a polytypic picture with an admixture of lymphocytes, plasma cells and an occasional eosinophil. Polymorphism and mitotic activity amongst the histiocytes adds to the pseudo-malignant appearance. Although the condition is not a form of ML the mortality is high, especially from the pulmonary involvement (in Liebow's series, 65% of the patients died). Further data on the lesion, derived from an updated analysis of the original Liebow series (Katzenstein et al., 1979) are given in Chapter 9 (p. 386).

*Arthropod bites* may produce notoriously pseudo-cancerous tissue reactions, either as pseudo-epitheliomatous hyperplasia or pseudo-lymphomatous infiltrates, well described by Allen (1948, 1967). Two guiding principles stand out: (a) arthropod bites are frequently single but may be multiple; lymphomatous lesions are frequently multiple but may be single; (b) 'eosinophil granuloma' of the skin should not be regarded as a final diagnosis; apart from bites it may be the presenting feature of, to name only the commonest, allergic angiitis (polyarteritis nodosa), histiocytosis X, juvenile xanthoma, and malignant lymphoma, especially HD. 'Bites' of this kind are naturally commoner in tropical and subtropical countries but, as with exotic disease as a whole, increasing foreign travel brings an equivalent increase in incidence elsewhere.

The explanation may be merely this smallness of number but I cannot recall an instance here where malignant lymphoma and arthropod granuloma have been reciprocally misdiagnosed. One of the two types of false positive diagnosis is, of course, much easier to detect than the other. The malignant lymphoma wrongly diagnosed as a bite granuloma, will certainly recur. The bite granuloma wrongly diagnosed as malignant lymphoma is harder to detect but would come to light as a malignant lymphoma of skin which, on review, had 'done surprisingly well'. The so-called eosinophil granuloma has almost always been identifiable for what it truly is (for example, ML or polyarteritis nodosa) and only a single example in our files, a relatively deep-seated lesion around the wrist, remains unexplained after many years; it resolved completely over some 3 months so there probably never will be an explanation. Of arthropods known to be the cause locally, trombiculid mites are the commonest. A single example of sea-urchin granuloma was of sarcoid, not eosinophil, type and in no way simulated a lymphoma.

The possibly related angiolymphoid hyperplasia with eosinophilia is considered later as one of the lesions of the vascular apparatus.

## Conclusions

1) The Pautrier micro-abscess is the most dependably diagnostic feature of MF (but see 6 below).

2) The infiltrate in MF is characterised by large atypical lymphoid cells ('mycosis cells') but they are neither peculiar to, nor diagnostic of, the lesion.

3) The presence in a dermal infiltrate of cells of many types (polytypia) is as common, if not commoner, in benign conditions as in MF.

4) The nonspecific chronic dermatitis that precedes MF gradually acquires the characters of MF. If histologically diagnosable with confidence as premycotic, it is already mycotic.

5) Sézary's syndrome is probably the leukaemic variant of MF. Both conditions (and 'lymphomatoid papulosis') may be T-cell lymphomas.

6) Significant simulators of cutaneous ML

are actinic reticuloid and insect bites. Actinic reticuloid may produce epidermal lesions closely simulating the Pautrier micro-abscess.

7) The eosinophil granuloma of skin has many causes.

8) ML should not be diagnosed on a single biopsy of skin.

## References

Ackerman AB, Tanski EV (1977) Pseudoleukemia cutis. Report of a case in association with molluscum contagiosum. Cancer 40: 813–817

Allen AC (1948) Persistent 'insect bites' (dermal eosinophilic granulomas) simulating lymphoblastomas, histiocytoses, and squamous cell carcinomas. Am J Pathol 24: 367–387

Allen AC (1967) The skin. A clinicopathological treatise. 2nd edn. Heinemann, London

Black MM, Jones EW (1972) "Lymphomatoid" pityriasis lichenoides: a variant with histological features simulating a lymphoma: A clinical and histopathological study of 15 cases with details of long term follow-up. Br J Dermatol 86: 329–347

Borrie PF (1969) Lymphomatoid papulosis. Proc R Soc Med 62: 159–160

Brehmer-Andersson E (1976) Mycosis fungoides and its relation to Sézary's syndrome, lymphomatoid papulosis, and primary cutaneous Hodgkin's disease. A clinical, histopathologic and cytologic study of fourteen cases and a critical review of the literature. Acta Derm Venereol (Stockh) 56: Suppl 75

Caro WA, Helwig EB (1969) Cutaneous lymphoid hyperplasia. Cancer 24: 487–502

Clark WH, Mihm MC, Reed RJ, Ainsworth AM (1974) The lymphocytic infiltrates of the skin. Hum Pathol 5: 25–43

Clendenning WE, Brecher G, Scott EJ van (1964) Mycosis fungoides: Relationship to malignant cutaneous reticulosis and the Sézary syndrome. Arch Dermatol 89: 785–792

Editorial (1972) Mycosis fungoides. Lancet II: 26–27

Epstein EH, Levin DL, Croft JD, Lutzner MA (1972) Mycosis fungoides: Survival, prognostic features, response to therapy, and autopsy findings. Medicine (Baltimore) 51: 61–72

Flaxman BA, Zelazny G, Scott EJV (1971) Nonspecificity of characteristic cells in mycosis fungoides. Arch Dermatol 104: 141–147

Greenberg BR, Peter CR, Glassy F, MacKenzie MR (1976) A case of T-cell lymphoma with convoluted lymphocytes. Cancer 38: 1602–1607

Harrington CI, Slater DN (1978) Mycosis fungoides with blast cell transformation. Arch Dermatol 114: 611–612

Ive FA, Magnus IA, Warin RP, Jones EW (1969) Actinic reticuloid; A chronic dermatosis associated with severe photosensitivity and the histological resemblance to lymphoma. Br J Dermatol 81: 469–485

Katzenstein A-LA, Carrington CB, Liebow AA (1979) Lymphomatoid granulomatosis. A clinicopathologic study of 152 cases. Cancer 43: 360–373

Kay S, Fu Y-S, Minars N, Brady JW (1974) Lymphomatoid granulomatosis of the skin: Light microscopic and ultrastructural studies. Cancer 34: 1675–1682

Liebow AA, Carrington CRB, Friedman PJ (1972) Lymphomatoid granulomatosis. Hum Pathol 3: 457–558

Long JC, Mihm MC (1974) Mycosis fungoides with extracutaneous dissemination: A distinct clinicopathologic entity. Cancer 34: 1745–1755

Lutzner M, Edelson R, Schein P, Green I, Kirkpatrick C, Ahmed A (1973) Cutaneous T-cell lymphomas: The Sézary syndrome, mycosis fungoides ,and related disorders. Ann Intern Med 83: 534–552

Macaulay WL (1968) Lymphomatoid papulosis: A continuing self-healing eruption, clinically benign —histologically malignant. Arch Dermatol 97: 23–30

Mach KW, Wilgram GF (1966) Characteristic histopathology of cutaneous lymphoplasia (lymphocytoma). Arch Dermatol 94: 26–32

Muller SA, Schulze TW (1971) Mucha-Habermann disease mistaken for reticulum cell sarcoma. Arch Dermatol 103: 423–427

Rappaport H, Thomas LB (1974) Mycosis fungoides: The pathology of extracutaneous involvement. Cancer 34: 1198–1229

Reed RJ, Cummings CE (1966) Malignant reticulosis and related conditions of the skin. A reconsideration of mycosis fungoides. Cancer 19: 1231–1247

Rosas-Uribe A, Variakojis D, Molnar Z, Rappaport H (1974) Mycosis fungoides: An ultrastructural study. Cancer 34: 634–645

Samman PD (1972) The natural history of parapsoriasis en plaques (chronic superficial dermatitis) and prereticulotic poikiloderma. Br J Dermatol 87: 405–411

Schein PS, Macdonald JS, Edelson R (1976) Cutaneous T-cell lymphoma. Cancer 38: 1859–1861

Schwarze E-W, Ude P (1975) Immunoblastic sarcoma with leukemic blood picture in the terminal stage of mycosis fungoides. Virchows Arch [Pathol Anat] 369: 165–172

# Part C    Melanocarcinoma

The term 'melanoma' should be banned. It causes confusion and sometimes needless alarm. Unqualified, in some clinics it means a cancerous lesion: elsewhere it does not, and the simple melanonaevus is sometimes referred to as a 'benign melanoma'. The term 'juvenile melanoma' is being gradually replaced by 'Spitz naevus' or 'spindle-celled naevus' thanks largely to the early campaigning of Ackerman and others (Kernen and Ackerman, 1960; Echevarria and Ackerman, 1967). If the user wishes to convey the meaning of a cancerous lesion, and still use the word 'melanoma', the term should be always 'malignant melanoma'. Despite some continuing uncertainty about the exact histogenesis, and until this is resolved, there is much to be said for removing ambiguity altogether by calling the lesion 'melanocarcinoma'. The use of the term 'superficial melanoma', and the confusion it may cause in the mind of the surgeon, has been criticised in an analytical article by DeCosse and McNeer (1969) that could be read with profit by all those who make use of the term.

Clearly enough, if this or any other lesion is to be discussed and classified for purposes of prognosis, it must be correctly diagnosed, and this is not always as easy in the case of melanocarcinoma as many writings would suggest. In probably any sizable series of melanotic lesions considered by a reasonably experienced pathologist as possibly melanocarcinoma, there will be borderline examples, and there must surely be few pathologists who, on showing such a lesion to colleagues, have not received quite different opinions; this at any rate has been my own experience. To be sure, the dermal pathologist will less frequently diagnose as melanocarcinoma the Spitz naevus, activated naevus, or cellular blue naevus, for example, but we are not all dermal pathologists and it is hard to believe that errors of this kind will not continue to be made. The size of the problem may be judged from some series of diagnostic reassessments from various clinics. Thus, in a series of 513 cases of malignant melanoma reviewed by Couperus and Rucker (1954), 40 were rediagnosed as not malignant melanoma. In 400 cases of melano-carcinoma analysed by Davis and his colleagues (1966), unanimity of diagnosis amongst a group of pathologists had been attained in 93%, yet there were, besides the 400 cases, a further 23 not included because they were 'borderline' cases. In another analysis, that of Truax and his associates (1966), a review was carried out on a series of 247 cases of 'long-term survivors', and in no less than 62 (25.1%) was the diagnosis found to be not melanocarcinoma (one effect of this, incidentally, was to lower the crude 5-year survival rate over a period of 20 years by 4.7%). Another account was that by Saksela and Rintala (1968), who reassessed 20 cases referred to a National Registry as prepubertal malignant melanoma: on review, only two were considered to be so. We have therefore to acknowledge that the pattern of some lesions will produce a diagnosis of 'benign' from some pathologists and 'malignant' from others.

That is one difficulty. Another is the notorious unpredictability of melanocarcinoma. Even amongst lesions agreed by all to have the pattern of an unequivocal melanocarcinoma, some lesions, shallow, small and excised with an ample margin will metastasise (that is, will already have metastasised) and kill. Others, large and deeply invasive, to everyone's equal surprise, will not. Our histoclinical correlation is disappointingly low. This unpredictability, particularly emphasised by Magnus (1973, 1977) in an analysis of nearly 3,000 cases, has frustrated, and still is frustrating, attempts at prognostically useful classification. The two difficulties are seen combined in the report by Delacrétaz (1969) of a lesion on the leg of a 14-year-old girl that was diagnosed as 'juvenile melanoma' yet was followed by inguinal nodal metastasis 5 years later. The original sections were shown to "plusiers histopathologistes particulièrement compétents" and all confirmed the diagnosis (probably independently, and possibly, at the outset, in ignorance of the clinical circumstances). The problems in the way of explaining the matter are obvious.

Electron microscopy, here as elsewhere, is

again a prognostic disappointment. In the words of Curran and McCann (1976), "Although electron microscopy is capable of showing in great detail within individual melanocytes many changes which are clearly associated with malignancy, the technique does not appear to offer significant advantages over light microscopy in determining the diagnosis and prognosis in this group of conditions".

## Local Series

As the opening paragraphs have shown, the diagnosis of melanocarcinoma still involves much uncertainty. Over the past 30 years or so, thanks to the studies of histopathologists, some formerly puzzling lesions have been recognised as separable entities, and to that extent tissue patterns formerly equivocal are now identifiable. At the same time, this has thrown even greater responsibility on the pathologist. In an earlier era he had to decide 'melanocarcinoma or not?' Now he may have to choose between, for example, Spitz naevus, cellular blue naevus, desmoplastic melanocarcinoma and lentigo maligna melanocarcinoma. Examples of these and other difficulties are included among the 24 cases (including 6 diagnosed as melanocarcinoma) comprising the local series. These were met during a period when 78 other cases were diagnosed firmly also as melanocarcinoma; that is, borderline problems arose on about one-third of the occasions when a possible melanocarcinoma or transected melanonaevus was in question.

### Summarised Totals

Doubt had been expressed for various reasons on the nature and possible behaviour of melanotic lesions in 24 instances.

*Junctional naevus*
1 case at age 26 (7.1): no sequelae

*Compound naevus with uncertainty*
1 apparently transected (7.2)  
2 unduly polymorphic (7.3, 7.4) } no sequelae  
1 unduly deep (7.5)

*Compound naevus or lentigo maligna*
1 still debatable (7.6): no recurrence before unrelated death 8 years later

1 case (7.7): unequivocal melanocarcinoma 18 years later

1 case (7.8): recurrence after 7 years, typically lentigo maligna

*Compound naevus, ? transected*
1 case (7.9): no sequelae

*Spitz naevus or melanocarcinoma*
2 cases (7.10, 7.11): no sequelae

*Cellular blue naevus, hypercellular*
1 case (7.12): no sequelae

*'? Neuronaevus'*
1 case (7.13): no sequelae

*'Naevus, ? nature'*
1 case (7.14): no sequelae

*Melanocarcinoma or not?*
2 cases 'superficial' melanocarcinoma (7.15, 7.16): fatal
3 cases 'superficial' melanocarcinoma (7.17, 7.18, 7.19): apparent cures
1 case (7.20): apparent cure
2 cases (7.21, 7.22): fatal
1 case with unusual sequel (7.23): unrelated death at 2 years
1 case of complex histology (7.24): fatal.

*Review has yielded:*
Appropriate diagnoses, 17
Underdiagnoses, 5
Overdiagnoses, 1
Inappropriate diagnoses, 1
The 24 cases regrouped in this way comprise Table 7.3

CASE DATA

*Case 7.1*

M (26 years) with nodule in palm slowly growing for 6 months. The specimen was extremely small, 5 × 3 mm skin ellipse with central 2-mm nodule.

Sections showed a 'junctional naevus' consisting of clear-cut, well-circumscribed spherical clusters of minimally pigmented naevus cells. They did not extend into the dermis in any significant way, and at most reached one-third of the distance within the epidermis towards the surface. The cells were uniform and rarely in mitosis.

The lesion was thus as histologically quiescent as a junctional naevus could be. However, its presence at age 26 was believed to warrant a caution that the patient be seen again within 1 year or so.

The patient emigrated shortly after the excision and has not been traced. Absence of enquiry since suggests that melanocarcinoma did not develop. The diagnosis was *appropriate*.

*Case 7.2*

F (38 years) with a 5 × 3 mm papilloma on the cheek, mildly pigmented, present since childhood, enlarging during the preceding 2 years.

The lesion was technically a 'compound naevus' though the junctional element involved no more than 1% of the epidermis. Cytologically there was considerable variation in naevus cell nuclear size, also occasional multinucleate masses and some four to six normal mitotic figures per whole section. The lesion was considered benign but the comment was made that an area of naevus cells had apparently been transected by the line of excision.

The area and the patient had remained trouble-free for at least the next 15 years; an *appropriate* diagnosis.

*Case 7.3*

F (45 years) with pigmented nodule on trunk, ? duration. The excised naevus was of 15-mm diameter, 3-mm depth.

It was an 'intradermal naevus' with one focus of junctional change; it showed moderate polymorphism with one to three mitoses per whole section. Some reservation had been voiced in the report, ". . . hesitate to call this tumour indubitably benign", mainly on account of the degree of polymorphism.

No further treatment was given and the patient was trouble-free at 12 years. The diagnosis was *appropriate* enough but a little unnecessarily alarmist.

**Table 7.3.** Twenty-four cases of equivocal melanocytic lesions.

| Case No. | Diagnosis on review | Treatment | Outcome |
|---|---|---|---|
| *5 cases under-diagnosed* | | | |
| 7.6 | Melanocarcinoma > LM | Excision | Unrelated death @ 8 yr |
| 7.7 | LM or me/carc. > cpd. naevus | Excision × 2 | Unrelated death @ 20 yr |
| 7.8 | LM > junctnl. naevus | Excision × 2 | Alive @ 10 yr |
| 7.21 | Me/carc. > metaplastic naevus | Excision | Death @ 4 yr |
| 7.24 | Eccrine carc. > SCC | Excision | Death @ 3 yr |
| *1 case over-diagnosed* | | | |
| 7.11 | Spitz naevus > me/carc. | Excision | Alive @ 8 yr |
| *17 cases appropriately diagnosed* | | | |
| 7.1 | Jnctnl. naevus @ 25 yr | Excision | Prob. alive @ 12 yr |
| 7.2 | Cpd. naevus transected | No further excision | Alive @ 15 yr |
| 7.3 | Cpd. naevus polymorphic ++ | Excision | Alive @ 12 yr |
| 7.4 | Cpd. naevus polymorphic ++ | Excision | Alive @ 2 yr |
| 7.5 | Cpd. naevus unduly deep | Excision | Alive @ 20 yr |
| 7.9 | I-derm. naevus transected | No further excision | Prob. still alive |
| 7.10 | Spitz naevus | Excision | Alive @ 11 yr |
| 7.12 | Cellular blue naevus | Excision | Unrelated death (prob.) @ 4 yr |
| 7.14 | Naevus ? nature, transected | No further excision | Alive @ 14 yr |
| 7.15 | Melanocarcinoma | Excision | Death @ 12 yr |
| 7.16 | Melanocarcinoma | Excision | Death @ 14 mo |
| 7.17 | Melanocarcinoma | Excision | Alive @ 8 yr |
| 7.18 | Melanocarcinoma | Excision | Alive @ 17 yr |
| 7.19 | Melanocarcinoma | Excision | Alive @ 15 yr |
| 7.20 | Melanocarcinoma (amelanotic) | Excision | Alive @ 14 yr |
| 7.22 | Melanocarcinoma (amelanotic) | Excision + lymphadenectomy | Death @ 4 yr |
| 7.23 | ? amelanotic me/carc. | Excision × 2 | Unrelated death @ 8 yr |
| *1 case inappropriately diagnosed* | | | |
| 7.13 | Histiocytoma > neuronaevus | Excision | Alive @ 7 yr |

LM, lentigo maligna; SCC, squamous-cell carcinoma

*Case 7.4*

M (32 years) with a 20 × 15 × 10 mm excoriated, pedunculated 'papilloma' in the groin. The excoriation was recent, and the main reason for consultation, but the duration, 'probably years', was uncertain.

The lesion was a 'compound naevus'. The facts considered in assessing prognosis were its relatively large size and pedunculated character; the fact that the junctional element was prominent, involving some 5% of the epidermis; a moderate degree of nuclear polymorphism mainly in the epithelioid component of what was a mixed epithelioid/spindle-celled pattern; the presence of mitoses with a frequency of approximately 1 per 10 hpf; and the apparent completeness of excision.

The abnormal features were considered insufficient to warrant diagnosis of melanocarcinoma but the reportedly greater menace of persisting junctional change was mentioned as a precaution or added warning.

The patient was known to be well 2 years later but contact thereafter was lost. The diagnosis and advice were *appropriate*.

### Case 7.5

F (20 years) with history of recent enlargement of a 'mole' present on the back since birth. The warty nodule, now 10 mm across, was excised.

The lesion was, apart from an occasional minute focus of junctional activity, an 'intradermal naevus' but uncertainty was noted about the future behaviour or prognostic significance of "tumour cells (that) penetrate rather deeply around skin appendages". However, the lesion had been completely excised and the naevus cells were in general uniform, not hyperchromatic and rarely in mitosis (no mitotic figures were seen in the whole of two sections). The recent enlargement could be correlated with a prominent subjacent granulomatous inflammatory reaction which had developed over a relatively large area into a frank abscess.

The patient was trouble-free 20 years later. The diagnosis and expression of caution still seem *appropriate*.

### Case 7.6

F (72 years) with pigmented spot on cheek, first noticed 1 year earlier and slowly growing since.

The lesion, an 8-mm warty nodule well cleared by the line of excision, was a mass of close-packed naevus cells, often streaming directly from a very ill-defined basal layer but nowhere reaching any deeper than the most superficial sweat glands. The cells were moderately polymorphic with a maximum incidence of mitoses in a few areas of 3 per hpf.

The epidermis showed prominent basal hyperpigmentation for some 3 mm beyond the edge of the cellular mass, while the peripheral 1 mm showed basal loosening or fraying that amounted virtually to junctional change. The epidermis was prominently hyperkeratotic. Nowhere was it being significantly invaded by migrating melanocytic or naevus cells, nor was it ulcerated.

In assessing the significance of the appearances, weighting had to be given, on the one side, to the polymorphism and mitotic activity of the naevus cells, and the presence of so much junctional activity around the margin, and, on the other, to the superficial location and lack of both ulceration and invasion of the epidermis.

A middle course was chosen: "If not a frank melanocarcinoma, this is certainly a 'highly active melanonaevus'. It has (apparently) been removed completely but whether metastasis may or may not have occurred is extremely difficult to assess . . . prognosis should be somewhat cautious".

No further treatment was given. There was no local recurrence, the area remaining healthy, as did the patient, until death from cerebral vascular disease some 8 years later.

This was perhaps an example of *underdiagnosis*; the lesion should perhaps have been diagnosed as an early melanocarcinoma developing in a lentigo maligna. No harm ensued, however.

### Case 7.7

F (70 years) with 10-mm dark plaque on cheek existing for 1 year. Biopsy was followed by the expected total excision.

The lesion comprised multifocal masses of variably pigmented or nonpigmented cells in the upper dermis though nowhere reaching deeper than hair follicles, and in many places in direct continuity with a notably open-work 'junctional change' type of basal layer. The clusters of cells varied in size and were sometimes separated by stretches of rather hyperpigmented but otherwise normal epidermis.

Figure 7.1 shows the edge of the lesion:

a) The basal layer of the epidermis is ill-defined over the lesion.

b) The dermis (right) is largely collagenous, otherwise (left) it appears highly cellular due to a mixture of large irregularly shaped pigment-bearing cells superficially, packed lymphocytes at the deep edge, and generally uniform pale cells elsewhere.

Figure 7.2 shows the open-work character of the basal layer, the large pigment-bearing cells and the background sheet of smaller, paler, nucleated cells.

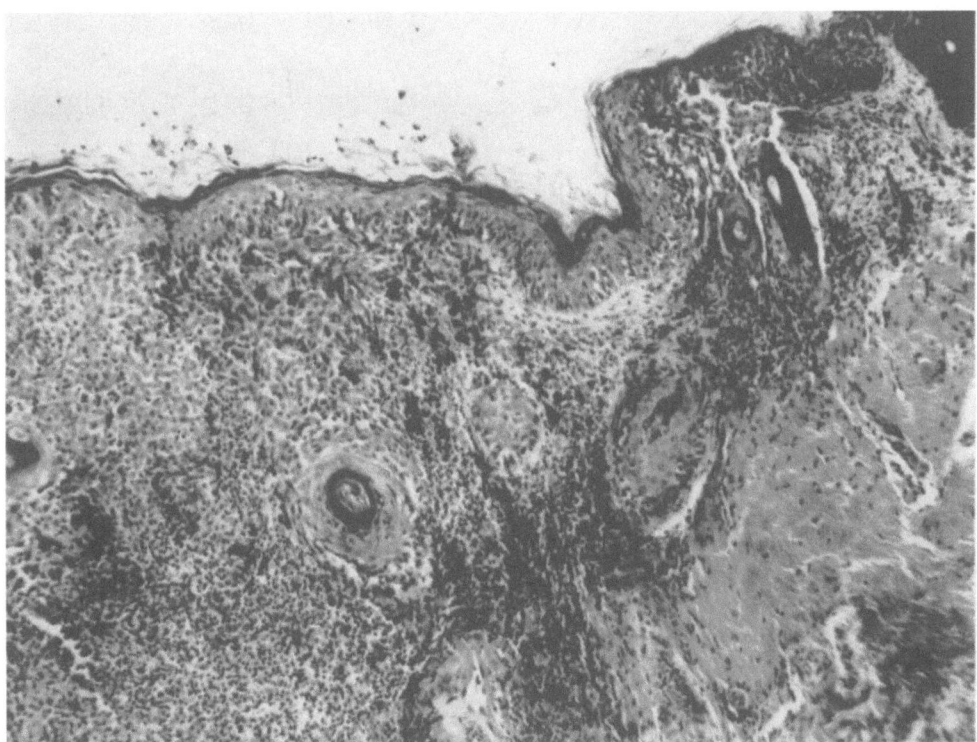

**Fig. 7.1.** See text. The lesion is clearly outlined by massed lymphocytes around the right-hand edge. H & E, × 123

Figure 7.3 shows the moderate degree of polymorphism and occasional mitotic figures, present, on average, at one per 20 hpf. Virtually every nucleus contained a 'red nucleolus'.

The lesion was reported as a 'compound melanonaevus', not malignant but almost certainly incompletely removed. No further excision, however, was performed.

The patient reappeared 18 years later. There had been slow growth of a dark patch at the same site ever since the original excision. The histological pattern of the now fully excised lesion was that of a frank melanocarcinoma. The patient died within the next 2 years, aged nearly 90, not from melanocarcinoma but from an unrelated cause. With little doubt the original lesion was at the least a lentigo maligna and could well have been diagnosed in some clinics as even then having become a frank melanocarcinoma. This, therefore, was an *under-diagnosis*. Whether total excision on the original occasion would have prevented its reappearance as an unequivocal melanocarcinoma 18 years later is speculative. At any rate, the outcome of events allowed the behaviour to be noted fortuitously over this relatively long period.

*Case 7.8*

F (59 years) with a 10-mm pigmented patch on the face, duration uncertain, considered clinically to be lentigo maligna.

Figures 7.4 and 7.5 show the essential abnormality, the loosened frayed appearance of the basal epidermis. The material received was a biopsy only, not the whole lesion, although the biopsy did in fact comprise most of the pigmented area.

These changes, though present throughout most of the biopsy, were nowhere more severe than this and the decision taken at the time was to designate the lesion as a 'junctional naevus', not lentigo maligna.

A point of prognostic interest was that in several places well-pigmented melanocytes were present (as individual cells rather than clusters) at all levels throughout the epidermis; they were even being desquamated either as still recognisably nucleated cells or as pigmented squames.

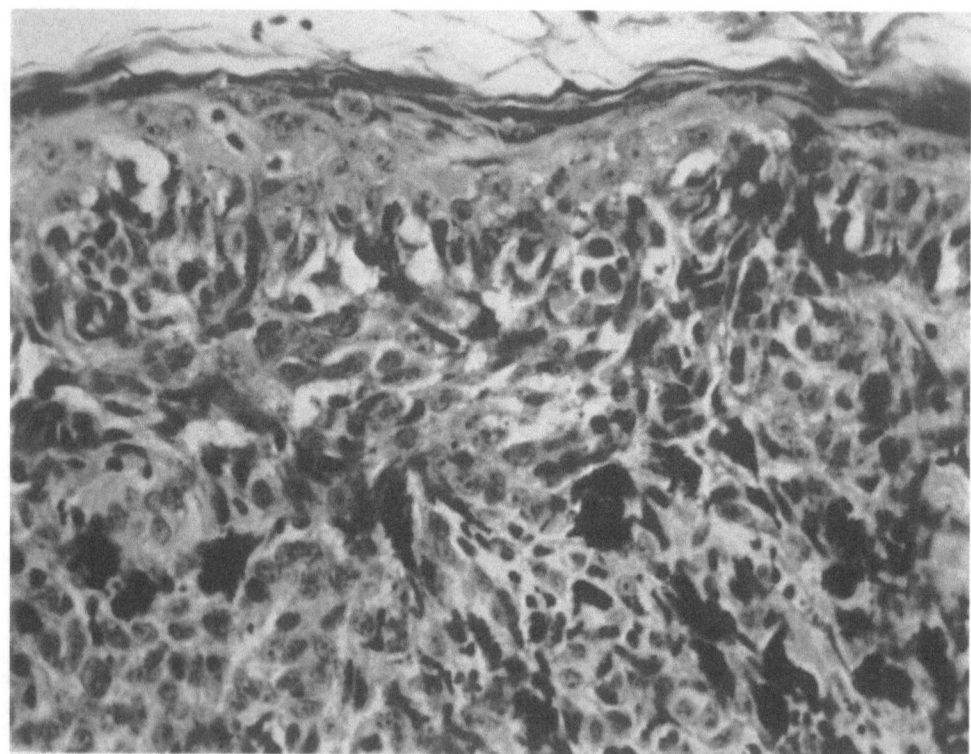

**Fig. 7.2.** See text. With cells as heavily pigmented as this, it is difficult to distinguish between melanophores and melanocytes. H & E, × 493

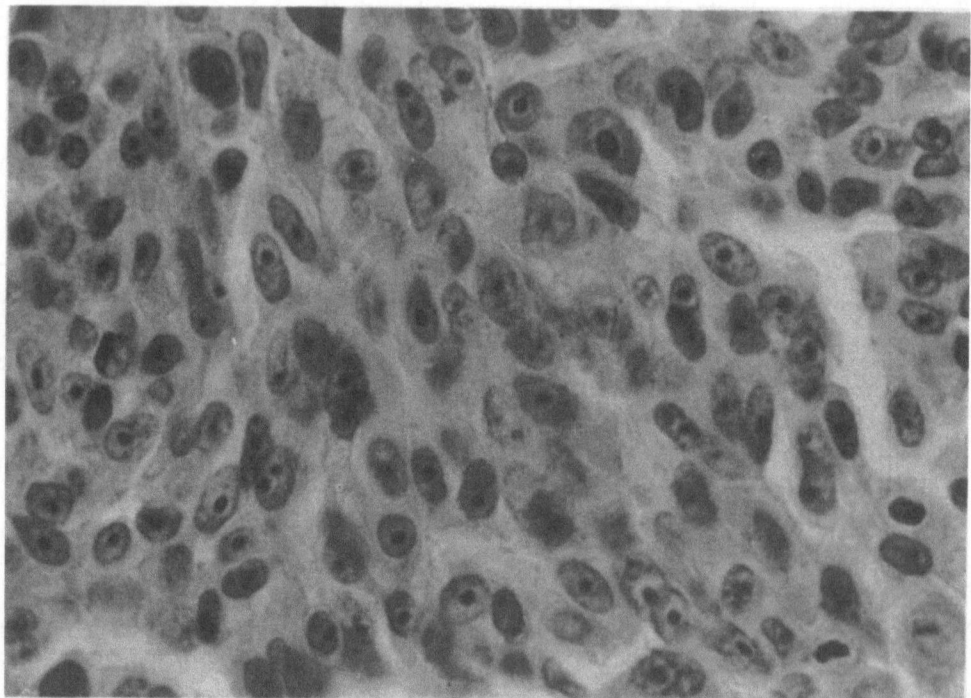

**Fig. 7.3.** See text. One cell here, lower right-hand corner, is in mitosis. The cells in Case 7.22, in which the patient died within 4 years, were remarkably similar to these. H & E, × 792

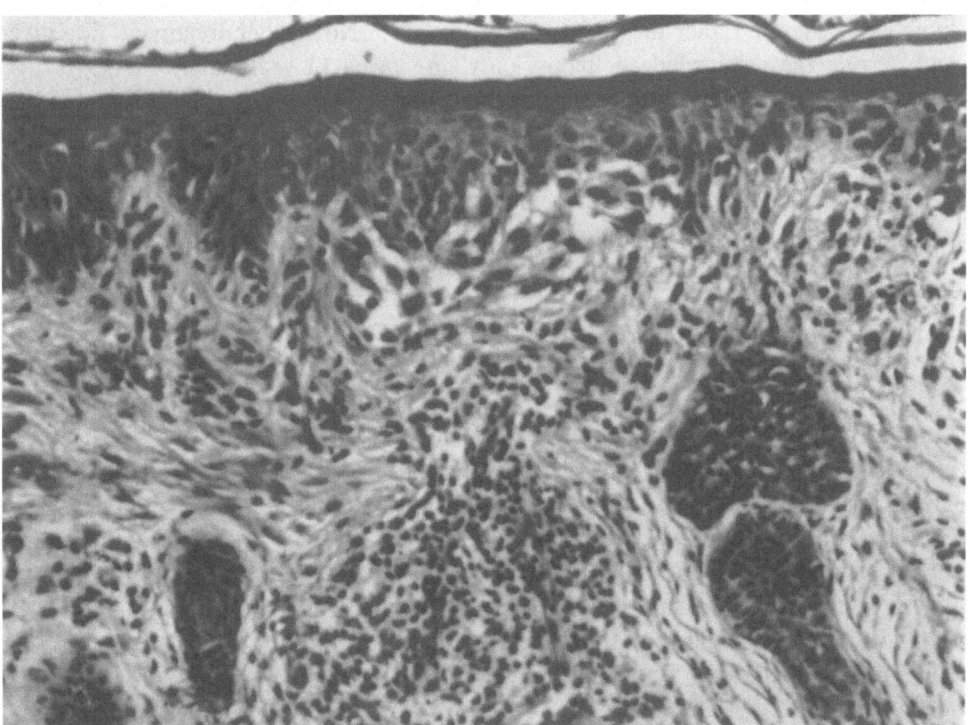

**Fig. 7.4.** The epidermis is obviously loosened along its lower margin, the appearance interpreted as amounting to junctional change. H & E, × 238

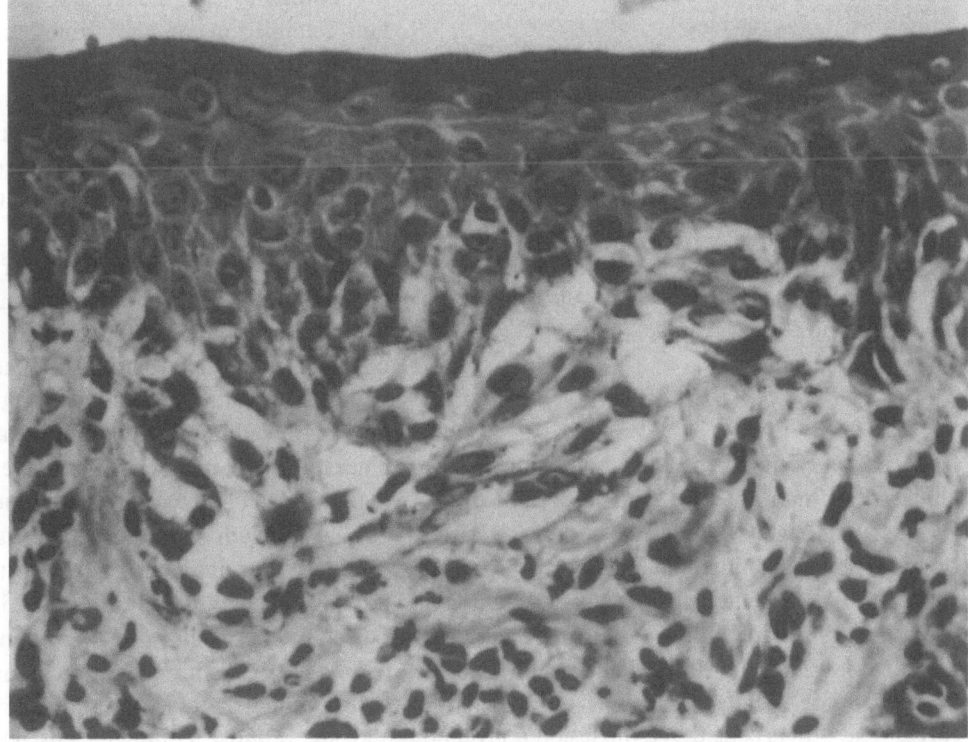

**Fig. 7.5.** Occasional, rather clearer cells within the epidermis appear to be mildly aberrant melanocytes making their way towards the surface. H & E, × 493

In view of the histological preference for 'junctional naevus' rather than 'lentigo maligna', and despite the acknowledged 'biopsy-only' incompleteness of excision, it was not further excised.

The patient reappeared 7 years later with evidently recurrent growth of pigmented tissue at the original site. This was completely excised, the specimen now showing more typically the features of a 'lentigo maligna'. The features were considered insufficiently aberrant to warrant diagnosis as melanocarcinoma. There was no sign of recurrence 3 years later.

In retrospect, the lesion should probably have been designated lentigo maligna at the outset. The original designation was an *under-diagnosis*. However, the decision that was taken allowed an opportunity to observe the later behaviour of incompletely excised tissue, and to assess the significance of permeation or 'invasion' of the epidermis by the at least mildly aberrant melanocytes.

### Case 7.9

F (34 years) with 10-mm nodule on forehead, growing slowly since its appearance three years previously; thought to be sebaceous cyst: "has numerous moles on face".

Histology showed the pattern of an 'intradermal naevus', almost certainly transected at one edge. This was mentioned in the report but no further excision was performed.

The area was healthy 3 months later, and the patient did not report again. The diagnosis was correct and *appropriate*. Such remnant naevus cells as there may have been would appear to have given no further trouble.

### Case 7.10

F (10 years) referred by school doctor for advice re 10-mm mole on outer aspect of thigh.

This was a highly cellular naevus characterised by widespread junctional change, polymorphism, spindle-cell and, much less frequent, giant-cell formation. Some pathologists, having examined the sections blind, considered the lesion one to be treated for practical purposes as a melanocarcinoma; others considered the lesion a juvenile melanoma; others a highly cellular spindle-form of compound naevus.

The diagnosis issued was 'juvenile melanoma'. No further treatment was given, and all was well 11 years later.

Those who had examined the sections not knowing of the patient's age and had considered the lesion benign, had done so mainly on the basis of scarcity of mitoses (on average two per whole section) and relative lack of hyperchromatism. The preferred diagnosis was *appropriate*.

### Case 7.11

F (45 years) with mole under chin gradually increasing in size for 5 years: it was received as a 12 × 6 × 6 mm nodule in the substance of a 4 × 1 cm ellipse of skin.

As seen in Fig. 7.6, the lesion comprised a moderately well circumscribed, almost spherical mass of variably pigmented cells lying in the subcutaneous fat but connected by a broad band or tract of similar though less numerous cells to the deep surface of the epidermis. It is the blunt summit of this broad band of cells that forms the bulge on the surface and flattening of the epidermal pegs.

Figure 7.7 shows the high cellularity of the deeper part of the tumour. The cells have a predominantly spindle-shaped nucleus and outline reminiscent of the 'blue' naevus, with a uniformity of pattern and scarcity of mitoses suggesting a less than highly aggressive nature. As may be seen, melanin is abundant though varying within cells from nil to enough to obscure the nucleus and most of the cytoplasm completely.

Figure 7.8 shows part of one of several areas of junctional change. The melanocytes, again of notably spindle-shaped outline, appear to be migrating into the dermis from the basal layer. Also, however, they are 'migrating upwards' into or invading the epidermis, and in a few places were being desquamated either as still-recognisable cells or as remnant melanin.

The problem here was to assess the significance, on the one hand, of the history of steady growth, the high cellularity, deep ingrowth, and especially permeation or invasion of the epidermis by aberrant melanin-containing cells, and, on the other, the essential uniformity of the cells and the almost complete absence of mitoses (some slides showed not one in the whole section).

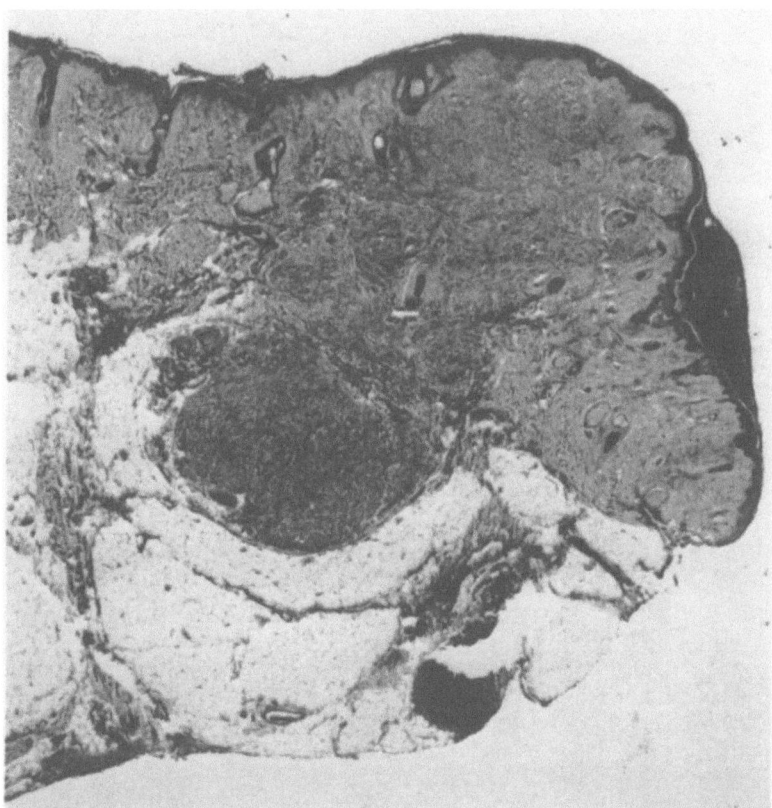

**Fig. 7.6.** See text. The main mass of abnormal cells lies within the dermis but extends obliquely upwards and to the right to the epidermis. H & E, × 15

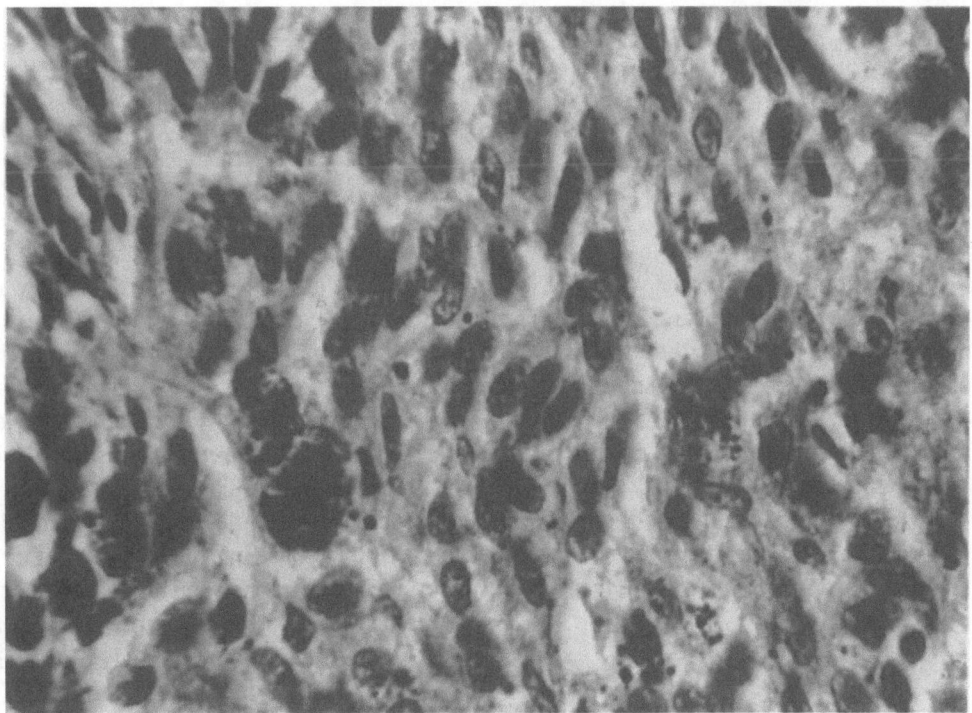

**Fig. 7.7.** See text. Relatively close-packed, spindle-shaped cells, variably pigmented and not unduly polymorphic. H & E, × 493

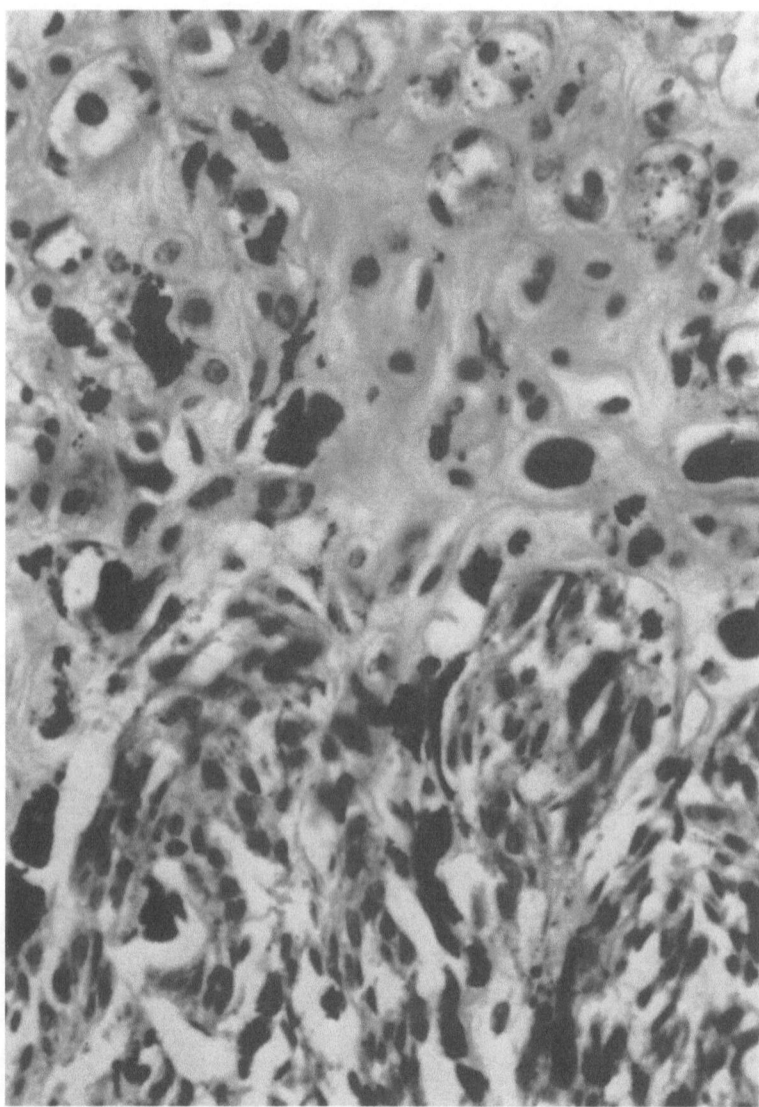

**Fig. 7.8.** See text. The permeation of the epidermis by aberrant melanocytes is evident. H & E, × 526

The lesion was reported as "For practical purposes . . . a melanocarcinoma" though with an added comment that the evidently adequate clearance might well prove sufficient treatment.

No further treatment was given, the area remained trouble-free, and was still so 8 years later.

In retrospect this can be designated with fair assurance as a 'Spitz naevus' of almost purely spindle-celled type. This was an *over-diagnosis*.

### Case 7.12

F (64 years) who was noted incidentally, while undergoing unrelated treatment, to have a 10-mm pigmented nodule on the wrist of uncertain, but of at least years' duration. It was diagnosed, clinically, as probably a blue naevus.

The only doubt raised by this lesion was on the significance of its high cellularity. It was examined initially without knowledge of the clinically favoured diagnosis and considered in fact, mainly because of a strikingly uniform cell pattern and fine diffuse pigmentation, to be a 'cellular blue naevus' (CBN) rather than an unusually compact and highly cellular intradermal naevus of orthodox type. There was no 'junctional' change and, in many of the whole sections examined, not a single mitotic figure.

The area was healthy when the patient was last seen (with cerebral vascular disease) 4 years later.

This was a fairly characteristic example of a CBN as described by Rodriguez and Ackerman (1968). The exceptions from their list of common features were patterns in many places that were appreciably epithelioid, and absence both of 'neuroid structures' and anything more than the mildest fasciculation. The diagnosis was *appropriate*.

### Case 7.13

F (43 years) with a 8-mm pedunculated nodule on side of nose; it had slowly grown over several years.

The bulk of the lesion was a mass of rather loose-textured, finely fibrillar and mildly oedematous fibrous tissue (Fig. 7.9). It showed two main abnormalities:

a) Many relatively large clear cells in the basal layers, one of which seemed very possibly to be in tri-polar mitosis (Fig. 7.10); also, there were scattered foci of loosened cell pattern closely similar to and perhaps quite truly 'junctional change' (Fig. 7.11).

b) Population of the stroma of the nodule by scattered multinucleated giant cells, most numerous in the subepidermal zone but present throughout (Fig. 7.9).

Without the epidermal changes the lesion would be acceptable with little question as a form of histiocytoma, and the giant cells, with their frequently peripherally placed nuclei, as of Touton type. However, the presence of unduly many and prominent cells of apparently melanocytic type, and of at any rate focal 'junctional change' of some kind, raised the question whether the lesion was essentially naeval or neuronaeval in type, the giant cells being multinucleated naevus cells, and the stroma representing the fibrous element of a neurofibromatoid overgrowth. It was reported as a 'neuronaevus'.

No further treatment was advised and the patient was well and trouble-free 7 years later.

Review of the sections suggests that the lesion was probably a 'histiocytoma' but the nature of the epidermal change remains uncertain; it may be no more than an expression of spongiosis and hydropic cell change in epidermis subject to repeated mild trauma (it had doubtless been powdered on countless occasions). Whether the apparent triaster was only that or was truly a mitotic figure remains unresolved; if it was truly

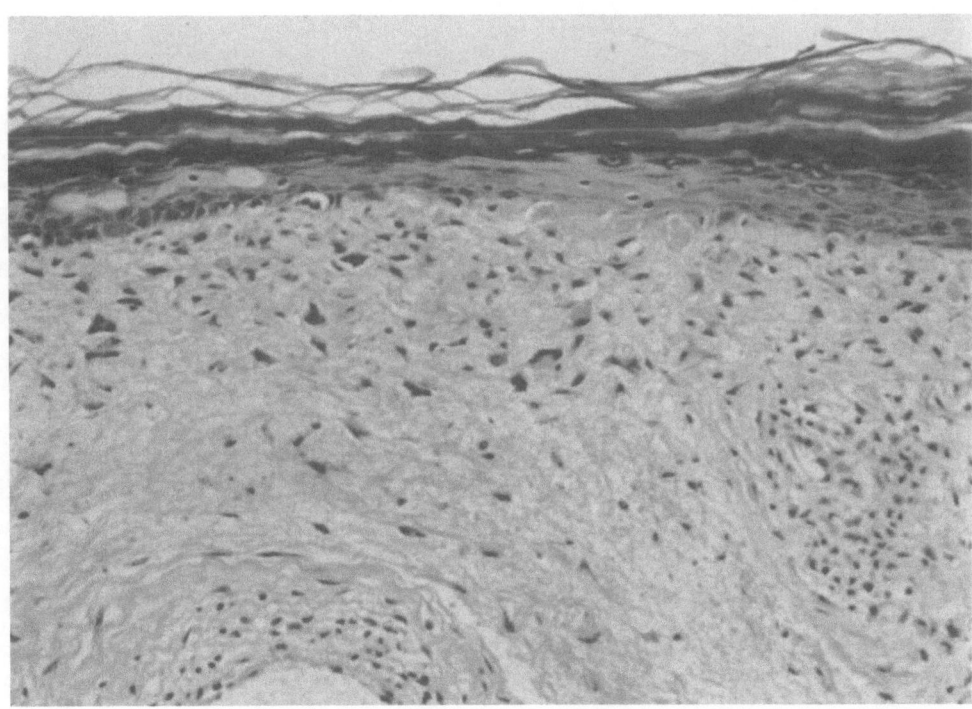

**Fig. 7.9.** See text. The larger masses in the upper dermis are multinucleated giant cells. H & E, × 176

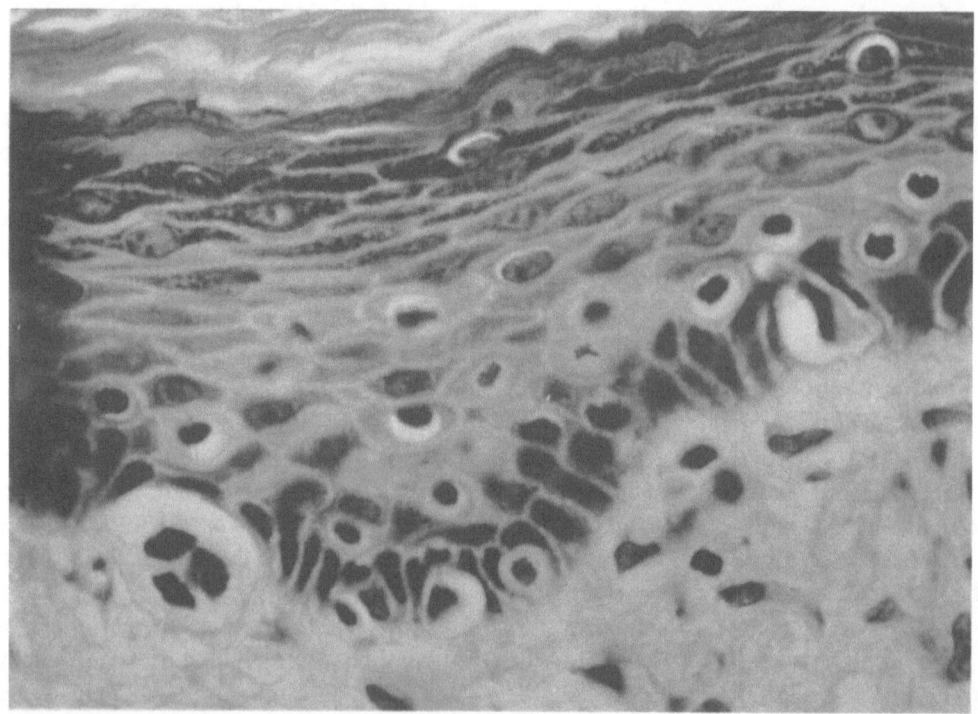

**Fig. 7.10.** See text. To the left is what appears to be a triaster mitotic figure. H & E, × 792

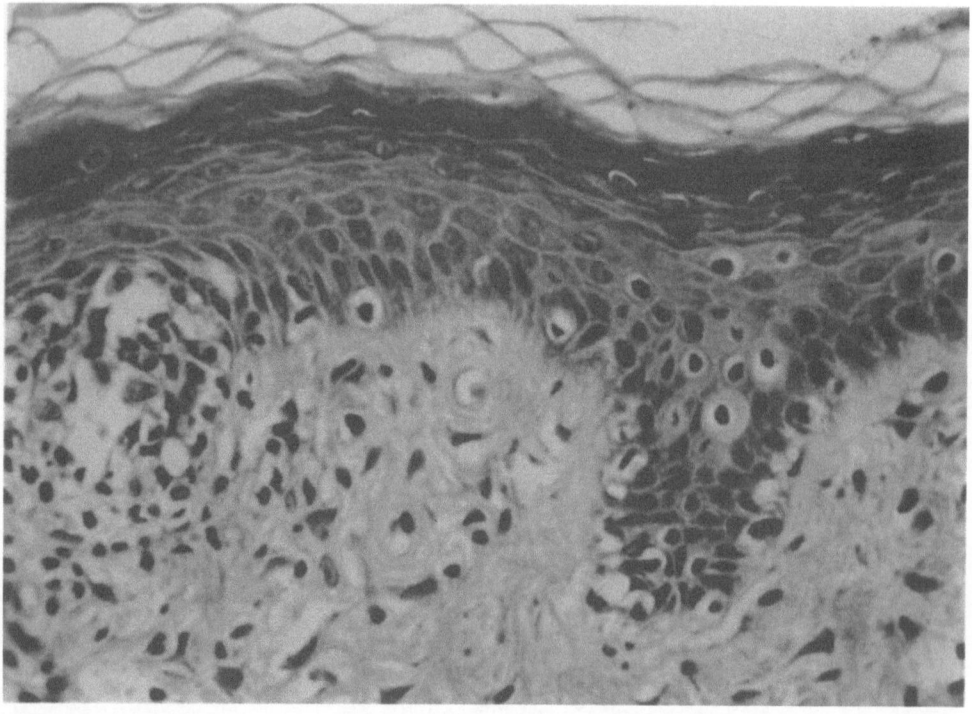

**Fig. 7.11.** Many hydropic cells are present in the basal layer. There is also, on the left, an area of what appears to be junctional change. H & E, × 432

an aberrant mitotic figure it had no ominous significance. The preferred diagnosis was probably *inappropriate* albeit harmlessly so.

### Case 7.14

M ('43 years) with small warty growth of 'some weeks' duration on roof of mouth at junction of hard and soft palates. Biopsy produced three fragments, the largest 5 mm across.

The largest fragment was a simple squamous papilloma sharing no feature in common with the relatively complex structure in the other two fragments. In these, the composition was of: (a) many small glandular acini within epithelium in direct continuity with the stratified squamous covering (Fig. 7.12); (b) swathes of melanin-containing cells, often heavily pigmented and of spindle shape. Some of the glandular cells contained mucin, a few contained melanin. It was regarded as "a naevus of some kind" and probably innocuous but its evidently incomplete removal was reported.

The area has remained trouble-free for 14 years, and to that extent the diagnosis was *appropriate*. However, the nature of the lesion remains uncertain. The melanin-containing cells appeared to be an integral part of the mass which could otherwise have been accepted as a simple salivary adenoma. The speculation remains that it may have some kinship with the melanotic epulis of infancy (Borello and Gorlin, 1966).

(This lesion, though not in skin, was considered more suitable for assessment in the present section than with lesions of the digestive tract.)

### Case 7.15

F (55 years) with 'pigmented mole' on right calf. The line of excision had achieved clearance by 5 to 10 mm.

Microscopy showed the lesion to be in essence a 10 × 2-mm disc of malignant cells covered, except for 4 mm of ulceration, by intact epidermis. It lay well above the sweat glands and even above a line joining the deepest-lying hair follicles at its margins.

Figure 7.13 shows several features of possible prognostic significance:

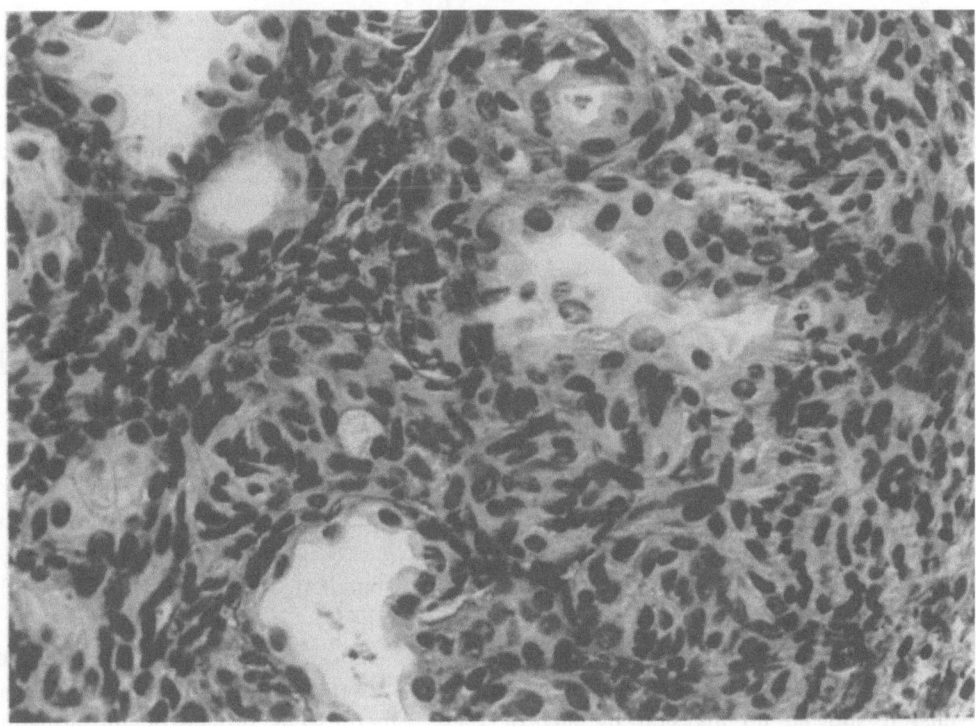

**Fig. 7.12.** Glandular acini with generally pale epithelium. Some of the epithelial cells contained mucin; others contained a sprinkling of melanin. Stromal cells elsewhere contained abundant melanin. H & E, × 493

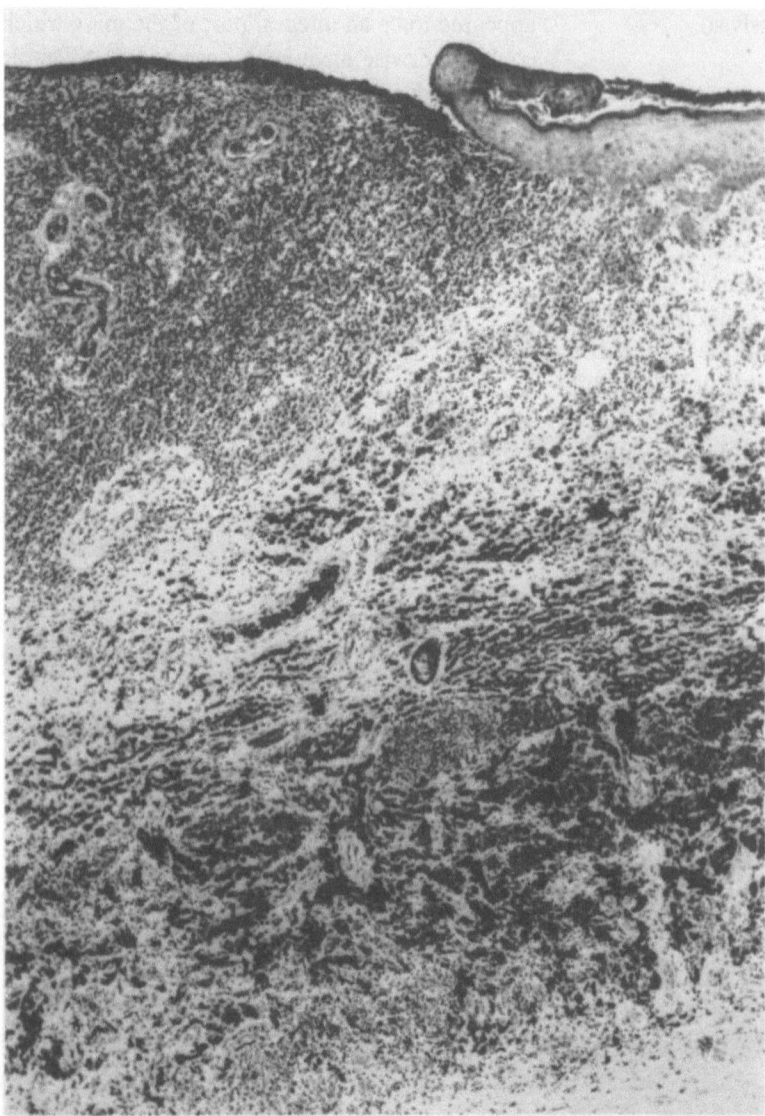

**Fig. 7.13.** See text. This shows the two different types of cell population: (a) relatively uniform and nonpigmented superficially, (b) polymorphic and pigmented in the lower dermis. H & E, × 66

a) There are two distinct cell populations, one superficial and composed of cells that were only moderately polymorphic but quite frequently in mitosis (3 per hpf) and only rarely pigmented, the other deep to this and composed of slightly larger and less polymorphic cells almost all heavily pigmented and only rarely in mitosis.

b) Although the epidermis was widely undermined by the pigmented cells and also, though to a much lesser extent, by the nonpigmented cells, it showed no invasion by any of these cells and not even any 'junctional' change.

c) Lymphocytic infiltration is considerable amongst the deeper pigmented cells, but almost completely absent amongst the superficial nonpigmented cells.

Figures 7.14 and 7.15 show, respectively, representative fields from the two cell populations described above: polymorphism, relatively small size, absence of melanin but mitotic activity in the one; relatively uniformity, larger size, abundant melanin and scanty mitoses in the other.

The lesion amply fulfilled the cytological criteria for a diagnosis of 'melanocarcinoma' but there were prognostically hopeful features in the notably superficial location, the apparent completeness of excision, the relatively small amount of ulceration and the absence of junc-

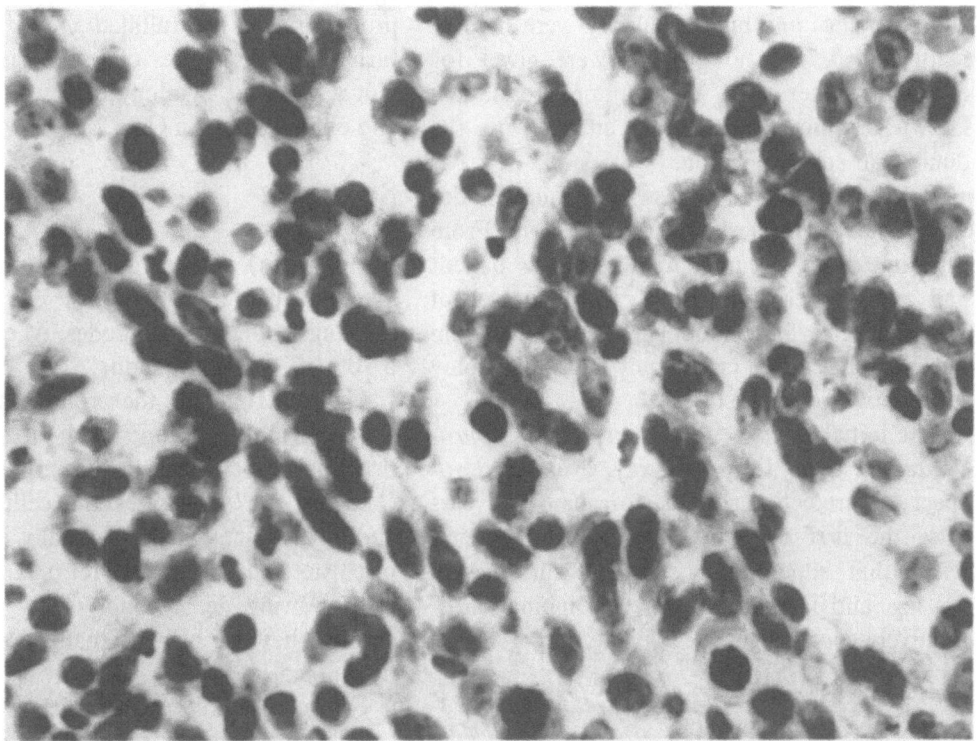

**Fig. 7.14.** Cells of population (a): moderately polymorphic and sometimes in mitosis; there are three mitotic figures here, top left, just below centre, and lower right. H & E, × 985

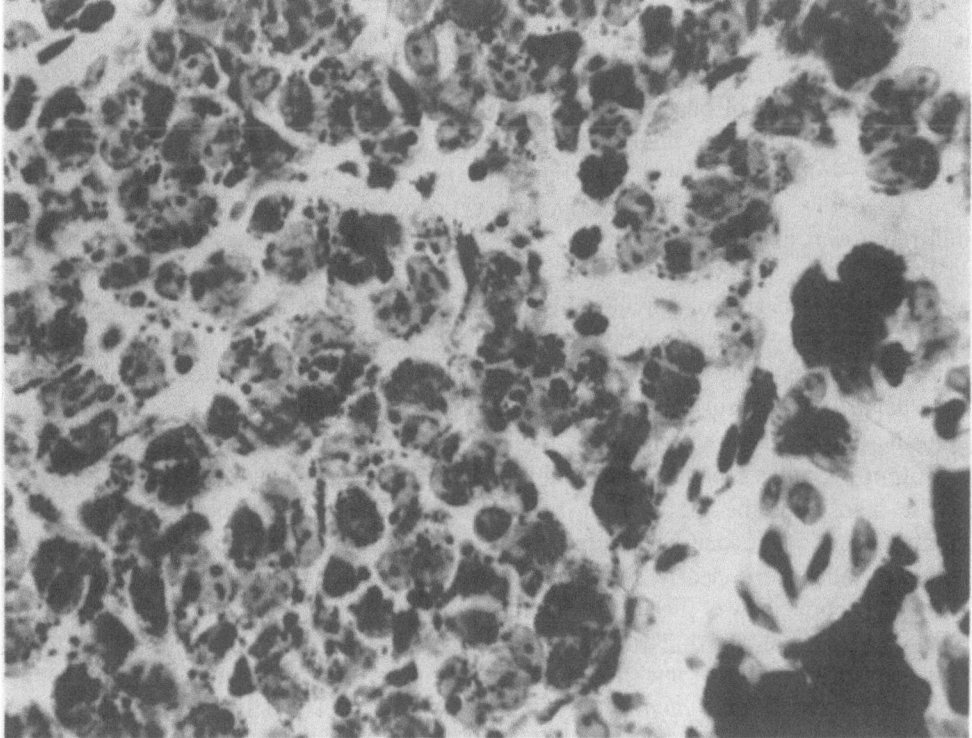

**Fig. 7.15.** Cells of population (b): larger and quite heavily pigmented. H & E, × 985

tional change elsewhere. However, the cytological characteristics and high cellularity were held to matter most, and no grounds were given for expecting other than a poor prognosis. No known significance could be attached to the dimorphic cell population.

Three years later, a mass of invaded nodes was removed from the inguinal region. From this time, for 9 years until death, the patient had many operations, mostly for removal of recurrent growths in the leg, thigh and groin but including also a craniotomy and laparotomy for removal of metastases.

The initial assessment was correct and *appropriate* but there seems no way, even in retrospect, of predicting survival for some 12 years after the first excision except in the general terms that superficial location, occurrence in the leg, and femaleness form a combination of relatively good prognosis.

### Case 7.16

F (45 years) with pigmented nodule on left ankle noticed 'for about 20 years', but slowly enlarging over past year: excision of dark, slightly raised plaque of 12 mm in diameter and 4 mm maximum depth: area grafted.

Cytologically there was little doubt that the lesion was a 'melanocarcinoma': it was highly cellular and moderately polymorphic, showed a mitotic frequency of one per hpf and permeation of the epidermis by malignant cells to the stage of desquamation though not frank ulceration (but this was imminent). Lymphocytic infiltration was almost negligible.

To offset this, however, in terms of prognostic assessment, the degree of polymorphism was, as stated, only moderate; no aberrant mitotic figures were seen; and the lesion was relatively superficial, the deep surface reaching no deeper than the uppermost sweat glands.

Within 7 months a small nodule had appeared at the margin of the graft. After a further 5 months (one year since the initial operation) inguinal nodes were clearly abnormal; excision and microscopy showed melanocarcinoma in all of the six nodes obtained. Two months later the patient died with signs of intracranial metastasis. The diagnosis was thus *appropriate*. The hope that the combination of female sex, site, superficiality and absence of mitotic aberrancy might

again, as in the previous case, indicate a good prognosis was not fulfilled. Also, to emphasise further the difficulties of prognosis in the individual case, the cytology here was less aberrant and ominous than in Case 7.15.

### Case 7.17

F (34 years) with pigmented nodule on upper anterior thigh for 9 months: there was 'slight swelling' of the inguinal nodes. At excision it was a $10 \times 7 \times 2$ mm plaque.

Figure 7.16 shows the prominently superficial situation of the lesion: none of it lies deeper than the deepest level of the original epidermis.

Figure 7.17 illustrates the cellularity of the abnormal tissue and its generally large alveolar or clustered architecture. Not only are abnormal cells growing deeply and widely into the epidermis, they are being actually desquamated or discharged.

Figure 7.18 represents fairly the degree of cellularity and polymorphism: neither is extreme. Where cytoplasmic outline was visible, cells were in equal proportion round and spindle-shaped. Some 5% of cells contained melanin. Mitotic figures were moderately frequent, one per 3 hpf, and none atypical. The pyknotic nuclei at the right edge and lower left are in mitosis.

As in Case 7.11 the histological evidence was equivocal. The invasion and, indeed, ulceration of the epidermis indicated aggressive malignancy. The notably superficial location, the wholly exophytic manner of growth and absence of aberrant mitoses indicated a much lesser degree of malignancy to the point when even highly activated naevus was entertained as a possible diagnosis. Spitz naevus was also seriously considered but rejected mainly because of absence of both telangiectasia and giant cells. Scattered foci of lymphocytes along the deep surface, mostly at the periphery but in more central areas also, supported the diagnosis of melanocarcinoma rather than Spitz naevus.

In practice, the lesion was diagnosed as 'melanocarcinoma' with an added comment that the adequate excision the lesion had evidently had was almost certainly also adequate treatment. The 'slightly swollen' inguinal nodes were not explored.

The patient reappeared 4 years after the

excision with a small, slightly dark swelling at the site of excision. It was found to be a mildly keloidal scar. She was known to be trouble-free 4 years later still.

The sections from the lesion have by now been seen by several pathologists, and almost all have diagnosed an unequivocal melanocarcinoma. A few have had a degree of reservation but concluded that for practical purposes the diagnosis would have to be melanocarcinoma. To this extent the diagnosis may fairly be judged *appropriate*.

### Case 7.18

F (35 years) with a 15-mm pigmented mass over mid-calf; it had increased in size during a recent pregnancy.

Sections showed a mainly exophytic mass that did not extend so deeply as to reach sweat glands. It was nevertheless highly cellular.

Figure 7.19 shows the high cellularity and the ulcerated surface; almost the whole of the surface was ulcerated. The relatively large black foci are deposits of melanin; it is a rather scantily pigmented lesion.

Figure 7.20 shows the quite highly cellular character of the lesion and the large alveolar-type pattern. The frequency of lymphocytes is fairly representative of the lesion as a whole.

Figure 7.21. No area was more polymorphic than this. Mitotic figures, of which one is included here, were moderately numerous at 1 per 4 hpf.

The high cellularity and presence of ulceration, with mitotic figures at the quoted incidence, favoured a diagnosis of 'melanocarcinoma', and this was the diagnosis given. However, the mainly exophytic character of the growth, and the fact that the absolute depth of penetration of the dermis was not great, led to advice that the evidently complete excision might be adequate treatment.

No further treatment was given and the patient was alive and trouble-free 17 years later.

No other diagnosis than melanocarcinoma would have been justified, and the diagnosis still seems *appropriate*, but the mild qualification induced by the superficial location was equally justified by events.

### Case 7.19

F (42 years) with pigmented nodule on calf since birth, often injured, recently 'pecked by hen' with much bleeding: excision of ellipse

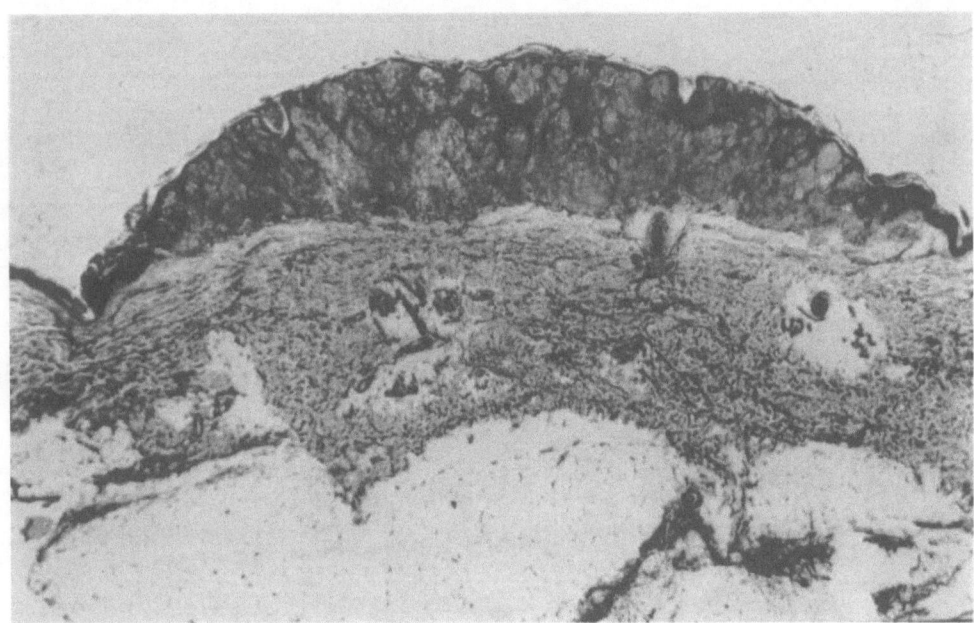

**Fig. 7.16.** Shows the superficial location of the mass. H & E, × 13

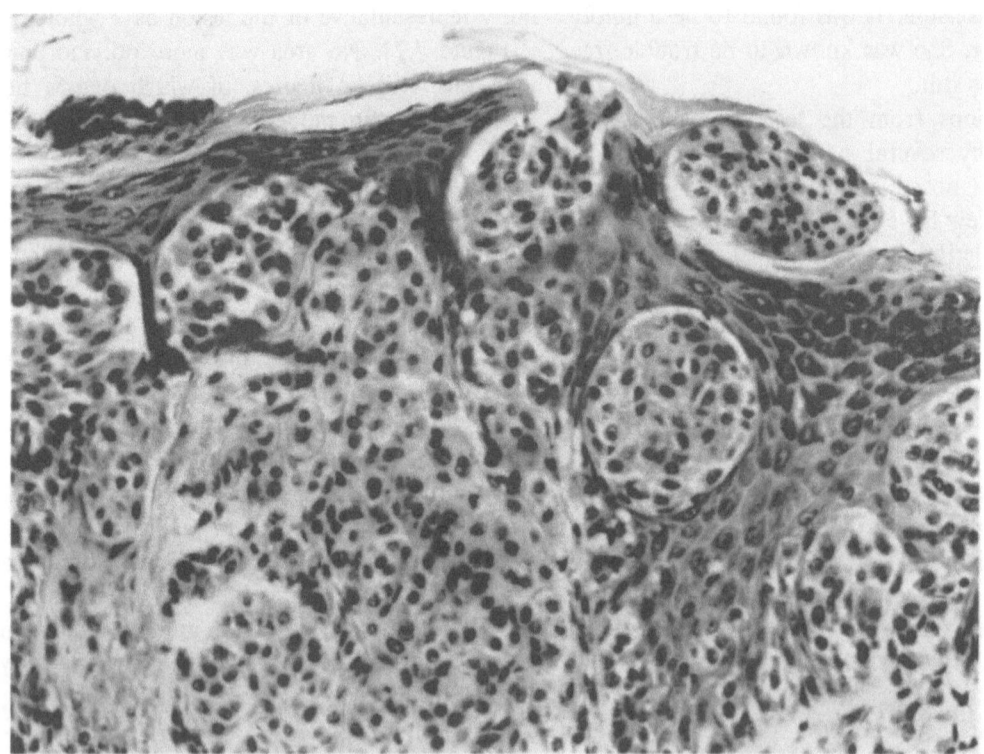

**Fig. 7.17.** The epidermis is widely permeated and in some places perforated by aberrant naevus cells. H & E, × 246

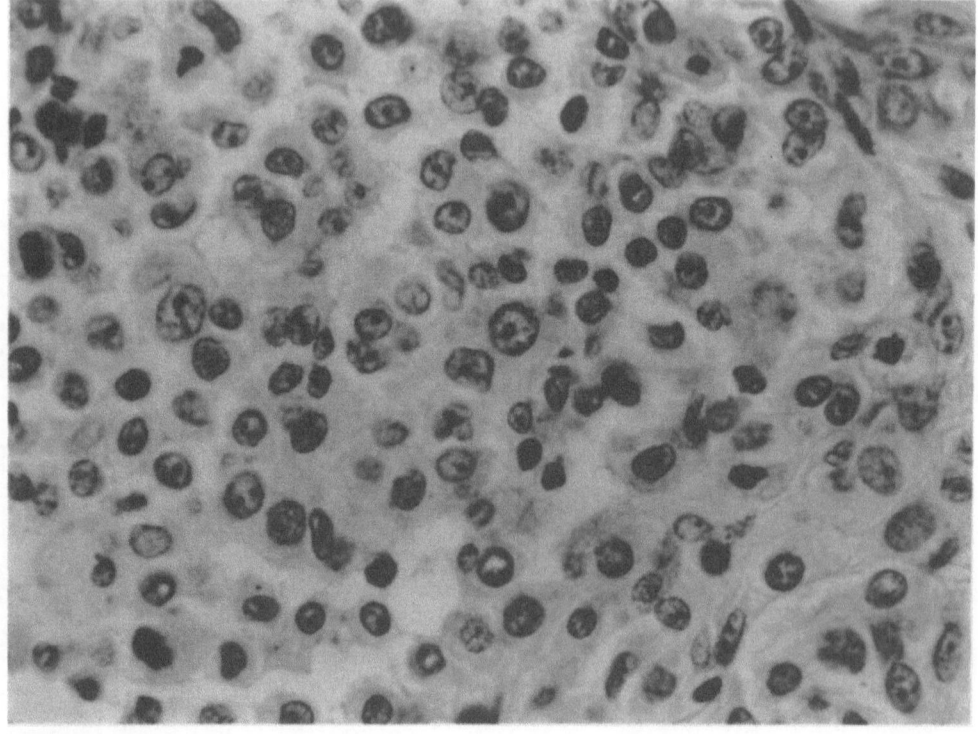

**Fig. 7.18.** See text, H & E, × 740

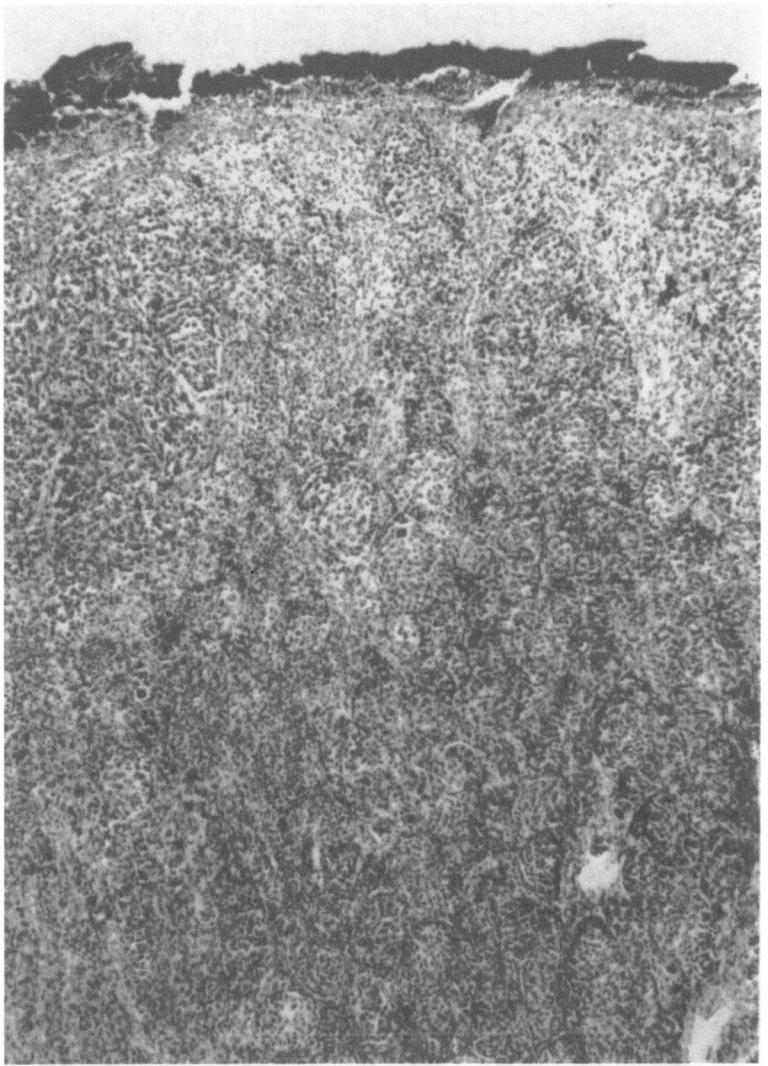

**Fig. 7.19.** See text. H & E, × 66

bearing flattened pigmented nodule 13 × 11 × 2 mm: excision apparently complete.

In general, the pattern was that of a highly cellular compound naevus with junctional change along its whole length and thinning of the epidermis throughout with ulceration over 5 mm. The naevus cells were notably polymorphic in the upper third of the mass but much more uniform in the lower two-thirds. They had penetrated deeply enough to surround the most superficial adnexa but no further. Mitotic figures were present but fewer than 1 per 10 hpf. Pigment was plentiful. Subjacent lymphocytic accumulation was scanty; infiltration amongst the mass of cells even less conspicuous.

Factors suggesting malignancy were the high cellularity, the extent of the junctional change, the ulceration and, particularly, the marked polymorphism in the superficial layers. For these reasons the lesion was diagnosed as "for practical purposes, melanocarcinoma". However, the scarcity of mitoses and the completeness of the excision were held to be prognostically favourable.

No further treatment was given, and the patient was well, having had no associated complications, 15 years later. In retrospect the diagnosis still seems *appropriate*. The features were not really those of a Spitz naevus.

## Case 7.20

F (24 years) presented with lump, ? wart, on the left calf, of 3 years' duration during which,

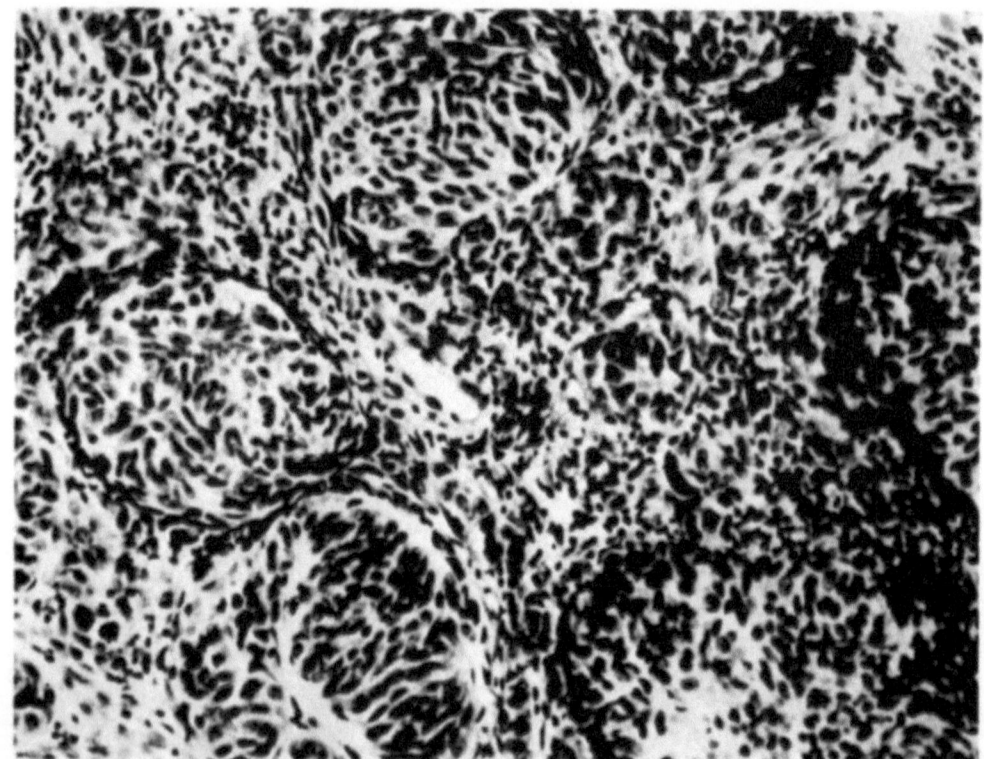

**Fig. 7.20.** The small dark nuclei, lymphocytes, are moderately numerous throughout. H & E, × 140

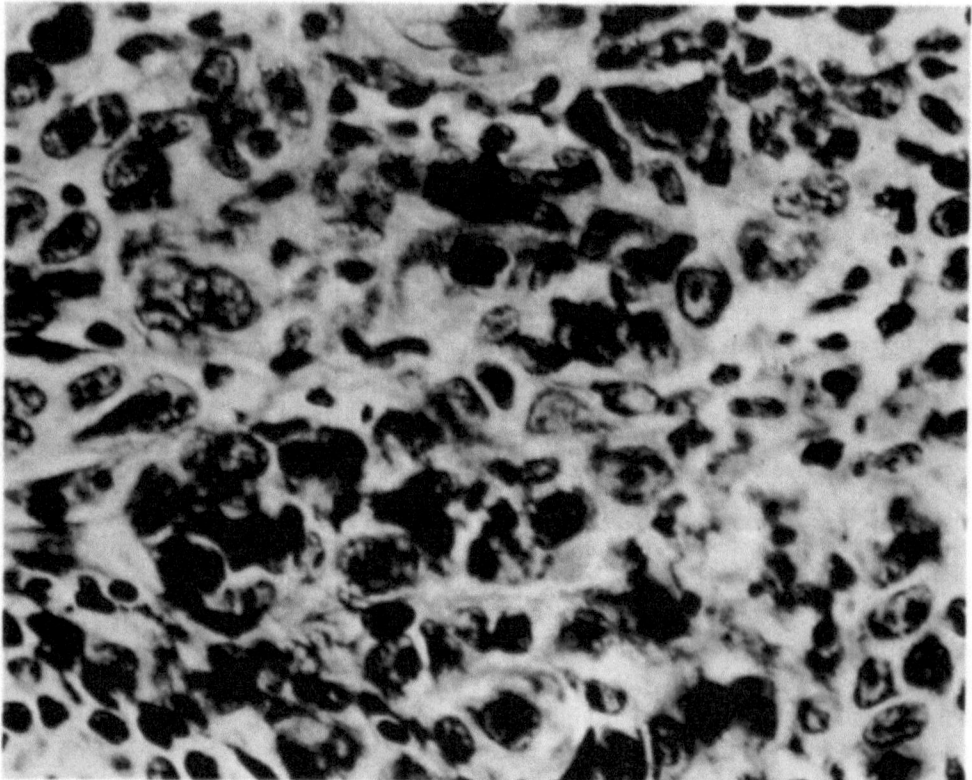

**Fig. 7.21.** Shows the mildly polymorphic though not hyperchromatic cells, and a mitotic figure upper centre. H & E, × 850

incidentally, it had received three applications of $CO_2$ snow.

Excision provided a 25 × 20 × 10 mm smooth, centrally ulcerated, reniform lump within a 50 × 40-mm ellipse of skin with subcutaneous tissue. The cut surface was firm, solid and pale pink.

Figure 7.22 shows the general pattern, a highly cellular spindle-celled neoplasm occupying the full depth of the dermis and flattening the epidermis. Here, as virtually throughout, the deep surface of the epidermis was smooth and uninterrupted except for the already mentioned area of ulceration and occasional relatively minute areas, involving no more than 10–20 cells in the 6-$\mu$m section where neoplastic cells

and basal cells merged. These seemed much more likely to be foci of early epidermal invasion by the neoplasm than foci of either junctional change or spindle-celled squamous carcinoma. Subcutaneous fat was being widely permeated by the neoplasm.

Figure 7.23 illustrates the notably whorled arrangement in many areas, particularly at the deeper levels. The darker plexiform area just below centre is reminiscent of Masson's neuroid structures.

Figures 7.24 and 7.25 are representative of the considerable polymorphism present almost throughout. In the centre of Fig. 7.25 is a pyknotic triaster, only one of many aberrant mitotic figures throughout the mass. The fre-

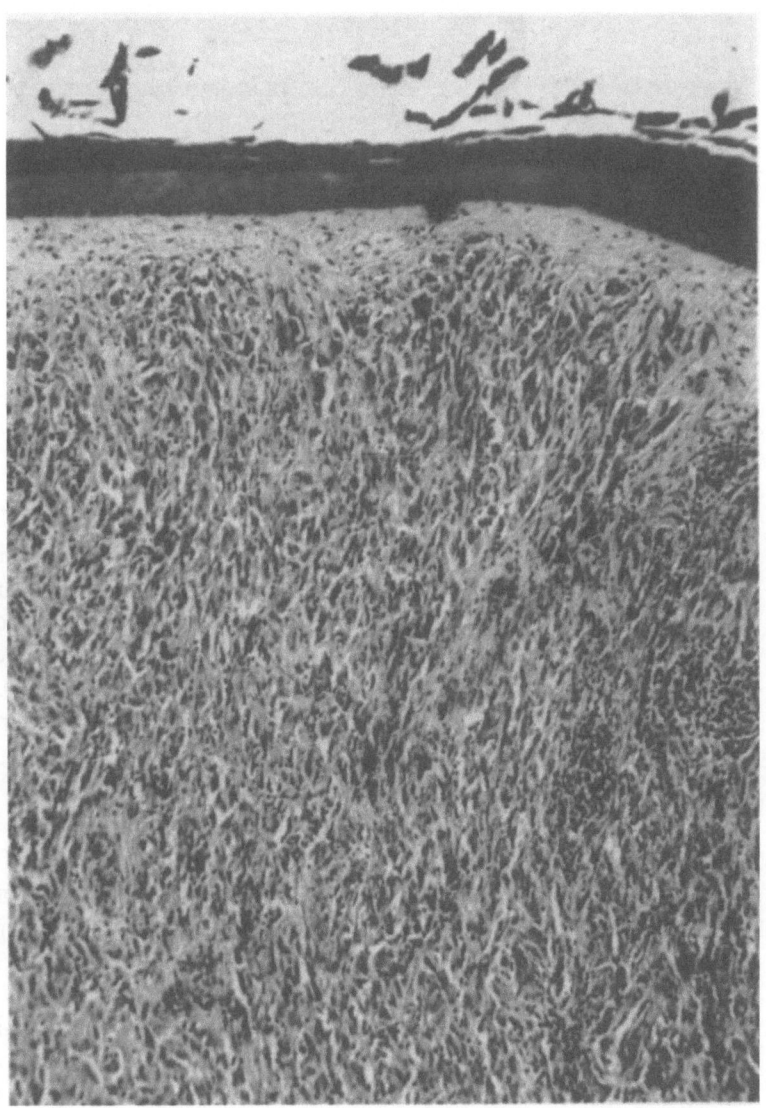

**Fig. 7.22.** See text. H & E, × 126

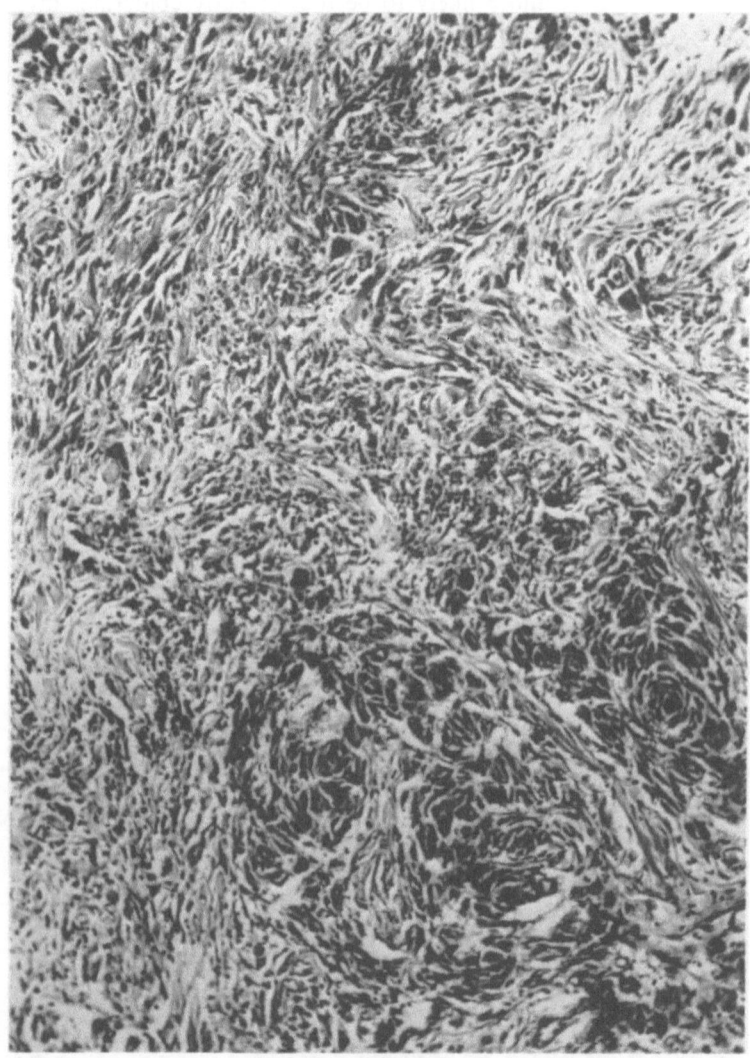

**Fig. 7.23.** See text. H & E,
× 126

quency of mitoses varied from place to place. At their most numerous they numbered approximately 1 per 4 hpf; of mitoses, 5% were aberrant. Cells with one or more 'red nucleoli' were frequent.

An occasional cell in the immediately subepidermal area contained melanin, otherwise all were nonpigmented.

No doubt was entertained but that this was a malignant neoplasm with the diagnostic combination of high cellularity, obvious invasiveness, polymorphism, many and aberrant mitoses. Doubt did exist, and still remains, about its histogenesis but the most likely designation was considered to be 'amelanotic melanocarcinoma'. The minimal involvement of the epidermis was admittedly a difficulty but it was a difficulty

equally in the way of both melanocarcinoma and what was regarded as the other most likely candidate, spindle-celled squamous carcinoma. Excision, if indeed total, had been achieved by no more than 0.5 mm in some places.

The patient remained free of trouble, locally and generally, and was in good health 14 years later.

Whatever its true nature, this lesion had all the histological features of a malignant neoplasm, relatively large and present for years. The possibility of its being a Spitz naevus remains but this was considered at the time and rejected largely on the grounds of the frequency and frequent aberrancy of mitotic figures. As was noted by Echevarria and Ackerman (1967), even normal mitotic figures are rare in Spitz naevus. The

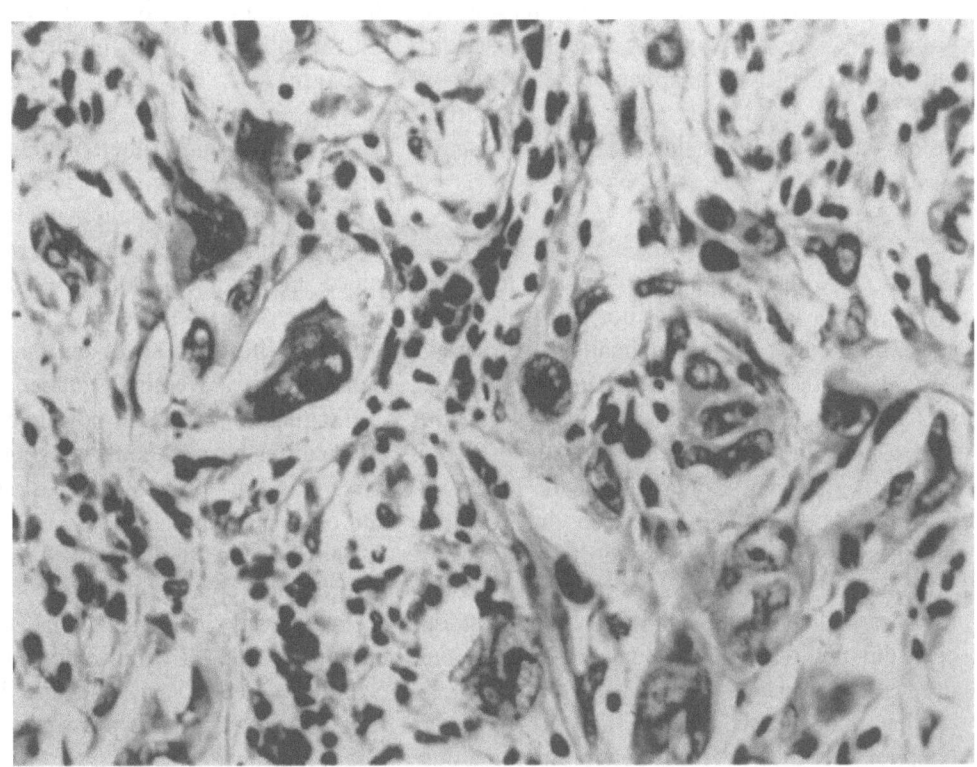

**Fig. 7.24.** Extreme polymorphism with giant cell formation is evident here. H & E, × 493

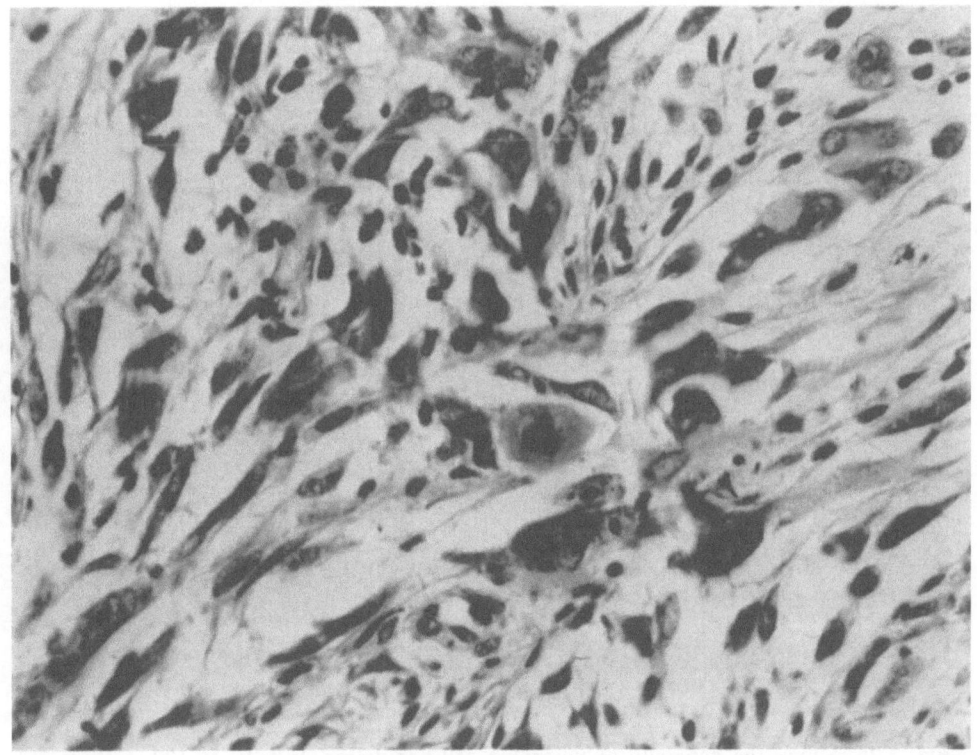

**Fig. 7.25.** Shows again the polymorphism with, centre, a triaster. H & E, × 493

diagnosis as given at the time may reasonably be regarded as *appropriate*. Simple excision, dubiously complete, was apparently curative.

It will be noted that, as in Case 7.18, the lesion was on the lower limb of a young woman.

### Case 7.21

F (39 years) sought advice about a mole on lower part of left leg. It was not biopsied at this stage, but liquid nitrogen applications were used. After 1 month biopsy was performed: the lesion was not ulcerated, nor did the history suggest that at any time it had been ulcerated.

Figure 7.26 shows one edge of the lesion. It was a plaque about 1 mm deep; half of this thickness lay above the surface of the adjacent skin; half represented occupation of the dermis by abnormal cells but even at their deepest these cells did not reach more than half-way to the deepest sweat glands.

The small nuclei at lower right are those of lymphocytes: they were nowhere more numerous than this and were only a thin scattering throughout the substance of the plaque.

Figure 7.27. The lesion comprises a mixture of large rounded and sometimes bi- or tri-nucleate cells and others similar but smaller though even they are much larger than lymphocytes which are the smallest nuclei of all in this view. About 1% of the abnormal cells contained melanin. Apart from simple flattening due to pressure, the epidermis appears essentially normal as it did in all of the many further sections that were eventually made.

Examination at higher powers gave little more information beyond confirming that mitotic activity was present but in occasional cells only, and of normal character.

The findings were regarded as equivocal but reported as representing most probably a form of 'metaplasia in a melanonaevus' consequent upon the liquid nitrogen treatment. Excision appeared to have been complete but continued supervision, against the possibility of at any rate local recurrence, was advised.

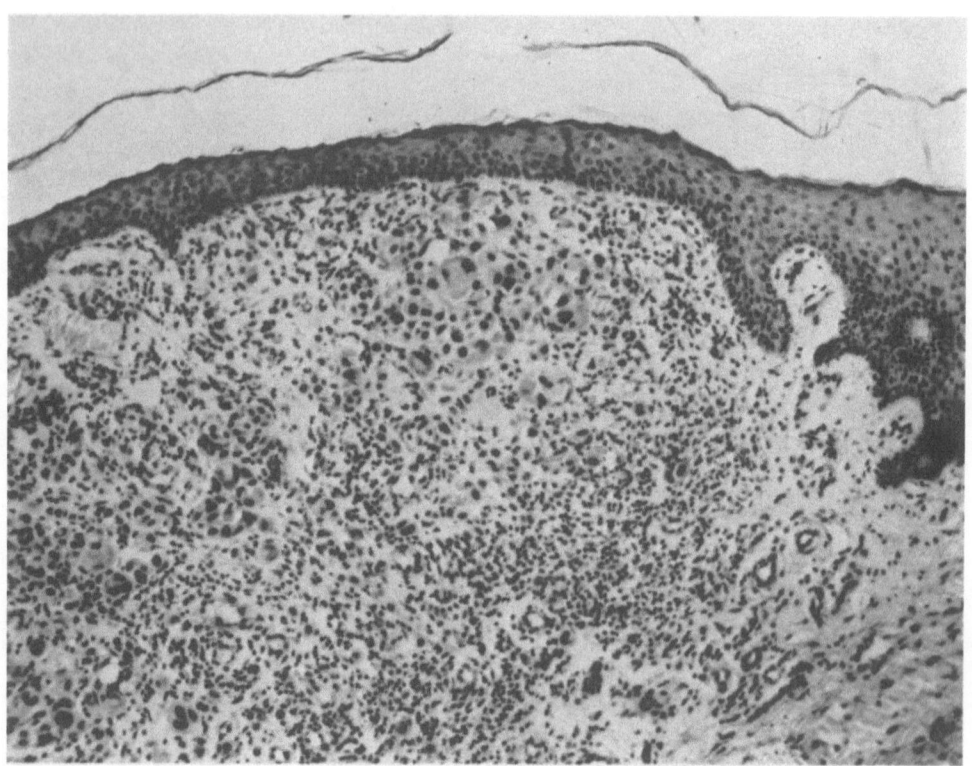

**Fig. 7.26.** Shows the generally polymorphic cell population. H & E, × 123

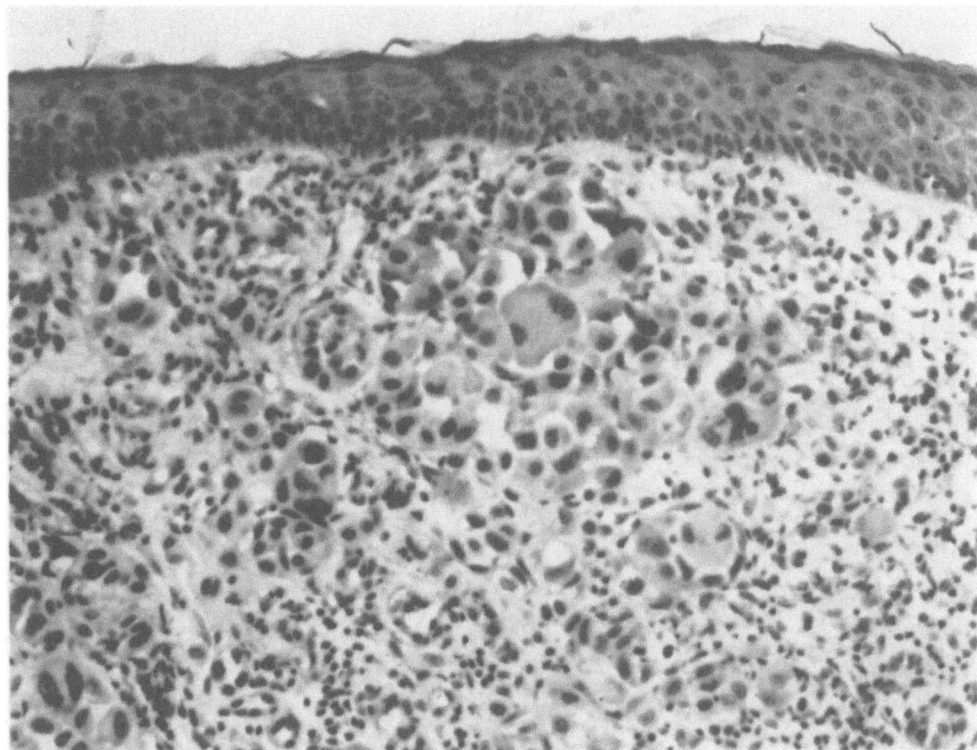

**Fig. 7.27.** Some cells are bi- or trinucleate and contain abundant cytoplasm. H & E, × 246

Within 6 months of the initial operation there was a 5 × 4 × 3 cm mass of nodes in the groin. Microscopy showed almost total replacement by obvious melanocarcinoma.

The patient died 4 years later after a succession of operations for removal of locally recurrent or metastatic lesions.

Examination of further sections from the original lesion, prepared on the occasion of the inguinal node biopsy and report, revealed a degree of polymorphism and mitotic activity that was so much more pronounced quantitatively and qualitatively as to establish the diagnosis beyond reasonable doubt, even allowing for the fact that reassessment was being made with the biassing advantage of hindsight.

These features are shown in Figure 7.28.

Two points merit mention. With the degree of doubt that was felt on the occasion of the original biopsy many more sections should perhaps have been examined, for unequivocally diagnostic abnormality did eventually emerge. However, the selected central block, taken along the full length of the plaque and quite properly believed to be fairly representative, was sectioned at seven levels. This was hardly inadequate coverage. The lesion had been reported as unusual and requiring continued observation, and it was unfortunate that the diagnostic area, cluster or clone had not been included in the original sections. Whether, had this happened, the outcome would have been different, is debatable. The report, however, must be accounted an *under-diagnosis*.

The second point is the integrity of the overlying epidermis, and also the total absence of 'junctional change' in any of the very many sections. It could be maintained that the epidermis 'must' have been destroyed by the earlier applications of liquid nitrogen, the presence of any pre-existing junctional change being thereby impossible to exclude. All one can say is that the absence of scarring over the lesion, and the orderly, well-differentiated pattern of the epidermis, make this seem unlikely. Whether an area of junctional change destroyed in this way would reappear as the epidermis regenerated, I do not know.

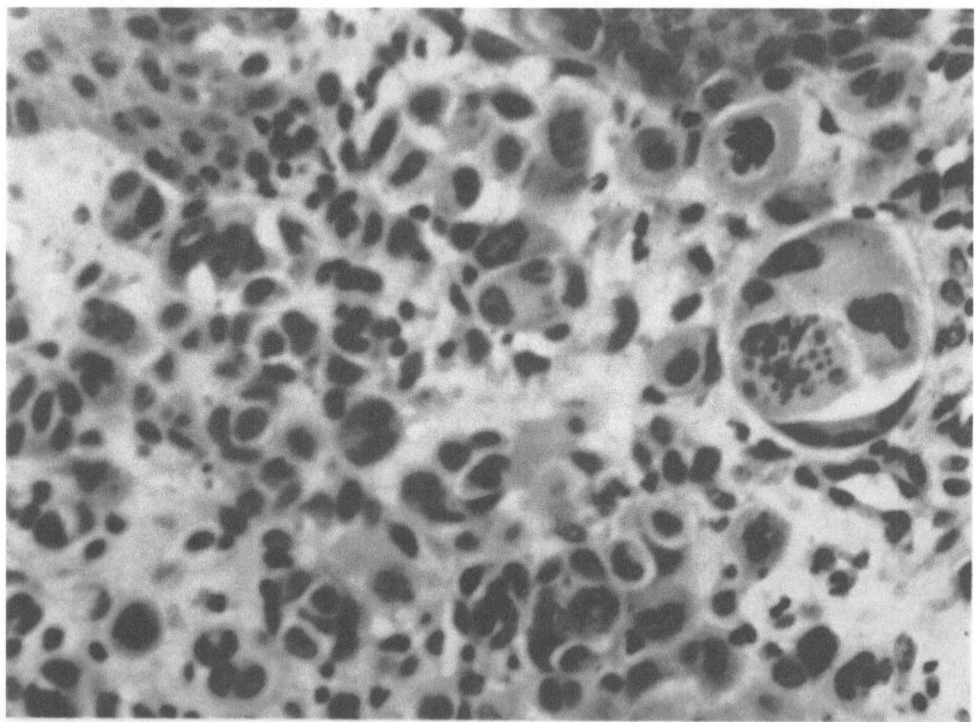

**Fig. 7.28.** Further sections from the original lesion yielded cells even more polymorphic than those in the earlier sections as seen above; aberrant mitotic figures had also appeared (*top right*). H & E, × 476

*Case 7.22*

M (49 years) with 'papule' on deltoid region for 2 years. It was itself red, was surrounded by a reddish 'flare', and was thought probably to be a pyogenic granuloma. It was received as a 15 × 12 mm domed or button-shaped nodule rising wholly above the surface of its surrounding ellipse of skin. As received, the edges of the ellipse were nowhere further than 2 mm from the base of the nodule.

Sections showed a partly ulcerated, quite highly cellular mass composed of relatively uniform, frequently nucleolated, nonpigmented cells, in mitosis occasionally though with a frequency of up to 2 figures per hpf in some places (they are now recognisable as bearing a close similarity to those seen in Case 7.7 and illustrated in Fig. 7.3). In some areas the abnormal cells were in direct structural continuity with the deep surface of the epidermis. In these areas, consequently, the basal layer as such had disappeared; in places elsewhere, not in continuity with intradermal ingrowths, it ap-

peared frayed. To this extent there was junctional change of a kind. As appeared likely macroscopically, none of the abnormal cells lay deeper than the adnexa of the surrounding skin but lymphocytes lay in dense aggregates across the whole of the deep surface.

Thought was given to the possibility of the lesion's being a mesodermal overgrowth of some kind, possibly even a histiocytoma, but the preferred diagnosis eventually was 'amelanotic melanocarcinoma'.

Receipt of the report led to further excision, grafting and axillary lymphadenectomy; none of the lymph nodes showed metastases. The patient, however, died 4 years later with evidence of systemic spread. There was no necropsy.

By the then available techniques, no decision was possible whether the lesion was melanocytic/amelanotic or of another nature. The more important decision was whether it was metastasisingly malignant or not. The deciding factors had been the direct mergence with, possibly origin from, the deep surface of the epidermis (see, however, Case 5.3), the high incidence of nucleoli and the relatively high incidence focally of mitotic figures. The diagnosis given as first preference was wholly *appropriate*.

### Case 7.23

F (52 years) from whose forearm a 5-mm nodule, duration uncertain, was removed.

Figure 7.29 shows a lesion of varying cell-density extending deeply into subcutaneous tissue (*lesion A*).

Figure 7.30 contains a single area of 'junctional' change, one of the few seen in many sections. The mass is thus technically a compound naevus though for practical purposes an intradermal naevus. There is a moderately uniform cell pattern apart from an occasional multinucleated giant cell of probably naevus-cell origin.

Figure 7.31 shows the deepest part of the lesion. The cells remain mostly uniform though still with an occasional giant cell, and there are no areas of prong-like infiltration of the stroma. Mitotic figures were few, at most 2 per section.

Figure 7.32 contains two multinucleated giant cells. These, and a scattering of others around the edge of the mass, differed from those of seemingly naeval origin in having a much closer resemblance to the Langhans type cell. Al-though none of the sections showed the familiar subnaeval granuloma, these giant cells seem almost certainly histiocytic nevertheless.

The mass was almost wholly devoid of melanin. No more than 20 Fontana-positive cells were present in the whole of any one of the sections. These do, however, support the view that the lesion was at any rate of melanocytic origin and probably an intradermal 'melano-naevus' albeit minimally pigmented. The possibility of melanocarcinoma was seriously considered but the benign diagnosis was finally preferred. Excision appeared to have been complete.

The patient re-appeared 6 years later with a subcutaneous nodular mass beneath the scar of the earlier excision.

Figure 7.33. The mass, 20 × 10 × 7 mm, had a lobular outline, was pink-white on the cut surface, rubbery and firm. The dark area to the left represents degenerative change akin to haemorrhagic infarction. Elsewhere for the most part the mass had a highly cellular character (*lesion B*).

Figure 7.34 shows the degree of cellularity and the generally plexiform or whorled pattern.

Figure 7.35 illustrates the spindle-shaped outline of cells and nuclei, the somewhat large-compartmented arrangement of the cells, and

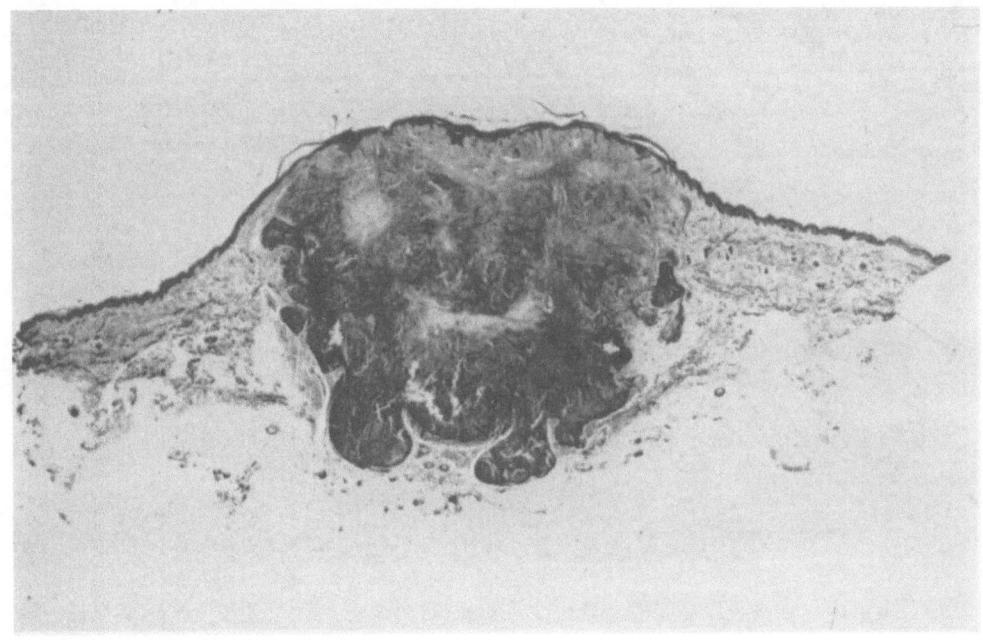

**Fig. 7.29.** Lesion *A*. See text. H & E, × 17

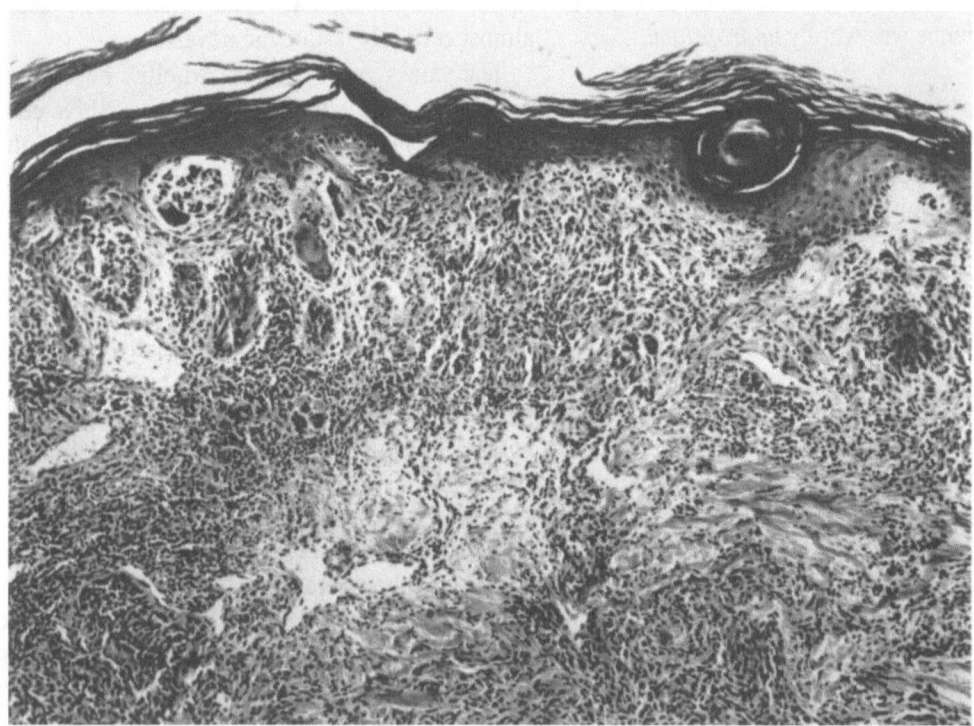

**Fig. 7.30.** Shows the predominantly intradermal location and distribution of the abnormal cells. H & E, × 119

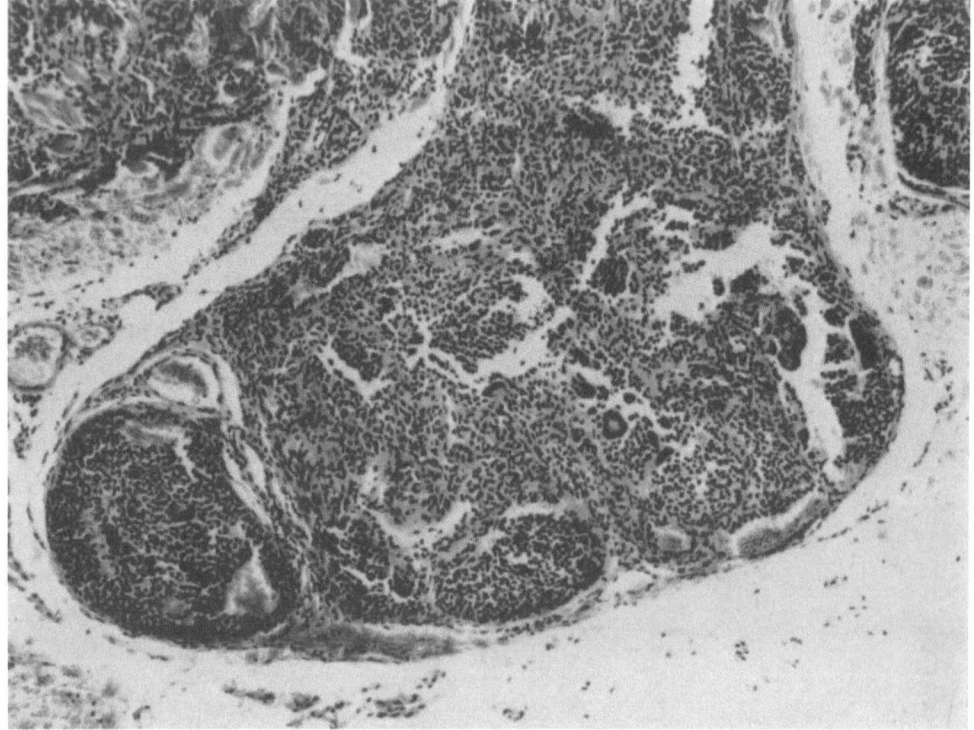

**Fig. 7.31.** The blunt front of the deepest area. H & E, × 123

the average frequency of cells. In this field there are four mitotic figures but the average was 1 per 3 hpf. About 10% of the mitotic figures were aberrant; one such and a more detailed view of cellular and nuclear detail is shown in Fig. 7.36. The prominent circular dark dots in so many of the nuclei are what appear in ordinary H & E preparations as 'red nucleoli'. Prolonged search revealed no melanin anywhere in several sections.

The histological pattern was straightforwardly that of a 'spindle-celled sarcoma' and none of many colleagues seeing the sections in ignorance of the clinical data has suggested otherwise. Understandably, views have differed on the likeliest type of sarcoma; most have suggested a 'neurogenic' origin. However, in the light of

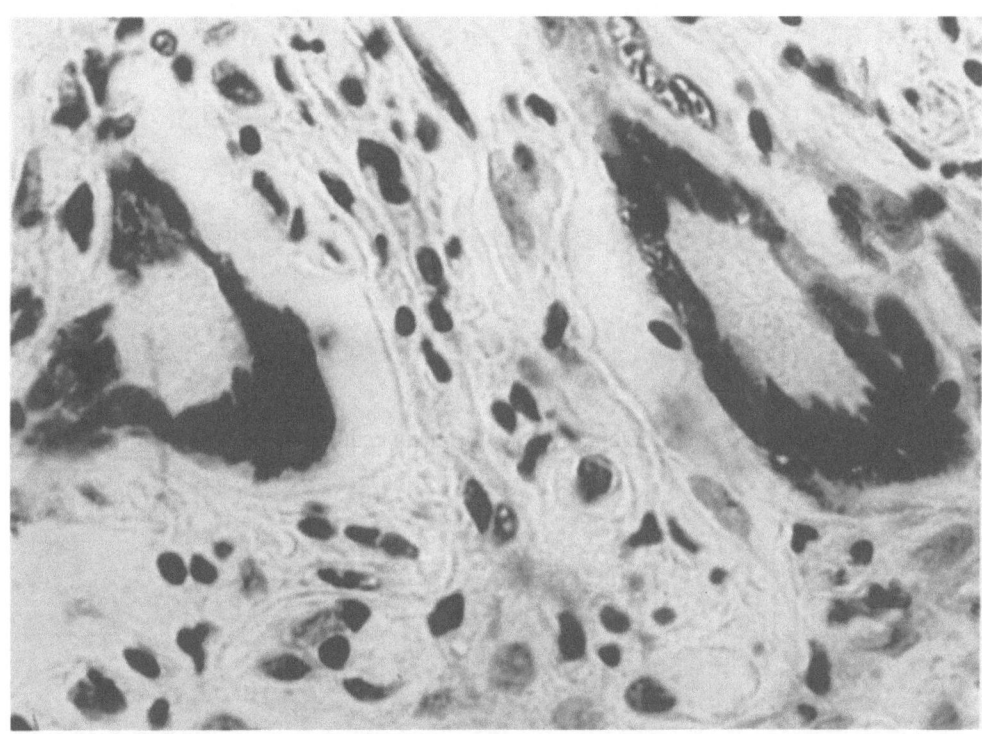

**Fig. 7.32.** Bizarre multinucleated giant cells, almost certainly histiocytic. H & E, × 985

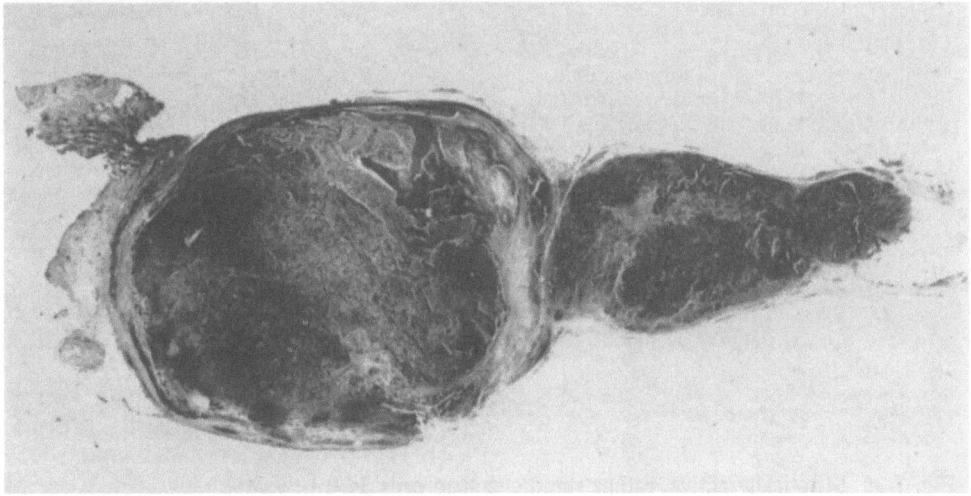

**Fig. 7.33.** Lesion *B*. The lobulate mass. H & E, × 6

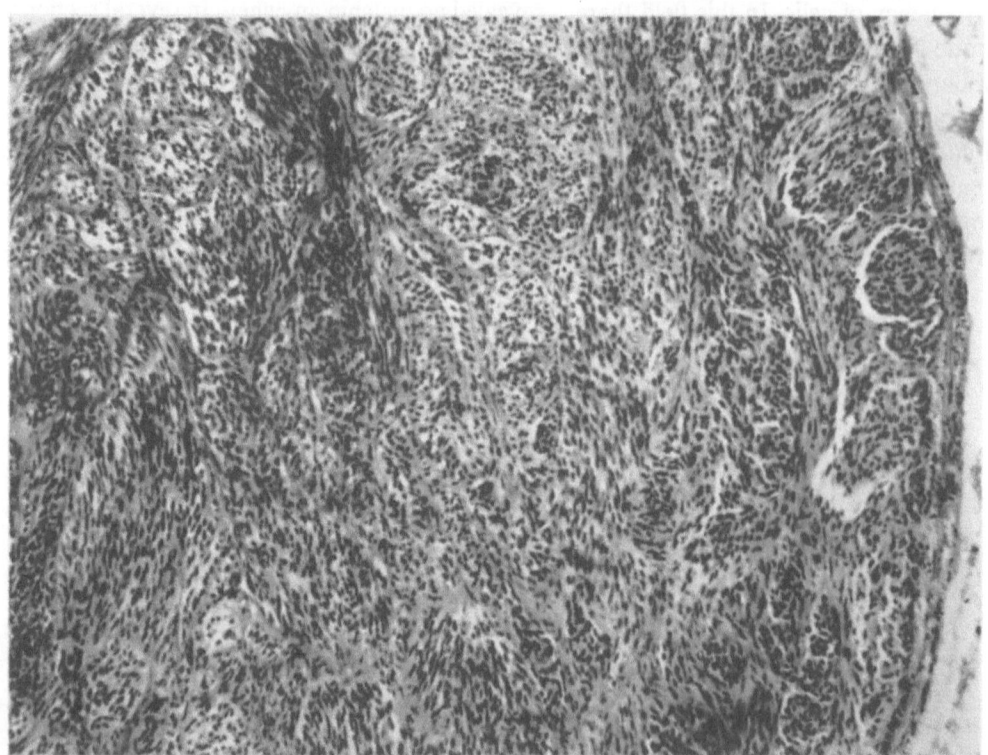

**Fig. 7.34.** The lesion is well circumscribed and highly cellular. H & E, × 70

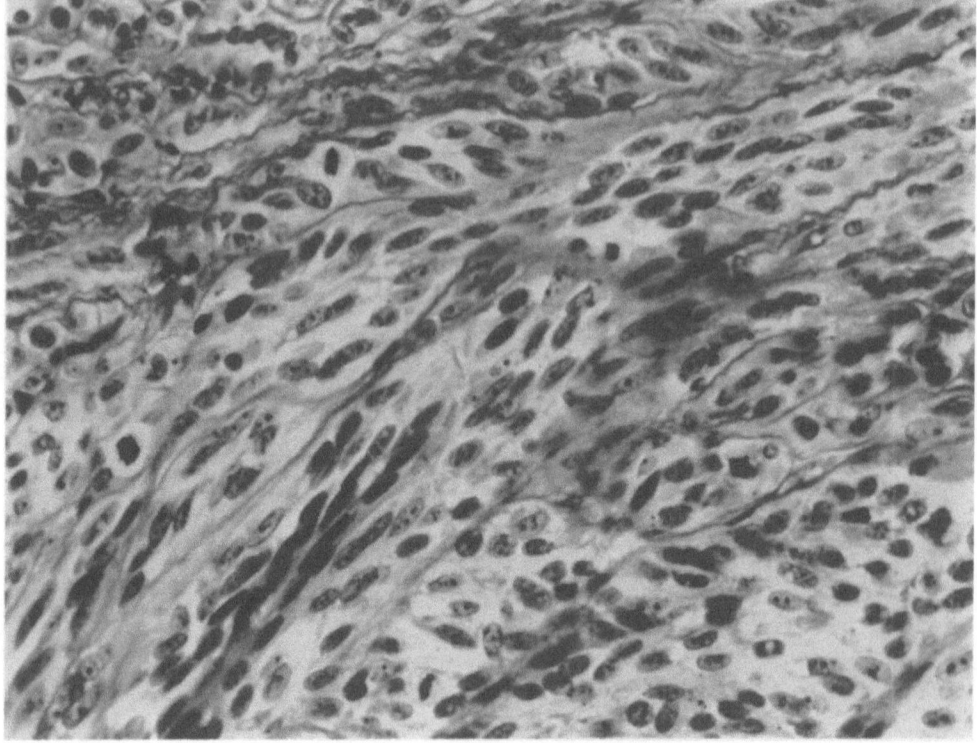

**Fig. 7.35.** Mitotically active, rather spindle-shaped cells. H & E, × 493

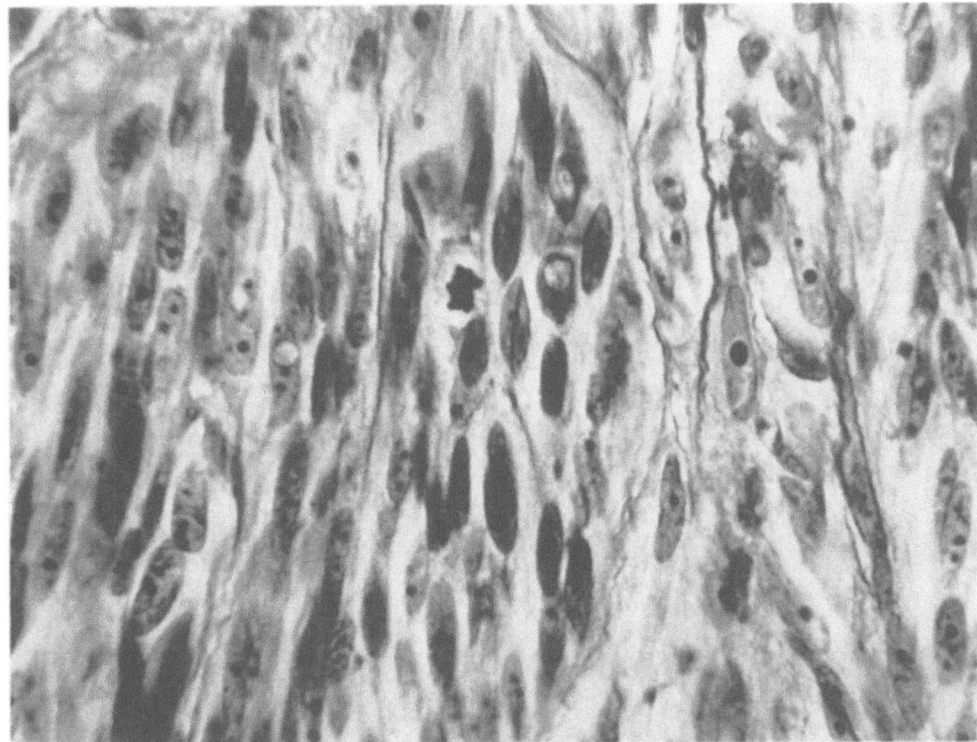

**Fig. 7.36.** One of the quite numerous aberrant mitotic figures (upper centre). H & E, × 985

the clinical circumstances, the origin may be other than this.

The patient died from an unrelated cause, inoperable colonic carcinoma, 2 years after removal of the recurrent subcutaneous nodule. There had been no further local recurrence, and the area had remained healthy. The colonic carcinoma was in no way unusual.

The problem posed here is: could Lesion B (Fig. 7.33) be related to Lesion A (Fig. 7.29), and, if so, how? Also, if related, what prognostic lessons does it teach? Lesion B is a spindle-celled histologically malignant neoplasm: could it, in view of the naeval character of the earlier-removed Lesion A, be a melanocarcinoma? I believe that it could, and that that was its nature, albeit non-pigmented (this belief is largely substantiated by the findings in another case, not in the present series but mentioned later, where a spindle-celled lesion created interest because of its diagnostic implications).

Even in retrospect, no features could be identified in Lesion A, the mildly equivocal naevus, that would have allowed an accurate prediction of the later events. In all the circum-

stances, the diagnosis of the original lesion may be deemed *appropriate*.

### Case 7.24

F (63 years) presented with warty nodule on back of thigh that had developed during past 2 years to present size of 35 mm in diameter.

Figure 7.37 shows the filiform papillary character of the lesion. It is not, however, a simple squamous papilloma but a histologically complex lesion.

Figure 7.38. The cores of the papillary projection were largely occupied by cells of unusual appearance; cells of quite the same character are present as sheets or shoals within the considerably thickened epidermis. They are shown in the next figure.

Figure 7.39. The cells are generally uniform, moderately hyperchromatic and only occasionally in mitosis. They have the appearance of slightly enlarged 'active' naevus cells, and some indeed contained a fine dusting of melanin.

Figure 7.40. Nests of cells in a more syncytial pattern, but again occasionally pigmented, lay in

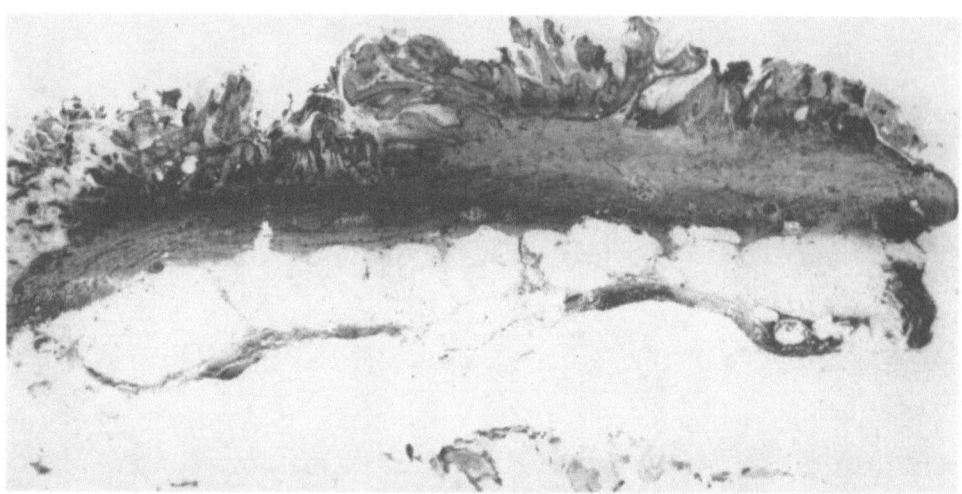

**Fig. 7.37.** The lesion was a filiform plaque. H & E, × 4

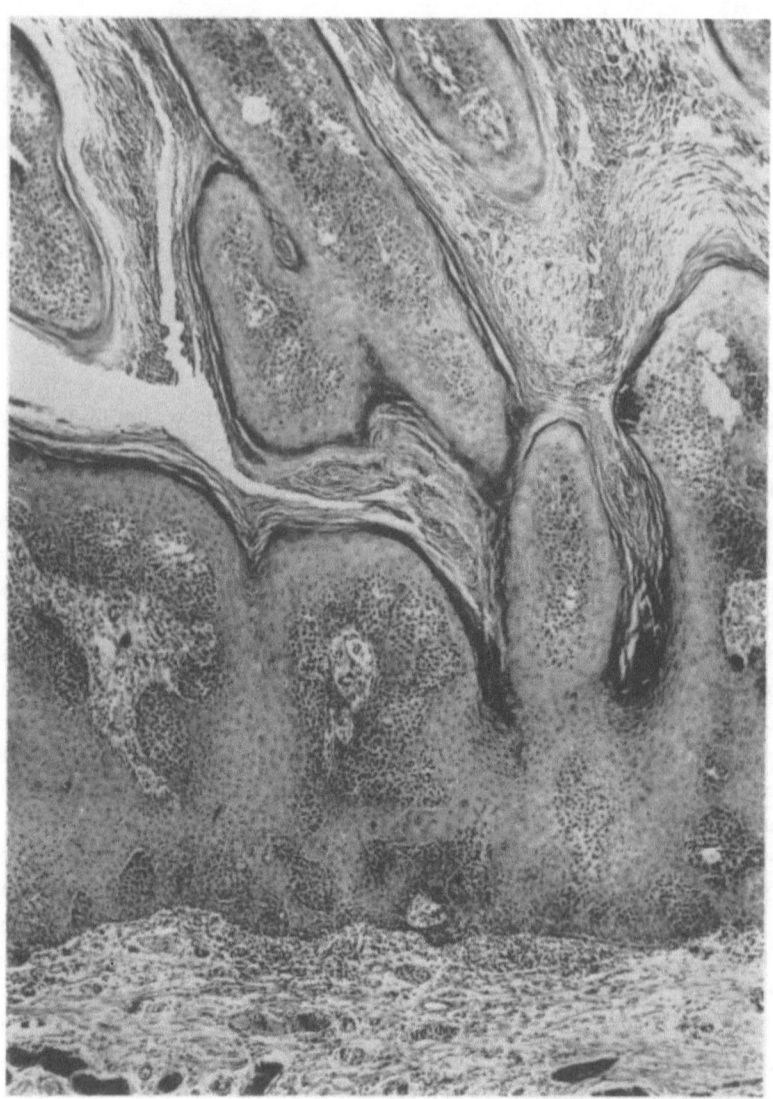

**Fig. 7.38.** The cells largely occupying the epidermis, whether papilliform or not, are mostly not prickle-cells but of the undifferentiated type seen in Fig. 7.39. H & E, × 66

some areas around the deep edge of epidermal downgrowths. This appeared to be a variant of the 'junctional change' pattern.

Figure 7.41 shows, in the centre, a rather long but normally differentiating and ultimately keratinising epidermal peg; to left, two solid areas of abnormal cells altogether lacking differentiation; and invasive growth into the dermis across the whole of the field.

Figure 7.42. The undifferentiated nature of the invading cells is evident; they occupy also the cores of epidermal pegs to right and left. The problem in their identification was that, while virtually identical with the 'core' cells, none contained melanin. It seemed likely, therefore, that they represented either undifferentiated

squamous-cell carcinoma or amelanotic melano-carcinoma with areas hinting also at basal-cell carcinoma and extra-mammary Paget's disease.

The diagnosis given for practical purposes was 'squamous-cell carcinoma'.

After 3 years ascites gradually developed: laparotomy revealed multiple nodules throughout the peritoneal cavity. Microscopy of three of these showed cells of exactly the same undifferentiated non-pigmented type as those seen earlier. It was still not possible to decide whether the lesion was undifferentiated squamous-cell carcinoma or amelanotic melanocarcinoma. The patient died soon after the operation and there was no necropsy.

Although the structure in some places closely

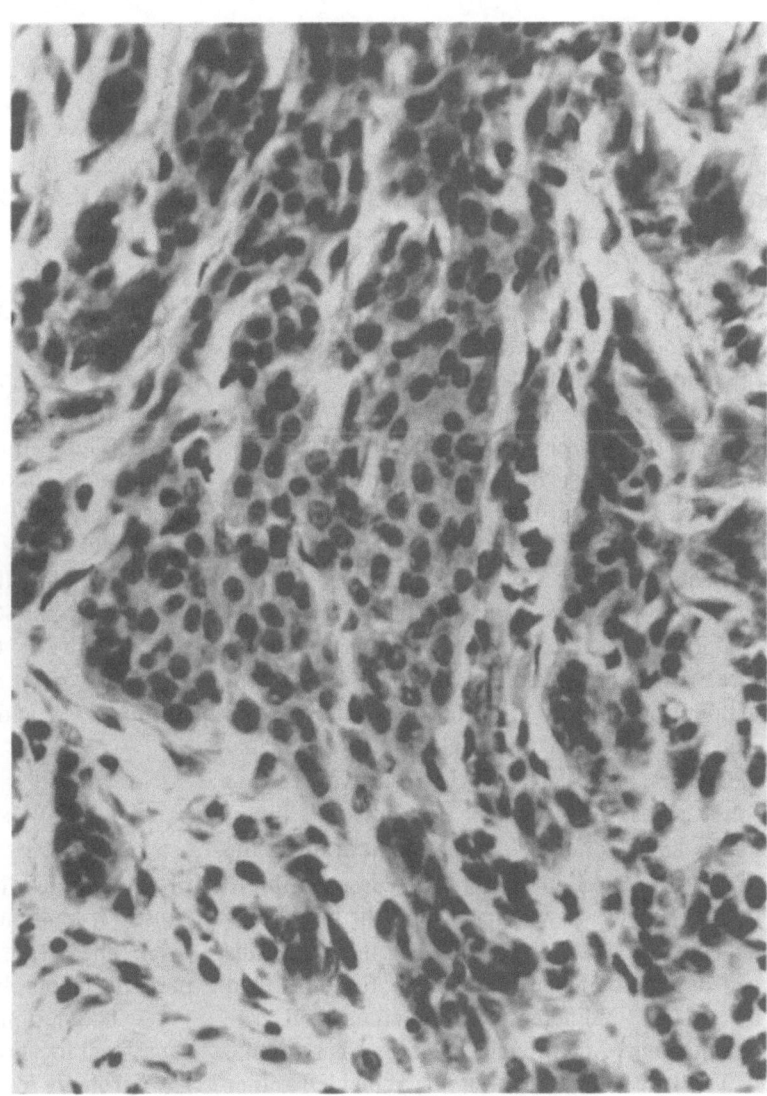

**Fig. 7.39.** The cells resemble naevus cells: some contained melanin. H & E, × 526

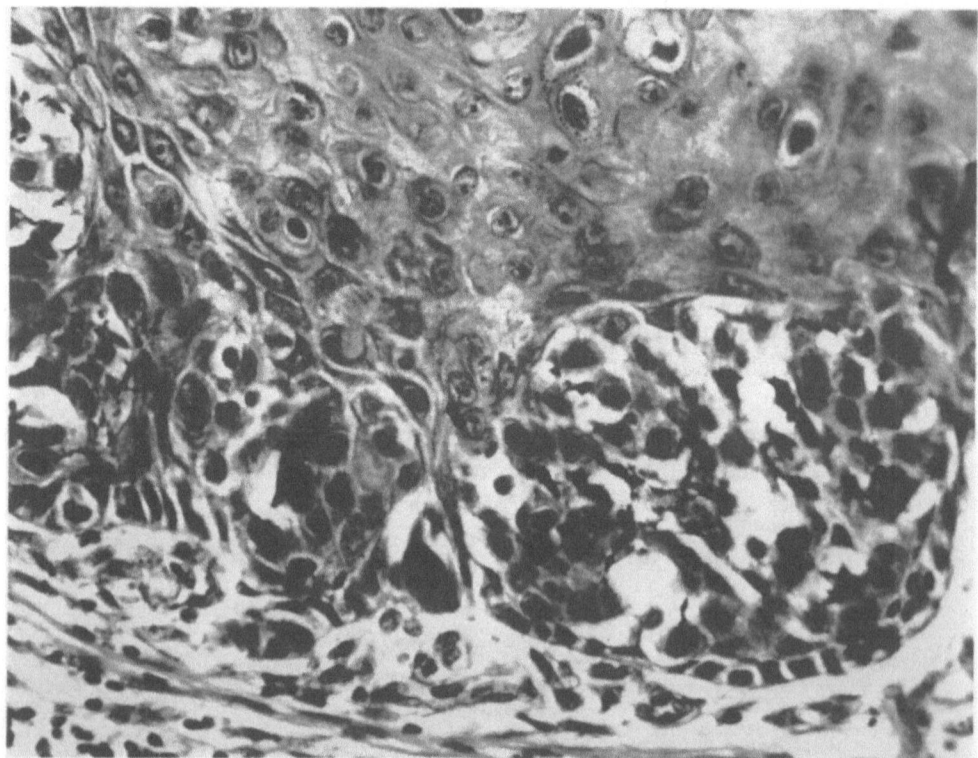

**Fig. 7.40.** This pattern is at least a form of junctional change. In this area the immediately adjacent cells are orthodox, if rather polymorphic, prickle-cells. H & E, × 493

resembled that of a basal-cell carcinoma, especially of morphoeic type, the character of the cells (and to some extent the complete absence of any peripheral 'palisading') suggested a nature of another kind; and this, in turn, at once gave the evident invasiveness a more sinister significance. The diagnosis of 'squamous-cell carcinoma' conveyed this assessment which was borne out, at least in terms of distant spread, by subsequent events.

Even so, this was unusual behaviour for an epidermal squamous-cell carcinoma with no local recurrence and no nodal involvement but with intraperitoneal spread. The acknowledged vagaries of melanocarcinoma with the associated melanosis and junctional-type change seen in some areas, albeit in the non-invasive areas, made amelanotic melanocarcinoma rather the likelier diagnosis in retrospect; unless the more comprehensive view is taken that the lesion was an expression of almost all that the epidermis can do in a carcinogenic climate. It would then be not an undifferentiated squamous-cell carcinoma but a multipotent epidermal carcinoma.

The true nature of the lesion remained rather a mystery until the description by Pinkus and Mehregan (1963) of an ultimately fatal carcinoma of skin which they regarded as an 'eccrine carcinoma' or 'malignant eccrine poroma', a rare and certainly aggressive neoplasm. The features in our local case match their description almost exactly, and with that the uncertainty was ended. The diagnosis of SCC may have been appropriate with its in-built warning of liability to metastasis but, so rarely does epidermal SCC metastasise, and by contrast so aggressive is the malignant eccrine poroma, the final verdict must be that this was both an *inappropriate* and an *under-diagnosis*.

COMMENTARY ON LOCAL SERIES

Prognostic uncertainty was expressed in 24 cases. Mostly it took one of three forms:

a) The lesion was a melanonaevus but apparently incompletely excised.

b) The lesion was a melanocarcinoma but superficial location and completeness of excision gave grounds for optimism.

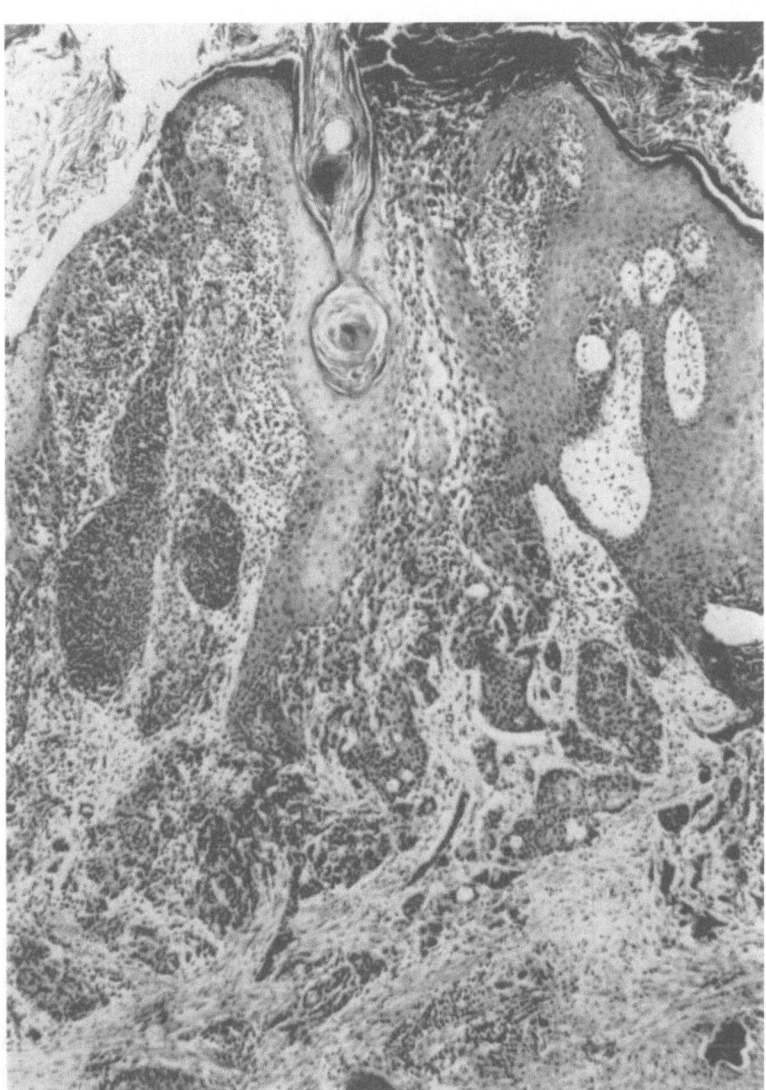

**Fig. 7.41.** See text. H & E, × 66

c) There was doubt whether the lesion was melanocarcinoma or a benign melanotic lesion.

*Melanonaevus but Incompletely Excised*

Three instances of this caused concern (Cases 7.2, 7.9, 7.14) but in none of the cases was further excision performed and none of the patients had further trouble. Histopathologists probably always comment on completeness or incompleteness of excision, and it seems reasonable that they should; even if incompleteness of excision carries a negligible risk of complication, knowledge of the fact gives the surgeon an extra datum by which his advice to the patient might be modified. It is clear in retro-

spect that the dangers supposed in earlier years to lie behind trauma to a melanonaevus were virtually nil; the impression that recurrent trauma or a single injury such as biopsy, cautery or partial excision could change a melanonaevus into a malignant melanoma was almost certainly based on the after-effects of these procedures in what was thought to be a benign melanonaevus but which was really a malignant melanoma from the start.

*Superficial Melanocarcinoma Totally Excised*

In five patients, all women, ages 55, 45, 34, 35, 42 (Cases 7.15–7.19 inclusive), the lesion was regarded as histologically unequivocal. All five

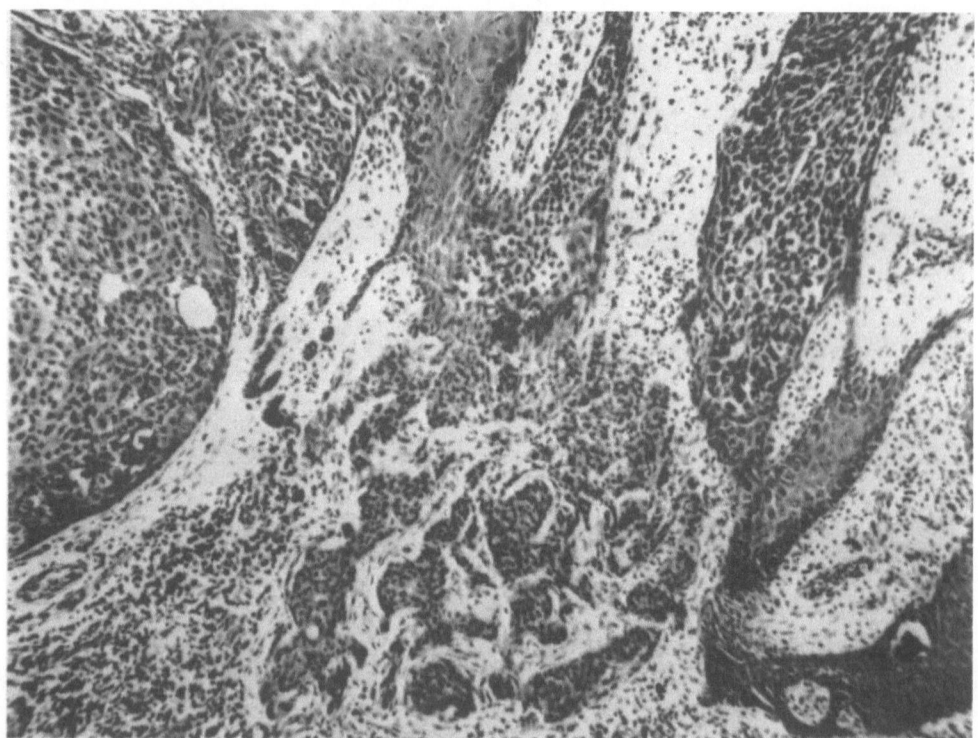

**Fig. 7.42.** See text. H & E, × 123

appeared to have been excised completely, yet two of the patients died with metastatic spread; the other three were cured. The limitations of histology as a predictor in the case of melanocarcinoma were well exemplified here but in these five patients the lesion had been so notably superficial that a note of cautious optimism did seem in order. Not a single feature, not even numbers of infiltrating lymphocytes, could in retrospect be identified as one that would in the future ensure a reliable distinction between the two lesions that were lethal and the 3 that were not.

### Melanocarcinoma or Not Melanocarcinoma?

As shown in the Summarised Totals (p. 275), this problem was posed, inter alia, by three 'compound naevi', two because of undue polymorphism, one because of undue penetration (Cases 7.3, 7.4, 7.5). Two of the patients were known to be well at 12 and 20 years after excision; the other was not traced but news of later trouble would almost certainly have arrived.

Three further lesions were highly cellular 'compound naevi' originally diagnosed as such

but in retrospect more accurately to be diagnosed lentigo maligna (all female, ages 59, 70, 72: Cases 7.6, 7.7, 7.8). The outcome in these cases, as shown earlier, was: no recurrence by time of unrelated death 8 years later; recurrence as typical lentigo maligna after 7 years; development of unequivocal melanocarcinoma 18 years later at age 88.

It may be that all lesions with the structure of a compound naevus over age 50 are, and should be treated as, malignant lentigines. If this be true, it provides another instance where melanocytes behave differently at different ages. The treatment of a compound naevus and of a lentigo maligna is essentially the same, namely, total excision, so the natural history of an untreated compound naevus at, say, age 30 is unknown. It is not, however, considered a lesion with the same connotations as the early lentigo of later ages that may be histologically identical. This may explain why lentigo maligna is virtually unknown before the age of 50; at younger ages such lesions are designated compound naevi, possibly more or less 'activated'.

Uncertainty was caused by two 'Spitz naevi'. The sections of one of these, from the thigh of a girl aged 10 (Case 7.10), when examined 'blind', were regarded by some as melanocarcinoma and by others as a Spitz naevus. Those favouring the benign diagnosis had done so mainly because of scarcity of mitotic figures and lack of hyperchromatism. In the case of the other patient, a woman of 45 with a nodule on the chin (Case 7.11), these features and also a general uniformity of pattern had led to a preferred diagnosis, at the time, of 'juvenile melanoma'. The presence of melanocytes 'invading' the epidermis, having been seen before in manifestly benign compound naevi, was not accepted as a criterion of malignancy.

Of the 12 cases where melanocarcinoma was either diagnosed or considered a strong possibility, the five superficial lesions have already been assessed. One other lesion, on the calf of a woman aged 24 (Case 7.20), remains debatable. Histologically it seemed an unequivocally malignant neoplasm, and only the complete absence of melanin precluded an outright diagnosis of melanocarcinoma. Whatever its true nature, whether amelanotic melanocarcinoma or not, and despite its extreme aberrancy, excision was evidently curative (trouble-free 14 years later).

The next lesion, on the leg of a woman of 39 (Case 7.21) was at the outset puzzling, and diagnosed as probably a metaplastic compound naevus partly because of recent topical therapy and partly because the epidermis was nowhere ulcerated. Further sections from the original lesion, prepared when the patient developed inguinal nodal metastases 6 months later, showed features by which the lesion should have been diagnosed as a melanocarcinoma at the beginning. There seemed no reason at the time to take further sections but in retrospect the degree of uncertainty that the lesion caused should of itself have been sufficient reason to do so.

The remaining three cases are less clinically than histologically puzzling. In one (Case 7.23), in which excision of a moderately highly cellular intradermal naevus from the forearm of a woman of 52 had been followed 6 years later by a subcutaneous spindle-celled sarcoma, the most likely explanation seemed to be late local development of a spindle-celled amelanotic melanocarcinoma. This, if true, is an unusual occurrence. The naevus was, however, itself rather equivocal and possibly in truth a melano-

carcinoma though it is difficult to be convinced of that even now.

In the next case, a filiform keratinising plaque on the thigh of a woman of 63 (Case 7.24), the picture was one of pan-epidermal malignancy with different areas having a main resemblance to squamous cell or basal cell or melanocarcinoma. An aberrant naevus cell pattern predominated but in the absence of melanin the lesion was diagnosed as squamous cell carcinoma. As mentioned in the case description, it was almost certainly the 'malignant eccrine poroma' of Pinkus and Mehregan (1963).

In one of the two remaining cases, the question of melanocarcinoma was raised indirectly and only in so far as the pattern of a cellular blue naevus may be mimetic. In this particular example (Case 7.12) the lesion was of typically high cellularity but notably uniform pattern and, in many sections, devoid of mitotic figures. The final case was a probable histiocytoma (Case 7.13) already described in some detail. It served to emphasise that not all that seems to be junctional change is so.

## General Commentary

The problems of melanocarcinoma become no less. Indeed, as offering one of the more hopeful roads for immunotherapists to travel, its precise diagnosis and definition grow steadily more urgent. Some of the still debatable matters are considered below.

### CLASSIFICATION

Many attempts have been made to frame a diagnostically useful classification of premalignant melanotic lesions, in particular those of recent years by Davis and his colleagues (1966), Bodenham (1968), Cochran (1968, 1969, 1969a), Clark and colleagues (1969) and McGovern (1970). It is very largely a summation of the opinions of these observers that comprises the recommendation of an international group (McGovern et al., 1973) on the approach to melanocarcinoma in terms of both classification and datum recording. The recommended scheme is essentially an extension of that of Clark and colleagues (1969) who subdivided melanocarcinoma into (i) lentigo maligna melanoma, (ii) superficial spreading melanoma, and (iii) nodular melanoma. It implicitly acknowledged also the logical attempt made by Cochran (1968) to assess the aggressiveness of a lesion by allocating a score to various factors such as situation, sex, depth and spread; with its reminder of many facts and features of the individual lesion that should be recorded, the scheme is of undoubted value scientifically. However, for the pathologist giving advice to the surgeon about a particular patient's lesion, there is much to be said for the simpler subdivision of Clark. Indeed, for practical purposes, there is much to be said for a simpler subdivision still into just (i) lentigo maligna, and (ii) with some prognostic assessment, melanocarcinoma. At the same time, we may note the recent experience of Larsen and Grude (1979). In analysing retrospectively nearly 700 cases of primary cutaneous malignant melanoma, clinical Stage I (". . . with no access to any clinical information, as usual."), these authors had to regard 20.5% of the lesions as unclassifiable: unanimity on classification could not be achieved.

The scoring system of Cochran, designed to estimate the aggressiveness of melanocarcinoma and later reassessed by him with colleagues (Mackie et al., 1972), showed that the combined clinical and pathological score could range from 10 to 55, and that the corresponding mortality rates covered the range 10%–90%. The local factors that mattered most in this and in many other series, for example that of Holmes and his associates (1976), were the depth of penetration and size (and the closely dependent ulceration) of the lesion. 'Depth of penetration', however, may have two meanings: either depth of penetration relative to the structural pattern of the skin (epidermis, papillary and reticular dermis), which is the basis of the scheme proposed by Clark and by McGovern and his international group; or depth of penetration from the granular layer of the epidermis, which is the measure recommended by Breslow (1975).

To the extent (a) that the disposition of papillary and reticular dermis is not always easy to distinguish (though fair reproducibility by 'levels' was achieved by Suffin and colleagues, 1977), and (b) that the total depth of penetration is relatively easy to measure objectively, the scheme proposed by Breslow is undoubtedly the simpler. Not only is it simpler and more reproducible, it has also been shown by the same

author (Breslow, 1977; Breslow and Macht, 1978) to have significant prognostic value. Lesions with a total depth of less than 0.76 mm are only exceptionally associated with recurrence or metastasis (one of 45 cases in Breslow's original series). Therefore, this observation has also therapeutic significance since, depending on local practice, regional lymphadenectomy might or might not be performed depending on the lesion's having or not having reached this depth (pathological technique is important, of course: blocks should be exactly orientated, and the artefact of oblique sectioning borne in mind, but this should not be a problem for any pathologist of reasonable experience).

The two schemes, the microanatomical and the purely mensural, were used in parallel in retrospective analysis of a series of 151 cases of melanocarcinoma of the extremities by Wanebo and his colleagues (1975). As could be expected, the predictive value of each was closely similar. However, the relative simplicity, objectivity and reproducibility of the Breslow scheme makes it attractive and worthy of wider trial. A fair assessment of the general position meantime vis-à-vis prognostic assessment seems to be that melanocarcinomas (i.e. unequivocal melanocarcinomas) of less than 1 mm total depth represent a risk of metastasis of some 5% or less, and that the risk increases progressively thereafter to a risk of some 75% or more at a total depth of 7 mm or more. The fact that the Breslow scheme has just received commendation from Dr. McGovern himself and his colleagues (1979), ". . . due mainly to excellent correlation of thickness with mortality", must make this now the favoured form of progmostic assessment. We should note, however, that there can be encouraging exceptions.

As a matter of possible interest, the Breslow technique was applied retrospectively to nine of the cases in the Local Series, namely, the eight melanocarcinomas 'appropriately diagnosed', and one of those 'underdiagnosed'; that is, Cases 7.15 to 7.23 inclusive. The results are as shown in Table 7.4. As may be seen, none of the tumours had a lesser depth than the 0.76 mm threshold of Breslow. However, all of the five survivors (including one unrelated death at 8 years) had lesions very much deeper than this, in one instance 11.02 mm. In each of the survivors, the lesion had been on a limb. In earlier days,

**Table 7.4.** Relation of depth of melanocarcinoma to clinical outcome (9 cases, Local Series)

| Case No. | Depth of Lesion |
|---|---|
| *Patients who died* | |
| 7.15 (F, 55, calf) | 1.68 mm |
| 7.16 (F, 45, ankle) | 2.70 mm |
| 7.21 (F, 39, lower leg) | 0.90 mm |
| 7.22 (M, 40, shoulder) | 6.30 mm |
| *Patients who survived* | |
| 7.17 (F, 34, thigh) | 1.35 mm |
| 7.18 (F, 35, calf) | 2.85 mm |
| 7.19 (F, 42, calf) | 1.95 mm |
| 7.20 (F, 24, calf) | 11.02 mm |
| 7.23 (F, 52, forearm) | 4.20 mm |

gravity of prognosis based on total depth of the lesion could have led to amputation; and this would have been unnecessary.

## CONSTITUENT CELLS

The well-known variation in type of constituent cell that may characterise a melanocarcinoma such as epithelioid, round, spindle and mixed, has been examined on many occasions (a good example is that of Bodenham, 1968, in his analysis of 650 cases) but no author has been able to establish any correlation of real prognostic value. In Bodenham's series, for example, little more could be said than that the 'mixed-cell' type had a rather better prognosis than the 'round-cell' type. Understandably, from its paradoxical morphology, the spindle-celled form has attracted particular attention. Spindle-cells may comprise part or virtually the whole of a lesion. In their morphological assessment of 89 cases of melanocarcinomas in general, Williams and his co-workers (1968) found that, with mitotically high-grade lesions, a significantly improved survival rate emerged in parallel with frequency of spindle-cells but, again, this is of limited value in the individual case.

Evidence that points in rather the opposite direction has been offered by Conley and his colleagues (1971) who separated from amongst the spindle-celled lesions a group that they named 'desmoplastic malignant melanoma'. In these, not only may the malignant melanocytes themselves be spindly, they appear also to stimulate a desmoplastic reaction and perhaps even themselves produce collagen. These authors give warning that lesions of this kind, frequently forming bulky subcutaneous masses, may be diagnosed as fibrosarcoma, as had happened in one of their seven cases (these seven cases form another example of the diagnostic pitfalls surrounding melanocarcinoma: in only one had the original diagnosis been melanocarcinoma: in only two others had the diagnosis been of a naevocytic lesion of some kind). They state also that ". . . melanin pigment was seen easily in association with the superficial dermal lesions but seldom in association with the deeper masses". Few pathologists will have the ultrastructural resources with which to identify the intracellular melanosomes and premelanosomes that these authors found diagnostic but attention can always be paid particularly to another feature that may clearly be of diagnostic significance, namely, the state of the epidermis covering any subjacent spindle-celled neoplasm. This matter was considered earlier in the context of histiocytomas of the dermis (Case 5.3).

Figure 7.43 shows part of a 6 × 5 × 3 cm firm white lymph node. It was as typically a 'spindle-cell sarcoma' as such a lesion could be: it even had an intimately pericellular reticulin pattern. Spindle-cell sarcoma within a lymph node should in any circumstances engender suspicion but there was no mystery here. The node, and others smaller, was removed from the axilla simultaneously with a finger bearing a straightforward though not heavily pigmented melanocarcinoma. Within the spindle-celled tissue an occasional minute area did show intracellular melanin, and so the diagnosis was established. However, some sections were wholly devoid of melanin. Had these been the only ones available for diagnosis, and the axillary nodal enlargement an isolated abnormality, there might have been a search for some deep-seated fibro- or leiomyosarcoma with the risk of some seemingly innocent mole's being overlooked. Hitherto, though troublesome for the patient, this would have been of little therapeutic consequence but, with the systemic treatment of melanocarcinoma at least a possibility in the near future, failure to recollect these histological vagaries could be therapeutically unfortunate. The frailties of reticulin staining as a diagnostic guide were sharply evident in this particular case.

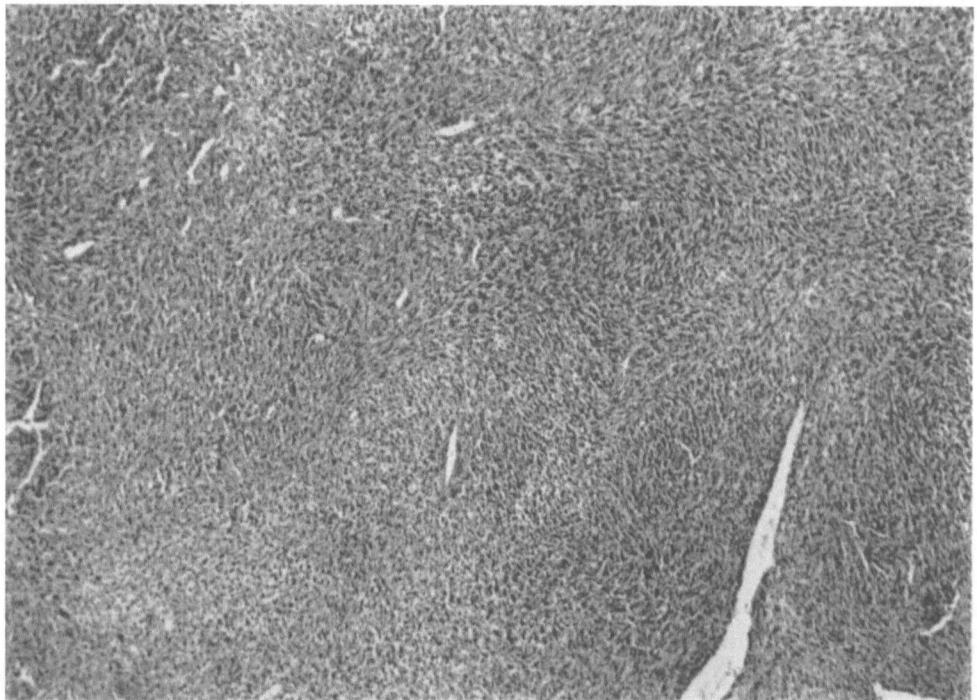

**Fig. 7.43.** Tissue of this pattern was completely occupying several axillary lymph nodes. An occasional minute area showed cells containing melanin. The source was a relatively orthodox paronychial melanocarcinoma. H & E, × 62

For whatever reason, the melanocarcinomas that arise from a lentigo maligna also commonly have a spindle-celled pattern (Clark and Mihm, 1969).

It seems right to recall the occasions on which *benign* melanotic lesions, too, may adopt a spindle-celled morphology, in particular the Spitz naevus and the cellular blue naevus, because of the danger of their being diagnosed as melanocarcinoma. This had happened in 5 of the 27 cases of spindle-celled naevi described by Kernen and Ackerman (1960), though fortunately without radical consequences, and must have happened many times before the lesions were adequately defined. This misinterpretation alone must have accounted for much of the great variability in survival rates or 'cure' rates amongst earlier series of cases of purported melanocarcinoma.

## Lentigo Maligna

The lentigo maligna (malignant freckle of Hutchinson; melanosis circumscripta precancerosa of Dubreuilh) is a relatively well-defined entity seen especially in those over 60 and probably the precursor of most melanocarcinomas developing in those over 70. This and other clinical features, well described by Davis and colleagues (1967) and Clark and Mihm (1969), distinguish it from the melanocarcinomas that develop in other ways, whether apparently from a pre-existing naevus or de novo, and Mishima (1967) has argued persuasively, in the main on ultrastructural evidence, that, however closely it may resemble a junctional naevus, it is basically a different entity. The lentigo maligna he regards as of 'melanocytic' origin, the junctional naevus as of 'nevocytic' origin, the corresponding carcinomas then being melanocytic melanocarcinoma and naevocytic melanocarcinoma (on ultrastructural evidence also, Anton-Lamprecht and his associates [1971] believe that the lentigo maligna has itself a recognisable precursor stage, the *stade éphélide*).

While all are agreed on the slow growth of the lentigo maligna, not all are agreed on the behaviour of the melanocarcinomas that may follow. In the experience both of Mishima

(1967) and Clark and Mihm (1969), they grow more slowly and are slower to invade and metastasise. In the opinion of Hartwell and his colleagues (1970), however, ". . . malignant melanoma arising in lentigo maligna is neither more nor less serious than the non-Dubreuilh form". At least, however, the characteristically slow growth of the lesion gives ample opportunity for diagnosis, and, if considered appropriate, prophylactic excision.

The distinction drawn by Mishima between 'melanocytic' and 'nevocytic' melanocarcinomas prompts a comment on the role of the mature naevus cell in relation to melanocarcinoma. It has become rather generally accepted that (non-ocular) melanocarcinomas arise only in areas of 'junctional' activity, so much so that melanocarcinomas *not* accompanied by junctional activity are regarded as with near-certainty metastatic. (I refer here to melanocarcinomas covered by unaltered intact epidermis, and adequately sampled: this excludes the easily invoked explanation with ulcerated lesions, that the junctional area had been destroyed.) This is tantamount to saying that melanocytes, when intradermal, never become malignant. As such they would be virtually unique among cells, and I know of no direct evidence to support this belief. Adequately sampled nonulcerated melanocarcinomas lacking junctional change may be rare but they do occur; Case 7.21 in the local series was almost certainly one such. When, in these circumstances, full search for a primary lesion elsewhere has been fruitless, credibility seems to me to be stretched further by insistence that such a lesion must still exist somewhere than to admit that the melanocarcinoma has arisen in situ by the transformation of mature naevus cells within the dermis.

The likeliest diagnostic error is misinterpretation of the lentigo maligna as a junctional or compound naevus, and this almost certainly applied in two, and possibly three, instances in the local series. In so far as it may cause delay, this is a serious misdiagnosis, and the local patient who developed a frank melanocarcinoma 18 years after the original diagnosis (Case 7.7) might have been spared this by more radical treatment at the outset. The two decisions, whether (a) a lesion is a simple melanonaevus or a lentigo maligna, and (b) whether a lentigo maligna has become a frank melanocarcinoma,

may equally be difficult, and useful guidance to their solution has been offered by all the groups of workers just cited. In the case of (b), whether a lentigo maligna has become a frank melanocarcinoma, the vexed question of 'invasion' is again to the fore. The difficulty in this particular context is well exemplified in illustrations in the already-mentioned article containing the recommendations of classification by the international group (McGovern et al., 1973). Their Fig. 10 shows part of a Hutchinson's melanotic freckle before invasion; their Fig. 13, of a "malignant melanoma, invasive", shows "single malignant melanocytes (that) have invaded the upper dermis"; yet abnormal cells have invaded the dermis twice as deeply from the freckle as from the invasive malignant melanoma. The problem at this stage is whether the lesion is to be regarded as invasive at all, and there can be no unanimity amongst pathologists on this. Yet there is still difficulty even where invasion is unequivocal, and unanimity on its existence could certainly be achieved. As mentioned above, mildly invasive lesions may kill, markedly invasive lesions may not (and an illustration firmly in mind is figure 29 in the early article by Allen [1949]; it shows part of a melanocarcinoma still wholly confined within the thickness of the epidermis, yet it had metastasised). Nevertheless, as with most other cancers, there is a broad correlation between depth of invasion and liability to metastasis, and, as already noted, most schemes of classification acknowledge the fact by noting the depth of invasion in relation to the adnexa and papillary and reticular dermis.

The problems posed by the lentigo maligna itself are not such as need cause the pathologist much worry, at least in the clinical sense; he is spared this by virtue of the fact that no radical or mutilating procedure such as amputation or even lymphadenectomy depends on his verdict. The culture or processing of malignant melanotic cells for production of an immune antiserum requires cells in far greater number than those present in even the most cellular of malignant lentigines. Therefore, if a lentigo maligna is considered as almost certain to become, or already to have become, a frank malignant melanoma, the subsequent totally excised specimen is not likely to be regarded by the immunotherapist as a very promising source of cells. Failure to diagnose correctly the excised lentigo maligna as being already in part a malignant melanoma would not, at present, be exposing the patient to any significantly increased danger.

## Spitz Naevus

This entity, formerly 'juvenile melanoma', is by now generally familiar, nevertheless it remains a possible candidate for misdiagnosis as melanocarcinoma, not least because it is not at all infrequent in the adult. In the series of 211 cases analysed by Weedon and Little (1977), for example, as many as 64 (31%) of their patients were aged 20 years or more. This analysis is so comprehensive that no further contribution could usefully be made here. It seems helpful, however, to reproduce the list of features that these observers found useful in distinguishing the lesion from melanocarcinoma. The possibility of Spitz naevus should not be entertained unless the cell pattern is of spindle or epithelioid character. Thereafter, features suggesting melanocarcinoma rather than the naevus are the presence of atypical mitoses; prominent upward epidermal spread of cells, particularly single cells, without overlying hyperkeratosis; lack of naevus cell maturity at the base of the lesion; nuclear hyperchromatism and clumping of chromatin in uninuclear cells; and destruction of collagen. They give a warning that vascular pseudo-invasion may be seen, and mislead: it was present in 6% of their cases.

A noteworthy comment apropos the diagnostic pitfalls around the Spitz naevus was made by Echevarria and Ackerman (1967) in the paper cited at the beginning of this section, thus:

> With the relative infrequency of malignant melanomas in early life, a diagnosis of benign lesion can be made in most cases. On the other hand, in adults malignant melanomas are more frequent than spindle cell nevi. There is then a danger here of mistaking a spindle cell nevus for a malignant melanoma, which may lead to radical surgery such as a lymph node dissection. It is important to keep in mind the existence of this rare benign neval lesion in adults.

While acknowledging the further comment of these authors, that there is no single criterion that allows a certain distinction between 'benign' and 'malignant', the danger they mention could at least be lessened by the pathologist's adopting the initially 'blind' approach or, if he himself is ineradicably biassed by foreknowledge of the patient's age, asking the opinion of colleagues still with an open mind.

## Diagnosis by Frozen Section

Understandably, the surgeon will seek help sometimes in frozen section diagnosis. An analysis of the value of this has been made by Little and Davis (1974) in the case of 329 pigmented lesions of skin of which 71% were melanocytic lesions either benign or malignant. An error was made in four cases, surgery was excessive or performed unnecessarily in 16 cases, and a diagnosis deferred in 19 cases. Coming from a specialist centre such as this, these figures may fairly be regarded as optimal. The authors calculate the accuracy of diagnosis as 98.8% but stated that this is after the 'diagnosis withheld' reports have been excluded, as has been the practice in analyses published by others that they quote where a similar figure has been claimed. When the point at issue is the very reliability and dependability of frozen section diagnosis, this seems strangely selective and does tend rather to obscure the issue. It seems fair to comment that if borderline cases are excluded from a survey of any diagnostic technique, the level of accuracy is bound to rise but any figure expressing the degree of accuracy then begins to become more apparent than real.

However, if these figures are regarded as encouraging enough to warrant continuance of the policy, it must be that the advantages to the many in the series have outweighed the disadvantages to the overtreated few. The pros and cons are obviously difficult to balance but there is at least an argument that the slender inconvenience of a 48-h delay is not too great a price to pay for the reduction by even a single case in the number overtreated. A rather different policy that goes some way to meet this difficulty is the selective one of Hughes (1975). In his experience, 'raised' lesions are either melanocarcinomas or not naevocytic lesions at all, and frozen section examination rarely raises problems; most pathologists would agree with this: 'flat' lesions under suspicion as melanocarcinoma are usually naevocytic and much likelier to cause diagnostic difficulty than the raised lesions. This difficulty is acknowledged by Hughes in his practice of excision with a 5–10 mm margin, the wound being left open thereafter pending arrival of the paraffin section report, all being well, within 48 h. This seems sound practice. It minimises the risk of a wrong diagnosis; it increases the likelihood of a correct diagnosis, and all else follows from this. The outcome may be at best no more than the suturing of the wound, and at worst, no more radical dissection than would have been required had the diagnosis of melanocarcinoma been made 48 h earlier. Any procedure that conduces to more accurate diagnosis, even if the further inconvenience to the patient were significant, which is not the case with the policy of Hughes, seems preferable.

There are many other debatable aspects of the melanocarcinoma that have a bearing on treatment and about which the pathologist may be consulted, including the risks of biopsy, the place of regional node dissection, the significance of pregnancy and childhood, the absent primary lesion and, closely parallel, delayed metastasis and spontaneous regression.

## Trauma

There are probably few now who believe that trauma, whether recurrent or in the form of a biopsy, provokes a benign melanotic lesion into a malignant one, and nowadays large naevi may be transected and removed in stages in a way that 30 years ago would have been regarded as virtually tantamount to malpraxis. A comparison was made by Epstein and his co-workers (1969) of the outcome in 115 patients with a biopsied lesion and 55 with immediately removed lesions; there was no difference. A survey of the prognostic value of various factors in 111 patients was made by Jones and his associates (1968) and they also concluded that biopsy was of no significance (size of lesion did appear to be significant: of patients with lesions greater than 3-cm diameter, only 9% survived 5 years; of those with lesions less than 3 cm in diameter, 49% had survived). In their account of 172 melanotic lesions in children, McWhorter and Woolner (1954) gave details of a juvenile melanoma, one half of which was excised at age one year and the other half at age eight years without complications. At the second operation, an adjacent nodule had a structure suggesting that it was also a juvenile melanoma but one that had matured histologically over the years.

Despite this and much other evidence of the harmlessness of biopsy, it possibly remains true, as was said by Allen and Spitz (1953), that "even those who are most positive in their denial of such an association (between trauma and malignant transformation) would probably recoil at the thought of repeatedly traumatising a suspicious lesion of their own". I have never, incidentally, had experience of a case where excision of a melanonaevus, unequivocally benign on microscopy, has been followed by the emergence of a melanocarcinoma at the same site: nor, despite frequently asking the question, have I met anyone who has. The nearest approach to this has been Case 7.22 of the local series but, as is evident, the position here remains obscure. With some preferring a diagnosis of melanocarcinoma for the original lesion, the criterion that benignancy be unequivocal has not been met.

The downgrading of trauma as a factor possibly provocative of malignancy is well illustrated in a publication by Kornberg and Ackerman (1975). These authors describe the histological features of eight lesions where repigmentation had developed at the site of earlier incomplete removal of intradermal melanonaevi by a surgical shaving procedure (and, in six of the eight patients, also by later electrodesiccation). The authors emphasise how closely the repigmenting areas of scarring may histologically resemble the superficial spreading melanocarcinoma, including permeation of the epidermis by atypical melanocytes both individually and in varyingly sized nests (melanocytes in mitosis, however, were few). The eight recurrent lesions, designated 'pseudo-melanoma', were regarded as recurrent melanocytic naevi, and as wholly benign: there was, however, no mention of the length of follow-up observation.

## Lymphadenectomy

Elective regional lymph node removal, its desirability or otherwise, whether in continuity or 'discontinuous' is still much in debate (see, for example, Southwick, 1976). The reason for this is evident: the lack of adequate 'control' information. It was rightly pointed out by Ballantyne (1970) that conclusions could properly be drawn from observed results only if the population whose treatment included prophylactic lymphadenectomy were compared with another population matched for age, sex, type and depth of lesion and other factors that might be relevant. The main difficulties in the way of doing this are evident, and they are in conflict. The surgeon will properly decide to treat an individual patient's lesion as he thinks appropriate to that particular patient, yet at the same time he will wish to avoid mutilation in the absence of any really convincing evidence that it is necessary. Yet so long as treatment is individualised, just so long will the accumulation of matched data be postponed. As things are, there are those, for example, Bodenham (1968), who believe that regional nodal excision should not be routinely performed, and those, such as Das Gupta and McNeer (1964) and Goldsmith and colleagues (1970), who believe that it should (for lesions on the limbs, Das Gupta and McNeer would omit the epitrochlear and popliteal nodes as areas only rarely involved). For superficial melanocarcinomas, that is, lesions limited to the upper one-third of the corium, Peterson and his associates (1964) suggest that routine node dissection should not be performed. It was noted by Milton (1969) that in 100 patients with recurrent or metastatic lesions, 76% developed secondary lesions at a potentially resectable site and that in only 24% was the reappearance first detected as metastatic foci in lungs, liver or brain: on this evidence he generally favours prophylactic lymphadenectomy. Further workers who have assessed the problem are Wilkinson and Paletta (1969), who broadly advocate lymphadenectomy (though for subungual melanocarcinoma on the foot, the results were so poor even with removal of nodes that they considered disarticulation at the hip would possibly be the better course) and Gläser and Graetz (1970) who advocate the use of pre-operative frozen sections of regional nodes, and lymphography especially for information on the status of retroperitoneal nodes. An earlier report on the use of lymphography by Cox and his colleagues (1966) had been far from encouraging; both false-negative and false-positive results were far too numerous.

The uncertainties of the whole position have been logically analysed by Conrad (1972) whose evidence indicated that it made little difference whether, in patients with melanocarcinoma and clinically uninvolved nodes, lymphadenectomy was performed or not, but that in those whose nodes did appear clinically to be involved the operation should be performed. This latter group was studied further by the same author (Conrad, 1972a) who showed clearly that some unexpectedly gratifying results could be obtained by the resection of involved nodes appearing some years after excision of the melanocarcinoma. Of 170 patients with metastatic cutaneous melanocarcinoma, 17% had survived for longer than 5 years after resection of their metastatic lesion; this report recalls the much earlier account of Allen and Spitz (1953) of three patients still alive 9, 11 and 12 years respectively after the excision of involved lymph nodes. Even yet, as Goldsmith (1979) makes plain, the pros and cons remain widely debatable.

It is important to note that melanin within a node draining the site of a melanocarcinoma does not always indicate the presence of malignant cells. Melanin may arrive there innocently in macrophages and present a difficult problem for the pathologist even in paraffin sections, let alone frozen sections: the volume of melanin may obscure cellular detail completely. Not only may melanin reach lymph nodes innocently: on occasion benign naevus cells may be found in the capsule of a node: examples have been reported by Johnson and Helwig (1969), Hart (1971) and McCarthy and associates (1974), and by Ridolfi and his colleagues (1977) who calculate that 46 examples have been reported so far. These cells, too, are harmless and should not be mistaken for metastatic melanocarcinoma. To this rather curious finding may be added the observation by Rodriguez and Ackerman (1968) of apparently naeval cells in the lymph nodes of 14 patients all of whom had had excision of a cellular blue naevus: all had survived without trouble for up to 16 years. Two similar cases were reported also by Azzopardi and colleagues (1977). Whatever the origin of such ectopic cells, whether metastatic or maldevelopmental, their presence is innocuous but, nevertheless, a possible cause of diagnostic concern. From their finding of naevus cells in 'endothelial lined channels' in five of 76 benign naevi (intradermal or junctional), Bell and his associates (1979) believe lymphatic deportation and thus innocent metastasis to be the likeliest explanation.

In the light of these findings, there cannot but be reservations about the comment of Hughes (1975) that "Frozen section diagnosis of melanoma in lymph nodes presents no difficulty". A rather bizarre contribution in this context is the report by Gérard-Merchant (1969) of the misdiagnosis of three cases of anaplastic carcinoma of the thyroid as melanocarcinoma: formalin pigment had been mistaken for melanin!

## PREGNANCY

The pathologist may be asked for information on the behaviour of melanocarcinoma during pregnancy, or on the possible influence of pregnancy on a patient who once did have a melanocarcinoma. Such information is available in the studies carried out specifically into the pregnancy/melanocarcinoma relationship by George and colleagues (1960) and White and colleagues (1961) and also, but more incidentally, in the reports of Bodenham (1968), on 650 cases, and Cochran (1969), on 165 cases, who referred to the matter in their analyses of melanocarcinoma in general. These authors were all agreed that the prognosis for a patient with melanocarcinoma is in no way affected by pregnancy.

However, even though these observations may have a general validity, individual cases occur sometimes when an explosive recurrence and spread of melanocarcinoma during pregnancy stretches belief in coincidence as the explanation almost beyond reason. Three such cases (one, however, was ocular), for example, were described by Cameron (1968) in an essentially clinical account of the lesion. Furthermore, a more recent appraisal of the matter by Shiu and his colleagues (1976) has somewhat modified this generally optimistic view. From a survey of 251 women aged 15–45 with melanocarcinoma they report a difference in prognosis when melanocarcinoma is considered in terms of clinical staging, whether at Stage I, "localized to the primary site" or Stage II, "metastases confined to the regional lymph nodes". Of their 165 patients in Stage I (36 nulliparous; 109 parous non-pregnant; 20 "admitted and treated during pregnancy") none of the sub-groups showed any significant difference in survival rate at 5 yrs from the other sub-groups; this at least

is in line with the earlier-cited reports. Of the 86 patients in Stage II, however, the group of 14 admitted and treated during pregnancy showed a significantly lower survival rate, 29%, than the nulliparous, 55%. Those not currently pregnant but who had experienced activation of a naevus during an earlier pregnancy fared even worse, with a survival rate of only 22%. There is much further information in this paper of great practical value to the pathologist approached for advice on the matter. An interesting peripheral point, illustrating the pitfalls of species difference, is that in experimental observations on the behaviour of the transplantable melanocarcinomas of hamsters and mice, the authors found that during pregnancy the growth and spread of these tumours was not enhanced but inhibited.

There is a belief, or at least suspicion, in some places that the contraceptive pill may activate melanonaevi but evidence is hard to find. In a brief case-report concerning the development and removal of a melanocarcinoma in a woman of 25 years on oral contraception, Ellerbroek (1968) remarked that "The experience reminds one of the enhancing effects of pregnancy or steroid treatments on the junctional nevus". No necessarily causal connection, however, was implied: and indeed, as Jelinek (1970) wrote in commentary on the case, "On statistical grounds, the occasional occurrence of a melanoma in a population of 7 million users is to be anticipated by chance". A former colleague, the late Professor John Milne of Glasgow, believed that some naevi could be activated by the 'pill' but, as his one-time associate, Dr A. McQueen (1979) has said in a personal communication, "Despite the strong feelings amongst workers (in this field) . . . there is very little hard evidence in the literature as yet". Some indirect and marginally relevant information lies in the observations by Smith and his colleagues (1977) on the possible interrelation between oral contraceptives and chloasma. They found that, in patients taking these substances, the plasma levels of immunoreactive $\beta$-melanocyte-stimulating hormone at least ". . . did not differ significantly from those in a group of age- and sex-matched controls". In view of its obvious clinical importance, the possible over-diagnosis of an activated naevus as a melanocarcinoma, further observations are much needed.

## INFLUENCE OF AGE

With little doubt, the earlier view that melano-carcinoma in children was curiously benign was due to misinterpretation as melanocarcinoma of the 'Spitz naevus'. As familiarity grew with the report by Spitz (1948), so, gradually, did the picture change. Melanocarcinoma in children is still rare but some 60 examples have by now been recorded, and, of these, about 25% have arisen in giant hypertrophic naevi (Lerman et al., 1970). Of the 12 patients described by Lerman, 8 died within 18 months: the 5-year survival rate was 33%. It may be, as Lowry (1974) suggests, that 'immunological factors' are concerned in the rarity of cancers as a whole in childhood, but, once established, their rate of progress seems little, if any, slower or less lethal than in the adult. In a case reported by Penman and Stringer (1971), a melanocarcinoma that developed in a giant naevus in a male infant, probably at age of about 12 months, had caused death by metastasis 16 months later.

## DELAY IN METASTASIS

Long-delayed metastasis is a well-known, even if fairly rare, feature of melanocarcinoma but probably occurs no more frequently than with, say, carcinoma of the breast. In his analysis of survival patterns in 216 patients with metastatic melanocarcinoma, Hendrix (1969) found that 35 of his patients (16.2%) treated for metastatic or recurrent lesions had survived for 5 years or longer: two had survived for 28 and 26 years respectively; and 1 patient died from the disease 21 years later. Comparison of various features, including age and sex, in these 35 patients, with those in the rest, however, yielded none of prognostic value.

Phenomena that are seen more commonly than with any other neoplasm except chorio-carcinoma are both spontaneous regression of a primary lesion and of metastases. As has been described by many authors, including Smith and Stehlin (1965), Bodenham (1968), Ballantyne (1970), McLeod and associates (1971), and Conrad (1972), widely disseminated melano-carcinoma with no demonstrable primary lesion is a well-recognised curiosity (in the McLeod series, it was exemplified by 5% of their 361 patients). It is true that the discovery, perhaps at necropsy, of a hitherto undetected lesion in some hairy part of the body has sometimes explained all, but this is altogether too rare to be a universal explanation. It has recently been suggested (Lewis and Copeman, 1972: Editorial, 1973) that the regression of a primary melano-carcinoma may have much in common with the regression seen in a 'halo' naevus, and that the halo naevus is in fact a 'frustrated malignant melanoma': that is, frustrated by some mechanism of immunity whose failure in lethal mel-anocarcinoma is itself so frustrating because so poorly understood.

## Conclusions

1) Of lesions histologically considered to be certainly or possibly melanocarcinoma, some 20% are at risk of being over-diagnosed or under-diagnosed.

2) Of histological criteria that may help to distinguish malignant lesions from benign, mitotic activity still seems the most useful. Upward migration of melanocytes through the epidermis may occur in benign lesions. Simulated vascular invasion may be seen in the Spitz naevus and probably other benign lesions.

3) Any spindle-celled neoplasm of skin should prompt thoughts of a melanocytic lesion, benign or malignant.

4) Naevus cells may metastasise to or be present within lymph nodes with innocence.

5) Melanin within melanophores in lymph nodes may be mistaken for metastatic melano-carcinoma.

6) On frozen section, any diagnosis less than 'unequivocally melanocarcinoma' is an indication for deferral of further action.

7) Benign naevus cells remnant after apparently incomplete excision seem rarely if ever to cause trouble.

8) Demonstration of melanosomes will enable diagnosis of an apparently amelanotic lesion, whether primary or metastatic, as melanotic but it is rarely prognostically helpful.

9) Prognosis in the individual case, even when malignancy is histologically unequivocal, remains difficult. In general, probability of metastasis lies between 5% or less with total depth of malignant tissue of 1 mm or less, and 75% or more with total depth of 7 mm or more.

# References

Allen AC (1949) A reorientation on the histogenesis and clinical significance of cutaneous nevi and melanomas. Cancer 2: 28–56

Allen AC, Spitz S (1953) Malignant melanoma. A clinicopathological analysis of the criteria for diagnosis and prognosis. Cancer 6: 1–45

Anton-Lamprecht I, Schnyder UW, Tilgen W (1971) Das "Stade éphélide" der melanotischen Präcancerose. Eine vergleichende klinisch-histopatholowisch-elektronenmikroskopisch Studie. Arch Dermatol Forsch 240: 61–78

Azzopardi JG, Ross CMD, Frizzera G (1977) Blue naevi of lymph node capsule. Histopathol 1: 451–461

Ballantyne AJ (1970) Malignant melanoma of the skin of the head and neck. An analysis of 405 cases. Am J Surg 120: 425–431

Bell MAE, Hill DP, Bhargava MK (1979) Lymphatic invasion in pigmented nevi. Am J Clin Pathol 72: 97–100

Bodenham DC (1968) A study of 650 observed malignant melanomas in the south-west region. Ann R Coll Surg Engl 43: 218–239

Borello ED, Gorlin RJ (1966) Melanotic neuroectodermal tumor of infancy—a neoplasm of neural crest origin. Report of a case associated with high urinary excretion of vanilmandelic acid. Cancer 19: 196–206

Breslow A (1975) Thickness, cross-sectional areas and depth of invasion in the prognosis of cutaneous melanoma. Ann Surg 172: 902–908

Breslow A (1977) Problems in the measurement of tumor thickness and level of invasion in cutaneous melanoma. Hum Pathol 8: 1–2

Breslow A, Macht SD (1978) Evaluation of prognosis in stage I cutaneous melanoma. Plast Reconstr Surg 61: 342–346

Cameron JRJ (1968) Melanoma of skin. Clinical account of a series of 209 malignant melanomas of skin. J R Coll Surg Edinb 13: 233–254

Clark WH, Mihm MC (1969) Lentigo maligna and lentigo-maligna melanoma. Am J Pathol 55: 39–67

Clark WH, From L, Bernardino EA, Mihm MC (1969) The histogenesis and biologic behavior of primary human malignant melanomas of the skin. Cancer Res 29: 705–727

Cochran AJ (1968) Method of assessing prognosis in patients with malignant melanoma. Lancet II: 1062–1064

Cochran AJ (1969) Malignant melanoma. A review of 10 years' experience in Glasgow, Scotland. Cancer 23: 1190–1199

Cochran AJ (1969a) Histology and prognosis in malignant melanoma. J Pathol 97: 459–468

Conley J, Lattes R, Orr W (1971) Desmoplastic malignant melanoma (A rare variant of spindle cell melanoma). Cancer 28: 914–936

Conrad FG (1972) Treatment of malignant melanoma. Wide excision alone vs lymphadenectomy. Arch Surg 104: 587–592

Conrad FG (1972a) Cures achieved in patients with metastatic malignant melanoma of the skin. Cancer 30: 144–147

Couperus M, Rucker RC (1954) Histopathological diagnosis of malignant melanoma. Arch Dermatol Syphilol 70: 199–216

Cox KR, Hare WSC, Bruce PT (1966) Lymphography in melanoma. Correlation of radiology with pathology. Cancer 19: 637–647

Curran RC, McCann BG (1976) The ultrastructure of benign pigmented naevi and melanocarcinoma in man. J Pathol 119: 135–146

Das Gupta T, McNeer G (1964) The incidence of metastasis to accessible lymph nodes from melanoma of the trunk and extremities—its therapeutic significance. Cancer 17: 897–911

Davis NC, Herron JJ, McLeod GR (1966) Malignant melanoma in Queensland. Analysis of 400 skin lesions. Lancet II: 407–410

Davis J, Pack GT, Higgins GK (1967) Melanotic freckle of Hutchinson. Am J Surg 113: 457–463

DeCosse JJ, McNeer G (1969) Superficial melanoma. A clinical study. Arch Surg 99: 531–534

Delacrétaz J (1969) Mélanome juvénile (mélanome de Spitz) a évolution maligne. Dermatologica 139: 79–83

Echevarria R, Ackerman LV (1967) Spindle and epithelioid cell nevi in the adult. Clinicopathologic report of 26 cases. Cancer 20: 175–189

Editorial (1973) The Halo Naevus and Malignant Melanoma. Lancet I: 982

Ellerbroek WC (1968) Oral contraceptives and malignant melanoma. JAMA 206: 649–650

Epstein E, Bragg K, Linden G (1969) Biopsy and prognosis of malignant melanoma. JAMA 208: 1369–1371

George PA, Fortner JG, Pack GT (1960) Melanoma with pregnancy. A report of 115 cases. Cancer 13: 854–859

Gérard-Marchant R (1969) Pseudo-mélanomes malins du corps thyroide (Apropos du pigment formolé). Bull Cancer (Paris) 56: 91–98

Gläser A, Graetz H (1970) Die Behandlung der malignen Melanome aus chirurgischer Sicht. Dtsch Gesundheitsw 25: 158–160

Goldsmith HS (1979) The debate over immediate lymph node dissection in melanoma. Surg Gynec Obstet 148: 403–405

Goldsmith HS, Shah JP, Kim DH (1970) Prognostic significance of lymph node dissection in the treatment of malignant melanoma. Cancer 26: 606–609

Hart WR (1971) Primary nevus of a lymph node. Am J Clin Pathol 55: 88–92

Hartwell SW, Anderson R, Hazard JB (1970) Superficial malignant melanoma. Clinicopathologic correlation. Plast Reconstr Surg 46: 425–428

Hendrix RC (1969) Unusual survival patterns of

patients with metastatic melanoma. Cancer 24: 574–576

Holmes EC, Clark W, Morton DL, Eilber FR, Bochow AJ (1976) Regional lymph node metastases and the level of invasion of primary melanoma. Cancer 37: 199–201

Hughes LE (1975) The place of frozen section in the practical management of melanoma. Br J Surg 62: 840–844

Jelinek JE (1970) Cutaneous side effects of oral contraceptives. Arch Dermatol 101: 181–186

Johnson WT, Helwig EB (1969) Benign nevus cells in the capsule of lymph nodes. Cancer 23: 747–753

Jones WM, Williams WJ, Roberts MM, Davies K (1968) Malignant melanoma of the skin: Prognostic value of clinical features and the role of treatment in 111 cases. Br J Cancer 22: 437–451

Kernen JA, Ackerman LV (1960) Spindle cell nevi and epithelioid cell nevi (so-called juvenile melanomas) in children and adults: A clinicopathological study of 27 cases. Cancer 13: 612–625

Kornberg R, Ackerman AB (1975) Pseudomelanoma. Recurrent melanocytic nevus following partial surgical removal. Arch Dermatol 111: 1588–1590

Larsen TE, Grude TH (1979) A retrospective histological study of 669 cases of primary cutaneous malignant melanoma in clinical stage I. 5. The consequences of a reclassification of the original group of lentigo maligna melanomas. Acta path microbiol Scand A 87: 255–260

Lerman RI, Murray D, O'Hara JM, Booher RJ, Foote FW (1970) Malignant melanoma of childhood. A clinico-pathologic study and a report of 12 cases. Cancer 25: 436–449

Lewis MG, Copeman PWM (1972) Halo naevus— a frustrated malignant melanoma? Br Med J I: 47–48

Little JH, Davis NC (1974) Frozen section diagnosis of suspected malignant melanoma of the skin. Cancer 34: 1163–1172

Lowry WS (1974) Passive immunity against childhood cancer. Lancet I: 602–603

McCarthy SW, Palmer AA, Bale PM, Hirst E (1974) Nevus cells in lymph nodes. Pathology 6: 351–358

McGovern VJ (1970) The classification of melanoma and its relationship with prognosis. Pathology 2: 85–98

McGovern VJ, Mihm MC, Bailly C, Booth JC, Clark WH, Cochran AJ, Hardy EG, Hicks JD, Levene A, Lewis MG, Little JH, Milton GW (1973) The classification of malignant melanoma and its histologic reporting. Cancer 32: 1446–1457

McGovern VJ, Shaw HM, Milton GW, Farago GA (1979) Prognostic significance of the histological features of malignant melanoma. Histopathol 3: 385–393

Mackie R, Carfrae DC, Cochran AJ (1972) Assess-

ment of prognosis in patients with malignant melanoma. Lancet II: 455–456

McLeod GR, Beardmore GL, Little JH, Quinn RL, Davis NC (1971) Results of treatment of 361 patients with malignant melanoma in Queensland. Med J Aust 1: 1211–1216

McWhorter HE, Woolner LB (1954) Pigmented nevi, juvenile melanomas, and malignant melanomas in children. Cancer 7: 564–585

Magnus K (1973) Incidence of malignant melanoma of the skin in Norway, 1955–1970. Variations in time and space and solar radiation. Cancer 32: 1275–1286

Magnus K (1977) Prognosis in malignant melanoma of the skin. Significance of stage of disease, anatomical site, sex, age and period of diagnosis. Cancer 40: 389–397

Milton GW (1969) Malignant melanoma and a study of some aspects of cancer. J R Coll Surg Edinb 14: 193–202

Mishima Y (1967) Melanocytic and nevocytic malignant melanomas: Cellular and subcellular differentiation. Cancer 20: 632–649

Penman HG, Stringer HCW (1971) Malignant transformation in giant congenital pigmented nevus. Death in early childhood. Arch Dermatol 103: 428–432

Peterson RF, Hazard JB, Dykes ER, Anderson R (1964) Superficial malignant melanomas. Surg Gynecol Obstet 119: 37–41

Pinkus H, Mehregan AH (1963) Epidermotropic eccrine carcinoma. A case combining features of eccrine poroma and Paget's dermatosis. Arch Dermatol 88: 597–604

Ridolfi RL, Rosen PP, Thaler H (1977) Nevus cell aggregates associated with lymph nodes: Estimated frequency and clinical significance. Cancer 39: 164–171

Rodriguez HA, Ackerman LV (1968) Cellular blue nevus. Clinicopathologic study of forty-five cases. Cancer 21: 393–405

Saksela E, Rintala A (1968) Misdiagnosis of prepubertal malignant melanoma. Reclassification of a cancer registry material. Cancer 22: 1308–1314

Shiu MH, Schottenfeld D, Maclean B, Fortner JG (1976) Adverse effect of pregnancy on melanoma: A reappraisal. Cancer 37: 181–187

Smith AG, Shuster S, Thody AJ, Peberdy M (1977) Chloasma, oral contraceptives, and plasma immunoreactive β-melanocyte-stimulating hormone. J Invest Dermatol 68: 169–170

Smith JL, Stehlin JS (1965) Spontaneous regression of primary malignant melanomas with regional metastases. Cancer 18: 1399–1415

Southwick HW (1976) Malignant melanoma: Role of node dissection reappraised. Cancer 37: 202–205

Spitz S (1948) Melanomas of childhood. Am J Pathol 24: 591–609

Suffin SC, Waisman J, Clark WH, Morton DL

(1977) Comparison of the classification by microscopic level (stage) of malignant melanoma by three independent groups of pathologists. Cancer 40: 3112–3114

Truax H, Barnett RN, Hukill PB, Campbell PC, Eisenberg H (1966) Effect of inaccurate pathological diagnosis on survival statistics for melanoma. Survey of cases in the Connecticut Tumor Registry. Cancer 19: 1543–1547

Wanebo HJ, Woodruff J, Fortner JG (1975) Malignant melanoma of the extremities: A clinicopathologic study using levels of invasion (microstage). Cancer 35: 666–676

Weedon D, Little JH (1977) Spindle and epithelioid cell nevi in children and adults: A review of 211 cases of the Spitz nevus. Cancer 40: 217–225

White LP, Linden G, Breslow L, Harzfeld L (1961) Studies on melanoma. The effect of pregnancy on survival in human melanoma. JAMA 177: 235–238

Wilkinson TS, Paletta FX (1969) Malignant melanoma: Current concepts. Am Surg 35: 301–309

Williams WJ, Davies K, Jones WM, Roberts MM (1968) Malignant melanoma of the skin: Prognostic value of histology in 89 cases. Br J Cancer 22: 452–460

# 8 Lesions of the Digestive Tract

The digestive tract has, in the years under review, produced many more biopsies than, for example, the skeletal system or lymph nodes, but many fewer borderline problems. With an adequately representative biopsy, and excluding for the moment unusual individual lesions, problems in the digestive tract form fairly well-defined groups, none essentially different from those met in other systems. They are: (a) the squamous epithelial overgrowths of the oral cavity; (b) dysplasia or carcinoma in situ in oesophagus, stomach and large intestine; (c) the fibrotic pancreas; (d) the adenomatous polyps of, predominantly, the large intestine. A problem of a different order impinges only partly on histopathology, that of sampling, and for understandable technical reasons it is relatively common in the gastrointestinal tract. The tissue submitted may be quite unrepresentative; a 'negative' report is likely then to confirm the surgeon's suspicion that it was so, and indicate a further biopsy. At other times, the tissue may have come from only the edge of a neoplasm where malignant changes may be still only in situ, or from a neoplasm proper but severely distorted (not infrequent with biopsies from the lower oesophagus). As endoscopy advances, so pathologists receive an increasing number of 1–2 mm biopsies. The procedure may enable the clinician to diagnose, say, an ulcer-cancer earlier than he otherwise could but, in parallel, it will produce for the pathologist more biopsies that are negative or borderline, and the difficulties may be great. Stringent discipline will be required to assess the correctness of diagnosis of gastro-oesophageal and colonic carcinoma reached on such specimens. Strict comparison of the biopsy report with the findings in the resected specimen is mandatory, otherwise the uncertainty that still surrounds carcinoma in situ of the cervix will emerge again here, and statistics will be suspect.

## Local Series

Diagnostic uncertainty or debate was raised by 26 cases. This is a minimum figure since (a) any chronic peptic ulcer of stomach is a borderline lesion to the extent that it may include an area of carcinoma or be the ulcerated part of a paucicellular linitis plastica (exemplified by Case 8.17), and (b) all adenomatous polyps of the large intestine are also in some degree borderline lesions (Case 8.20 has been included as a single representative example). Taking into account these sizeable reservations, comparison may be made between these 26 cases and the incidence of carcinoma of stomach diagnosed during the same time, approximately 20 cases a year or nearly 500 in all.

### SUMMARISED TOTALS

The appropriateness or otherwise of the original diagnosis could be reasonably assessed in 25 of the 26 cases: early death precluded long-term assessment in one (a probable leiomyosarcoma of stomach).

*Review has yielded:*
Under-diagnoses, 4
Over-diagnoses, 2
Appropriate diagnoses, 20

The cost of the four under-diagnoses was, in one case (8.2), an unnecessary number of excisions for the eventually complete removal of a verrucous carcinoma of alveolus: in the three other cases, death from carcinoma which would, however, almost certainly not have been prevented even if the diagnosis had been made correctly earlier.

The cost of the two over-diagnoses was a course of radiotherapy for a benign lympho-epithelial lesion in palate, though the patient was still trouble-free 21 years later (Case 8.4); and the loss of a pancreas for a hamartoma of duodenum, though the patient was well 7 years later (Case 8.19).

Data of the 26 cases are reproduced in Table 8.1.

CASE DATA

*Case 8.1*

F (67 years) with 10-mm ulcerated swelling of left upper alveolus.

**Table 8.1.** Twenty-six cases of equivocal lesions of digestive tract.

| Case No. | Diagnosis on review | Treatment | Outcome |
|---|---|---|---|
| *4 cases under-diagnosed* | | | |
| 8.1 | Carcinoma > papilloma (alveolus) | Radiotherapy | Death @ 16 yr |
| 8.2 | Verrucous ca. > papilloma (alveolus) | Excision × 3 | Unrelated death @ 3 yr |
| 8.9 | Carcinoma > 'disquieting' (oesophagus) | Resection | Death @ 3 yr |
| 8.23 | Angiosarcoma > 'vascular papilloma' (gall bladder) | Excision × 3 | Death @ 2 wk after laparotomy |
| *2 cases over-diagnosed* | | | |
| 8.4 | Benign lymphoepithelial lesion > 'polyblastoma' (palate) | Radiotherapy | Alive @ 21 yr |
| 8.19 | Hamartoma > carcinoma (duodenum) | Excision + pancreatectomy | Alive @ 7 yr |
| *20 cases appropriately diagnosed* | | | |
| 8.3 | Carcinoma (palate) | Radiotherapy | Unrelated death @ 5 yr |
| 8.5 | Salivary carcinoma (lip, aged 10 yr) | Excision | Alive @ 14 yr |
| 8.6 | Pseudo-sarcomatous carcinoma (pharynx) | Excision | Death @ 3½ yr |
| 8.7 | 'Lymphoepithelioma' (tonsil) | Radiotherapy | Death (but from related sq. carc.) @ 18 yr |
| 8.8 | Chronic tonsillitis | Excision | Alive @ 8 yr |
| 8.10 | Oesophagitis | Conservative | Alive @ 15 yr |
| 8.11 | 'Suspicious' (oesophagus) | Resection | Death @ 11 yr (carcinoma) |
| 8.12 | 'Almost certainly carcinoma' (oesophagus) | Resection | Death @ 3 wk (carcinoma) |
| 8.13 | 'Abnormal' (oesophagus) | Resection | Death @ 7 mo (carcinoma) |
| 8.14 | Leiomyosarcoma (stomach) | Partial gastrectomy | Alive @ 15 yr |
| 8.15 | Leiomyosarcoma (stomach) | Partial gastrectomy | Unrelated death @ 5 months |
| 8.16 | Carcinoid tumour (stomach) | Partial gastrectomy | Alive @ 15 yr |
| 8.17 | Chronic peptic ulcer (stomach) | Partial gastrectomy | Prob. unrelated death @ 28 months |
| 8.18 | Chronic PU + carc. (stomach) | Partial gastrectomy | Unrelated death @ 4½ yr |
| 8.20 | Carc. in-situ (polyp, rectum) | Resection | Alive @ 12 yr |
| 8.21 | Mucoid carcinoma (anus) | Resection | Death @ probably 35 yr (carc.) |
| 8.22 | Metaplastic polyp (rectum) | Excision | Alive @ 12 yr |
| 8.24 | Omental metastasis (carcinoma) | Palliative | Death @ 5 months |
| 8.25 | Serosal metaplasia (adnexal) | Excision | Alive @ 5 yr |
| 8.26 | Carcinoma > endometriosis | Excision | Postoperative death |

The 8-mm biopsy showed stromal tissue widely permeated by bands and strands of neoplastic, nonkeratinising, stratified squamous epithelium. It was reported as a 'highly cellular papillomatous tumour . . . with numerous mitotic figures'. A firm diagnosis of malignancy was considered to be unwarranted but the advice was given that the lesion should be treated as if it were malignant.

The patient was treated by radiotherapy but died 16 years later, essentially from the effects of the lesion, a 'carcinoma of maxilla'.

The problem originally was 'highly cellular papilloma or carcinoma?' Re-examination of the sections shows so much mitotic activity, with so many of the figures aberrant, that this has to be regarded as a *significant under-diagnosis*. However, on the advice offered, appropriate treatment was used and was associated, at any rate, with 16-year survival.

## Case 8.2

M (69 years) with craggy ulcerated 15-mm swelling on left upper alveolar margin. It was excised by diathermy.

Sections showed an extreme degree of squamous epithelial hyperplasia, and the lesion was reported descriptively only. The lesion had recurred within 4 months and was re-excised, on this occasion including clearance on the deep surface down to bone. The tissue was of essentially similar pattern though now recognisably more papillary. Squamous papilloma, at the least, would have been a more appropriate diagnosis but the lesion was reported as 'a rather exuberant denture hyperplasia'.

Again the mass re-grew and a more radical maxillary resection was performed, again to yield a relatively large amount of tissue in the form of a warty mass, 32 × 20 × 15 mm. This was now reported as a highly cellular 'squamous papilloma', more cytologically aberrant in some places than before, and apparently transected through some of the more aberrant areas. Yet further clearance was attempted, and similarly hyperplastic tissue obtained, and still there was doubt about adequacy of resection.

No further resection or other treatment was used, and the patient was known to be alive and trouble-free (in this respect) 2 years later. He was reported as having died '2 or 3 years' after that, almost certainly from an unrelated cause.

In all respects, in its mode of presentation, gross and microscopic appearance and behaviour, this is recognisable now as a typical 'verrucous carcinoma'. To the extent that the lesion was apparently finally excised in toto, the first formal diagnosis of hyperplastic squamous papilloma, if not wholly appropriate was at any rate not inappropriate. However, to the extent that the lesion was extirpated only after several resections, the original diagnosis was an *under-diagnosis*. Had the diagnosis of verrucous carcinoma been made originally, as it might have been, radical excision would have followed at once and the patient spared the succession of operations described.

A subsidiary aspect raised by the histology on review is that stretches of epithelium at the edge of the lesion show a 'saw-tooth' pattern and general disposition extremely like that of lichen planus. The questions this raises are (a) is the lesion essentially hypertrophic lichen planus, and the answer to this is almost certainly 'no': (b) if not that, or no longer that, is this a verrucous carcinoma that arose from a hypertrophic LP? This last may be so but the question cannot be answered with certainty. If it could be answered, and had been answered, treatment would still have had to be the same. The practical implications are thus minimal, but the point is raised since I recall an instance where, after enquiry by a dermatologist, a lesion reported as SCC was found on review certainly to be hypertrophic LP.

## Case 8.3

M (79 years) with a 10 × 8 mm polypoid nodule on free edge of soft palate.

As in Case 8.1, this was a papillary mass of hyperplastic stratified squamous epithelium. Here, however, almost the whole of the tissue was epithelium; stroma was minimal. Also, the overgrowth was highly differentiated, with orderly maturation of the convoluted bands of epithelium from basal layer, through well-formed prickle cells, to nonkeratinising squames. The disquieting feature was an exceptionally high frequency of cells in mitosis, in some places up to 6 per hpf. Almost all, however, were in the basal half of the epithelial bands, and none was convincingly aberrant. Nevertheless, advice was offered that the lesion should be regarded as a squamous-celled carcinoma.

The nodule was treated by radiotherapy, and the patient died 5 years later with pernicious anaemia, and no recurrence of the palatal lesion.

Again, as in Case 8.1, the diagnosis lay between highly cellular papilloma and carcinoma but there was none of the aberrant mitotic activity that should have made the diagnosis in the earlier case one of unequivocal malignancy. In the present case the degree of activity was high, and there was no certainty that it would subside. In the circumstances therefore, this seems in retrospect an *appropriate diagnosis*.

### Case 8.4

F (56 years) with 15 × 10 mm swelling of 1-year duration on side of soft palate.

Sections of the ten irregular fragments, up to 5 mm across, showed glands and ducts thinly scattered throughout a background of lymphoid tissue. The lesion was regarded as probably neoplastic and malignant, and given the unusual designation 'polyblastoma': both elements, the lymphoid and the epithelial, had presumably, therefore, been regarded as malignant.

Reassessment, however, shows that many of the ducts and glands, of both mucous and mixed salivary types, are structurally and cytologically regular. Many others have become variably hypercellular, often with obliteration of tubular or acinar outline, and now appear as larger or smaller islands of still uniform cellularity, with an occasional cell in (normal) mitosis. The background or infiltrate is almost purely lymphocytic but there is a sprinkling of cells with much larger and paler nuclei, not identifiable further than as reticulum cells; they, too, were occasionally in normal mitosis. Review finds the complex pattern of tissue almost certainly an example of the so-called 'benign lymphoepithelial lesion' of salivary tissue.

On the original diagnosis, the patient was treated by irradiation. Enquiry found her asymptomatic and well 21 years later. This was a significant *over-diagnosis*.

### Case 8.5

M (10 years) with an 'ulcer in the mouth' present for 6 months. The ulcer was 18 × 5 mm on the inner surface of the upper lip opposite the right premolar teeth. After biopsy and diagnosis the lesion was excised by wedge-resection of a piece of tissue 35 × 30 × 25 mm. The ulcerated area was now 20 × 7 mm and beneath it, as shown in Fig. 8.1, obviously abnor-

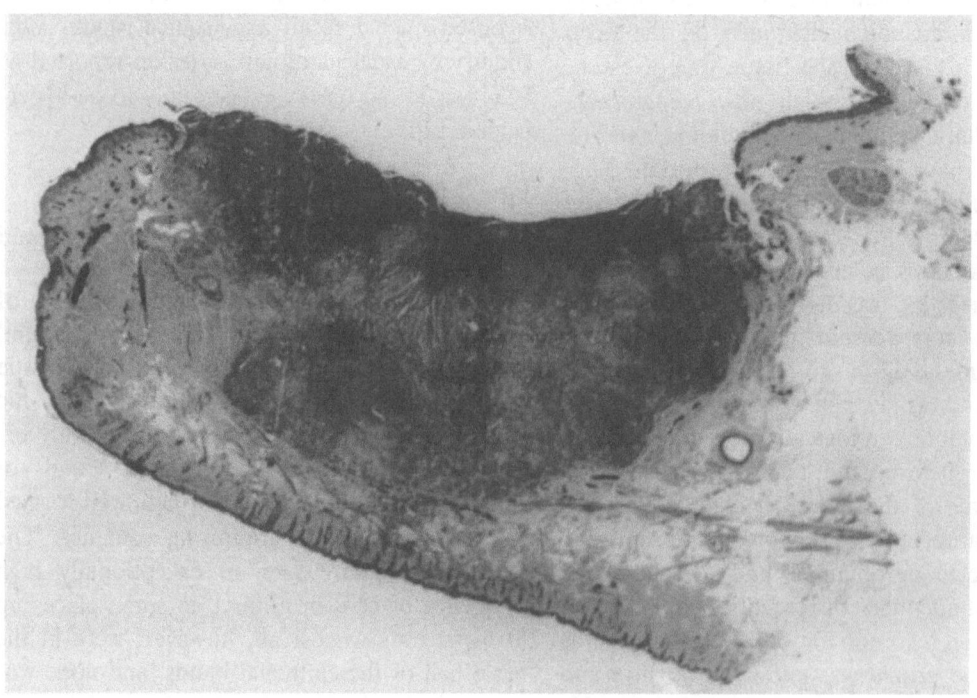

**Fig. 8.1.** Occupation of almost the full thickness of the lip by hyperchromatic tissue. The upper (buccal) surface is totally ulcerated. H & E, × 5

mal tissue occupied almost the full thickness of the lip.

The abnormal tissue was glandular carcinoma widely infiltrating muscle bundles (Fig. 8.2) and varying in its degree of differentiation. In some places acinar formation was prominent, so much so that in some areas, as seen in Fig. 8.3, where the acini were filled by brightly eosinophilic secretion, the possibility was considered that the tissue was metastatic thyroid carcinoma. In other places, especially at the edge where epidermis was being infiltrated and destroyed (Fig. 8.4) the tissue was quite undifferentiated and disposed in sheets. Figure 8.5 shows that the nuclei were relatively uniform though mitotic figures were not infrequent.

The lesion was considered most probably to be a 'salivary carcinoma' and, as such, unlikely to have already metastasised and, with the evident completeness of excision, very possibly to have been eradicated in toto. The question of radiotherapy was considered but, in view of the certainty of damage of the teeth and possibly temporo-mandibular joint, rejected.

All was well for 16 months until the patient was found to have a 12-mm palpable node at the lower anterior edge of the parotid on the affected side. This was excised and found to be essentially normal. There was no further trouble, and all was well 14 years later.

The course of events showed that the carcinoma, despite its extensive invasion, had not yet had the capacity to metastasise. Its restricted aggressiveness largely confirms the view that it was of salivary-gland origin: an *appropriate* diagnosis.

## Case 8.6

F (65 years) with complaint of dysphagia, nasal regurgitation, and nasality of speech. Examination showed a smooth globular mass, 30 × 30 × 15 mm, in the hypopharynx. This lesion was the subject of a case report (Glover and Park, 1971) when it was described and designated a 'leiomyosarcoma'. Subsequent events showed that this diagnosis was almost certainly wrong; or, at least, that the mass was in retrospect identical with the lesion described earlier, and later by others, for example Sherwin and colleagues

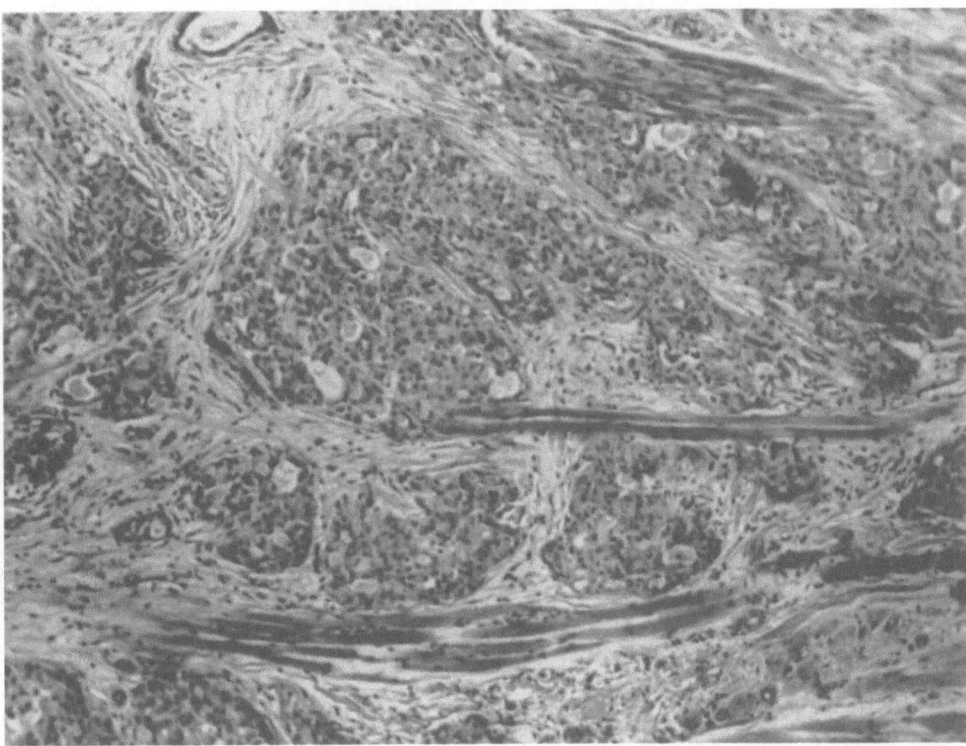

**Fig. 8.2.** Disruption of muscle by recognisably glandular carcinoma. H & E, × 62

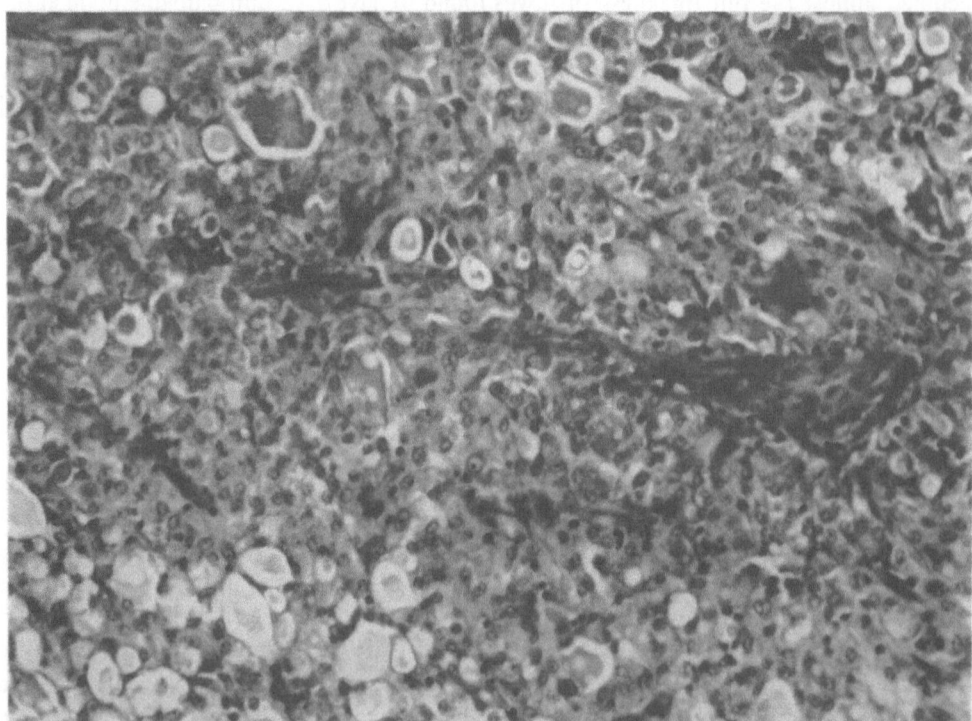

**Fig. 8.3.** A mixture of highly differentiated and almost completely undifferentiated tissue. H & E, × 246

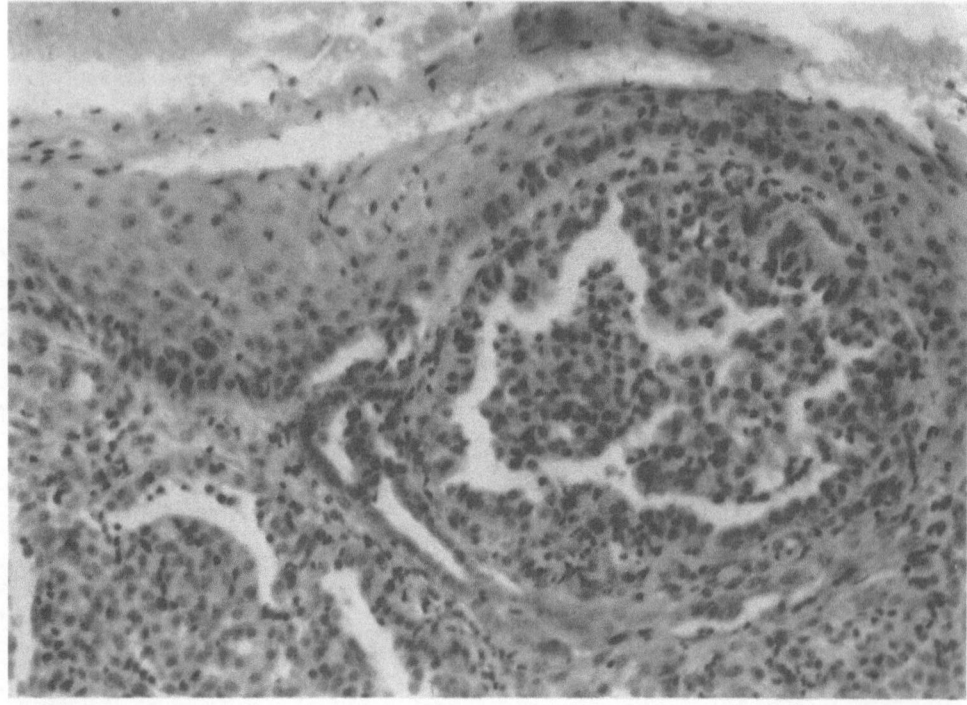

**Fig. 8.4.** Undifferentiated carcinoma is undermining the epidermis. The large circular mass was not convincingly within a vessel. H & E, × 246

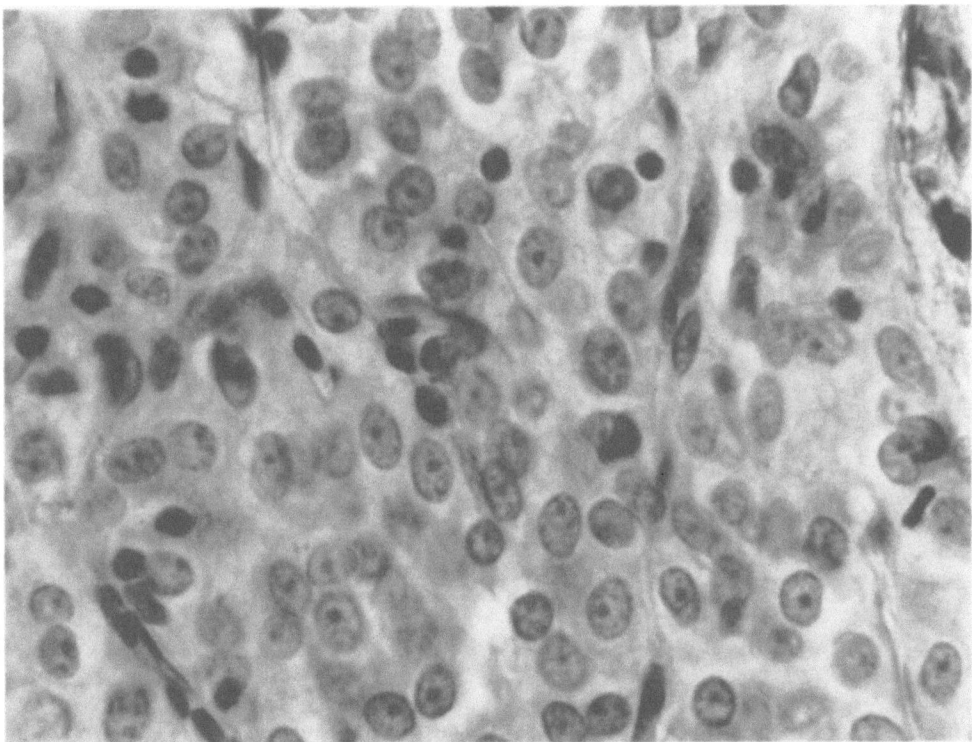

**Fig. 8.5.** The cells are generally uniform. A mitotic figure lies at the upper left-hand corner. H & E, × 985

(1963) and Enrile and associates (1973), as a polypoid pseudo-sarcomatous carcinoma.

After diagnosis of the mass as a sarcoma, a further definitive excision was performed, in essence a wider excision of the tissue around the base of the pedicle. This yielded fragments of tissue showing, unexpectedly, what seemed with little doubt to be 'carcinoma in situ' in the adjacent epithelium. The relation of this lesion to the other was an obvious problem.

The mass as a whole and its highly polymorphic, mitotically aberrant character are shown in Figs. 8.6–8.10. Reassessment now, with particular attention paid to the surface of the mass immediately beside the pedicle, where any possibly derivative association with the pharyngeal epithelium might still have been evident, shows no transitional pattern that could reasonably be interpreted as indicating an origin from the epithelium. Also, although distortion from the cauterisation that was part of the second operation was considered as the possible explanation for the unexpected finding, the area that seemed with little doubt to be carcinoma in situ

still looks most plausibly to be exactly that.

Three years later the patient reappeared with an extensive ulcerating lesion at the site of the previous lesion. Biopsy showed unequivocal 'invasive squamous-celled carcinoma'. This removed the last doubts about the earlier lesion having been carcinoma in situ. Despite various forms of therapy she died 4 months later.

In terms of total probability, 'pseudo-sarcomatous carcinoma' is almost certainly the correct diagnosis for the initial polypoid lesion. In terms of histology, this example at least remains devoid of structural evidence, as seen, for instance, with reticulin staining, that would justify a diagnosis of carcinoma. It remains a histological oddity: its diagnosis as a malignant neoplasm was *appropriate* even if nosologically inaccurate.

### Case 8.7

This case is included only because the unexpected reappearance of the patient at age 87 years, 17 years after the diagnosis of 'lympho-epithelioma' of the tonsil, gave rise to doubt

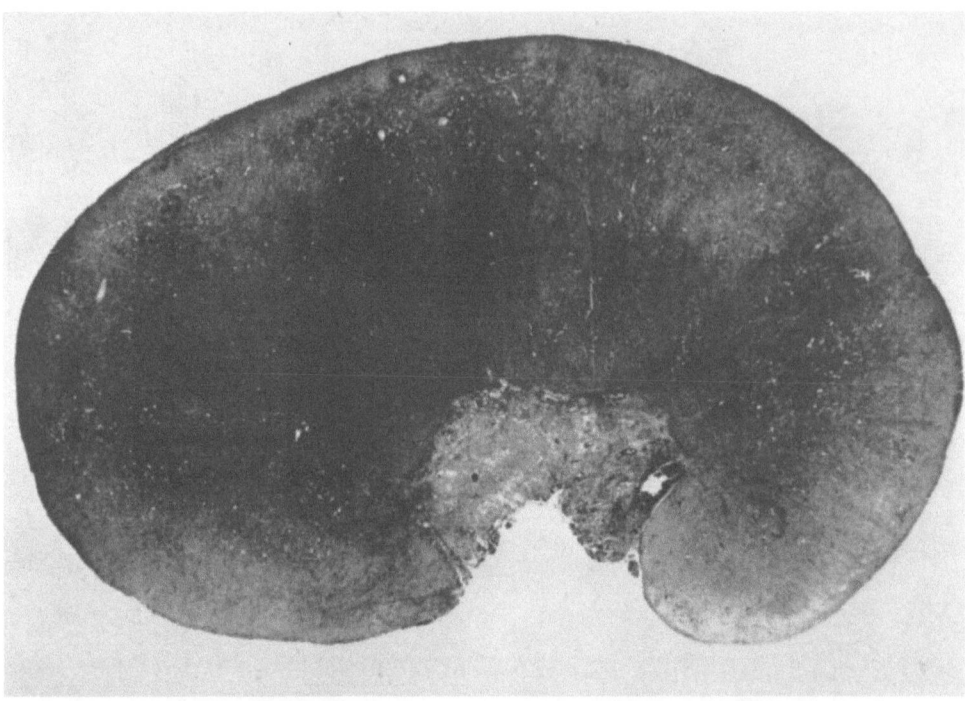

**Fig. 8.6.** The smooth-surfaced globular mass. Such pedicle as there was had shrunk into the 'hilum'. The surface retained a covering of epithelium that showed no area of transition to the polymorphic tissue beneath. H & E, × 4

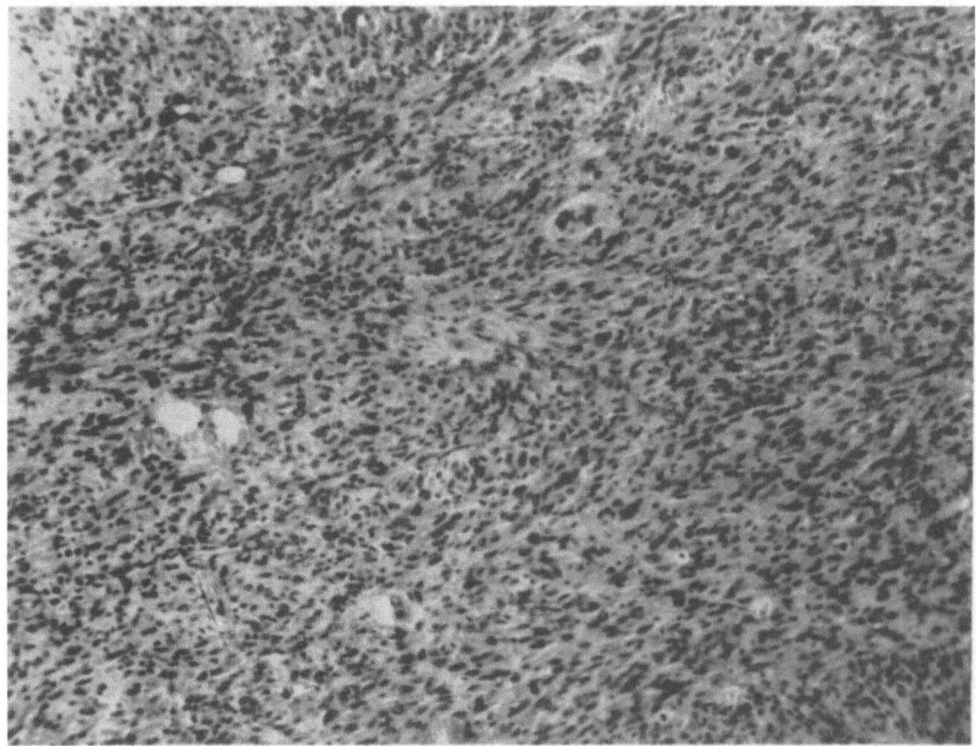

**Fig. 8.7.** A fasciculate pattern acceptable as that of a leiomyosarcoma. H & E, × 123

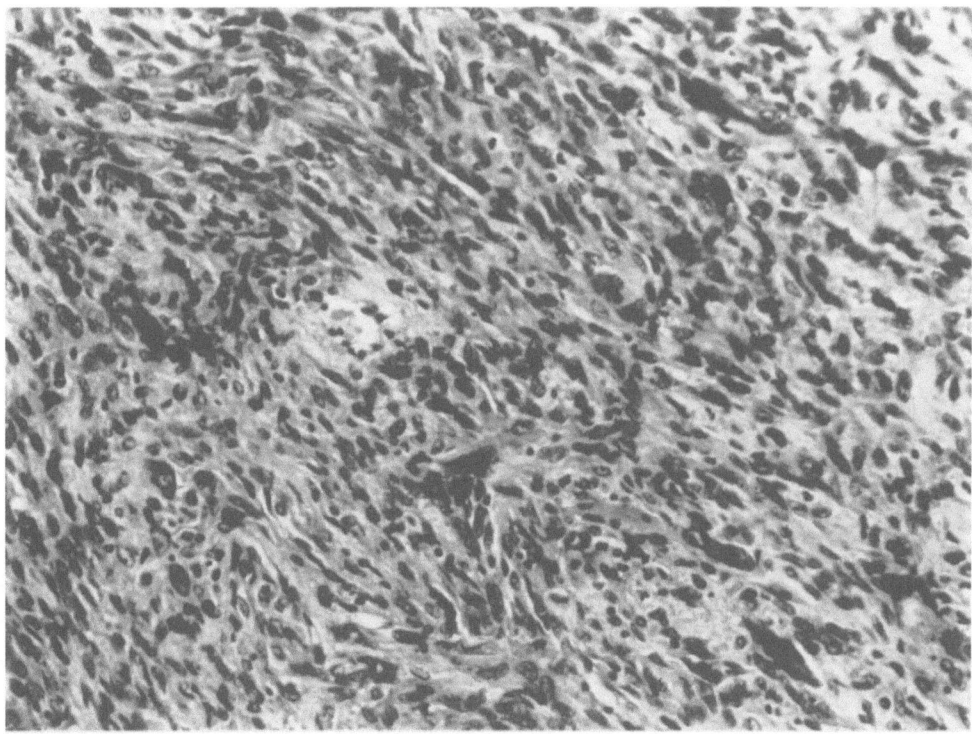

**Fig. 8.8.** An area of moderate polymorphism. The pyknotic masses could be degenerative nuclear substance. H & E, × 238

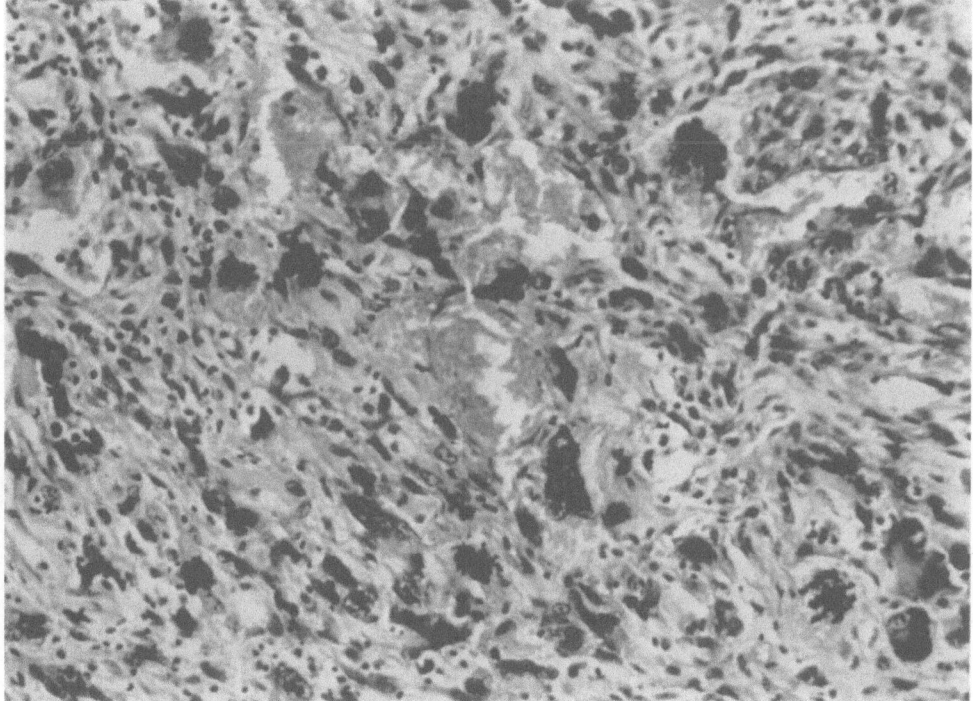

**Fig. 8.9.** It was difficult to decide in areas like this whether, in some instances, the pyknotic masses were irregularly swollen degenerate nuclei or nuclei in mitosis. The spiky mass at the lower right corner seemed certainly to be a multipolar mitosis. H & E, × 238

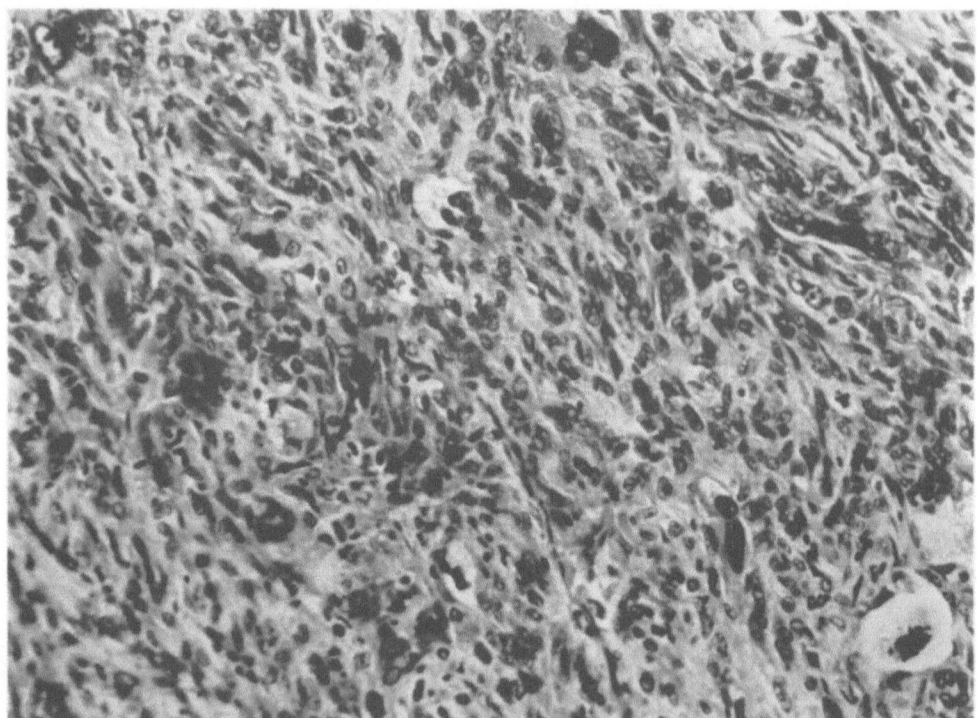

**Fig. 8.10.** Two cells here appeared certainly to be in aberrant mitosis, the clear cell at the lower right corner and the smaller clear cell with pyknotic bar just above 6 o'c. H & E, × 238

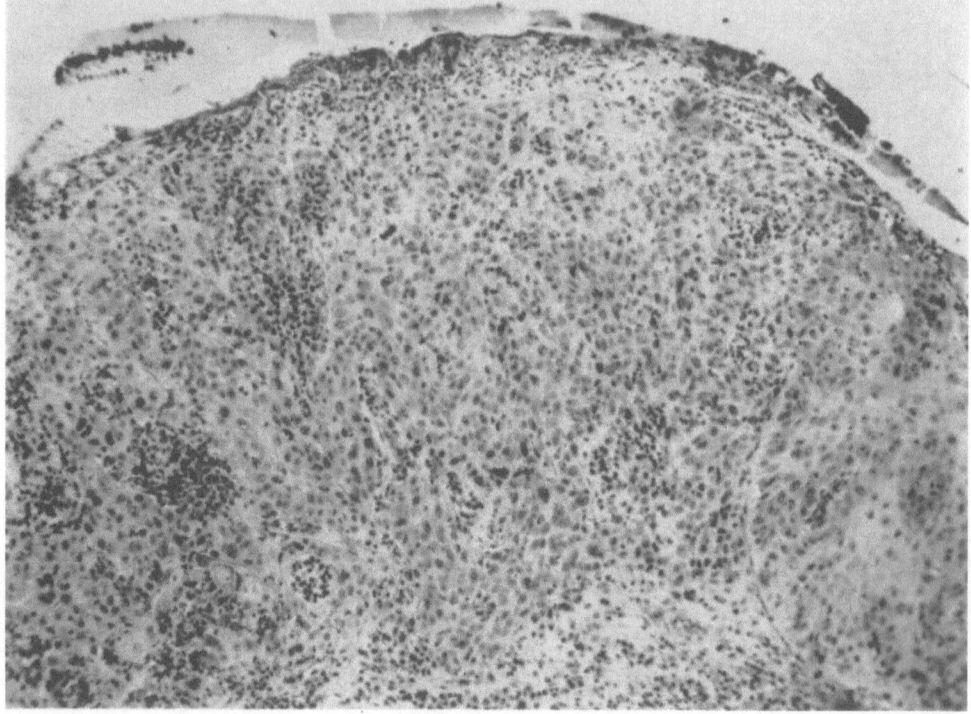

**Fig. 8.11.** A representative part of the original lesion showing an ulcerated mass of highly cellular tissue. The edge of remnant pharyngeal or tonsillar epithelium lies at right edge. H & E, × 119

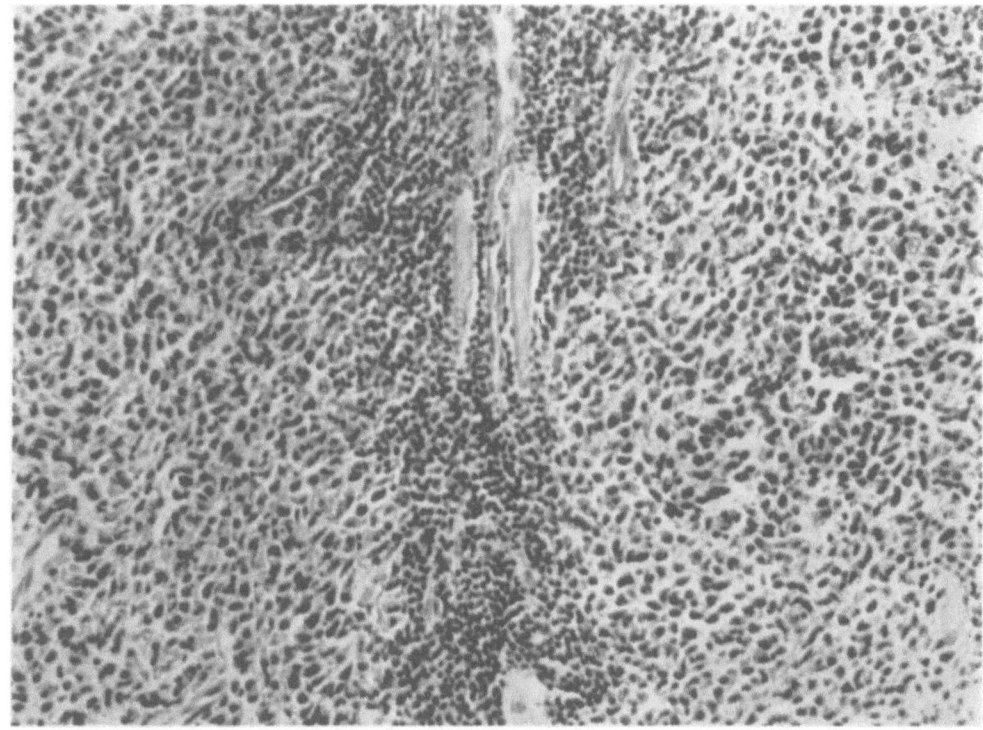

**Fig. 8.12.** The cells are polymorphic and larger than the lymphocytes along the edges of a one-time tonsillar crypt in the centre. H & E, × 238

about the correctness of the original diagnosis.

The complaint was dysphagia, and biopsy of the tonsillar mass showed virtually total replacement by a mass of polymorphic cells (Figs. 8.11, 8.12), obviously neoplastic and malignant. The appearances would now more probably be diagnosed as undifferentiated carcinoma than lymphoepithelioma but that has no significant bearing on the matter. The mass was irradiated.

As just said, to general surprise she reported 17 years later, again complaining of dysphagia and again with an ulcerated mass at the same site. Biopsy on this occasion showed the lesion to be a poorly differentiated 'squamous-celled carcinoma' (Fig. 8.13). Despite further radiotherapy the lesion rapidly grew until death 10 months later. Rather than invoke coincidence, it seems more reasonable to regard the lesion as a post-irradiation carcinoma. There must be few patients with undifferentiated carcinoma of the nasopharynx who survive long enough to be at risk from this possible complication. The original diagnosis was in the circumstances *appropriate*.

*Case 8.8*

F (38 years) with recurrent attacks of sore throat. Biopsy of one of the enlarged tonsils performed.

Lymphoid follicles were relatively few, most of the biopsy comprising stromal tissue densely infiltrated by lymphocytes and, frequently in mitosis (up to 6 per hpf in some areas), large mononuclear cells. The overlying epithelium was in many places wholly permeated by both types of cell. Some concern was expressed on account of these features, and examination of the blood, including serology, was recommended before the proposed tonsillectomy. This was done, with negative results, and the diagnosis remained as 'chronic tonsillitis'.

The tonsils were removed, and the patient was well and trouble-free eight years later. This was an *appropriate diagnosis*.

*Case 8.9*

M (46 years) with dysphagia for past 2 months. A first biopsy at oesophagoscopy showed chron-

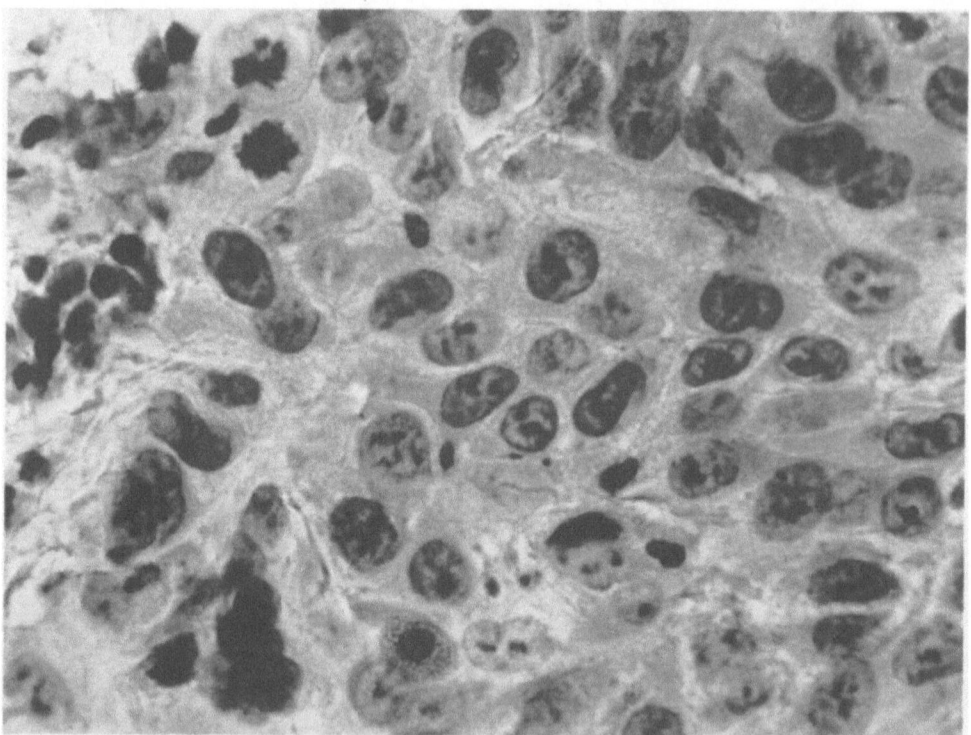

**Fig. 8.13.** A field from the lesion recurrent at the site 17 years later; abundantly mitotic and moderately polymorphic squamous-celled carcinoma. H & E, × 952

ically inflamed, partly metaplastic, gastric-type mucosa, and no evidence of malignancy. Further biopsy was recommended and performed 1 week later.

Appearances, as expected, were generally similar to those seen earlier but now two additional features were present, erosion of the surface with replacement of the mucosa by granulation tissue extending as far as the edge of the muscularis propria, and a considerable degree of nuclear polymorphism and mitotic activity in some of the deeper-lying glands. These last features comprised the 'borderline' element: they were regarded as 'disquieting' but not so abnormal as to warrant a diagnosis of carcinoma (Figs. 8.14, 8.15).

Symptoms persisted, and 10 months later a further biopsy was carried out. It showed unequivocal 'glandular carcinoma'. Resection the next day produced a specimen 7-cm long of which the proximal 4 cm was a relatively rigid tube with 10-mm fibrotic wall and almost totally occluded lumen. Sections showed apparent transection of widely spreading glandular carcinoma

at the proximal end but evidently ample (2 cm) clearance at the distal end.

In retrospect, in the second biopsy, the rather distorted glands with their appreciably polymorphic cells and not infrequent mitotic figures were almost certainly components of a well-differentiated glandular carcinoma. The pattern was to that extent *under-diagnosed*, and treatment therefore delayed for some 10 months. This reassessment is now, and after the definitive resection was, easy but that is with hindsight. In prospect, the histology remains a problem. On occasion, distorted glands almost indistinguishable from those in the present case may be seen around the cardia in association with nonspecific inflammation and fibrotic scarring; in the present series, Case 8.10 was one such where, after some concern about the appearances on biopsy, the lesion was thought to be probably benign and the patient was unmutilated and trouble-free 15 years later.

The difference between the two cases is subtle, based as it is on degree of nuclear polymorphism and frequency of cells in mitosis, a situation in

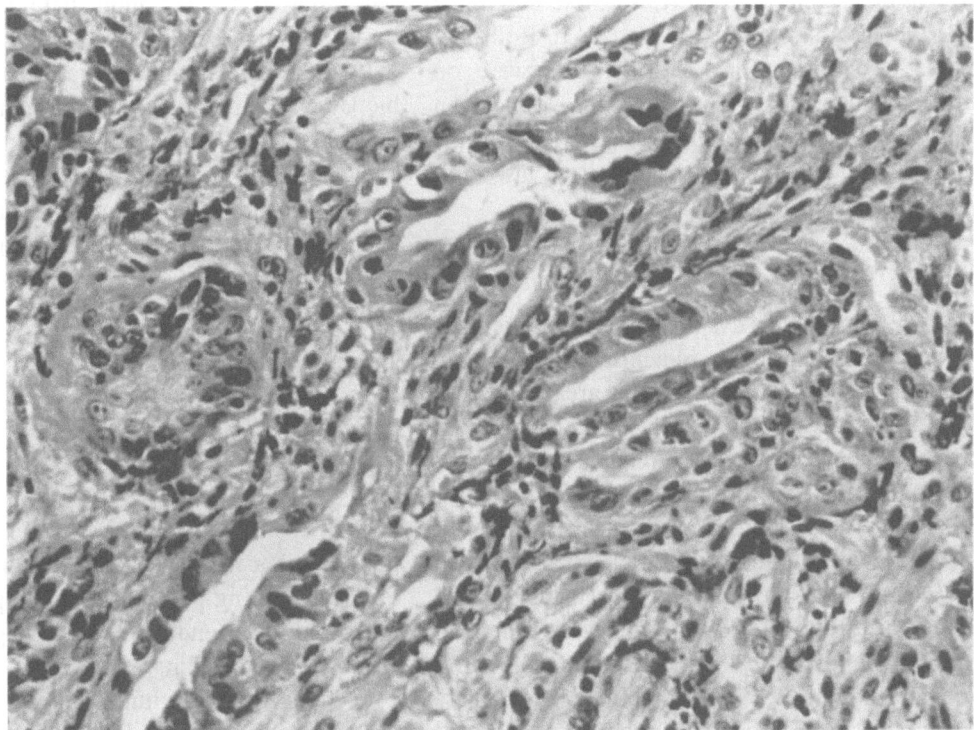

**Fig. 8.14.** Distorted glands lined by cells showing a moderate degree of polymorphism. The appearances were regarded as suspicious but not beyond the capacity of long-standing inflammation and scarring to produce. H & E, × 340

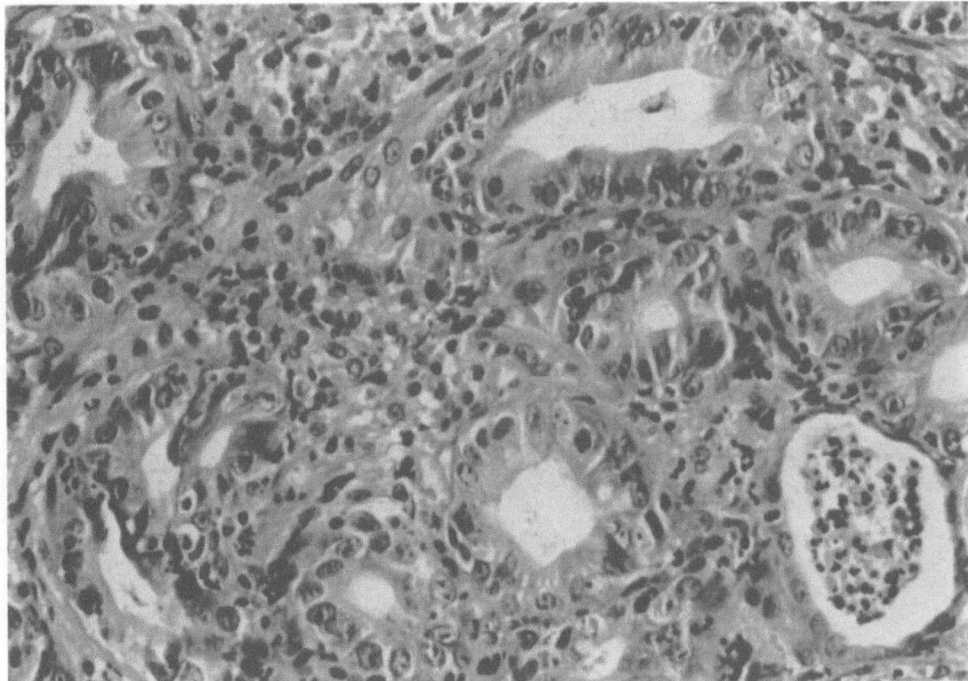

**Fig. 8.15.** Further glands lined by rather more polymorphic cells, some in mitosis (the uppermost elongated gland contains two, the lower central gland one). This area also was not considered diagnostic. H & E, × 340

which diagnostic decision rests on the individual pathologist's morphological threshold. Both features, as shown in Figs. 8.14 and 8.15 were, on direct comparison, rather more pronounced in the present case wherein, though well for the next 18 months, the patient died from his carcinoma after a further 18 months.

### Case 8.10

M (71 years) with dysphagia for 6 weeks. The lower oesophagus was inflamed and stenosed, and a biopsy was taken from this area.

The biopsy contained many glands within which goblet cells were frequent. These are normally not a feature of either oesophageal or gastric cardiac glands and, especially in the absence of villi of small intestinal type, suggested large intestinal metaplasia. The glands showed some distortion, a tendency towards confluent growth, mild nuclear polymorphism and fairly numerous cells in mitosis (Fig. 8.16). These features were regarded with some suspicion, and as possibly indicating a frank carcinoma nearby,

but reported as, for immediate practical purposes, 'not malignant'.

Conservative treatment was used, no further biopsy was performed, and the patient was well 15 years later. It seems likely that epithelium changed to an intestinal type by metaplasia may be allowed the same amount of mitotic activity as normal intestinal epithelium without raising a significant degree of suspicion of carcinoma. The appearances here may be compared with those in Case 8.9 where the ultimate outcome was diagnosis as unequivocal carcinoma and death. The diagnosis as nonmalignant in the present case was *appropriate*.

### Case 8.11

F (49 years) with dysphagia, vomiting, and loss of weight during past 6 weeks. Biopsy from the narrowed lower end of the oesophagus was difficult owing to bleeding.

Sections from the initial biopsy showed only glandular epithelium amid which were occasional glands of "a rather suspicious appearance, but

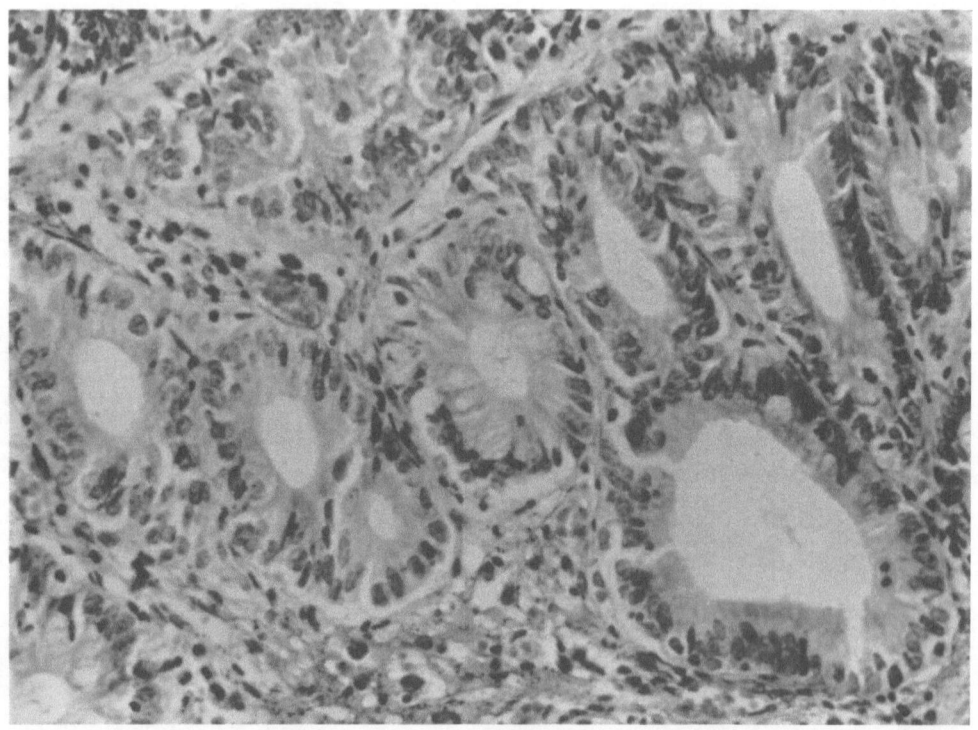

**Fig. 8.16.** The gland elements are again distorted but their cells, though sometimes crowded, are less polymorphic than in the previous case. Mitotic figures, however, are evident: there are four in this field, the most easily seen a diaster at the lower right corner and a pyknotic bar just above centre. H & E, × 320

no more than that". Further biopsy was recommended but the clinical features were such as to indicate a formal operation as the next procedure. Resection of the lower oesophagus and proximal stomach showed an obvious and widely permeating 'glandular carcinoma'. The lines of resection had cleared the edges of the carcinoma but in much of the central part of the oesophageal segment the muscularis propria had been permeated throughout its full thickness: foci of carcinoma beyond its outer edge seemed almost certainly to be within lymphatics.

The patient remained generally well for 11 years after which dysphagia and the other earlier symptoms recurred. A further biopsy revealed lower oesophageal carcinoma, glandular as before, palliative intubation was performed, and the patient died shortly thereafter.

Review of the first biopsy confirmed the mild aberrancy in some of the glands. The degree of nuclear polymorphism and mitotic activity was similar to, but less marked than, that in Case 8.9 and would not of itself, even in retrospect, warrant a diagnosis of early carcinoma. In this particular instance, nothing was lost by the failure to confirm the diagnosis on the first biopsy. Clinical evidence clearly indicated the presence of a destructive and obstructive lesion demanding exploration whatever its nature. In view of the blatant malignancy and extensive infiltration found to be present when adequate tissue did become available, the 11-year survival is remarkable. The original diagnosis expressing only suspicion still seems *appropriate*.

### Case 8.12

M (63 years) with dysphagia for 4 months.

The tissue pattern to be assessed in the biopsy is that shown in Fig. 8.17. The difficulty it presented is that, while the 'invasiveness' of the central mass of epithelium is not in question—there are minute clusters of cells already amongst the subjacent muscular layers—its cytology is remarkably bland. At higher magnification there was some nuclear aberrancy and rather more mitotic activity than would be present in a comparable area of wholly normal epithelium but

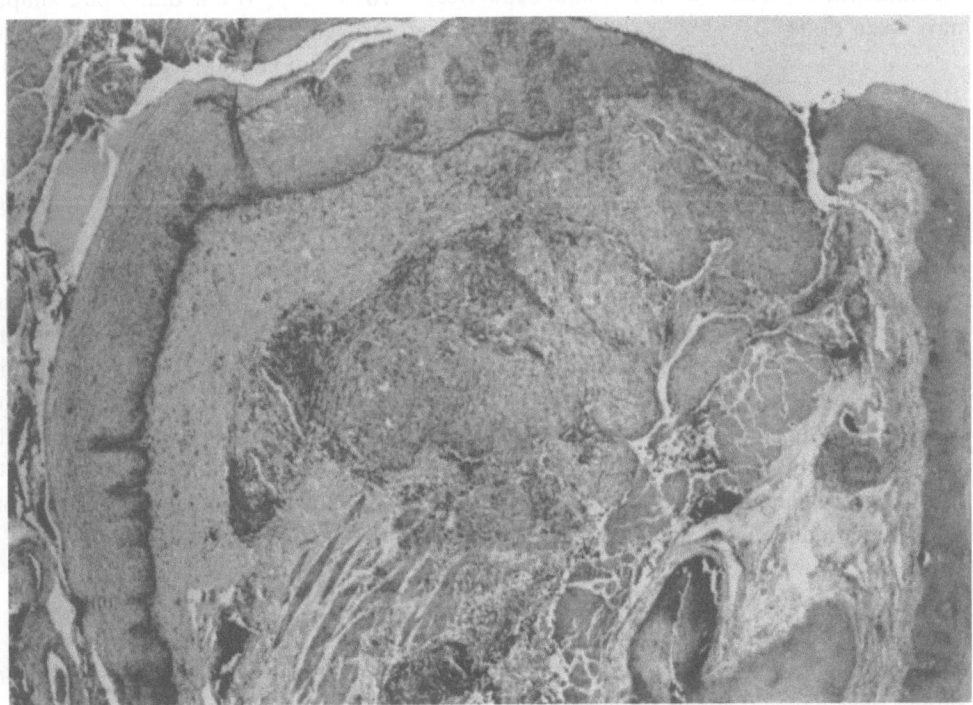

**Fig. 8.17.** There are two main abnormalities; (a) the short stretch of darker epithelium to left of the cleft at upper right-hand corner was typically carcinoma in situ; (b) there is well-differentiated and cytologically almost normal stratified squamous epithelium already infiltrating bundles of muscle in the lower left quadrant. H & E, × 32

neither feature was present in significantly greater amount than in adjacent epithelium still confined to the surface. That is, there were areas in the superficial epithelium that merited classification as carcinoma in situ; how aggressive was the deeper-lying and evidently invasive but cytologically much less aberrant epithelium likely to be?

The procedure adopted was to report the lesion as 'almost certainly squamous carcinoma' and to advise a further biopsy should there be continuing clinical suspicion.

The patient died 3 weeks later, apparently from 'carcinoma of the oesophagus'; there was no necropsy.

The initial report was, in retrospect, over-cautious; in prospect, many would agree that it was correctly cautious. There was no scarring or significant inflammatory reaction in company with the ingrowing epithelium such as might have explained its location, and its disposition probably was almost certainly a truly malignant invasion. Nevertheless, discrepancy between 'invasiveness' and cytological character is sometimes a real obstacle to accurate prognosis.

The qualified diagnosis was *appropriate*. Had the patient not died so soon after the biopsy, the recommended further biopsy would doubtless have been done.

### Case 8.13

M (60 years) with dysphagia for 6 weeks. Biopsy was taken from an area of what was believed to be gastric mucosa in a proven hiatus hernial sac.

Each of the three 8-mm particles showed the two epithelia of the squamo-columnar junction, and in each 3 the glandular element was aberrant. The glands were, in general, smaller than normal (i.e. smaller than normal for fundal but not cardiac glands) and more variable in outline; also their epithelial cells were more polymorphic and more frequently in mitosis than normal. In short, the problem was essentially the same as that presented by the lesions in Cases 8.9, 8.10 and 8.11. The biopsy was reported as abnormal but not diagnostic of malignancy, and further biopsy was recommended. However, so suspicious were the various clinical features by themselves that the mere expression of suspicion on biopsy was enough to determine the decision to perform resection.

The resected specimen contained a large carcinoma with proximal edge at the gastro-oesophageal junction: many adjacent nodes were invaded.

The patient died 7 months later with inoperable recurrent growth.

As was clear from the resected lesion, with a further or larger biopsy there would have been little or no difficulty; there was ample diagnostic tissue within 10 mm of the original biopsy. When seen in smooth continuity with the obvious carcinoma, the tissue at the edge, as seen in the biopsy, was so clearly also carcinoma as to make the initial hesitation surprising and virtually an under-diagnosis. Even yet, however, on 'blind' review, there are those who would have recommended a further biopsy rather than at least to have had their own gastro-oesophageal junction resected. In all the circumstances, this may fairly be judged an *appropriate diagnosis*.

### Case 8.14

M (61 years) developed melaena, without symptoms, while in hospital under investigation for ? infective arthritis. Partial gastrectomy yielded a $10 \times 6 \times 6$ cm dumb-bell shaped mass, half projecting towards the spleen, the other half markedly elevating the (partly eroded) mucosa of the fundus.

The mass was a highly cellular fasciculate neoplasm with numerous mitoses (Fig. 8.18). Of the discrete pyknotic masses in Fig. 8.19, three were mitoses, and this is a reasonably representative area. In several samples there was no 'palisading' to suggest a neurilemmoma: therefore, and in view of the high mitotic frequency, the lesion was diagnosed as a 'leiomyosarcoma'.

Apart from his rheumatoid arthritis, the patient was well 15 years later. Despite its size and abundance of mitotic activity, this sarcoma clearly had a limited capacity for metastasis: an *appropriate* diagnosis.

### Case 8.15

F (69 years) complaining of tiredness and loss of weight. A mass was palpable in the right epigastrium. Partial gastrectomy yielded a $6 \times 6 \times 4$ cm ulcerated mass in the posterior wall of the stomach.

The mass was a highly cellular, spindle-cell

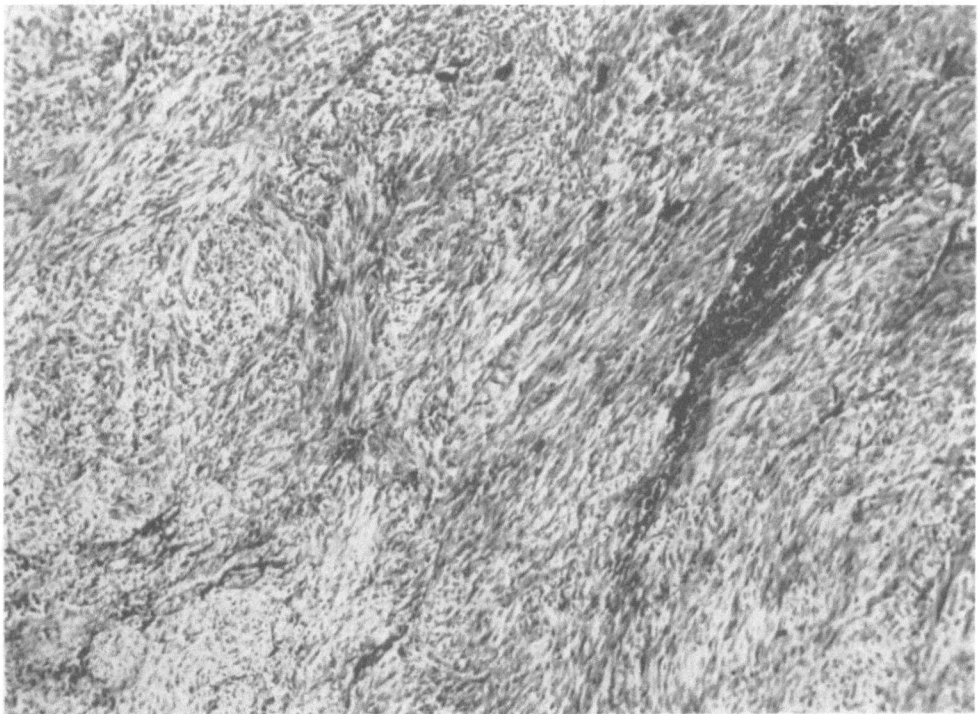

**Fig. 8.18.** A fasciculate neoplasm of high cellularity including occasional pyknotic masses. H & E, × 123

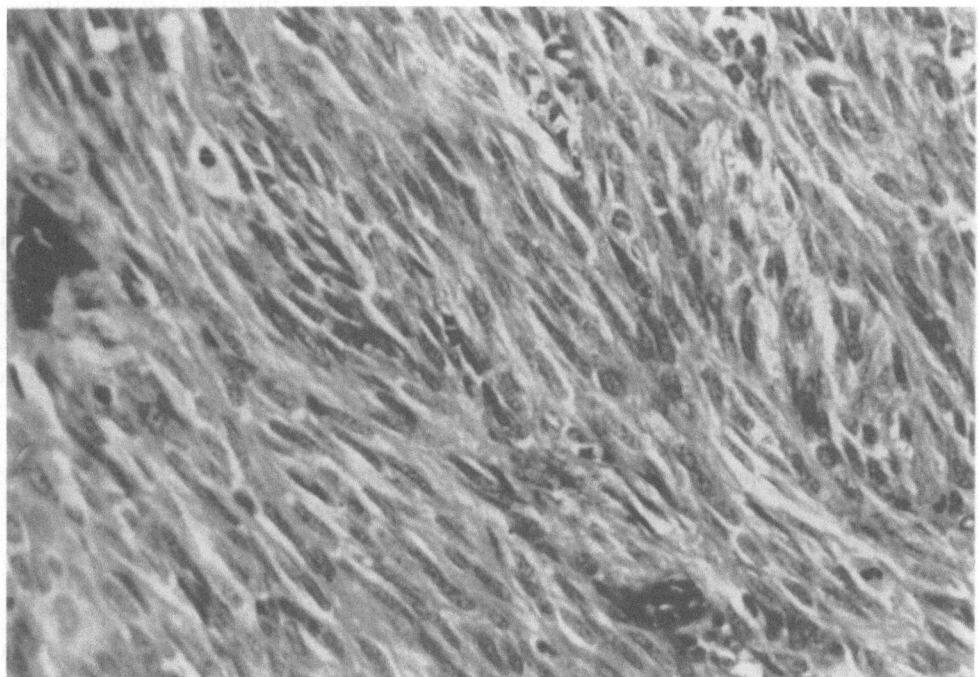

**Fig. 8.19.** This area shows the spindled outline of the nuclei and is representative of the mitotic frequency. The pyknotic masses at lower right and upper left corners, and one of those more centrally, were mitotic figures. The dark mass at left-hand edge consisted of chromatin and was presumably a cluster of degenerate nuclei. H & E, × 493

neoplasm. With mitoses in places up to 4 per hpf the possibility of its being a leiomyosarcoma rather than leiomyoma was considered but it was reported as still 'probably benign'.

The patient died 5 months later of tuberculous bronchopneumonia; necropsy showed no residual or recurrent neoplasm in the stomach. Even if the supporting evidence is largely negative, the diagnosis may reasonably be regarded as *appropriate*.

### Case 8.16

F (45 years) reoperated upon (partial gastrectomy) as part of treatment for a postanastomotic stomal ulcer. The short (2 cm) length of duodenum in the specimen was mildly distorted and fibrotic.

One of the sections from the pyloroduodenal end contained a 3-mm partly acinar, partly undifferentiated mass of tissue extending from halfway up the mucosa and through the full thickness of the submucosa to the edge of, but not into, the muscularis propria. This aroused considerable suspicion, for there was some polymorphism and nuclear irregularity amongst the cells, and their 'invasiveness' was not in question. However, the possibility of the lesion's being a 'carcinoid tumour' was realised, and this diagnosis was confirmed by the silver-staining reactions.

The patient was known to be well 15 years later. The diagnosis was correct and *appropriate*.

### Case 8.17

M (78 years) having had partial gastrectomy for chronic gastric ulcer, which was radiologically diagnosed and seen, after partial gastrectomy, to be on the lesser curvature: it was 15 × 5 mm in outline, 10 mm deep, and attended by dense fibrosis. Microscopy showed interruption of the muscularis propria and the other typical features of a 'chronic peptic ulcer'.

Recovery was satisfactory but symptoms recurred and a further laparotomy was performed 16 months later. The gastric remnant, 14 cm long, had now the appearance of a leather-bottle stomach, and there were enlarged nodes along the curvature and in the hilum of the spleen.

The original lesion, as mentioned above, was regarded as a simple chronic peptic ulcer. The later specimens, both stomach and nodes, showed diffuse infiltration by highly cellular neoplastic

tissue; its nature was in doubt, and so also, obviously, was the status of the original apparently simple peptic ulcer.

In neither the granulation/fibrous tissue of the ulcer nor the rather polymorphic undifferentiated neoplastic cells of the gastric remnant or nodes was any mucin demonstrable. The reactions of a group of pathologists to the sections of the peptic ulcer and one of the later-obtained nodes, both examined 'blind' and at the same meeting, were interesting and instructive. The preferred diagnosis for the node was 'lymphosarcoma' (though some considered Hodgkin's disease a possibility): the ulcer aroused some suspicions, as many a chronic peptic ulcer will, but none was prepared to pronounce it 'malignant': furthermore, although both sections were examined and discussed at the same meeting, none present associated the two.

There was no evidence of metastasis to liver or peritoneum at the time of operation, and no evidence of skeletal metastasis during an investigation of unexplained diarrhoea 4 months later. However, the patient died after a further 4 months with a strong presumption that the neoplasm was the cause (no necropsy).

All chronic peptic ulcers of stomach are potentially borderline lesions to the extent that the paucicellular scirrhous carcinoma, the linitis plastica, is always a possibility all too easily overlooked. Had this happened here? The stringent review just mentioned made this possibility seem most unlikely. The neoplastic tissue in the gastric remnant and nodes was so suggestively lymphomatous and so unlike the pattern in the partial gastrectomy specimen that coincidence seems the likeliest explanation; that is, the peptic ulcer *was* benign, the later lesion *was* a malignant lymphoma, and the diagnoses thus *appropriate*.

At all events, the features in this case served well to recall the notorious difficulty sometimes presented by the probable or possible linitis plastica.

### Case 8.18

M (55 years) with dyspepsia and a demonstrable peptic ulcer on lesser curvature of pyloric antrum.

Sections from four areas around the deep 4-cm ulcer showed typical appearances with no evidence, not even marginally suggestive evi-

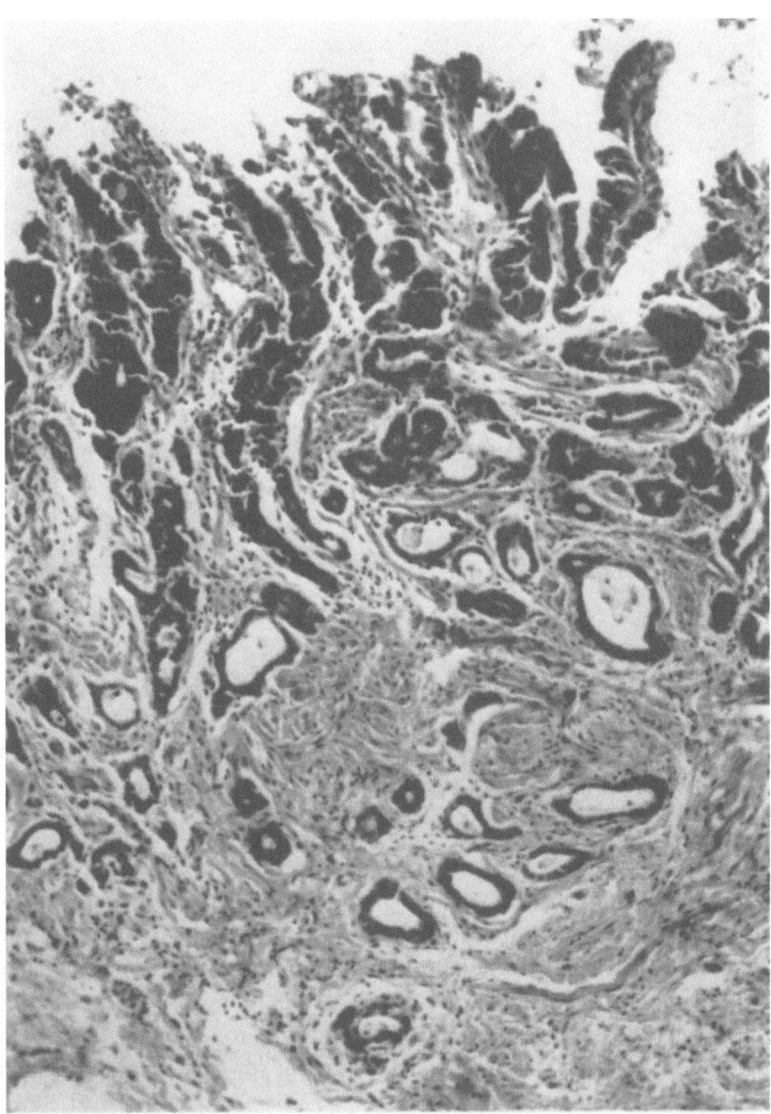

**Fig. 8.20.** The initially unsuspected carcinoma. The epithelial basophilia identifies the lesion and shows the carcinoma to be still mostly in situ. H & E, × 132

dence, of malignancy, and the report was issued accordingly: 'benign peptic ulcer'.

However, within days, a colleague with an interest in gastric exfoliative cytology reported that a smear preparation from the antral region showed malignant cells. Further blocks were then taken from the (not visibly abnormal) antrum with the results here illustrated. Figure 8.20 shows undue basophilia of the superficial epithelium, microscopically carcinoma in situ, and also glandular elements of varying size amid and beyond the frayed muscularis mucosae. Not only this, as seen in Fig. 8.21 there were polymorphic glandular structures within the muscularis propria, i.e. *infiltrative glandular carcinoma*.

The partial gastrectomy already performed

was deemed adequate treatment and nothing further was done (two adjacent nodes showed no carcinoma).

The patient remained well for 4 years, when an episode of 'bronchitis' was followed by a persistent cough. The presence of an inoperable broncial carcinoma was confirmed on biopsy of both bronchus and pleura, and the patient died some 4 months later. The histological appearances in both biopsies were those of a moderately well-differentiated 'squamous-celled carcinoma'. Had the lesion been glandular, the possibility of metastasis from the gastric carcinoma would have been hard to exclude. The course of events demonstrates that a gastric carcinoma, even though extensively permeating the muscular

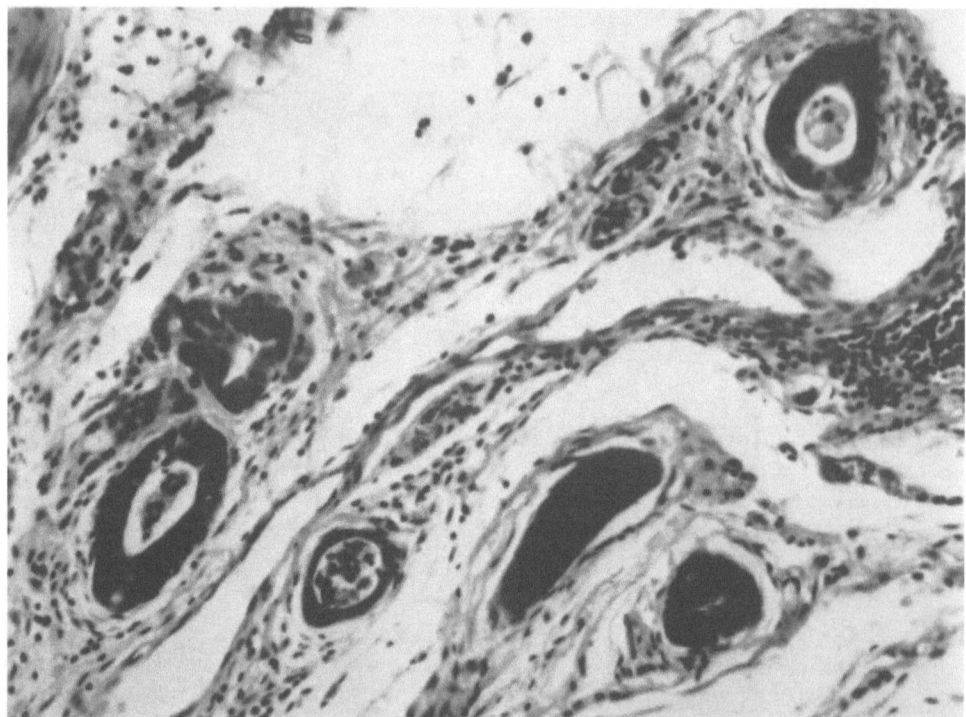

**Fig. 8.21.** Small well-differentiated elements of glandular carcinoma within the oedematous muscularis propria. H & E, × 238

layers of the gastric wall, need not simultaneously be capable of successful metastasis. The diagnosis as infiltrative carcinoma was histologically wholly *appropriate*. However, the fact that the lesion was discovered at all owed nothing to orthodox block-selection but to fortuitous cytology.

*Case 8.19*

M (62 years) with obstructive jaundice which was increasing. Operation comprised pancreatectomy with simultaneous removal of pyloric antrum, duodenum, part of jejunum, and lower part of common bile duct.

Dissection showed, around the ampulla of Vater and bulging into the lumen of the duodenum, a 20 × 15 mm cyst surmounted by an almost spherical 6-mm nodule of solid tissue. The mucosa covering the abnormal structure was smooth and intact. The general architecture of the area is shown in Fig. 8.22.

Serial gross sections were made through the cyst + nodule and produced the appearances seen in Figs. 8.23 and 8.24. The nodule was

itself finely cystic, the size of the cysts and the proportion of stromal connective tissue varying considerably at different levels. The epithelium lining the spaces was uniform and apparently benign but prognostic worry was caused by the evident extension or 'invasion' of glandular elements into the submucosa at the edges of the lesion. This fine permeation, or seeming permeation, is seen in Fig. 8.25 where the mucosa is being extensively undermined.

There was uncertainty whether the lesion was purely a hamartoma or, in view of the intimate permeation of adjacent tissue, a well-differentiated carcinoma. Unanimity was not achieved but the lesion was eventually labelled 'carcinoma'.

The patient remains well 7 years later; almost certainly, therefore, the lesion was not a carcinoma but a *hamartoma*. However, it did have to be removed, and we may doubt whether either an exploratory laparotomy with preliminary biopsy or a cryostat section at the time of definitive laparotomy could have excluded the possibility of carcinoma with enough assurance to save the pancreas. The uniformity of the cells might be held sufficient to offset the apparent invasiveness;

on the other hand, most pathologists will have seen examples of undoubted scirrhous carcinoma of the pancreas where the cells in many areas have been, in isolation, strikingly and misleadingly 'benign'.

This was almost certainly an *over-diagnosis*.

*Case 8.20*

M (53 years) with complaint of intermittent diarrhoea, occasionally accompanied by loss of blood, over past 2 years. Sigmoidoscopy showed a pedunculated papillary mass at 14 cm.

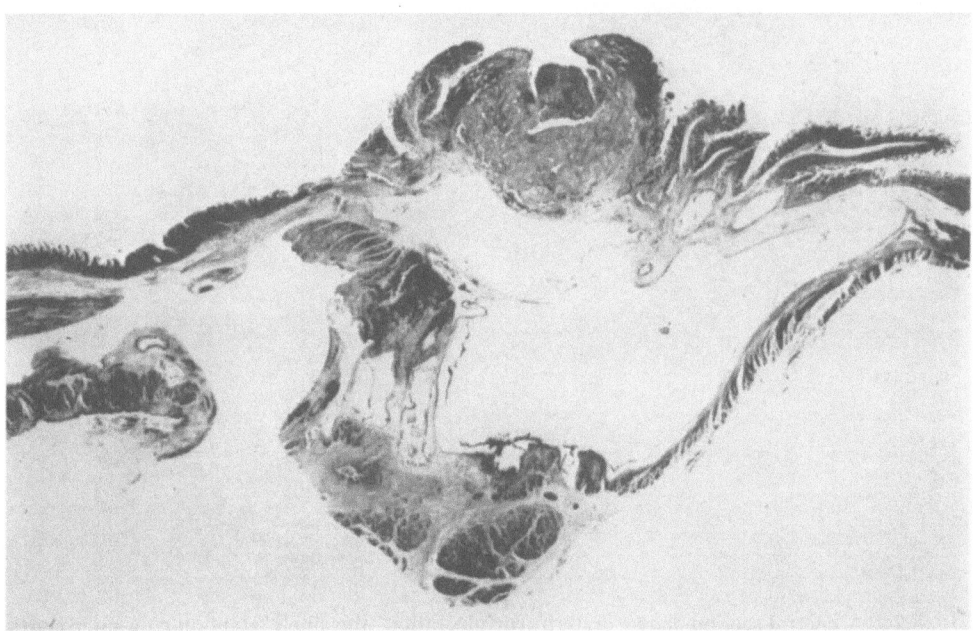

**Fig. 8.22.** A nodule of relatively solid tissue surmounting a cyst in the wall of the duodenum. H & E, × 6

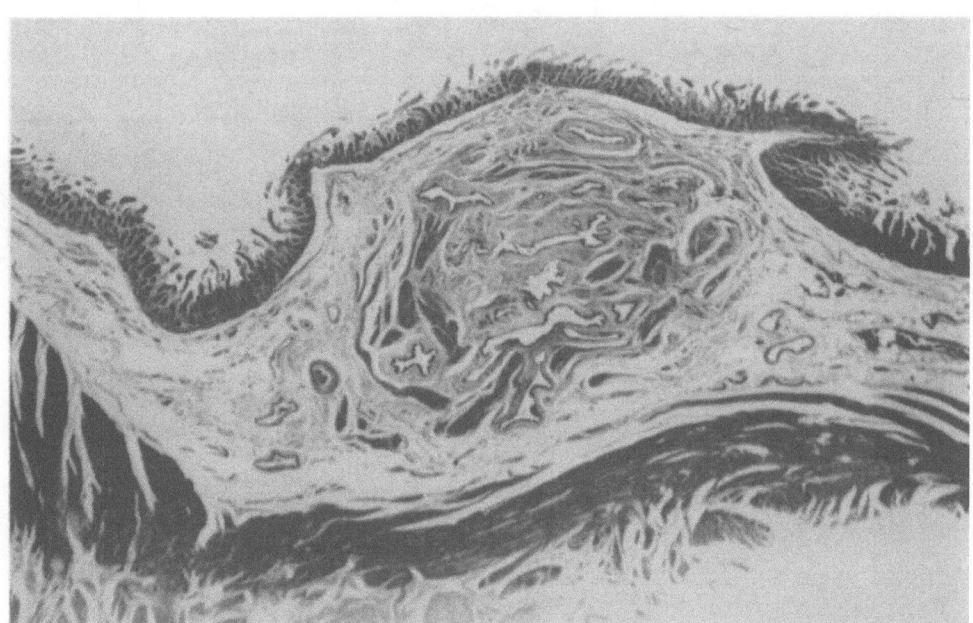

**Fig. 8.23.** A tangential section shows the peripheral part or shell of the nodule to be in fact microcystic or finely trabecular. The band of dark tissue beneath is not hyperplastic muscularis mucosae but the muscularis propria. H & E, × 17

The biopsy fragments consisted largely of highly cellular, obviously neoplastic, glandular tissue. The aberrancy was sufficient to warrant diagnosis as carcinoma rather than adenoma (nowhere did the pattern suggest a villous papilloma); the question was, In what degree a carcinoma? The appropriate designation was held to be 'carcinoma in situ'. A further biopsy produced

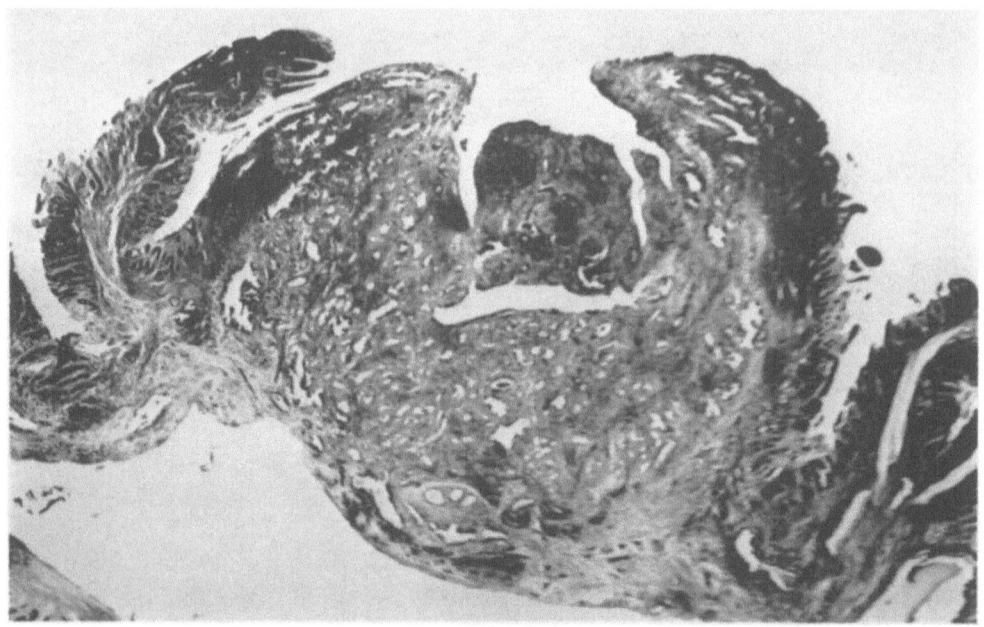

**Fig. 8.24.** A central section shows crateriform ulceration, the finely glandular or microcystic structure of the mass and the roof of the subjacent cyst. H & E, × 17

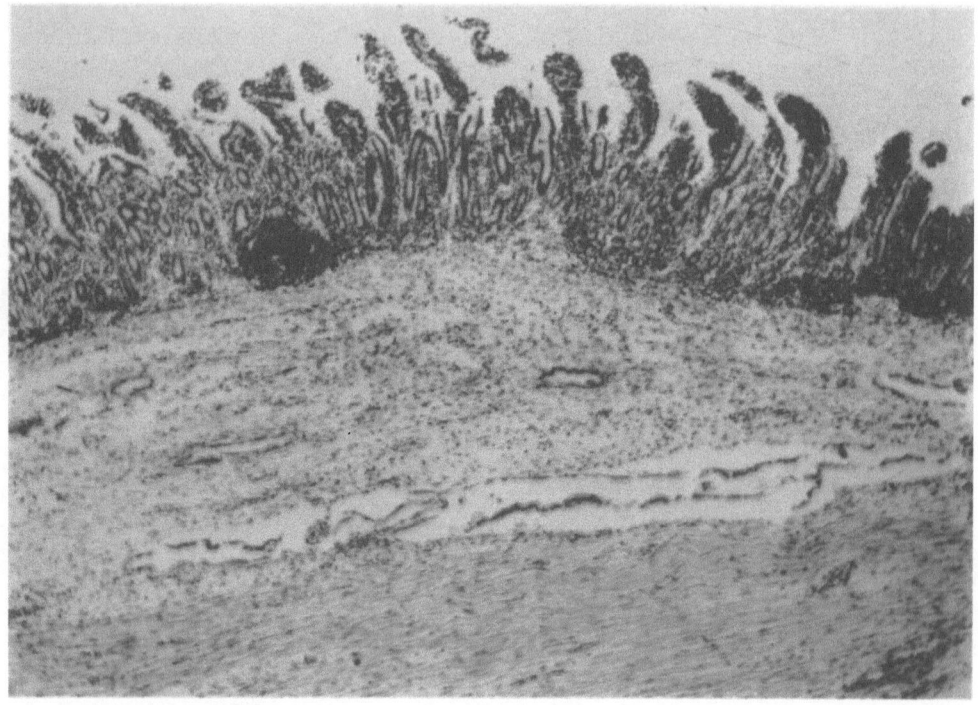

**Fig. 8.25.** Many fine glandular structures of this type permeated the submucosa around much of the margin of the mass. H & E, × 60

fragments of tissue of exactly the same kind; the diagnosis therefore also remained the same with an added statement that segmental resection, if technically feasible, should be adequate treatment.

Segmental resection was not feasible; the patient had to lose anus, anal canal, rectum and some 10 cm of colon. The rectum contained a 30-mm spherical polypoid mass, freely mobile and held by a soft 20-mm pedicle. It was diagnosed as a 'highly cellular, noninvasive, potentially malignant papilloma'.

The patient was alive and well 12 years later. To the extent that such malignant potential as the lesion may have had was obviously nullified, the diagnosis was *appropriate*.

This case has been included as a typical example of an almost standard problem, namely, assessment of an intestinal adenomatous polyp wherein tissue is clearly neoplastic but not obviously carcinoma; and, for practical purposes, this problem at once reduces itself to the possible outcome, resection + colostomy or not? It matters relatively little to the patient with a polyp in the colon whether the pathologist decides aggressive adenoma, carcinoma in situ or frank carcinoma; there is little long-term difference between a 10-cm segmental resection or a hemicolectomy. In the rectum the difference is obviously crucial.

### Case 8.21

M (53 years) admitted for excision of a perineal sinus, said to have been discharging for 35 years. The excised tissue comprised two fibrofatty masses, the bulkier 3 × 3 × 2 cm.

As expected, various areas showed granulation tissue with scarring, distortion of architecture, ulceration of epidermal epithelium and granulomatous foreign-body type inflammatory reaction; one area showed a flake of seemingly metaplastic bone. What was not expected was the presence of clusters of mucus-secreting cells scattered at random amongst the scar tissue. They were too aberrant to be simply muciphages, and no other conclusion could be reached than that, despite the 35-year history and fortuitous finding, this was 'mucoid carcinoma'. In the hope that local excision had been achieved, as seemed possible with such an apparently indolent lesion, a 'wait and see' policy was adopted.

Three years later the lesion recurred, and resection of rectum was performed. The pararectal tissues were manifestly involved. The patient died after a further 4 years, of pelvic obstruction and eventual uraemia; many forms of palliation had been tried over the years. Clearly enough, the diagnosis was *appropriate* but it may be that the excision of rectum should have been performed when the carcinoma was first diagnosed. Yet, in view of the infiltrative nature of the lesion one suspects that even this would have been inadequate. When, during the evolution of the lesion, the malignant growth began, or whether it had been a carcinoma during the whole of the 35 years, we cannot know.

The mucus-containing phagocyte, whether in lamina propria or a lymph node, may at times be very difficult to distinguish from a mucus-containing malignant cell (cf. the similar problem with the melanophage) but the number and distribution of the mucus-containing cells in the tissues here was explicable only in terms of carcinoma.

### Case 8.22

M (51 years) with recurrent attacks of diarrhoea over 9 years. Three fragments of tissue were taken from a 10-mm area of rectal mucosa thought possibly, on sigmoidoscopy, to be an angioma.

Two of the three fragments showed hyperplasia and microcystic dilatation of glands in the superficial mucosa (Fig. 8.26). The other fragment was normal and a useful control (Fig. 8.27). The pattern indicated aberrant differentiation and raised the question of whether it represented any long-term neoplastic threat. However, the cells were in no way aberrant, and the lesion was regarded as a form of 'hamartoma' of no preneoplastic significance. Review has found it to be a 'metaplastic polyp', not recognised as such at the time of reporting.

No further treatment was given, the symptoms were relieved and the patient was still trouble-free 12 years later. The relief of symptoms suggests that the 'diarrhoea' was the result of excessive production of mucus by the hyperplastic epithelium; functional activity like this is unusual in a metaplastic polyp. To the extent that such lesions may be malformations, the diagnosis, if not quite accurate, was reasonably *appropriate*.

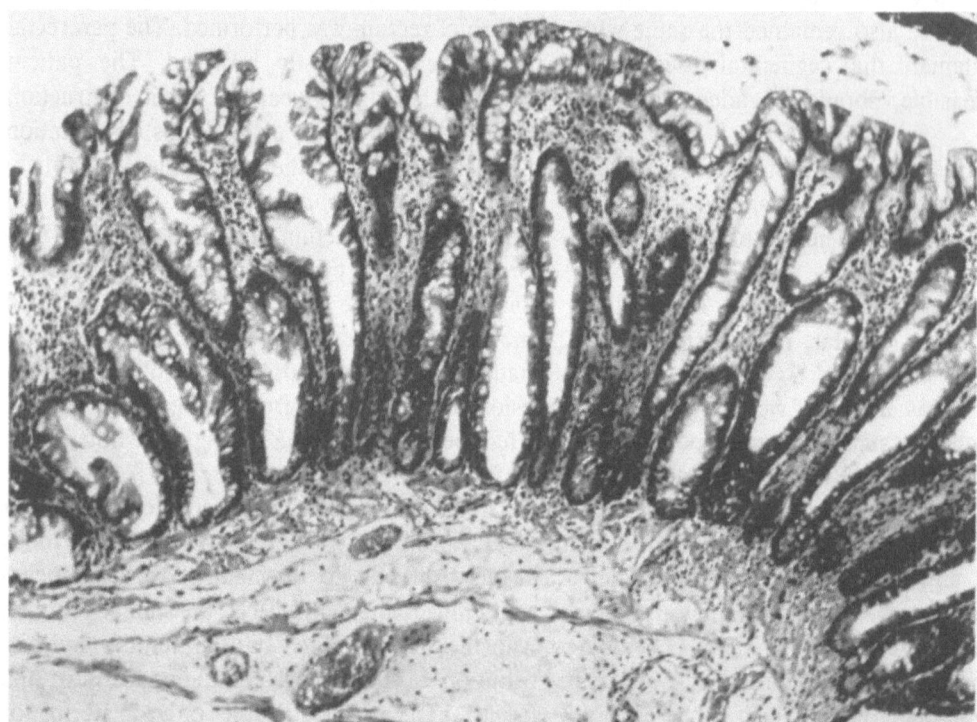

**Fig. 8.26.** The mucosal aberrancy is best appreciated by comparison of this view with the normal mucosa in Fig. 8.27. Some of the glands are verging on the cystic with (to left) delicate intraluminal papillary projections. H & E, × 82

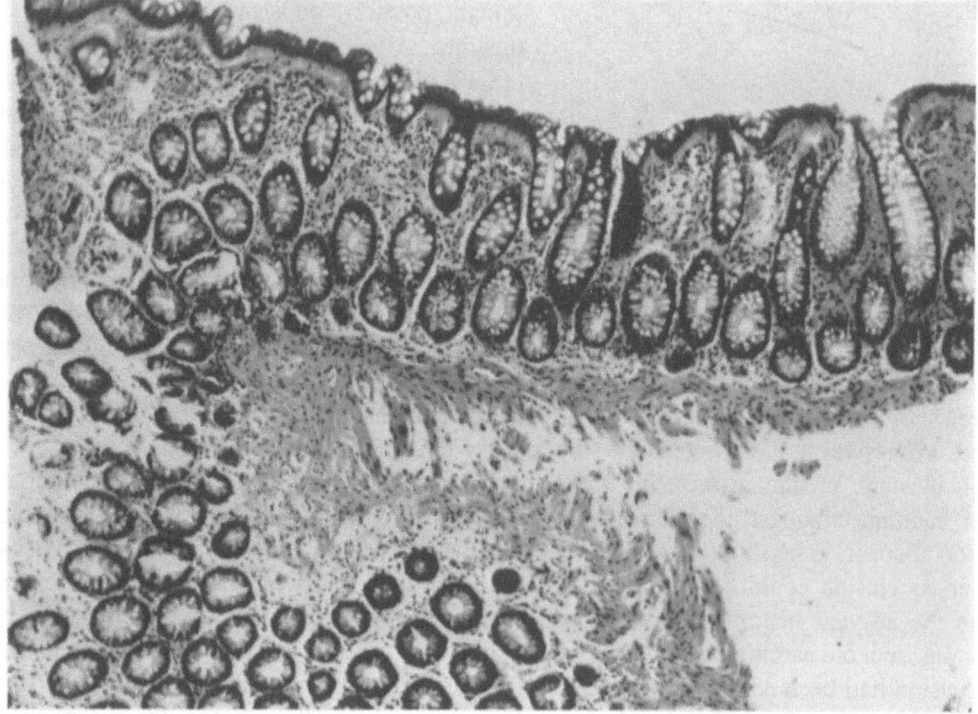

**Fig. 8.27.** See Fig. 8.26. H & E, × 82

*Case 8.23*

F (69 years) with signs and symptoms leading to cholecystectomy. The wall of the gall-bladder was up to 8 mm thick: the mucosal surface was irregularly 'bumpy'.

Sections showed, besides the leucocytic infiltration and fibrosis of chronic cholecystitis, occupation of much of the wall of the gall-bladder by a fine meshwork of sinusoidal spaces, some containing blood (Fig. 8.28). The cells lining the sinusoids were mostly uniform but sometimes formed small solid clusters (Fig. 8.29). The irregularity of the mucosal surface was largely due to this underlying abnormal tissue which had been regarded as 'vascular papilloma'.

The patient became jaundiced 2 months later. Laparotomy showed a 2-cm mass surrounding the upper part of the common bile duct. Sections showed an essentially normal mucosa but infiltration of the considerably thickened wall by tissue substantially the same as that seen in the gall-bladder; that is, for the most part loosely sinusoidal (Fig. 8.30) but focally more compact and, with its considerable polymorphism and mitotic activity, almost certainly malignant (Fig. 8.31). The lesion was now diagnosed as a carcinoma of bile duct.

The patient's condition failed to improve. Yet another laparotomy showed, besides much fibrosis from the earlier operations, nodules in the omentum; one of these is shown in Fig. 8.32. It was hollow and contained blood; the wall was a sponge-work of spaces almost all also containing blood (Fig. 8.33). Foci of compact cellularity were fewer than in the mass surrounding the bile duct but there was still much mitotic activity amongst the cells lining the vascular spaces. In any context the pattern would have raised the question of malignancy; here, it made virtually certain the diagnosis of 'angiosarcoma'. The patient died 2 weeks later.

Both elements of the final diagnosis had been identified on the earlier occasions, first as 'vascular papilloma', then as 'carcinoma': in all, however, this was a significant *under-diagnosis*. The final diagnosis had been considered earlier by some but not until examination of the omental metastasis was it firmly established.

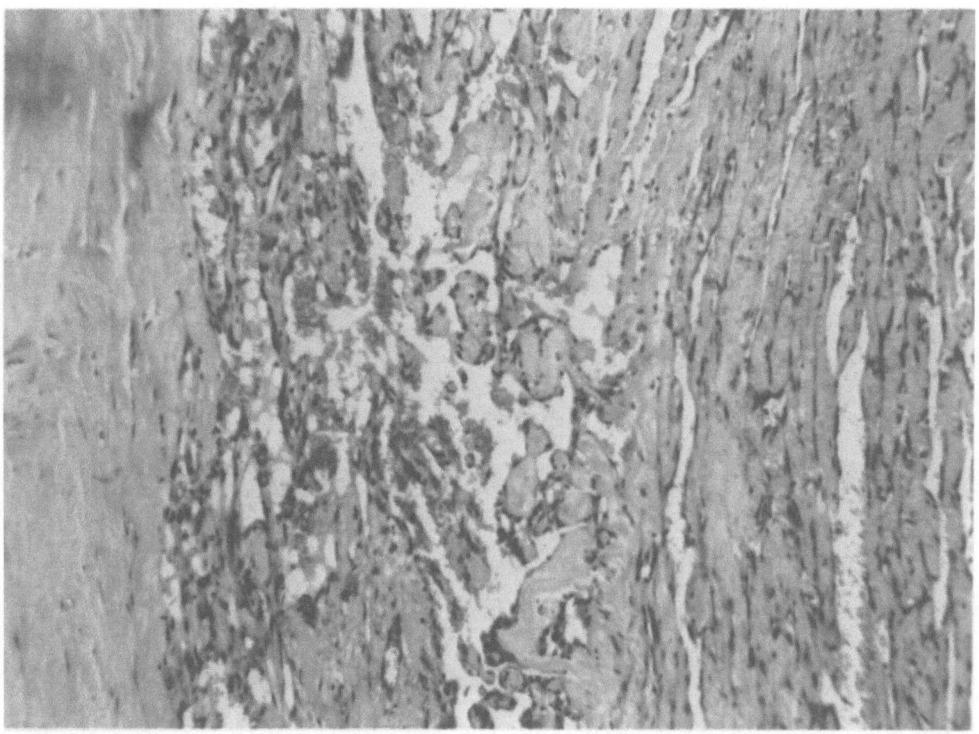

**Fig. 8.28.** Shows the meshwork of vascular spaces responsible for the thickening of the wall of the gall-bladder. H & E, × 123

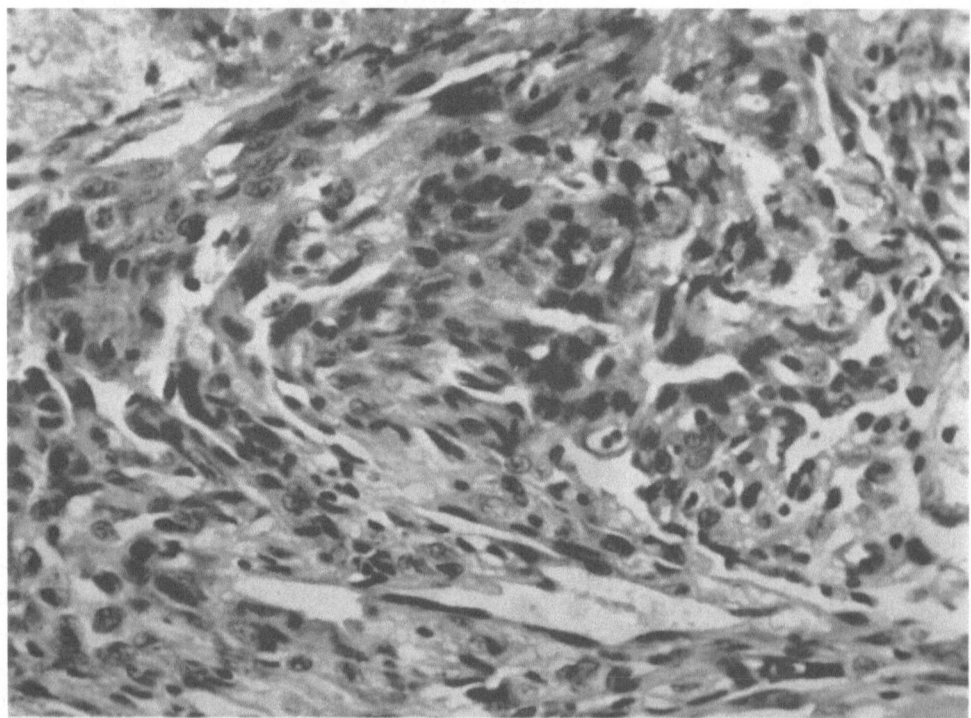

**Fig. 8.29.** In scattered areas there were foci of abnormal cells, apparently a condensation or concentration of the cells otherwise lining the sinusoidal spaces. They were mildly polymorphic and occasionally in mitosis. H & E, × 476

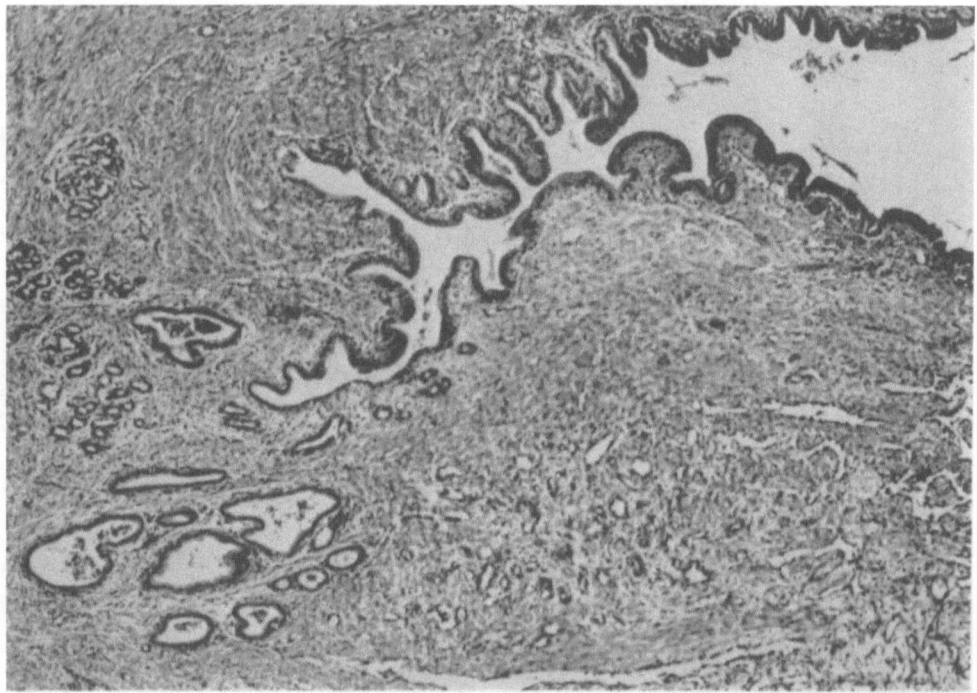

**Fig. 8.30.** Shows part of the wall of the bile duct with (*upper left*) included glands and (*lower right*) the same type of sinusoidal meshwork as that seen in the wall of the gallbladder. H & E, × 60

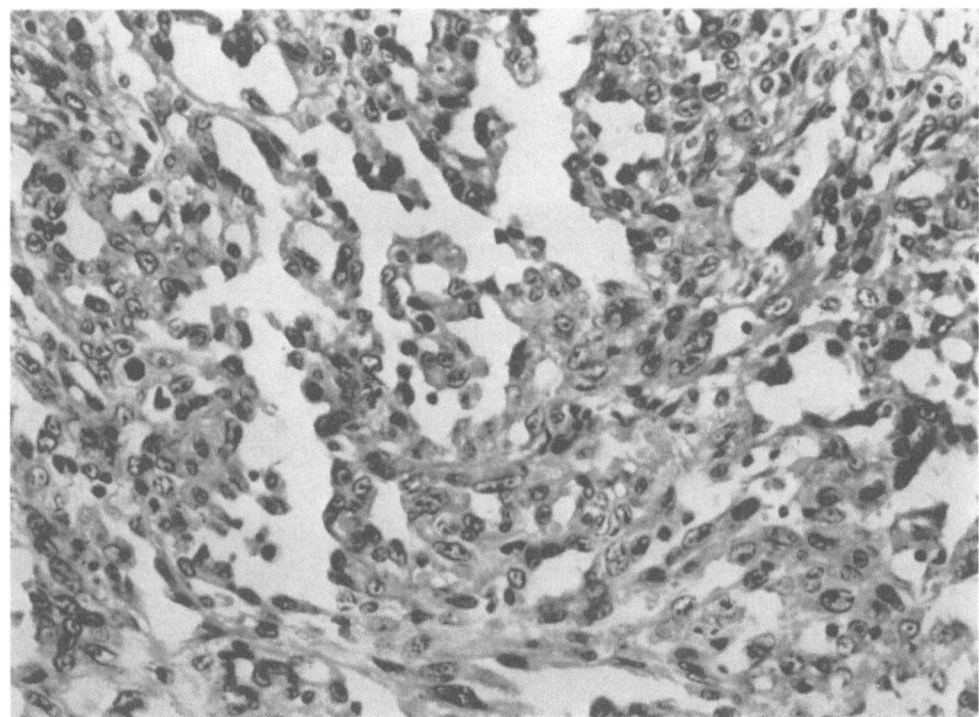

**Fig. 8.31.** The trabecular or sinusoidal pattern is maintained even at this magnification. In this field there are five cells in mitosis. H & E, × 340

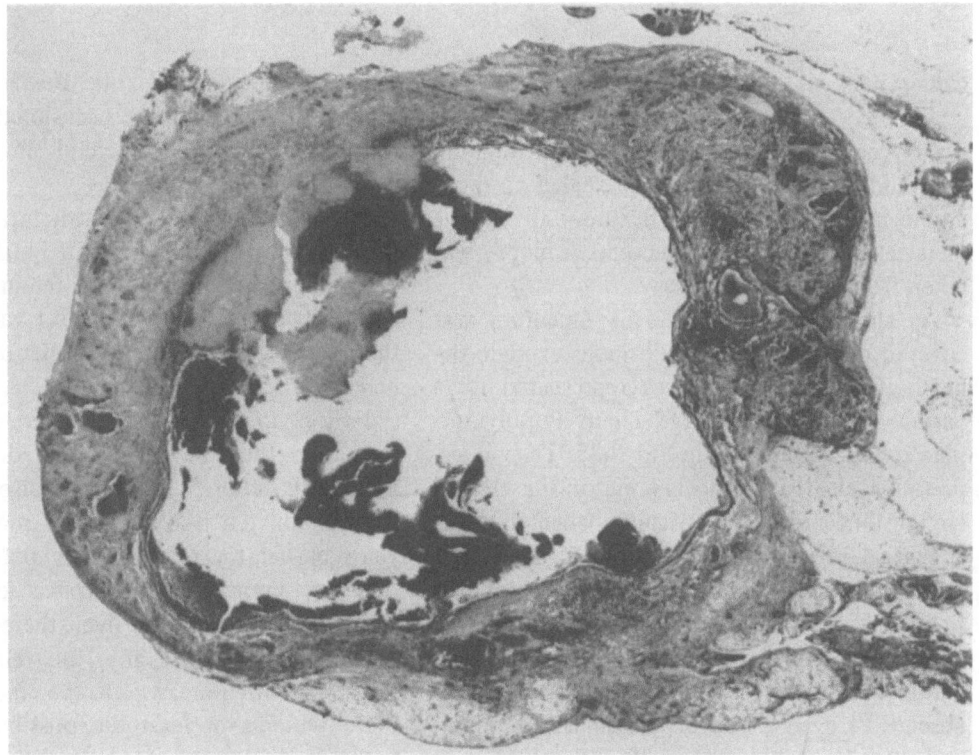

**Fig. 8.32.** A cystic blood-filled mass from the omentum. H & E, × 11

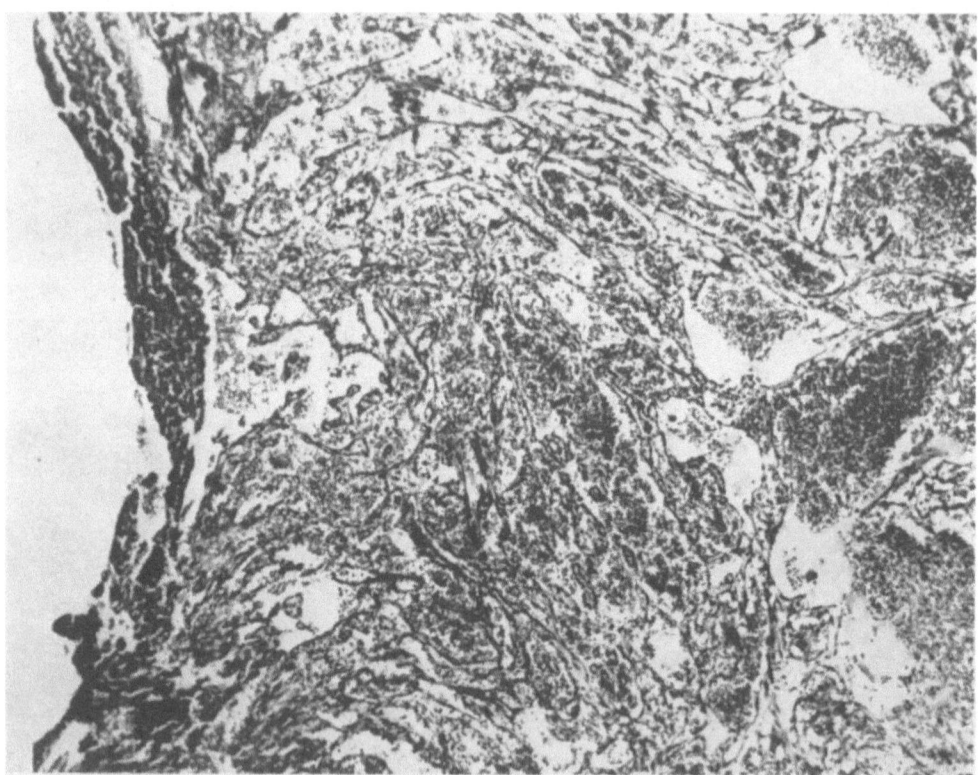

**Fig. 8.33.** An area from the wall of the mass in Fig. 8.32. It consists of a sponge-work of vascular spaces. The cells lining the spaces showed the same degree of polymorphism and mitotic activity as those in the original lesion in gall-bladder. H & E, × 62

*Case 8.24*

F (63 years) with abdominal pain, constipation and mild ascites. Laparotomy revealed an inoperable mass at the splenic flexure with hepatic metastases and nodular omentum. A biopsy was taken from the omentum only.

As shown in Fig. 8.34, the omentum was covered by a thin layer of fibrinous exudate beneath which the serosa was represented by a variably thick layer of large, relatively polymorphic cells seen in detail in Fig. 8.35. Their interpretation clearly had no bearing on the clinical circumstances in this particular patient but has a general relevance to the problem sometimes posed by transformed or metaplastic serosal cells as may be seen in association with simple inflammation (see, for example, Case 8.25). The matter was further complicated by the complete absence of even a hint of glandular differentiation such as could reasonably be expected in association with the presumed glandular carci-

noma of the splenic flexure. Besides their polymorphism, the cells were occasionally in mitosis but that also may be seen in simple 'reactive' serosa.

It was decided, on their structural detail, that the cells were of undifferentiated malignant character, their lack of glandular features having to be ascribed merely to structural variation. Further possibly relevant information, however, emerged.

Follow-up enquiry revealed the expected information that the patient had died not long afterwards, after 5 months. It also yielded the information that she had had a mastectomy 16 years earlier for removal of a poorly differentiated carcinoma. In the absence of any tissue from either the colon or liver, there is no means of knowing what, if any, the relation of the mammary carcinoma was to the other lesions but there remains at least the possibility that the tissue in the omentum represented carcinoma metastatic after 16 years from the breast.

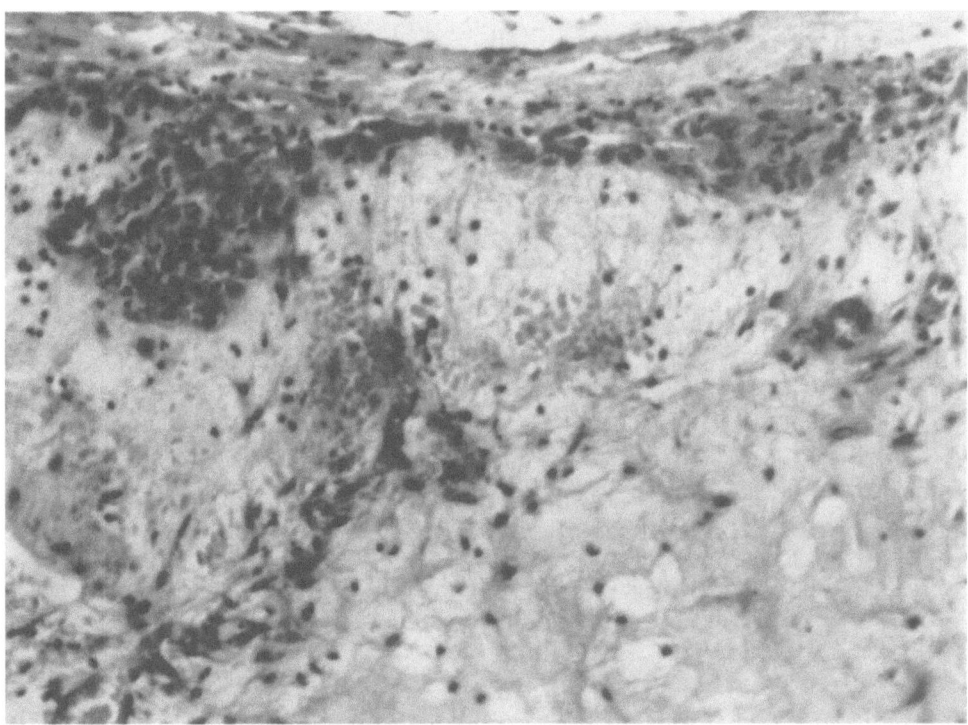

**Fig. 8.34.** The uppermost layer, with free border, is fibrinous exudate. The variably thickened cellular layer beneath represents the serosal epithelium; beneath is the oedematous subserosa. H & E, × 238

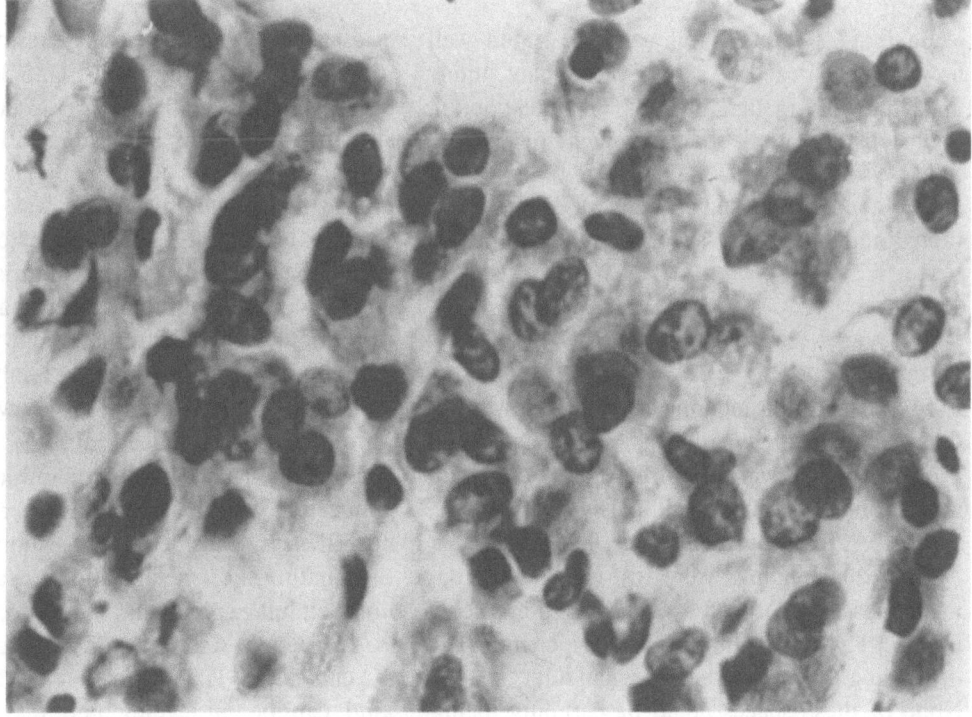

**Fig. 8.35.** A cluster of cells interpreted as carcinomatous rather than as metaplastic serosal or subserosal cells. H & E, × 985

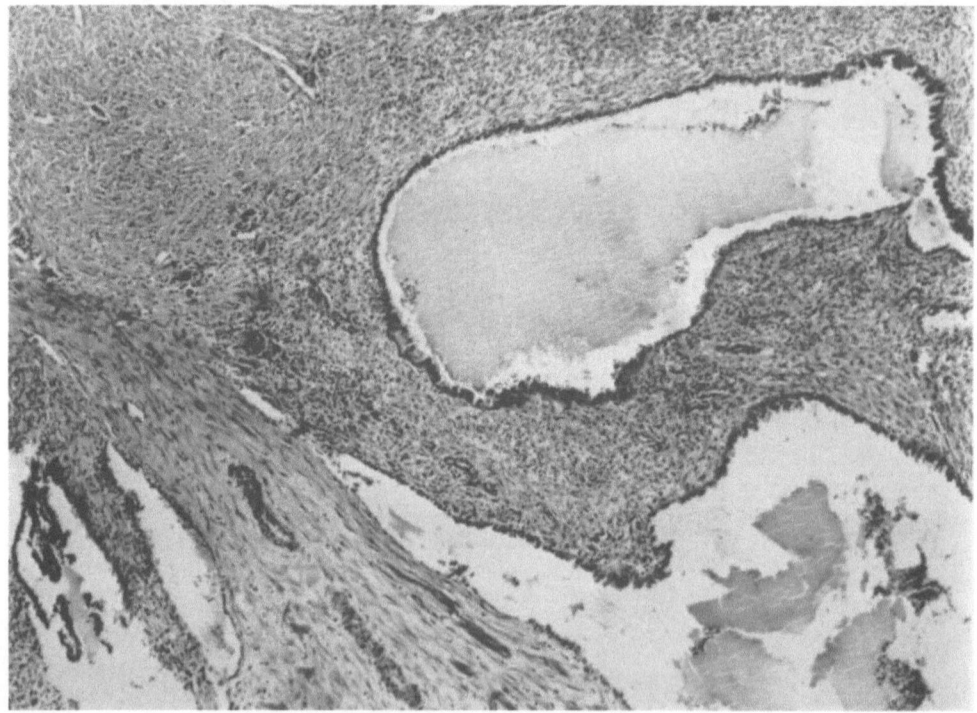

**Fig. 8.36.** Glandular structures with only one associated area of dubiously endometrioid stroma (beneath the concavity of the upper structure). Between the two largest glandular formations are occasional other small gland-like structures of which further examples are shown in Fig. 8.37. H & E, × 60

Be that as it may, this case illustrated well how closely reactive serosal cells can mimic metastatically malignant cells. The distinction may depend entirely on assessment of the detailed cytology.

The conclusion reached here was *appropriate* though immediately of academic interest only.

### Case 8.25

F (44 years) with menometrorrhagia, lower abdominal pain and an adnexal mass. Operation produced an outwardly normal uterus and right adnexa but firm brownish partly cystic mass, 7 × 4 × 2 cm, representing the left adnexa.

Abnormal findings were restricted to the adnexal mass. It consisted essentially of a markedly fibrotic stroma including leucocytic infiltrate, organising haematomas and glandular spaces. None of these spaces could be certainly identified as endometriotic but the most appropriate diagnosis was, nevertheless, considered to be

'presumptive endometriosis'. Besides the well-formed spaces, as shown in Fig. 8.36, there were other smaller epithelial or pseudo-epithelial structures, singly or in clusters (Fig. 8.37) that at least raised the question of glandular carcinoma. The possibility of this was reinforced to some extent by the detailed cytology. Figure 8.38 shows the cells, those comprising the acini and also those lying singly or in small aggregates, to be notably hyperchromatic and polymorphic, though mitotic figures were certainly scarce.

Almost all these formations lay well within the fibrous mass, as indeed did the much larger 'glands' in Fig. 8.36. None showed any certain connection with the investing serosa but this was, nevertheless, considered to be almost certainly their nature, i.e. 'metaplastic serosal inclusions', not glandular carcinoma.

The patient was well and trouble-free at least 5 years later. Histological appearances of this kind can be misleading and may be wrongly diagnosed as carcinoma, primary or secondary. The diagnosis was *appropriate* and correct.

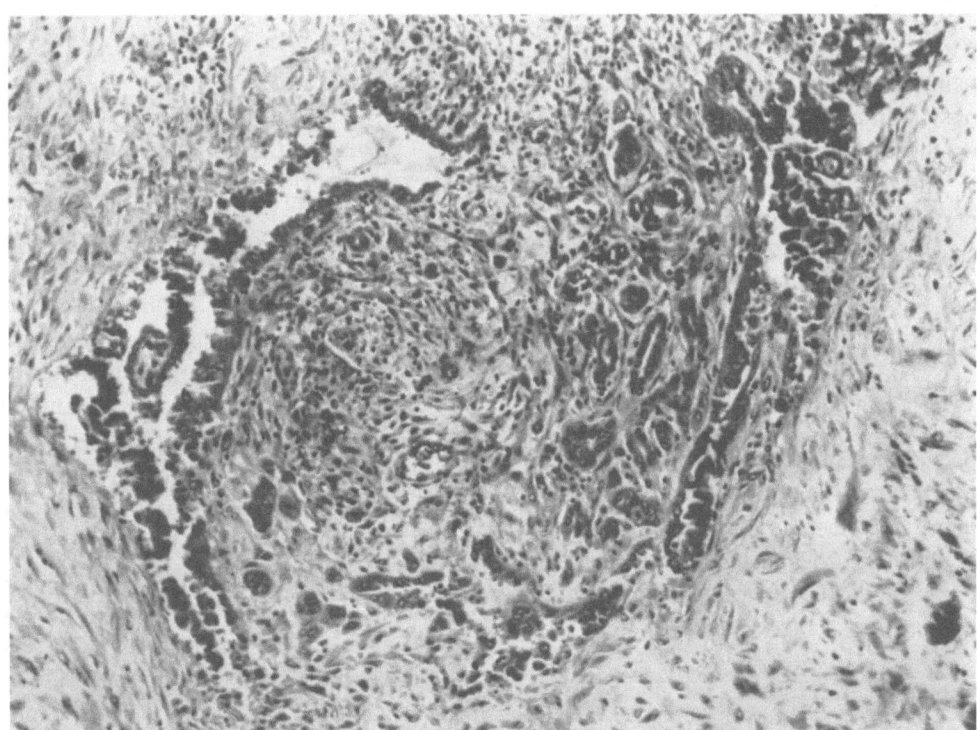

**Fig. 8.37.** Glandular or pseudoglandular formations in the inflammatory adnexal mass. H & E, × 246

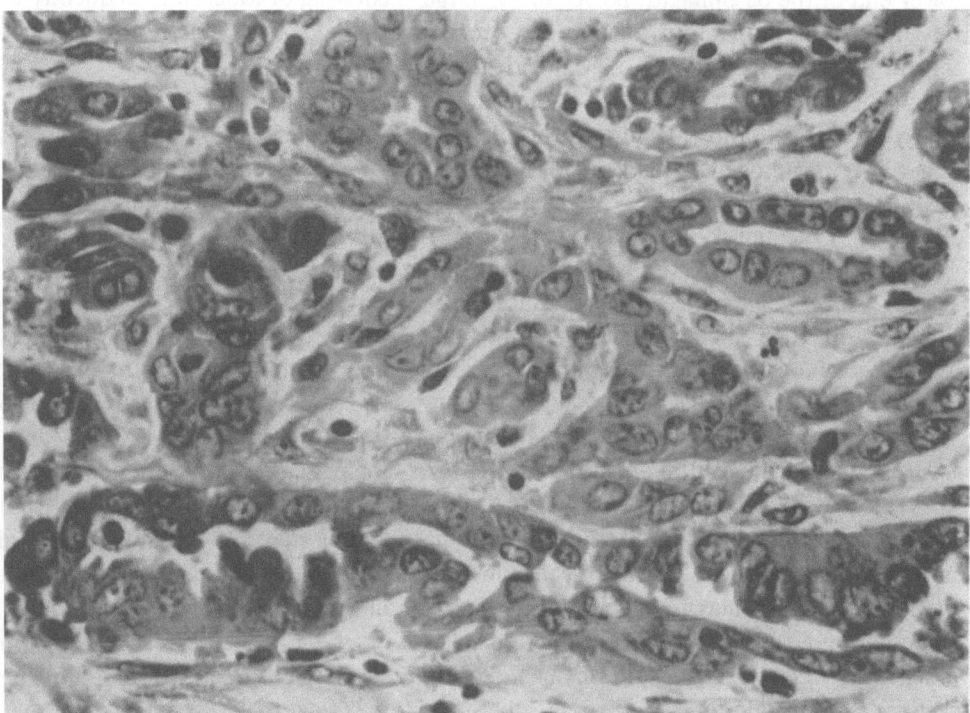

**Fig. 8.38.** The nuclei of the cells comprising the formations in Fig. 8.37 are large and appreciably polymorphic but only rarely in mitosis. The polymorphism is little less than that in Figs. 8.14 and 8.15 (of oesophagus) where the lesion was almost certainly carcinomatous. H & E, × 352

*Case 8.26*

F (41 years) with lower abdominal and pelvic pain, thought possibly to be appendicitis. A biopsy was taken from a small area of puckering on the surface of the rectum.

The 6-mm particle consisted of fibrous tissue permeated by glandular structures of various sizes and shapes. There seemed little doubt that they were 'carcinomatous' but mention was made of an outside possibility of their representing endometriosis.

Further investigation, including a second (trans-sigmoidoscopic) biopsy, revealed the expected 'carcinoma'. The rectum was excised but the patient died of bronchopneumonia 7 days later. The lesion in the rectum was a deeply penetrating 25-mm ulcer with many associated lymph nodes largely replaced by carcinoma. The diagnosis had been *appropriate*.

COMMENTARY ON LOCAL SERIES

With occasional exceptions, the sources of diagnostic difficulty were hyperplastic stratified squamous epithelium; glandular distortions at the lower end of the oesophagus; polyps of the large intestine; and aberrantly reactive peritoneal serosa. There is no example in the series of a diagnostically difficult biopsy of pancreas; the still controversial problems inherent in this context will be mentioned in the General Commentary nevertheless.

Of the exceptions, the pharyngeal pseudosarcoma (Case 8.6) was misdiagnosed at the outset but the error almost certainly exercised little influence on either the treatment or the outcome. The leucocytic permeation of epithelium overlying a tonsil (Case 8.8) had added some concern but proved innocuous. A salivary carcinoma (Case 8.5) was unusual in appearing at the age 10 years but has not reappeared during the 14 years since excision. The glandular hamartoma in duodenum (Case 8.19) was resected in continuity with the pancreas on clinical evidence. In terms of simple probability, carcinoma was much the likelier diagnosis; whether frozen-section examination at the time of operation would have allowed a firm diagnosis of non-malignancy is dubious. An instance of lymphoid polyp of the rectum, overdiagnosed as lymphosarcoma, was mentioned earlier (Case 4.24).

# General Commentary

## ORAL CAVITY

### *Verrucous Carcinoma*

The overgrowths of stratified squamous epithelium provide their problems in the mouth and pharynx just as they do elsewhere. One form, the *verrucous carcinoma* (Ackerman, 1948) was mentioned earlier in connection with the skin. The lesion occurs most commonly in the oral cavity (77 of the 105 cases analysed by Kraus and Perez-Mesa, 1966) and, by its relentlessly recurrent and destructive character, presents a formidable therapeutic problem. The experience of Kraus and Perez-Mesa, and of Fonts and his colleagues (1969) who described ten examples, was that irradiation is likely to induce an aggressively anaplastic change in the carcinoma and possibly provoke metastasis. Surgical excision is always the treatment of first choice. A further 55 examples were described by Goethals and his associates (1963), and a single example, evidently effectively controlled by oral methotrexate, by Kanee (1969). An association with the chewing of tobacco is frequently mentioned.

### *'Leukoplakia'*

Implications of *epithelial leukodystrophy* (white patches or the clinician's 'leukoplakia') differ little in the mouth from its implications in other areas. An analysis of its precancerous status was made by Einhorn and Wersäll (1967) in the case of 782 patients. Their analysis showed that the percentage cumulative probability that carcinoma would develop after a postdiagnosis period of 2, 5 and 15 years was (*a*) for patients whose lesion was removed, 1.6, 2.3 and 4.6, and (*b*) for patients whose lesion was not removed, 0.4, 1.1 and 2.5 respectively. The rather unexpected figures may, as the authors explain, be due to selection of patients: the apparently greater risk of carcinoma in those operated upon might result from the selection of only the more clinically suspicious for operation. A further difficulty in the way of prognostic assessment, well illustrated in this series but common to most, is that in only one-third of the cases was biopsy performed and the diagnosis microscopically confirmed. The prognostic assessment of Cawson

(1969) for 'leukoplakia' is that, while the incidence of carcinoma is probably 50 to 100 times greater than in the normal mouth, over 90% of patients with it will not develop carcinoma within 5 years of detection. Multifactorial analysis of many histological criteria by computer is believed helpful by Kramer (1975) as a means of distinguishing lesions of particularly precancerous potential. However, in a somewhat comparable study of oral carcinoma by Friedman and his associates (1973), growth rate and cell kinetics in general were found to be of no value as predictors of response to treatment.

### Papillary and Pseudo-epitheliomatous Overgrowths

The behaviour of the four papillary epithelial lesions of the buccal cavity in the local series indicates that overgrowths of this kind, whatever their histology, should not be underestimated. The need for 100% resection should be emphasised since any such growth may be a verrucous carcinoma at an early stage. At the same time, it is essential to make the distinction between the papillary overgrowths and 'denture hyperplasia'. At one stage of its evolution, the verrucous carcinoma in Case 8.2 was thought to be an example of this condition. Denture hyperplasia has a pattern of epithelial overgrowth much more akin to the spiky variety of pseudo-epitheliomatous hyperplasia, as seen, for example, around a chronic varicose ulcer; it does not have the exophytic or fungating character of the true papilloma or verrucous carcinoma.

Pseudo-epitheliomatous hyperplasia characterises two further lesions that may be over-diagnosed as carcinoma. The ducts and glands of salivary tissue in the hard palate may undergo extensive and marked squamous metaplasia to produce a pattern closely mimetic of carcinoma, a condition described by Abrams and his associates (1973) as "necrotizing sialometaplasia": excision, even if only partial, had proved curative. The other potentially misleading condition is 'glossitis rhombica mediana', the largely self-explanatory designation for a diamond-shaped area of roughened and possibly ulcerated mucosa in the mid-line of the posterior quarter of the tongue. Originally believed to be a developmental anomaly (Martin and Howe, 1938), it has more recently been interpreted as a manifes-

tation of long-standing candidiasis (Cooke, 1975). However, in two local cases, candida was not demonstrable.

## SALIVARY TISSUE

### Adenomas and Carcinomas

*Salivary neoplasms* present problems of classification rather than diagnosis. The notoriously recurrent tendency of the pleomorphic adenoma of the parotid is a product almost certainly of incompleteness of excision: the surgeon balances the integrity of the facial nerve against the minimal risk of metastasis and understandably favours the former. In a series of 1678 tumours of the parotid, Eneroth and his colleagues (1968) classified only 21 as malignant. On the evidence of long duration of a mass before, and short survival of the patient after, diagnosis and treatment of these 21 cases, the authors concluded that carcinoma arises by transformation of a pre-existing adenoma. On the other hand, Gerughty and his associates (1969), from observations on 134 salivary tumours, believe that the salivary carcinoma is a malignant lesion ab initio. All 134 tumours had been classified originally as 'malignant mixed tumors': on review, 35 were reclassified as " 'benign' mixed tumors (all varieties)", i.e. a revealed rate of over-diagnosis of 26%. Of the 99 remaining cases, only 25 were confirmed as satisfying the histological criteria of both 'malignant' and 'mixed'. Of ten patients experiencing local regrowth, seven developed metastases. Lesions showing nuclear aberrancy were associated with metastasis in 66% of cases; of ten lesions showing focal necrosis, nine metastasised; of eight showing focal calcification, all metastasised.

Informative data on prognosis, derived from a study of 288 cases of parotid carcinoma (50% muco-epidermoid), are provided by Spiro and his colleagues (1975). Survival rates at 5 years ranged from 86% for low-grade muco-epidermoid carcinoma to only 19% for high-grade adenocarcinoma. At the same time, these observers stress the shortcomings of the 5-year interval as a measure: for their group of 'malignant mixed' carcinomas, the survival at 5 years was 63% but at 10 years 39%. The corresponding figures in the just-mentioned series of Gerughty and colleagues had been 50% and

30% (and 20% at 15 years). Apropos treatment, both Rafla (1977) and Fu and co-workers (1977) conclude that radiotherapy has more to offer in the treatment of malignant lesions of salivary glands than has been generally believed hitherto.

Salivary neoplasms in children, of which Case 8.5 was an example, are believed by Krolls and his associates (1972) to behave in no significantly different way from the same lesions in the adult, though a follow-up period of at least 20 years is advised. Of their 430 cases, 54 were malignant: of these, 35 were epithelial (20 mucoepidermoid carcinoma).

### Benign Lymphoepithelial Lesion (Mikulicz Disease)

This lesion of salivary tissue is an entity prone to over-diagnosis as malignant, as happened in Case 8.4. An account of 55 cases, inter alia, was given by Bernier and Bhaskar (1958). The lesion is regarded by them as a nodular or diffuse inflammatory reactive hyperplasia of lymphoid tissue with an admixture of islands of epithelium of various sizes and shapes (the 'epimyoepithelial islands' of Morgan and Castleman, 1953) that arise by proliferation, metaplasia and hyalinisation of the epithelium of ducts in consequence, to some extent, of their occlusion. The conclusion of Morgan and Castleman was that the lesion was 'chronic and benign'. However, the process is not always innocuous; in the opinion of Azzopardi and Evans (1971), ". . . probably all cases of benign lymphoepithelial lesion have a degree of malignant potential though the degree of risk has still to be determined". Their own five cases were MLs, in one instance HD. These authors describe, as features suggesting malignancy, tracts of immature lymphoid cells; unexplained foci of necrosis; focal or diffuse histiocytic background; and absence of the epithelial islands over relatively wide areas of tissue. Carcinoma also has been described as a consequence, by Gravanis and Giansanti (1970) in three cases.

### PALATE

#### Mucoepidermoid Carcinoma

Neoplasms of the palate have been extensively studied by Eneroth and co-workers (1970,

1972), in particular, in these articles, the mucoepidermoid carcinoma. So highly differentiated may the lesion be that, in their earlier paper, this group of observers raised the question whether the most highly differentiated form might be a benign neoplasm. In their later paper, however, on the evidence of highly differentiated tissue in metastases, they concluded that a benign equivalent of mucoepidermoid carcinoma does not exist.

### PHARYNX

#### Pseudo-sarcomatous Lesions

Problematical lesions in the pharynx include the so-called pseudo-sarcomatous tumours of the upper digestive and respiratory tracts, especially of the oesophagus. The first formal descriptions of the lesion were given by Stout and Lattes (1957), two cases in the oesophagus; and by Lane (1957), ten cases in mouth, fauces and larnyx. Since then, at least a further six accounts have appeared (Hay-Roe et al., 1960; Sherwin et al., 1963; Hughes and Cruickshank, 1969; Razzuk et al., 1971; Shields et al., 1972; Enrile et al., 1973). A further single example of what is certainly the same lesion was described by Glover and Park (1971) but, in error (Park, 1979), as a pharyngeal leiomyosarcoma (local Case 8.6).

The lesion is typically a polypoid mass of spindle-celled but commonly also bizarre and monstrously polymorphic tissue, mitotically active and often aberrantly so, and invariably accompanied by a squamous-celled carcinoma even though the carcinoma may at the time of diagnosis be still at the in situ stage. However, in patients who have died, the lethal element has almost always been the carcinoma, not the morphologically much more alarming stromal element, hence the term *pseudo*-sarcoma. From this, the important practical point emerges that, whatever the implications of the pseudo-sarcoma per se, the presence of apparently sarcomatous tissue in a biopsy from this anatomical region must be taken as a warning that the patient almost certainly harbours a carcinoma as well. As Lane (1957) said, the pseudo-sarcoma may be the 'smoke-screen' concealing a carcinoma.

This curious lesion naturally raises many questions: What is its nature? What is its relation to the underlying carcinoma? Why has it arisen, and is it always only 'pseudo'? There is a firm answer to the last of these questions only.

The nature of the lesion and its relationship to the carcinoma were fully and carefully analysed by Lane who, recalling the sometimes bizarre behaviour of cells in healing fractures, muscle and connective tissue, and in organising haematomas and thrombi, concluded that the pseudo-sarcomatous morphology is ". . . in the nature of an exuberant, reparative connective-tissue response, and that the carcinoma may possibly be acting as the stimulus". Inevitably, the problem has in it much of the problem of the spindle-celled carcinoma. In their ultrastructural analysis of 13 examples of the 'spindle-cell variant of squamous carcinoma', Lichtiger and his colleagues (1970) regarded the 10 cases of Lane (1957) as being of this nature. However, of the cases in the Lichtiger series, four were on lower lip and two on the skin of the face, while eight of the 13 were growths recurrent after radiotherapy. It may be, as Woyke and his colleagues (1974) suggest, that the examples examined by Lichtiger and his associates were not, or at least were not all, the same as the pseudo-sarcoma of Lane. The present position was fairly stated by Woyke and his colleagues namely, that ". . . post-irradiation sarcoma (or pseudosarcoma) of the skin, spindle cell carcinoma of the lower lip, and polypoid 'pseudo-sarcoma' of the upper respiratory and digestive systems are not a single entity, and therefore the conclusions drawn from the observation of one of them cannot be applied to the others". From his ultrastructural studies on spindle-cell carcinoma, Battifora (1976) concluded that ". . . the pseudosarcomatous component of SCC (spindle cell carcinoma) originates from mesenchymal metaplasia of squamous cells and that collagen is produced by these metaplastic cells".

Is the pseudo-sarcoma always only 'pseudo'? This is the question that matters in practice. Certainly, the sarcomatoid tissue seems rarely if ever to metastasise: in that sense 'pseudo-sarcoma' is justified. However, as in the case described by Hughes and Cruickshank, it may invade, destroy and kill. This single example is probably insufficient reason for abandoning the term altogether but we should bear in mind that many of the reported patients have died of their carcinoma within 13 months and that reports of survival longer than five years are few (only two of Lane's ten patients achieved this): perhaps, with more tissue, the pseudo-sarcoma would truly show itself as sarcoma. It seems wise to heed the advice of Hughes and Cruickshank that the lesion should not be underestimated: an over-conservative approach with inadequate removal may cost a life.

*Leucocytic Infiltration*

Permeation or invasion of the epithelial covering of tonsils or adenoids by lymphocytes, and usually also some monocytes, has sometimes been considered a pointer to possible malignancy: the pattern was prominent in Case 8.8 and proved innocuous. The occurrence is the analogue of 'transgression of the capsule' in lymph nodes: that is, common in the MLs but not unusual also in simple chronic inflammation. The morphology of individual cells is the better guide.

Dense accumulations of plasma cells appear with what seems to be disproportionate frequency in response to chronic inflammation in the oro-naso-pharynx as, for example, in chronic sinusitis and the dental and otitic granulomas (with immunological implications as yet uncertain): therefore, the problem 'plasmacytoma or not?' is correspondingly frequent. The matter has been considered already with lesions of the skeletal system, and will be considered again presently in relation to the gastrointestinal tract where special circumstances entail special assessment.

OESOPHAGUS

Biopsies from the lower oesophagus may present great diagnostic difficulty. The combination of ulceration, scarring and metaplasia may produce distorted tissue patterns of great complexity. Sampling errors apart, and after semiserially sectioning the block (which should always be done; it may save the patient a further intubation), and no matter how experienced the pathologist, evidence may still be equivocal. However, a report to this effect will often, of itself, be enough to induce resection. Diagnosis on clinical grounds alone appears to be extremely accurate, and occasions are few when a specimen resected on only 'suspicious' biopsy evidence does not contain carcinoma. As always in such circumstances, when confronted by some degree of nuclear aberrancy, mitotic activity and possible invasion, the pathologist cannot do better than decide whether, were the biopsy his own, he would have his lesion resected.

The rare recurrent *benign papillomatosis* (Waterfall et al., 1978) and the *verrucous carcinoma* (Minielly et al., 1967) have been described in the oesophagus where the clinical and pathological implications are essentially the same for both lesions as apply elsewhere. This holds equally for *carcinoma in situ* of the oesophagus although this lesion will be seen most usually in company with an already frank carcinoma, either at the edge or as an independent focus. Endoscopy is already yielding an increasing number of biopsies of stomach showing carcinoma in situ: the same trend may appear with oesophageal disorders. A possible source of confusion, perhaps a discrepancy in successive biopsies, is that a carcinoma of oesophagus may rarely show a combined pattern, that of typically squamous-celled carcinoma in company with typically glandular carcinoma, and either may be still at the in situ stage.

## STOMACH

### Polyps

Gastric polyps raise the question of precancer just as may polyps anywhere in the gastrointestinal tract. From analysis of series of 106 and 97 examples respectively, Berg (1958) and Tomasulo (1971) each concluded that the polyp indicates a precancerous tendency. A histological subdivision was made by Tomasulo into hyperplastic and adenomatous forms, essentially on the basis of epithelial atypia. The hyperplastic forms were distributed at random throughout the stomach. The adenomatous forms, more usually antral in site, were regarded as analogous to adenomatous polyps of the colon, and only in them was marked atypia or carcinoma in situ seen. Follow-up observations (one patient developed a polypoid carcinoma) suggested that excision was adequate treatment unless polyps were either multiple or more than 2 cm in diameter.

### Early Gastric Cancer

Endoscopy directs growing attention to early gastric cancer, designated EGC by Fevre and his colleagues (1976) and defined by them as "... carcinoma confined to mucosa or submucosa without infiltration into the muscularis propria". The cure rate for carcinomas of this extent they calculate as 95%. For carcinoma in situ, with no involvement of even the lamina propria, the rate might be even nearer to 100%. The analogy with carcinoma in situ of the cervix uteri is pathologically exact; if routine screening of well persons became established, the analogy would be wholly exact and carry with it the same uncertainties.

A recent article (Editorial, 1976) analyses the problems posed by the reported finding of unsuspected carcinoma in association with gastric ulcer in as many as 6.4% of cases, and supplies the interestingly provocative reply that "... indiscriminate gastrectomy is not the answer; diagnosis of three or four early cancers does not justify a hundred unnecessary operations with the occasional operative death". That is, to approach the problem in one way, 33 or 25 partial gastrectomies may or may not be considered a worthwhile price to pay for saving one patient from carcinoma. To approach it in another way; if, as Sano and associates (1972) calculate, EGC may be present for 5–10 years before advancing beyond the muscularis mucosae, partial gastrectomy might well be advised in the young but not in the elderly. The pathologist, given a representative biopsy, can supply the diagnosis and help to assess the probabilities but only the clinician can prescribe the treatment. The main obstacle to diagnosis remains the unreliability of biopsy by endoscope; even multiple specimens may fail to include an area of carcinoma, hence the finding by Segal and co-workers (1975) that merely the macroscopic appearance of an ulcer was a better indicator of malignancy than the particles obtained on biopsy (this is not, as the just-cited Editorial [1976] suggested, a failure of histology but a failure of biopsy). Here, perhaps more than anywhere in the context of cancer, a negative biopsy 'means nothing'.

### Carcinoma

The above problem is generated by changes in superficial gastric mucosa. The problems with deeper tissue have long been familiar, namely, the difficulties of deciding whether small distorted glanduliform structures around the depths of a chronic peptic ulcer represent carcinoma or not.

Opinions can legitimately vary, and to that extent differences in the reported incidence of carcinoma in peptic ulcer will also vary. With general awareness of the problem, the one-time appreciably high rate of over-diagnosis of ulcer-cancer has greatly decreased. For the histologist, an intrinsically greater difficulty is that of deciding whether, in some cases of ulceration, shallow or deep, a diffusely cellular stromal infiltrate is leucocytic, mainly histiocytic, or neoplastic. A local case (not in the present series) illustrates the problem. Partial gastrectomy had been performed for an apparently simple peptic ulcer; sections were reported as showing no more than that. One year later the patient returned with a nodule in the laparotomy scar; sections showed diffusely scirrhous carcinoma. 'Blind' review of further sections from one of the original blocks of the ulcer by a group of pathologists produced different opinions; some thought 'simple', others 'malignant'. The scanty cells that contained mucin (mucicarmine + ve) had appeared to some to be muciphages; to others they were carcinoma. The later events showed the original lesion to have been certainly an ulcerated linitis plastica but the difference in opinions it produced was instructive. A frozen section is sometimes requested on a gastric lesion (if there is any possibility of the lesion's being a lymphoma, frozen section should always be requested): the section may allow recognition of a lymphoma but identification of a linitis plastica can be extremely difficult if not, in view of the difficulties with paraffin sections, virtually impossible.

The outlook for patients with fully developed gastric carcinoma is improving, and useful information towards better prognostic assessment is available. The 5-year survival rate in a relatively early series of 1264 patients, of whom 457 were operated upon, was reported by Ransom (1953) as 7.8%. In a recent series of 903 cases described by Serlin and his colleagues (1977) the corresponding figure was 26%. These authors found their cases to fall into three groups; those cured, and those uncured with either slow-growing or rapidly-growing lesions, and 26 months or 8 months median survival respectively. The whole of the excess mortality had occurred within 5 years of resection; the difference in mortality from a normal population was maximum at 5 years. Three factors had proved valid predictors of recurrence within 3 years, namely, involve-

ment of nodes, penetration of the serosa and resection of the oesophagus. Three other more particularly histological features, lymphoid infiltrate, nuclear grade and follicular hyperplasia, were assessed as predictors by Black and his associates (1971). Presence of all three features was associated with a 5-year survival of some 75%, and of any two with a survival of 45%–65%; absence of all three was associated with a nil survival at 5 years (and at 1 year only 50%). Sinus histiocytosis, often emphasised by Black and his various associates as a useful predictor in axillary nodes draining a carcinoma of breast, had been surprisingly rare in nodes draining a carcinoma of stomach.

A contributor to the longer-term survivals in many series may be the lesion described by Brander and his co-workers (1974) as 'indolent' mucoid carcinoma. Of 574 gastric carcinomas, 50 were defined as mucoid, and, of these, 6 were 'well-differentiated' and associated with a mean survival of 9 years, even though nodal metastasis had been present in two of the patients.

*Sarcoma*

Sarcomas (nonlymphomatous) of the stomach have been recently analysed by Appelman and Helwig (1977) who divided their 44 examples into 24 'epithelioid leiomyosarcoma' (of either spindle-celled or round-celled forms), 1 liposarcoma, 1 possible rhabdomyosarcoma and 18 'heterogeneous' sarcomas. Distinction between spindle-celled-myoma and -sarcoma was made on the basis of mitotic incidence, namely, 5 figures or fewer and 20 figures or more per 50 hpf respectively (values between 5 and 20 thus remaining as the borderline zone). In the case of the round-celled variety, larger cells were taken to indicate '-myoma', smaller cells, especially when densely packed, to indicate '-sarcoma'. The size of the tumours was also predictive: of sarcomas less than 6 cm in diameter, 20% metastasised: of those more than 6 cm in diameter, 85% metastasised. Mitotic incidence had been similarly used as a discriminator by Crocker (1969) and, in assessing smooth muscle tumours also of the intestinal tract and retroperitoneum, by Ranchod and Kempson (1977).

## SMALL INTESTINE

Duodenal lesions of the type diagnosed on review as a *hamartoma* in Case 8.19 are not unduly rare but they are more likely to be found in infancy, when obstruction will cause problems with feeding, than in the adult.

*Periampullary carcinomas* seem often to be unusually slow to metastasise, and probably many pathologists, at necrospy of a patient who has died after the extensive resection that carcinomas involving the duodenum require, will have found few if any metastases in nodes or liver. Until the reassessment of the lesion in Case 8.14, a hamartoma, it, too, was a seeming example of a nonmetastasising periampullary carcinoma. However, the extent to which over-diagnosis of this type contributes to the impression of slowness to spread is probably small.

The possibility exists that prognostic problems may be raised in the small intestine by potentially precancerous changes in the mucosa. In a case report by Warner (1979), a woman of 89 years is described as having developed mucosal hyperplasia, dysplasia and carcinoma in situ, as well as multifocal carcinoma, in the upper jejunum 18 years after the ingestion of [131]I (toxic goitre). As Warner explains, [131]I is rapidly absorbed in the upper small intestine and may be recycled in the enterohepatic circulation.

## LARGE INTESTINE

### Juvenile Polyps

Some forms of polyp of the large intestine are generally acknowledged as innocuous, namely, the juvenile (retention, hamartomatous), the metaplastic (hyperplastic) and the inflammatory. Their identification as such will exclude the risk of over-diagnosis as premalignant, if not actually malignant, but the slightly atypical cytology and degree of mitotic activity the epithelium may show can at times mislead. In one of three examples of the hamartomatous variety reported by Allen (1966), over-diagnosis had led to excision of the rectum. An account of 124 juvenile retention polyps, none associated with carcinoma, has been given by Silverberg (1970). Problems of prognosis are raised particularly by the adenomatous and villous forms. One problem is essentially statistical and concerns the degree of risk represented by such a polyp or polyps: the other is more purely histological and concerns a misleading tissue pattern.

### Adenomatous Polyps and Carcinoma

In the opinion of Muto and his colleagues (1975), ". . . at least half of all cancers of the colon and rectum arise from previously benign adenomatous polyps or villous adenomas", probably all having passed through stages of increasingly severe atypia before becoming invasive: the duration of this progression they estimate at 5–10 years. Further, from their data, they conclude that the risk of subsequent carcinoma represented by a single polyp less than 10 mm in diameter extends from 1% with the adenomatous polyp, through 4% for the intermediate adenomatous/villous mixed form, to 10% for the purely villous. Polyps up to 2 cm in diameter show no prognostic variation with histological type; with larger polyps, however, the malignant potential is greater with the villous forms.

The reported incidence of 'carcinoma' in polyps varies widely. The diagnosis is not often one of panel-decision; rather, as McDivitt (1974), in citing series where the figure varied from 20% to 0.3%, has said, it ". . . seems to depend principally on the reporting pathologist's histologic criteria for diagnosing carcinoma". The likelihood that a focally aberrant *adenomatous* polyp, even if showing what most pathologists would concur in calling focally invasive carcinoma, will already, at the time of diagnosis, have metastasised to nodes, is small. Examples have been reported (refs. in McDivitt, 1974) but they are extremely few. The individual *villous* polyp, on the other hand, is much likelier at the time of diagnosis, not only to contain areas of frankly invasive carcinoma but also already to have metastasised. The importance of a polyp of either variety, even if histologically benign, is its role as a warning of danger. From analysis of their data, Muto and his colleagues (1975) provide the further useful calculations: (a) that ". . . at least 1 in 5 of all patients with neoplastic disease of the large bowel, when first seen, have more than one benign or malignant tumor somewhere in the colon or rectum"; and (b) that "The risk of a patient developing a second tumor is at least 1 in 10 . . .". The need for possibly lifelong follow-up is evident.

The fact that carcinoma in villous polyps may be focal is important: it may be responsible for false-negative diagnosis, to the extent of 50% in the series of Quan and Castro (1971), and responsible also, if not for 'false' negative diagnosis, at least for the biopsy's appearing, from examination after excision, to have removed the whole of the carcinomatous area from a polyp.

### Pseudo-malignant Pattern in Polyps

The more purely histological hazard inherent in polyps of the intestine is that some, though wholly benign, may show a misleadingly pseudo-malignant displacement of epithelium through the muscularis mucosae and into the submucosa. The pattern was seen by Muto and his associates (1973) in 2.4% of 2341 polyps, mostly from the sigmoid colon: during the same period, 4.7% of the 2341 showed unequivocally invasive carcinoma. The same phenomenon was described also by Greene (1974) in 3.2 % of 637 polyps: of the 21 polyps concerned, 18 had been diagnosed as malignant; two as having a "possibly premalignant potential"; one correctly as artefact due to the plane of section; and all the patients had undergone at least partial resection. The displacement of glandular elements is believed by Muto and his associates (1973) to be due to traumatic twisting, haemorrhage and associated inflammation, the disruption of normal architecture thus allowing the pseudo-carcinomatous migration of tissue through the muscularis mucosae. Diagnostic pointers offered by these observers are deposits of haemosiderin and areas of granulation tissue in the stalk and around the glands in the submucosa, an excessive amount and branching of the muscularis mucosae and much cystic distension of the glands in the affected areas. The dangers of mistaking hypertrophied muscularis mucosae for muscularis propria are mentioned later in connection with the intestinal lymphomas and pseudo-lymphomas.

The same type of misleading pattern has been reported in polyps of the Peutz-Jeghers syndrome by Bolwell and James (1979). As these authors remark, "This entity of pseudoinvasion may explain some of the reported cases of malignancy associated with Peutz-Jeghers syndrome and it needs recognition as an entity because of the implications with regard to management".

A pattern of morphological and histochemical changes sometimes seen adjacent to carcinomas of colon and designated 'transitional mucosa' has borderline significance to the extent that it has been regarded as a precancerous change. However, the demonstration by Isaacson and Attwood (1979) of the same type of pattern in relation to benign ulcers and colostomies indicates that it does not have premalignant significance.

### Carcinoma in Ulcerative Colitis

Carcinoma is likely to develop in some 3%–5% of patients with ulcerative colitis: that is, the risk to a patient with the disease is some five to ten times greater than for the rest of the population (Morson, 1966). Diagnostic difficulties met by the pathologist are essentially the same as those raised by polyps, with the obviously added complication af a variably inflammatory, distorted and scarred background. The observations of Morson and Pang (1967) indicate that, like carcinoma in situ in many tissues, carcinoma in ulcerative colitis passes through stages of dysplasia en route to carcinoma in situ and is subject to the same diagnostic uncertainties, whether arising in a polypoid lesion or in flat mucosa. As well as having to evaluate a rising gradient of glandular overgrowth, loss of goblet cells, cytological aberrancy and mitotic activity, the pathologist may have to assess here also, as with adenomatous polyps in the otherwise normal colon or rectum, the significance of glandular elements within the submucosa. It is reassuring to the nonspecialist pathologist that Morson and Pang, from their great experience, conclude that a distinction between chronic inflammatory distortion and malignancy is "sometimes impossible".

Hitherto, only some 40% of the area most likely to develop such lesions has been accessible for biopsy, via the sigmoidoscope (Hinton, 1966). The practice of colonoscopy will increase this figure but will also, from the small size of the biopsies, increase the difficulties of diagnosis. The same limitation applies in relation to diagnosis of the lymphoid lesions of the large intestine. As mentioned later, the presence of a well-differentiated lymphoid follicle may determine a preference for a benign diagnosis rather than a malignant, and a biopsy may be too small to include one.

### CARCINOID TUMOUR

Debate whether the lesion should be called carcinoid tumour or argentaffin carcinoma is needless: the term carcinoid tumour is familiar and unambiguous, and its general implications are well understood. The main problems posed by the neoplasm are: (a) whether it can always be distinguished from a glandular carcinoma, and (b) whether, when correctly identified, its histology can indicate likely behaviour.

*Structural Variants*

The morphology of the lesion varies considerably, to the point where Soga and Tazawa (1971) have proposed a subdivision into six histological types (without, however, offering correlations with clinical behaviour). The consequences of this structural variability are two. First, some carcinoids of mildly follicular appearance may be misinterpreted as poorly differentiated glandular carcinoma (as happened initially with local Case 8.16): of an original series of 38 apparent carcinoids of the rectum described by Genre and his colleagues (1971), three were rediagnosed on review as glandular carcinomas. Second, some lesions seeming certainly to be glandular carcinomas may contain a mixture of argentaffin cells and mucous cells, and be possibly atypical carcinoids (Soga and Tazawa, 1971; Soga et al., 1971). With lesions of either these follicular or mixed-cell types, a false-positive diagnosis of carcinoma is possible. At the same time, as emphasised and illustrated by Genre and his colleagues (1971), there is a possibility of false-negative diagnosis: a glandular carcinoma may occasionally consist partly or predominantly of quite undifferentiated carcinoma simplex with cells so uniform and sheet-like as to suggest a carcinoid.

The silver-staining reactions should be studied in any gastrointestinal glandular carcinoma that resembles in any part a carcinoid tumour. In the single case of 'argentaffin cell adenocarcinoma of the stomach' reported by Soga and his co-workers (1971), none of 47 nodes contained malignant tissue: therefore, even a partial component of silver-staining cells may indicate a prognosis better than expected. The fact that, for no well-understood reason, carcinoids of the rectum usually fail to react to specific stains is no reason for not making a search, rather the reverse.

A lesion closely comparable to that just mentioned but occurring in the appendix has been designated 'adenocarcinoid' by Warkel and his colleagues (1978) who describe 39 cases. As the name indicates, the neoplasm possesses features of both adenocarcinoma and carcinoid: its behaviour is correspondingly intermediate. The 5-year survival rate for the series was close to 80%. For pure adenocarcinoma these authors cite the figure of 33%; for the pure carcinoid, survival is better than 99%. Prognosis with such a borderline lesion presents a problem, but Warkel and his colleagues offer the useful advice that, while appendicectomy will be adequate treatment for most examples, hemicolectomy is indicated for those that show ". . . atypical foci, a high mitotic count (1–5 per 10 hpf), or spread beyond the appendix".

*Prediction of Metastasis*

The behaviour of classical or typical carcinoids in respect of metastasis can be predicted with fair accuracy but not on their intrinsic histology. In the opinion of Orloff (1971), "There is usually no way of predicting the likelihood of metastases from the cytologic pattern . . .", and also of Zakariai and his colleagues (1975), "Histologic diagnosis per se of the carcinoid is unreliable in distinguishing between benign and malignant or . . . non-metastasizing and metastasizing carcinoids". However, these authors are agreed that the depth of penetration towards the serosa is a useful indicator. From their analysis of the tumours in 107 patients, Zakariai and his colleagues found that, of their 45 patients whose lesion had extended to or through the serosa, only 5% had survived beyond 5 years; of the 72 patients whose lesion was still 'intramural', 85% had survived 5 years. To the criterion of penetration to or through the serosa as an indicator of likely metastasis, Orloff added, as an equally reliable indicator, size of the mass; a tumour diameter of 2 cm or more. By this criterion there were but 4% false-negative and 7% false-positive predictions of metastasis. Similarly, using the criterion of mural incursion, in only one of 14 cases was penetration of the muscularis propria not associated with nodal spread, while, where nodal metastasis had occurred, invasion of the muscularis propria was invariable.

On essentially the same criteria, 6 of the 35 cases of rectal carcinoid analysed by Genre and his colleagues (1971) were judged malignant and all metastasised (from the circumstances in two other patients, these authors considered the possibility that nodal metastases from at least a rectal carcinoid may become dormant or even regress after removal of the primary lesion).

### Requirements of Biopsy

The gastrointestinal carcinoid is a classically borderline growth: in general, in cases not yet metastatic, the histology directly determines the treatment. Evidence cited above shows that the correlation is high betwen penetration of the muscularis propria and metastasis. Penetrating lesions therefore demand more radical excision than the nonpenetrating. In much of the gastrointestinal tract this may matter little, but in stomach or rectum it is crucial. Therefore, a biopsy must be deep enough to include the muscularis propria, and this need is ordinarily rarely met. Therefore, if a first biopsy shows a lesion of stomach or rectum to be a carcinoid but does not include the muscularis propria, a further and deeper biopsy should be the next step. Assessment of penetration should be quite possible on frozen section. The surgeon could then proceed at once either to local excision or, perhaps, to excision of the rectum (in practical terms, the position and implications are similar to those wherein mastectomy may or may not immediately follow diagnosis of a breast lump on frozen section as carcinoma).

The carcinoid of the vermiform appendix still represents a challenge to the general correlation between mural invasion and likelihood of metastasis, a paradox still in as much need of explanation as the negative staining reactions of and nonproduction of the carcinoid syndrome by the rectal carcinoid.

### Malignant Lymphoma and Pseudo-lymphoma

Malignant lymphomas of the gastrointestinal tract are less common than reported figures would indicate for they are greatly prone to over-diagnosis. In many cases the lesion has been a highly mimetic benign overgrowth of lymphoid tissue, a pseudo-lymphoma. Six such examples (all in association with idiopathic ulceration of the small intestine) were described by Artinian and his colleagues (1971). The initial diagnosis in three had been HD, in two, RCS, and in one, anaplastic carcinoma. Three patients had died, two with no neoplasm present at necropsy (no necropsy in one); three, including the patient diagnosed as having carcinoma, were well at 10, 10 and 12 years. The misleading elements had been the pleomorphism of the inflammatory reaction and ". . . many bizarre reticulum cells" (believed on ultramicroscopic evidence to be phagocytic reticulum cells, not R–S cells). In an analysis of pseudo-lymphomas of the gastrointestinal tract (and of lung), Saltzstein (1969) stated, of apparently lymphomatous tumours of the stomach, that ". . . between one-fourth and one-half have been found to be pseudolymphomas" but acknowledged that there probably is a gradient of change up to the point of frank ML. Assessment of diagnostic accuracy is made difficult by the tendency the true lymphomas may have towards late recurrence; a 10-year follow-up period is recommended. In the experience of Saltzstein, pseudo-lymphomas are rare in the small intestine but relatively common in the large intestine, especially in the rectum. Most examples in the stomach are seen in association with peptic ulceration, as, for example, in the accounts given by Eras and Winawer (1969) and Kobayashi and co-workers (1970). The occasional presence of many eosinophil polymorphonuclear cells has earned for some lesions the term 'eosinophil granuloma' (Hardy and Elesha, 1968). A similar lesion has been described also in the rectum by Klein and Baumgartl (1970).

A prognostic assessment of gastric ML (including HD) has been given by Lim and his colleagues (1977) on the basis of experience with 50 cases, all followed for at least 6 years. Survival rates for the various types ranged from nil to 100% with overall figures of 51% at 5 years and 37% at 10 years; that is, appreciably higher rates than for established carcinoma. Stage-for-stage, however, there was little difference; the better overall survival was due essentially, as the authors remark, to the fact that ". . . only a small proportion of patients had tumors extending through the serosa involving lymph nodes or metastasizing beyond the perigastric nodes". ML, when primary within the stomach, thus appears to be intrinsically much less aggressive than carcinoma.

A series of 100 cases of 'benign lymphoma' of

the rectum was described by Cornes and co-workers (1961). All consisted of well differentiated lymphoid tissue showing follicle formation, and all were benign and believed to be a response to inflammation ('pseudo-lymphoma' would therefore appear to be the better term: the implication of 'lymphoma', even if benign, is clearly neoplastic). Lesions of this kind are not uncommon and so represent a correspondingly frequent risk of over-diagnosis; in earlier series cited by Cornes and co-workers about half of the cases had been diagnosed as ML. Case 4.24 in the local series typified both the lesion and the risk. A possibly misleading feature is the frequent presence of lymphoid infiltration in adjacent submucosa; this is innocuous. The much rarer extension of lymphoid tissue into the muscularis propria, however, does more seriously raise the possibility of malignancy; and there is here a further diagnostic trap. In association with such lesions, the muscularis mucosae is often unduly hyperplastic and may be mistaken for the muscularis propria; awareness of the phenomenon should itself be a sufficient safeguard. The unmasking as benign of a lesion once widely regarded as malignant carries the reciprocal risk of under-diagnosis of those lesions that truly are malignant, and that possibility applies here. In the experience of Cornes and his co-workers, 3 of 19 MLs of the rectum had been initially regarded as benign lymphoid infiltrations.

## Plasma Cell Lesions

Difficulties of assessment almost exactly comparable with those just described for the lymphoid overgrowths attend the focal plasma cell infiltrations of the digestive tract. They were clearly recognised by Soga and his colleagues (1970) in reporting an example within the stomach, and by Henry and Farrer-Brown (1977) whose 125 reported examples were distributed between stomach (51), small intestine (53) and large intestine (21). The main causes of difficulty experienced by Henry and Farrer-Brown in distinguishing between an inflammatory and a neoplastic plasma cell lesion were the many types of cell resident normally within the gastrointestinal mucosa (a better term for this than 'pleomorphic' would be 'pleotypic'), frequent fibrosis, the superficial resemblance of multinucleated and giant forms of plasma cell to the R-S cell, and simple artefact such as shrinkage and distortion of cells and tissue. These authors found reticulin staining unhelpful, thus, "The reticulin content of these tumours is very variable and is of no assistance in the diagnosis of this group of tumours or for that matter of any of the gastrointestinal lymphomas, with the exception of follicular lymphomas". The case-report by Soga and colleagues (1970) includes a table of eight features which will aid distinction between the plasma cell granuloma and the plasmacytoma, based on the scattered distribution of the cells, their maturity, lack of mitoses, frequent fibrosis and Russell bodies, and pleocytic infiltrate of the benign lesion, and, in contrast, the aggregated distribution, immaturity of cells, presence of mitoses, scanty fibrosis, scarcity of Russell bodies and of cells of other kinds in the plasmacytoma.

## Pancreatic Biopsy

"Biopsy of the pancreas at the time of operation is advocated by some and condemned by more" (Cohn, 1976). The debate concerns the likelihood of frequency of postbiopsy complications such as death (3.8% of 159 patients in the series of Schultz and Sanders, 1963), fistula, peritonitis and haemorrhage. Besides this, in dealing with a biopsy, the surgeon is confronted by problems of sampling, the pathologist by problems of interpretation. The problem for each is created by the frequency with which a carcinoma of pancreas is surrounded by or associated with areas of chronic pancreatitis. The essence of the difficulty, however, is that of distinguishing histologically between chronic pancreatitis and carcinoma. There is no case of this in the local series but two examples have been seen more recently when, in a group of pathologists, unanimity could not be achieved on whether sections represented the one lesion or the other. Foci of distorted glandular tissue may lie within and appear to be infiltrating fibrous tissue in a way that exactly simulates the pattern of carcinoma. 'Stromal invasion' is then irrelevant as a criterion, and judgement has to depend on assessment of individual cellular morphology.

Despite the difficulties of interpretation, some remarkably accurate results of pancreatic biopsy have been reported. An analysis has been published by Isaacson and his associates (1974) of biopsy in 527 patients (by needle, wedge, both or unknown techniques). Diagnosis in all cases was made by frozen section, the tissue cut on a $CO_2$ freezing microtome and stained by polychrome methylene blue. In only one of the 527 sections (85 diagnosed as normal, 116 as benign, 326 as malignant) was the diagnosis changed on later paraffin sections; one biopsy diagnosed as benign was changed to malignant. In technical contrast to this series is that of George and her colleagues (1975) in which, in biopsies on 47 patients, frozen section was used only once. Further, in this series, ". . . no errors of interpretation were found". However, the authors add the circumspect comment, of the non-malignant diagnoses, that ". . . only time will show the final accuracy of the biopsies".

In investigation of the pancreas, as elsewhere, endoscopy is being used in an attempt to achieve at least earlier if not more accurate diagnosis. A recent account describes the value of assay of CEA activity in pancreatic juice obtained by cannulation of the pancreatic duct (Sharma et al., 1976). The values obtained in patients with carcinoma were notably higher than in patients with either no pancreatic disease or chronic pancreatitis.

A borderline problem other than 'infiltrating carcinoma vs. distorting fibrosis' is the atypical hyperplasia, whether papillary or non-papillary, of the pancreatic duct(s). Aberrant overgrowth of this kind was found at necropsy in just over 1% of 1174 patients by Kozuka and his colleagues (1979): also, it was present in nearly 30% (7/24) of pancreases containing infiltrating carcinoma but in less than 1% (5/713) of those not containing carcinoma. The change is equated by these authors with carcinoma in situ. Similarly, the lesion is regarded as premalignant by Ferrari and his co-workers (1979) in whose patient it had caused ductal obstruction and, clinically, simulated carcinoma. The problem has the same implications vis-à-vis diagnostic thresholds, therapy, and frequency of incidence and curability as has 'dysplasia vs. carcinoma in situ' at any site.

## SEROSAL METAPLASIA

Two examples of uncertainty induced by peritoneal aberrancy were included in the local series (Cases 8.24, 8.25). The phenomenon is not uncommon and has varying clinical significance. In a patient known certainly to have an intra-abdominal carcinoma, equally certain knowledge whether the omentum is or is not involved might have some bearing on the therapy. Decision here would depend on the assessment of detailed cytology and a parallel search for mucin within the cells. The problem is more serious when the serosal change may be the only hint of malignancy that there is, as may happen, for example, in the omentum in association with a benign but 'leaking' dermoid cyst of the ovary (where, however, the accompanying granulomatous lipophagic reaction will suggest the correct diagnosis) or in association with cirrhosis of the liver and long-standing ascites (where, incidentally, remarkably bizarre cells may be seen in the effusion).

The most suggestively glandular expressions of serosal metaplasia, as shown in Figs. 8.37 and 8.38, have been seen most frequently in my own experience in the pelvis, usually in lesions of the adnexa. Their significance vis-à-vis a possible carcinoma is essentially the same as that just outlined for the omental occurrence; in addition, there is in an adnexal mass the possibility of extension from an immediately adjacent primary source, the ovary, in a way that obviously does not apply to the omentum.

Awareness of the proliferative capacity and structural versatility of the serosa is the best safeguard against an erroneous diagnosis of malignancy.

## ENDOMETRIOSIS

Endometriosis is mentioned here because of its not infrequent involvement of the intestine and the threat it represents of over-diagnosis as carcinoma (one such case, long ago and not in this hospital, where the rectum was excised, remains indelibly in the mind). Clinically, with its fibrosis, induration and distortion of the gut wall, endometriosis may mimic carcinoma almost exactly. As with serosal metaplasia, all that may be required to make the correct microscopic diagnosis is awareness or recollection of the possibility. Endometriosis should be always in mind with every biopsy of the gut whether large or small. A relevant and educative case report has been published by Britton and Thomson (1979).

## Conclusions

1) The verrucous form of carcinoma may occur in the oral cavity and oesophagus. Though benign histologically it is as potentially destructive as basal cell carcinoma. Radiotherapy may provoke metastasis.

2) Pseudo-epitheliomatous lesions that require to be distinguished from early carcinoma are denture hyperplasia, necrotising sialometaplasia and glossitis rhombica mediana.

3) In salivary adenomatous neoplasms, nuclear aberrancy, focal necrosis and focal calcification are indicative of possible malignancy. Lesions at first dubiously malignant may not reveal themselves as carcinoma for at least 10 years or, in children, 20 years.

4) The 'benign lymphoepithelial lesion' of Mikulicz disease is usually benign but markedly prone to over-diagnosis as a malignant lymphoma. Unequivocally malignant lymphoma may, however, be rarely concerned.

5) The pseudo-sarcoma of the oesophagus or pharynx probably always accompanies and may overshadow a coexistent carcinoma.

6) Any suspicion at laparotomy that a gastric mass may be a malignant lymphoma should prompt a request for frozen section.

7) Mitotic incidence remains the best indicator of malignancy in nonlymphomatous sarcomas of the stomach.

8) As many as 50% of lesions diagnosed as malignant lymphoma of the gastrointestinal tract may not be so but, instead, florid inflammatory reactions, i.e. pseudo-lymphomas.

9) Malignant lymphomas are slower to spread than carcinomas. Invasion of the muscularis propria by a malignant lymphoma is prognostically ominous. In pseudo-lymphomas (and in some other benign lesions) the muscularis mucosae may be abnormally hyperplastic and thick; it should not be mistaken for the muscularis propria.

10) Distinction between plasma cell granuloma and plasmacytoma presents the same histological problem in the gastrointestinal tract as elsewhere.

11) Neoplastic polyps of the large intestine, depending on their structure, represent a risk of subsequent carcinoma of between 1% and 10%. Epithelium may be misplaced innocuously into the submucosa of polyps and be mistaken for malignant invasion.

12) In ulcerative colitis, a certain distinction on biopsy between inflammatory distortion and carcinoma is sometimes impossible.

13) Prognosis with carcinoid tumours is based empirically on size of the lesion and/or penetration of the muscularis propria.

14) The role of the pancreatic biopsy remains controversial. Certain distinction on biopsy between chronic pancreatitis and carcinoma is sometimes impossible.

15) Endometriosis in the wall of the gut may exactly simulate carcinoma macroscopically, and may be mistaken for carcinoma microscopically.

## References

Abrams AM, Melrose RJ, Howell FV (1973) Necrotizing sialometaplasia. A disease simulating malignancy. Cancer 32: 130–135

Ackerman LV (1948) Verrucous carcinoma of the oral cavity. Surgery 23: 670–678

Allen MS (1966) Hamartomatous inverted polyps of the rectum. Cancer 19: 257–265

Appelman HD, Helwig EB (1977) Sarcomas of the stomach. Am J Clin Pathol 67: 2–10

Artinian B, Lough JO, Palmer JD (1971) Idiopathic ulcer of small bowel with pseudolymphomatous reaction. A clinicopathological study of six cases. Arch Pathol 91: 327–333

Azzopardi JG, Evans DJ (1971) Malignant lymphoma of parotid associated with Mikulicz disease (benign lymphoepithelial lesion). J Clin Pathol 24: 744–752

Battifora H (1976) Spindle-cell carcinoma. Ultrastructural evidence of squamous origin and collagen production by the tumor cells. Cancer 37: 2275–2282

Berg JW (1958) Histological aspects of the relation between gastric adenomatous polyps and gastric cancer. Cancer 11: 1149–1155

Bernier JL, Bhaskar SN (1958) Lymphoepithelial lesions of salivary glands. Histogenesis and classification based on 186 cases. Cancer 11: 1156–1179

Black MM, Freeman C, Mork T, Harvei S, Cutler SJ (1971) Prognostic significance of microscopic structure of gastric carcinomas and their regional lymph nodes. Cancer 27: 703–711

Bolwell JS, James PD (1979) Peutz-Jeghers syndrome with pseudoinvasion of hamartomatous polyps and multiple epithelial neoplasms. Histopathol 3: 39–50

Brander WL, Needham PRG, Morgan AD (1974) Indolent mucoid carcinoma of stomach. J Clin Pathol 27: 536–541

Britton DC, Thomson JPS (1979) Rectal endometriosis. J R Coll Surg Edinb 24: 30–33

Cawson RA (1969) Leukoplakia and oral cancer. Proc R Soc Med 62: 610–615

Cohn I (1976) Cancer of the pancreas. Detection and diagnosis. Cancer 37: 582–588

Cooke BED (1975) Median rhomboid glossitis: Candidiasis and not a developmental anomaly. Br J Dermatol 93: 399–405

Cornes JS, Wallace MH, Morson BC (1961) Benign lymphomas of the rectum and anal canal: A study of 100 cases. J Pathol Bacteriol 82: 371–382

Crocker DW (1969) Smooth muscle tumors of the stomach. Ann Surg 170: 239–243

Editorial (1976) When is a gastric ulcer really a cancer? Lancet I: 233–234

Einhorn J, Wersäll J (1967) Incidence of oral carcinoma in patients with leukoplakia of the oral mucosa. Cancer 20: 2189–2193

Eneroth C-M, Blanck C, Jakobsson PA (1968) Carcinoma in pleomorphic adenoma of the parotid gland. Acta Otolaryngol (Stockh) 66: 477–492

Eneroth C-M, Hjertman L, Moberger G (1970) Muco-spidermoid carcinoma of the palate. Acta Otolaryngol (Stockh) 70: 408–418

Eneroth C-M, Hjertman L, Moberger G, Söderberg G (1972) Muco epidermoid carcinomas of the salivary glands. With special reference to the possible existence of a benign variety. Acta Otolaryngol (Stockh) 73: 68–74

Enrile FT, Jesus PO de, Bakst AA, Baluyot R (1973) Pseudosarcoma of the esophagus (polypoid carcinoma of esophagus with pseudosarcomatous features). Cancer 31: 1197–1202

Eras P, Winawer SJ (1969) Benign lymphoid hyperplasia of the stomach simulating gastric malignancy. Am J Dig Dis 14: 510–515

Ferrari BT, O'Halloran RL, Longmire WP, Lewin KJ (1979) Atypical papillary hyperplasia of the pancreatic duct mimicking obstructing pancreatic carcinoma. N Engl J Med 301: 531–532

Fevre DI, Green PHR, Barratt PJ, Nagy GS (1976) Review of five cases of early gastric carcinoma. Gut 17: 41–47

Fonts EA, Greenlaw RH, Rush BF, Rovin S (1969) Verrucous squamous cell carcinoma of the oral cavity. Cancer 23: 152–160

Friedman M, Nervi C, Casale C, Starace G, Arcangeli G, Page G, Ziparo E (1973) Significance of growth rates, cell kinetics and histology in the irradiation and chemotherapy of squamous cell carcinoma of the mouth. Cancer 31: 10–16

Fu KK, Leibel SA, Levine ML, Friedlander LM, Boles R, Phillips TL (1977) Carcinoma of the major and minor salivary glands. Analysis of treatment results and sites and causes of failures. Cancer 40: 2882–2890

Genre CF, Roth LM, Reed RJ (1971) "Benign" rectal carcinoids: A report of two patients with metastases to regional lymph nodes. Am J Clin Pathol 56: 750–757

George P, Brown C, Gilchrist J (1975) Operative biopsy of the pancreas. Br J Surg 62: 280–283

Gerughty RM, Scofield HH, Brown FM, Hennigar GR (1969) Malignant mixed tumors of salivary gland origin. Cancer 24: 471–486

Glover GW, Park WW (1971) Pharyngeal leiomyosarcoma. J Laryngol Otol 85: 1031–1038

Goethals PL, Harrison EG, Devine KD (1963) Verrucous squamous carcinoma of the oral cavity. Am J Surg 106: 845–851

Gravanis MB, Giansanti JS (1970) Malignant histopathologic counterpart of the benign lymphoepithelial lesion. Cancer 26: 1332–1342

Greene FL (1974) Epithelial misplacement in adenomatous polyps of the colon and rectum. Cancer 33: 206–217

Harly TG, Elesha W (1968) Eosinophilic granuloma of the stomach (a report of three cases). Am Surg 34: 296–299

Hay-Roe V, Hill RL, Civin WH (1960) An unclassifiable tumor of the esophagus. A case report. J Thorac Cardiovasc Surg 40: 107–113

Henry K, Farrer-Brown G (1977) Primary lymphomas of the gastrointestinal tract. I. Plasma cell tumours. Histopathol 1: 53–76

Hinton JM (1966) Risk of malignant change in ulcerative colitis. Gut 7: 427–432

Hughes JH, Cruickshank AH (1969) Pseudosarcoma of the oesophagus. Br J Surg 56: 72–76

Isaacson P, Attwood PRA (1979) Failure to demonstrate specificity of the morphological and histochemical changes in mucosa adjacent to colonic carcinoma (transitional mucosa). J Clin Pathol 32: 214–218

Isaacson R, Weiland LH, McIlrath DC (1974) Biopsy of the pancreas. Arch Surg 109: 227–230

Kanee B (1969) Oral florid papillomatosis complicated by verrucous squamous carcinoma. Treatment with methotrexate. Arch Dermatol 99: 196–202

Klein H, Baumgartl E (1970) Eosinophiles Granulom des Rektums. Munch Med Wochenschr 112: 1141–1144

Kobayashi S, Prolla JC, Kirsner JB (1970) Reactive lymphoreticular hyperplasia of the stomach. Arch Intern Med 125: 1030–1035

Kozuka S, Sassa R, Taki T, Masamoto K, Nagasawa S, Saga S, Hasegawa K, Takeuchi M (1979) Relation of pancreatic duct hyperplasia to carcinoma. Cancer 43: 1418–1428

Kramer IRH (1975) Computer-aided analysis in diagnostic histopathology. Postgrad Med J 51: 690–694

Kraus FT, Perez-Mesa C (1966) Verrucous carcinoma: Clinical and pathologic study of 105 cases involving oral cavity, larynx and genitalia. Cancer 19: 26–38

Krolls SO, Trodahl JN, Boyers RC (1972) Salivary gland lesions in children. A survey of 430 cases. Cancer 30: 459–469

Lane N (1957) Pseudosarcoma (polypoid sarcoma-like masses) associated with squamous-cell carcinoma of the mouth, fauces, and larynx: Report of ten cases. Cancer 10: 19–41

Lichtiger B, MacKay B, Tessmer CF (1970) Spindle-cell variant of squamous carcinoma. A light and electron microscopic study of 13 cases. Cancer 26: 1311–1320

Lim FE, Hartman AS, Tan EGC, Cady B, Meissner WA (1977) Factors in the prognosis of gastric lymphoma. Cancer 39: 1715–1720

McDivitt RW (1974) "Early" large bowel cancer. A morphologist's dilemma. Cancer 34: 904–908

Martin HE, Howe ME (1938) Glossitis rhombica mediana. Ann Surg 107: 39–49

Minielly JA, Harrison EG, Fontana RS, Payne WS (1967) Verrucous squamous cell carcinoma of the esophagus. Cancer 20: 2078–2087

Morgan WS, Castleman B (1953) A clinicopathologic study of 'Mikulicz's disease'. Am J Pathol 29: 471–503

Morson BC (1966) Cancer in ulcerative colitis. Gut 7: 425–426

Morson BC, Pang LSC (1967) Rectal biopsy as an aid to cancer control in ulcerative colitis. Gut 8: 423–434

Muto T, Bussey HJR, Morson BC (1973) Pseudo-carcinomatous invasion in adenomatous polyps of the colon and rectum. J Clin Pathol 26: 25–31

Muto T, Bussey HJR, Morson BC (1975) The evolution of cancer of the colon and rectum. Cancer 36: 2251–2270

Orloff MJ (1971) Carcinoid tumors of the rectum. Cancer 28: 175–180

Park WW (1979) Letter to Editor. J Laryngol Otol 93: 103

Quan SHQ, Castro EB (1971) Papillary adenomas (villous tumors): A review of 215 cases. Dis Colon Rectum 14: 267–280

Rafla S (1977) Malignant parotid tumors: Natural history and treatment. Cancer 40: 136–144

Ranchod M, Kempson RL (1977) Smooth muscle tumors of the gastrointestinal tract and retroperitoneum. A pathologic analysis of 100 cases. Cancer 39: 255–262

Ransom HK (1953) Cancer of the stomach. Surg Gynecol Obstet 96: 275–287

Razzuk MA, Urschel HC, Race GJ, Nathan MJ, Paulson DL (1971) Pseudosarcoma of the esophagus. A case report. J Thorac Cardiovasc Surg 61: 650–653

Saltzstein SL (1969) Extranodal malignant lymphomas and pseudolymphomas. Pathol Annu 4: 159–184

Sano R and others (1972) cit. Fevre et al. 1976 (q.v.)

Schultz NJ, Sanders RJ (1963) Evaluation of pancreatic biopsy. Ann Surg 158: 1053–1057

Segal AW, Healy MJR, Cox AG, Williams I, Slavin G, Smithies A, Levi AJ (1975) Diagnosis of gastric cancer. Br Med J 2: 669–672

Serlin O, Keehn RJ, Higgins GA, Harrower HW, Mendeloff GL (1977) Factors related to survival following resection for gastric carcinoma. Analysis of 903 cases. Cancer 40: 1318–1329

Sharma MP, Gregg JA, Loewenstein MS, McCabe RP, Zamcheck N (1976) Carcinoembryonic antigen (CEA) activity in pancreatic juice of patients with pancreatic carcinoma and pancreatitis. Cancer 38: 2457–2461

Sherwin RP, Strong MS, Vaughan CW (1963) Polypoid and junctional squamous cell carcinoma of the tongue and larynx with spindle cell carcinoma ("pseudosarcoma"). Cancer 16: 51–60

Shields TW, Eilert JB, Battifora H (1972) Pseudosarcoma of the oesophagus. Thorax 27: 472–479

Silverberg SG (1970) "Juvenile" retention polyps of the colon and rectum. Am J Dig Dis 15: 617–625

Soga J, Tazawa K (1971) Pathologic analysis of carcinoids. Histologic re-evaluation of 62 cases. Cancer 28: 990–998

Soga J, Saito K, Suzuki N, Sakai T (1970) Plasma cell granuloma of the stomach. A report of a case and review of the literature. Cancer 25: 618–625

Soga J, Tazawa K, Aizawa O, Wada K, Tuto T (1971) Argentaffin cell adenocarcinoma of the stomach: An atypical carcinoid? Cancer 28: 999–1003

Spiro RH, Huvos AG, Strong EW (1975) Cancer of the parotid gland. A clinicopathologic study of 288 primary cases. Am J Surg 130: 452–459

Stout AP, Lattes R (1957) Tumors of the Esophagus. Atlas of tumor pathology, sect 5, fasc 20. Armed Forces Institute of Pathology, Washington, D.C.

Tomasulo J (1971) Gastric polyps. Histologic types and their relationship to gastric carcinoma. Cancer 27: 1346–1355

Waterfall WE, Somers S, Desa DJ (1978) Benign oesophageal papillomatosis. A case report with a review of the literature. J Clin Pathol 31: 111–115

Warkel RL, Cooper PH, Helwig EB (1978) Adenocarcinoid, a mucin-producing carcinoid tumor of the appendix. A study of 39 cases. Cancer 42: 2781–2793

Warner TFCS (1979) Iodine-131 and malignancy. Lancet I: 38

Woyke S, Domagala W, Olszewski W, Korabeic M (1974) Pseudosarcoma of the skin. An electron microscopic study and comparison with the fine structure of the spindle-cell variant of squamous carcinoma. Cancer 33: 970–980

Zakariai YM, Quan SHQ, Hajdu SI (1975) Carcinoid tumors of the gastrointestinal tract. Cancer 35: 588–591

# 9 Lesions of the Respiratory Tract

Many of the borderline problems met in the respiratory tract are substantially the same as those occurring at other sites and already noted, as, for example, overgrowths of stratified squamous epithelium, including the verrucous carcinoma, pseudo-lymphoma and the curious pseudo-sarcoma of Lane (1957). However, even of these, some have particular relevance within, and others are peculiar to, the respiratory system: some such are mentioned in more detail later.

In comparison with most other systems or organs, the respiratory tract is not the site of many lesions as intrinsically borderline as, say, the adenomas of thyroid, nodular fasciitis, or bizarre uterine myomas. For understandable technical reasons, mainly concerning access, most everyday problems arise from inadequate or unrepresentative sampling of suspect lesions (and the pathologist will remember that many a patient may be spared a further endoscopy by the examination of deeper sections from the original biopsy).

## Local Series

With relatively little material available, and therefore many problems unrepresented, final analysis of local data in terms of over-diagnosis and under-diagnosis is not warranted. Six local cases only are described: points raised by them are included in the general commentary.

### Case Data

*Case 9.1*

F (36 years) had a left nasal polypectomy. The removed mass was typically grey, translucent and gelatinous, 10 × 6 × 3 mm.

The appearances were unusual in two respects: first, the mucoid matrix contained an unusually large amount of fibrin; second, it also contained a scattering of strikingly large aberrant cells of the types shown in Figs. 9.1 and 9.2. They were frequently multinucleate or, if mononucleate, multilobular; some nuclei were 50 $\mu$m in diameter. None, however, was seen in mitosis. Their nature was (and still is) uncertain. Occasionally, one contained a globule of mucin; to this extent there was a suggestion of a macrophagic and RE nature but beyond this no clues. In view of this uncertainty, some concern was expressed about their nature and possible implications: at the same time, comment was proffered on two specific matters that might have been relevant. The patient had been receiving antiepileptic medication for many years: it remains uncertain whether the various drugs concerned could have produced this degree of cellular atypia. Also, the suggested assay of serum folate levels showed a level in the low normal range; this also was possibly contributory.

The patient has had recurrent troubles of various kinds during the years since the polypectomy but none productive of any further biopsy. There have, at least, been no neoplastic developments nor has any folate-deficiency anaemia appeared.

*Case 9.2*

M (62 years) with complaint of hoarseness for 2 years. The left cord showed papillary excrescences.

Biopsy showed the appearances illustrated in Figs. 9.3, 9.4 and 9.5. There was marked overgrowth of epithelium with polymorphism and aberrant mitotic activity amongst the cells but along the whole length of all the fragments a

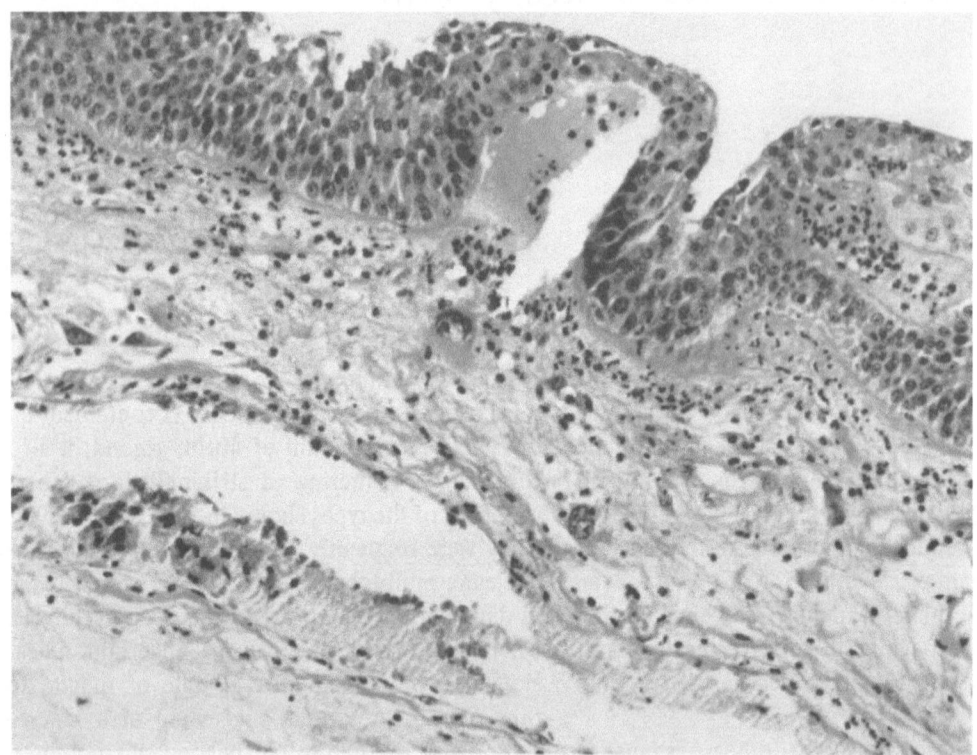

**Fig. 9.1.** Oedematous stromal tissue contains scattered lymphocytes and many abnormally large cells with irregularly shaped nuclei. H & E, × 217

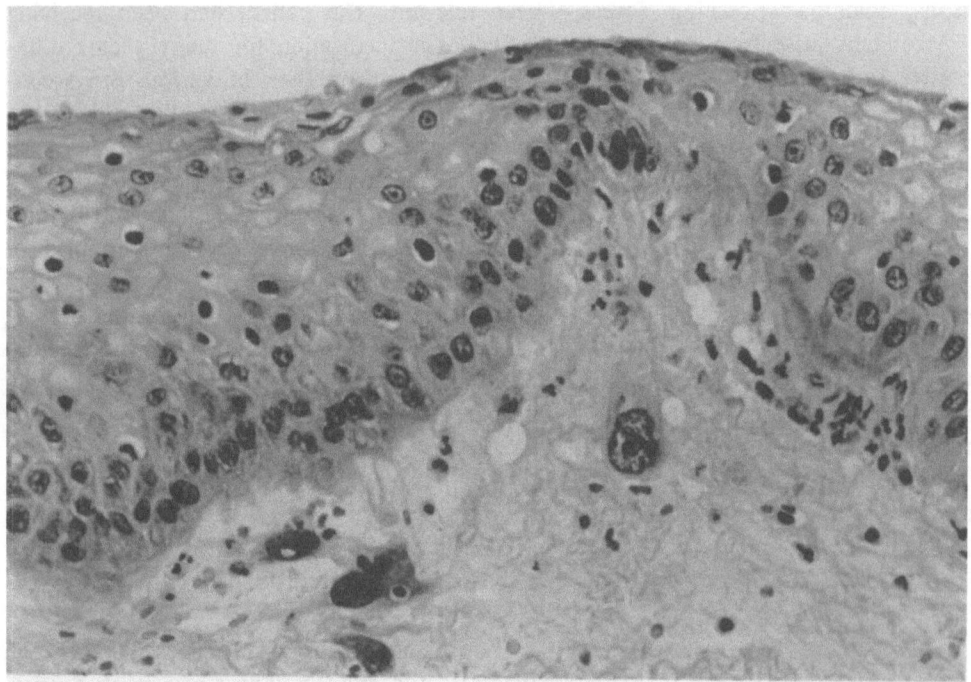

**Fig. 9.2.** Shows five of the large aberrant cells. The three to the left and the one virtually within the basal layer of the epithelium, just to right of centre, have a multilobular nucleus. The cell in the stroma vertically below is mononuclear and has a strikingly large nucleolus. H & E, × 328

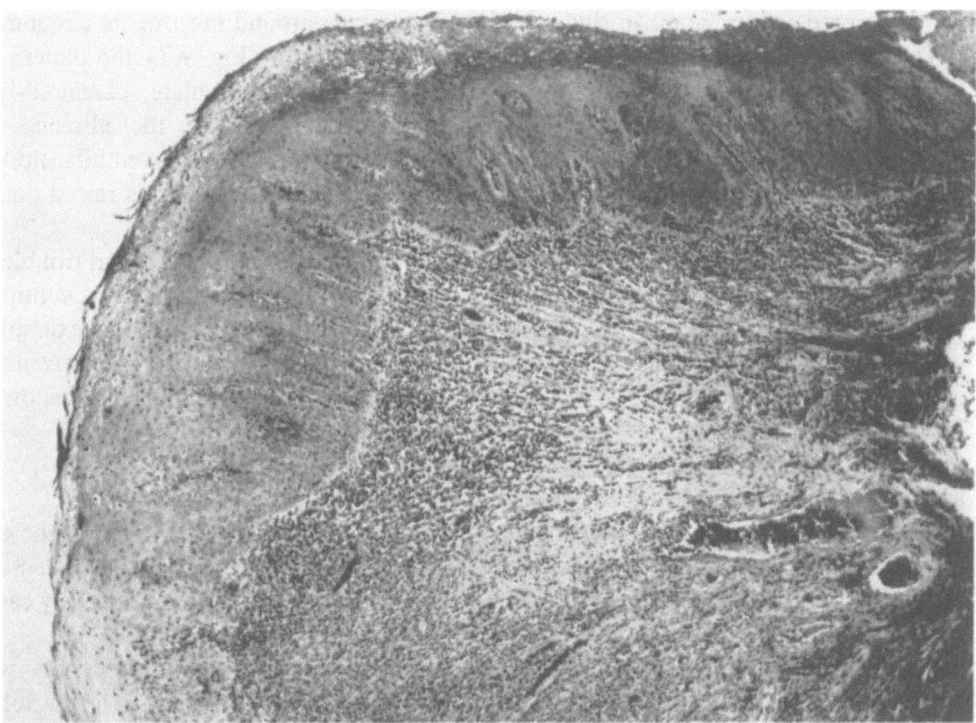

**Fig. 9.3.** Greatly thickened epithelium overlying a stroma heavily infiltrated by chronic inflammatory cells. H & E, × 62

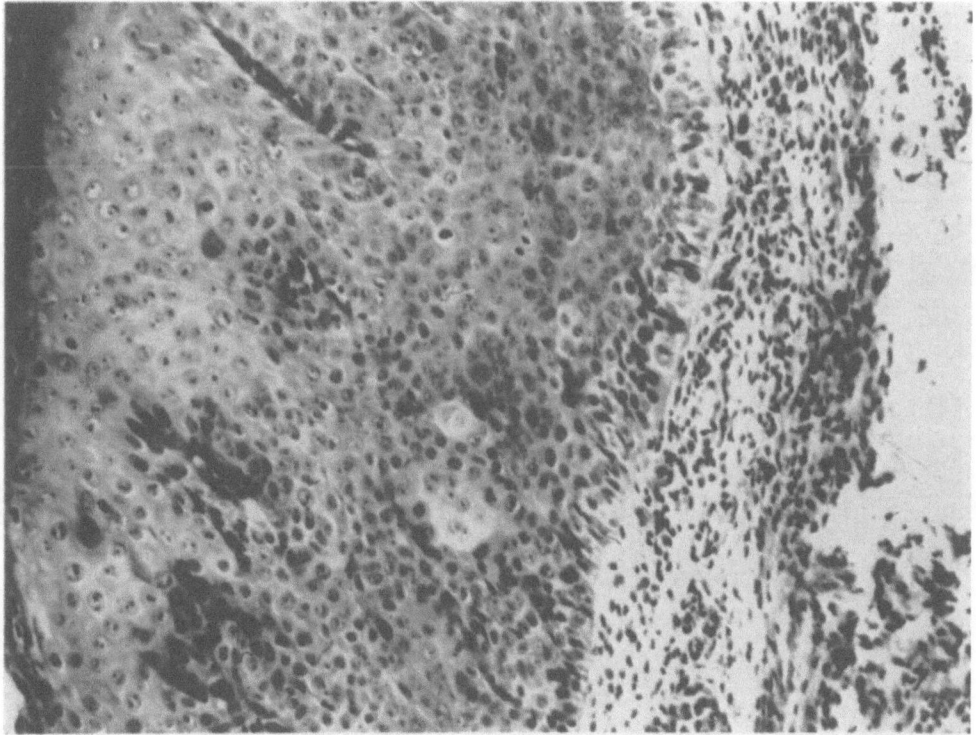

**Fig. 9.4.** The cytology of the epithelium is notably aberrant with mitotic figures closely approaching the surface. H & E, × 246

still quite sharply defined lower edge. The lesion was diagnosed as 'carcinoma in situ'.

The larynx was treated by radiotherapy. Thirteen years later, in another country, laryngectomy was performed: no details are available but the presumption must be that invasive carcinoma had supervened. An artificial larynx was fitted, and to this the patient adapted well. He was known to be active and well at least 4 years after the laryngectomy.

### Case 9.3

M (19 years) admitted for investigation of haemoptysis for past two months. Bronchoscopy and biopsy showed 'bronchial adenoma'. Lower lobectomy and removal of an 8-mm hilar node followed.

The mass was 25 mm in diameter, largely blocking the lumen of the main lower lobe bronchus, with much distal inflammation. Figure 9.6 shows the total destruction of part of the bronchial wall, the near-total occlusion of the lumen and the deep extension into adjacent parenchyma. Although macroscopically fairly well circumscribed, the mass had little compression-

capsule and seemed to be permeating the parenchyma around most of its circumference.

In detail (Fig. 9.7) the pattern was typically that of a trabeculate, carcinoid-type bronchial adenoma. Despite the absence of metastatic tissue within the removed hilar node, the obvious infiltrability of the mass raised doubts about the future.

The patient was well and trouble-free 21 years later. Despite its evidently continuing invasion of surrounding tissues, this example at least had not behaved with the aggressiveness that others of the same size and type may show.

### Case 9.4

F (71 years) with a lesion found incidentally in a lung at necropsy. It is included as an example of a well-known lesion that may cause prognostic difficulty during life.

The lesion was a 5-mm firm, whitish nodule in an otherwise normal lower lobe. As shown in Figs. 9.8, 9.9, 9.10, the nodule consisted of a cluster of glandular or pseudoglandular structures in a moderately dense fibrous stroma variably infiltrated by lymphocytes. The terminal

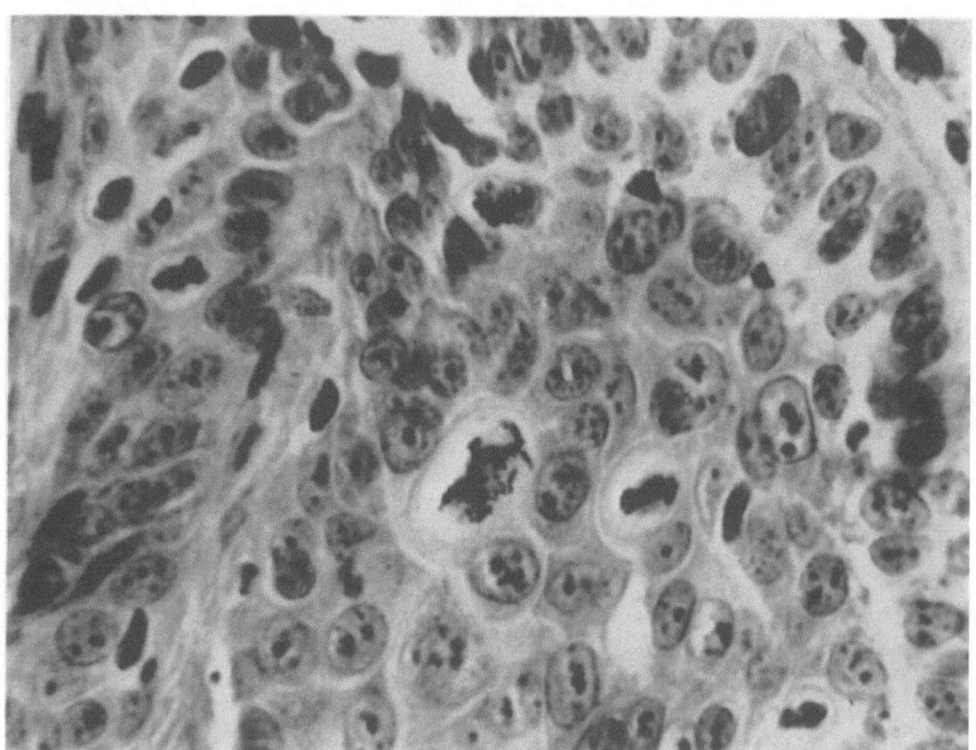

**Fig. 9.5.** Abundant mitotic activity including one obviously aberrant form. H & E, × 985

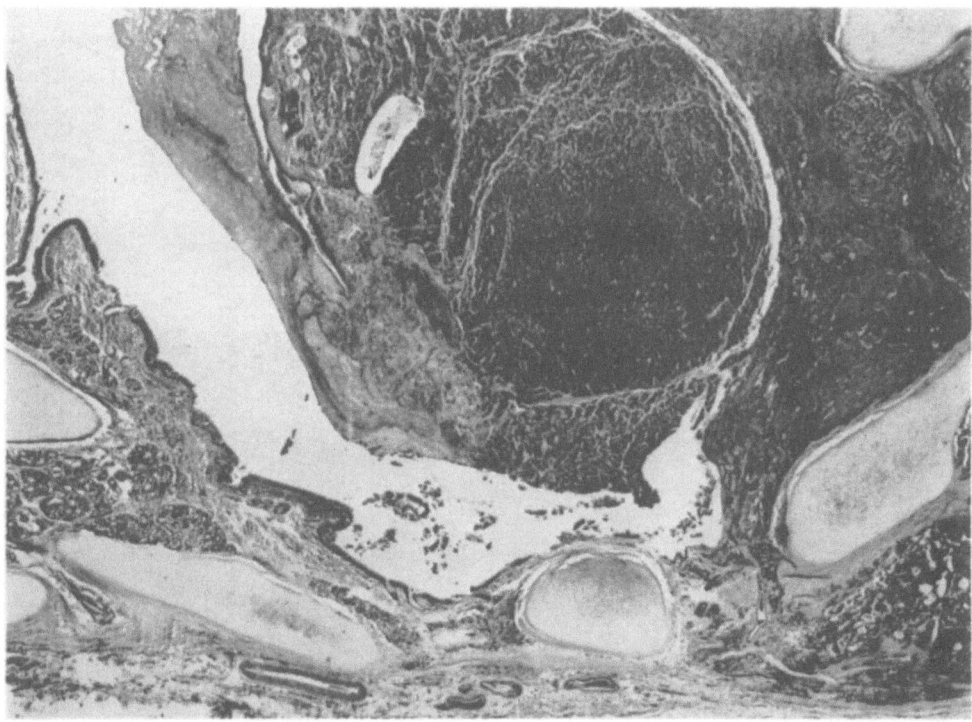

**Fig. 9.6.** The bronchus enters from above left and is narrowed by the highly cellular adenoma (over which the bronchial epithelium has become totally eroded). H & E, × 10

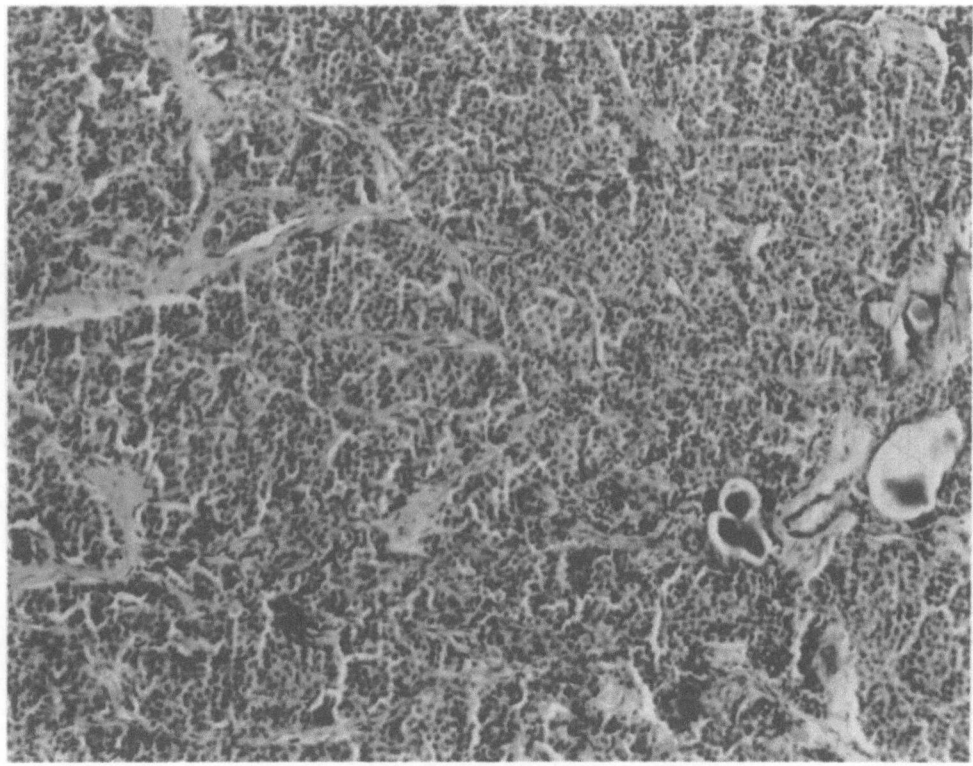

**Fig. 9.7.** Generally uniform cells in trabecular and microacinar pattern. H & E, × 119

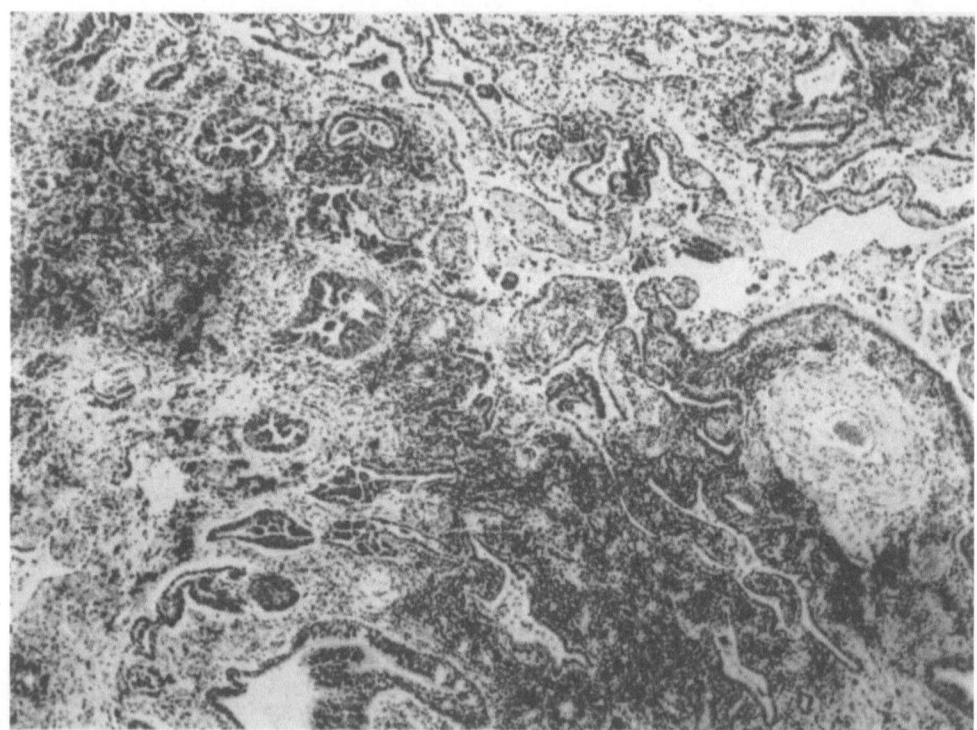

**Fig. 9.8.** Acinar structures of variable size surround the terminal part of a bronchiole (*entering upper right*). H & E, × 62

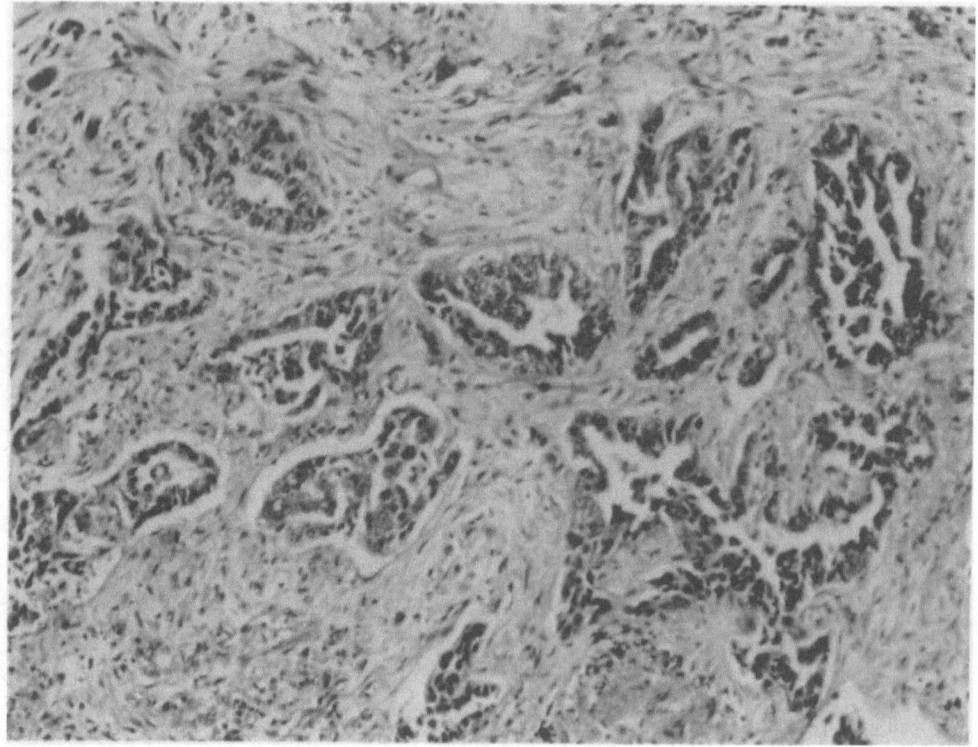

**Fig. 9.9.** Irregularly formed acinar structures lie in a fibroblastic stroma. H & E, × 187

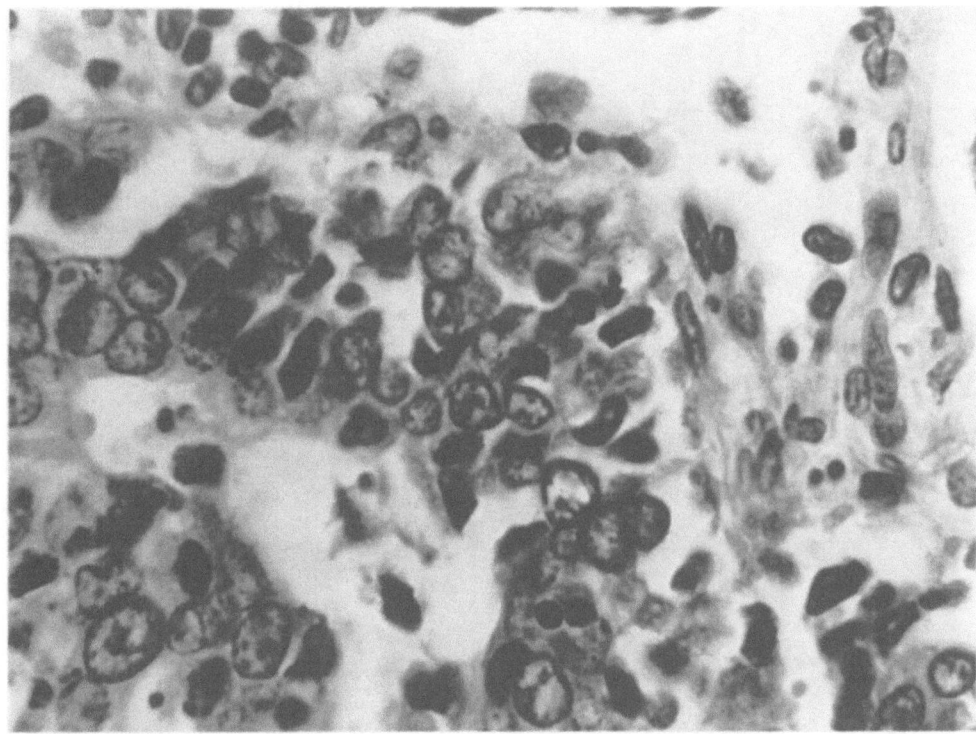

**Fig. 9.10.** The epithelial lining of the acinus is multilayered, and its nuclei are polymorphic. Two cells in the lower part of the lining are in mitosis. H & E, × 985

part of a bronchiole is seen right in Fig. 9.8: from the further branchings of this it was possible to trace a transition through metaplastic epithelium from the normal mucosa to some of the pseudo-glandular structures. Elsewhere, however, as illustrated, they were totally independent and seemingly permeating the stroma. Their cells were relatively large and rather polymorphic (Fig. 9.10).

The lesion is a form of 'tumourlet'. Although associated with, and thus seemingly arising via, bronchiolar epithelial metaplasia, not only is it not associated with an area of bronchiectasis or other form of parenchymal damage, its cells are polymorphic and much larger than those of even metaplastic respiratory epithelium. It offers little suggestion of either a carcinoid or a chemodectoma, and may be an early peripheral *glandular carcinoma*.

### Case 9.5

F (57 years) experiencing loss of weight and a feeling of fullness in epigastrium. Palpable mass in left hypochondrium was thought probably to be spleen. Laparotomy revealed, instead,

an 18 × 18 × 12 cm (1700 g) retroperitoneal mass. It was almost wholly necrotic, pultaceous and orange-yellow but retained a 5–10 mm subcapsular rim of probably viable tissue: an adjacent 8-mm node was also removed.

The cells were large and prominently granular (Fig. 9.11) and, as the reticulin pattern emphasises (Fig. 9.12), arranged in a clearly trabecular pattern. Mitotic activity was slight at one figure per 30 hpf. Occasional figures, however, were aberrant, and this was the main reason for the lesion's being diagnosed as 'adrenal carcinoma' rather than adenoma. The report added that "Recurrence and/or metastasis is less common with these lesions than their cellularity would suggest". The lymph node was not invaded.

At a routine follow-up examination 3½ years later a shadow was discovered in the right upper lobe. Lobectomy showed a sharply circumscribed yellowish mass, 17 × 15 × 12 mm near the hilum; its histology is shown in Figs. 9.13 and 9.14. Its cells were as large as those in the adrenal lesion, sometimes less granular but otherwise equally so and disposed in the same trabecular fashion.

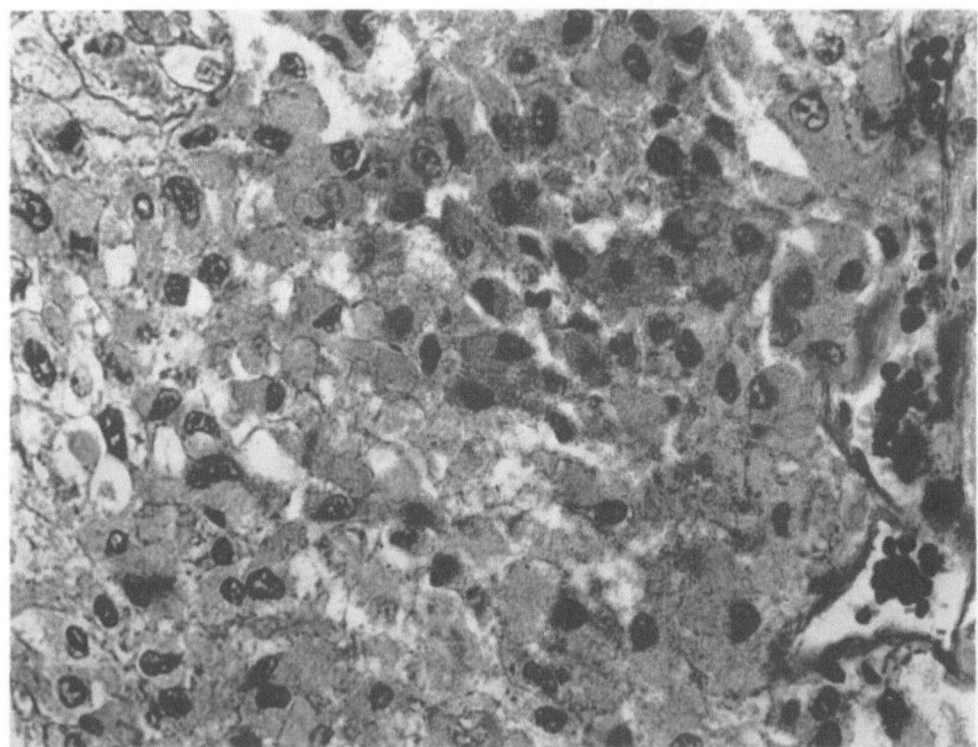

**Fig. 9.11.** The large prominently granular cells of the adrenal mass. H & E, × 493

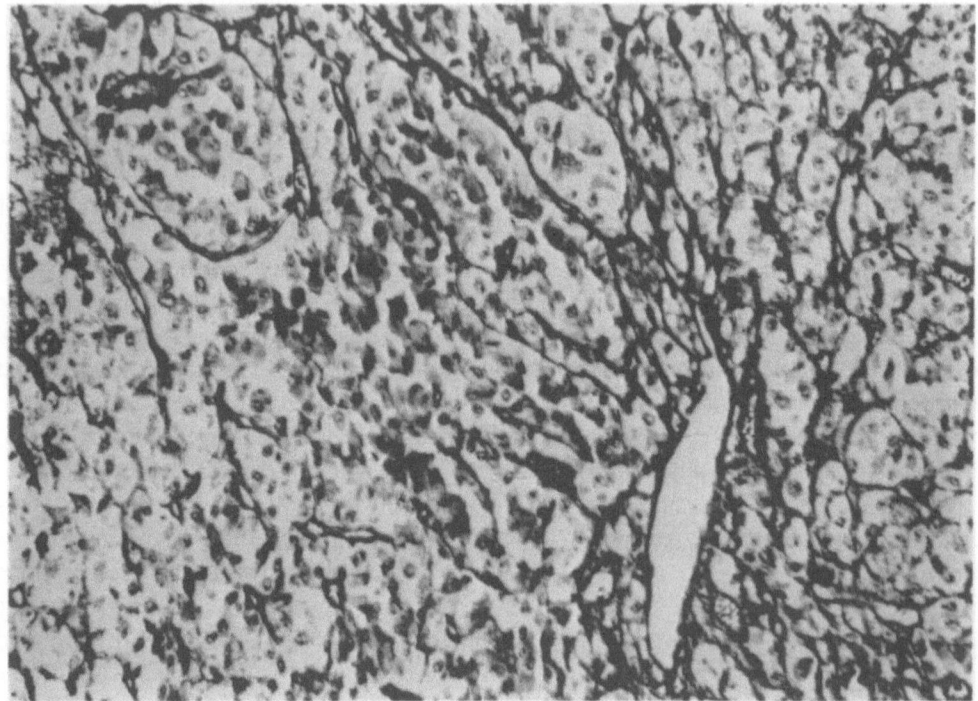

**Fig. 9.12.** Reticulin staining emphasises the trabecular pattern. Reticulin, × 238

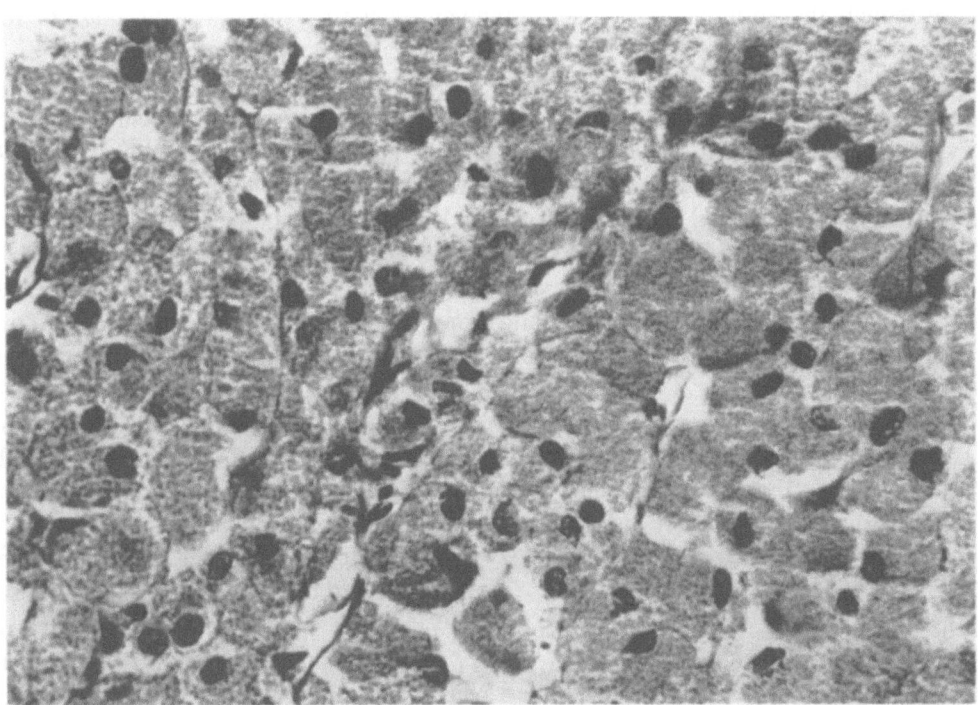

**Fig. 9.13.** A representative area from the pulmonary mass. By itself the morphology would raise the possibility of a so-called oncocytoma. It is nevertheless virtually identical with that of the adrenal lesion. H & E, × 493

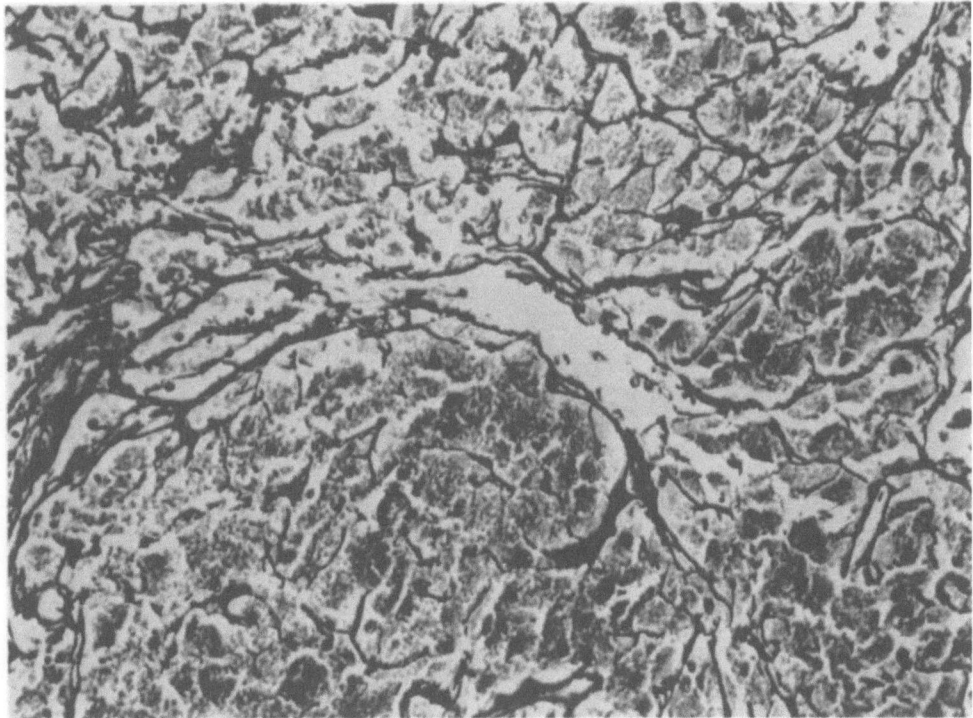

**Fig. 9.14.** Again, the reticulin pattern is virtually identical with that of the adrenal lesion. Reticulin, × 238

Although the eosinophilia and less granular appearance in much of the mass allowed it to qualify for designation as an 'oncocytoma', this was virtually certainly a *metastasis*, and the only evident metastasis, from the adrenal carcinoma.

The note apropos restricted malignancy was based on earlier personal experience of the finding at necropsy, in an elderly woman who had suddenly collapsed and died from haemorrhage into an adrenal mass of essentially identical appearance but even larger. Though also almost identical histologically it had produced no metastases.

The patient now in question remained fit and active for a further four years then died from a myocardial infarction.

*Case 9.6*

F (74 years) with complaint of right chest pain. X-ray showed an opacity in right lower zone. Segmental resection produced, within a 10 × 8 × 6 cm piece of lung, a 4 × 3 × 2 cm smooth yellowish white mass of relatively well-circumscribed outline.

The nodule was essentially a mass of lymphocytes, less sharply circumscribed than had appeared on gross section (Fig. 9.15). Other components were plasma cells, not at all intermingled with the lymphocytes but mostly forming small sheets in the compressed or collapsed parenchyma among the foci of lymphocytes; cuboidally metaplastic alveolar epithelium; and fairly numerous macrophages, again mostly in the collapsed parenchyma (Figs. 9.16, 9.17).

Though generally scattered, the individual foci of lymphocytes were mostly well circumscribed, the cells themselves of almost monotonous uniformity and rarely in mitosis (fewer than 1 per 50 hpf). The lesion was nevertheless diagnosed as 'lymphosarcoma'.

The patient received a course of irradiation and remained well for 7 years when she died of an unrelated cause with no indication anywhere of recurrence or extension of the original lesion.

The question of pseudo-lymphoma, later considered, is clearly raised by these events.

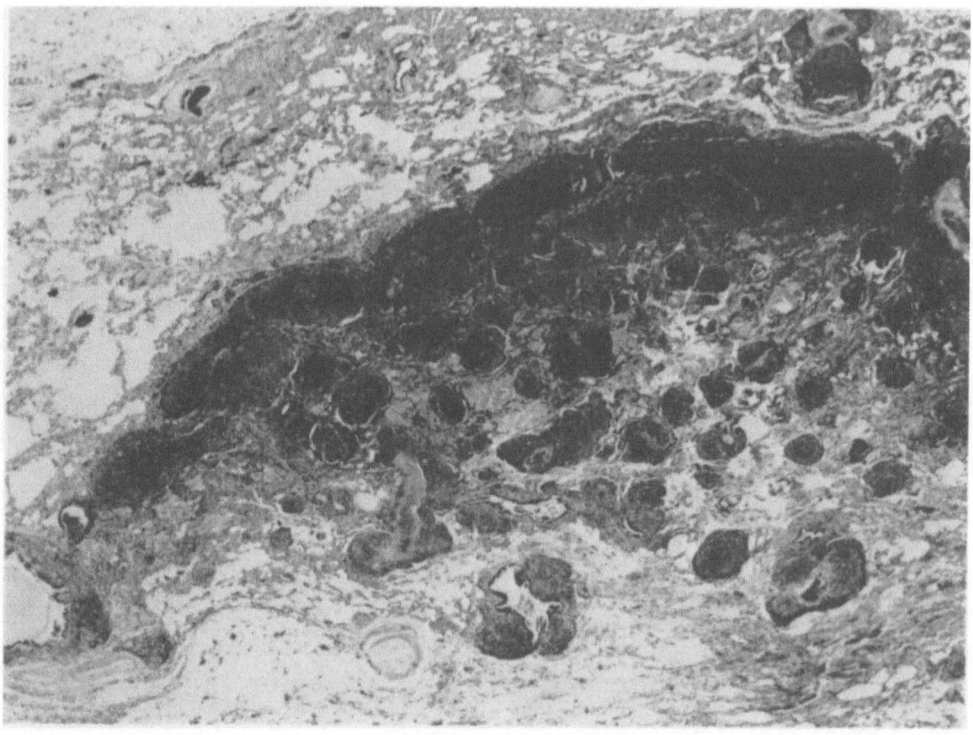

**Fig. 9.15.** The lymphocytic tissue is disposed in clusters of varying size with satellite foci around the main mass. H & E, × 12

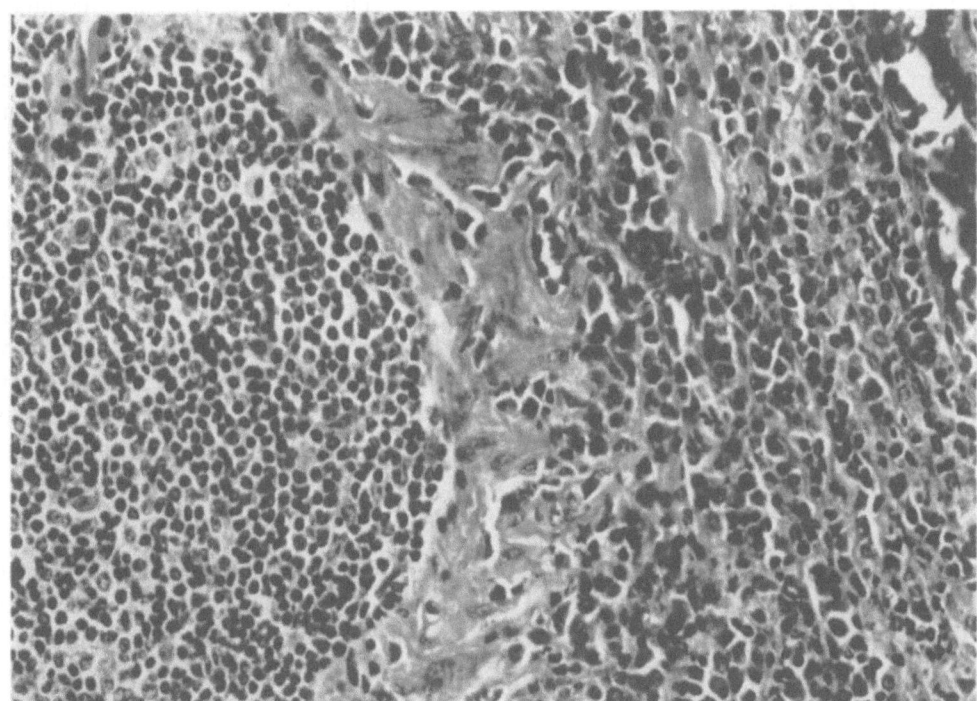

**Fig. 9.16.** Shows the edge of one of the foci of lymphocytes and an adjacent area of plasma cells. The lymphocytes are notably uniform, as was the case throughout. One of the rare mitotic figures is included in this field (*towards top left corner*). H & E, × 328

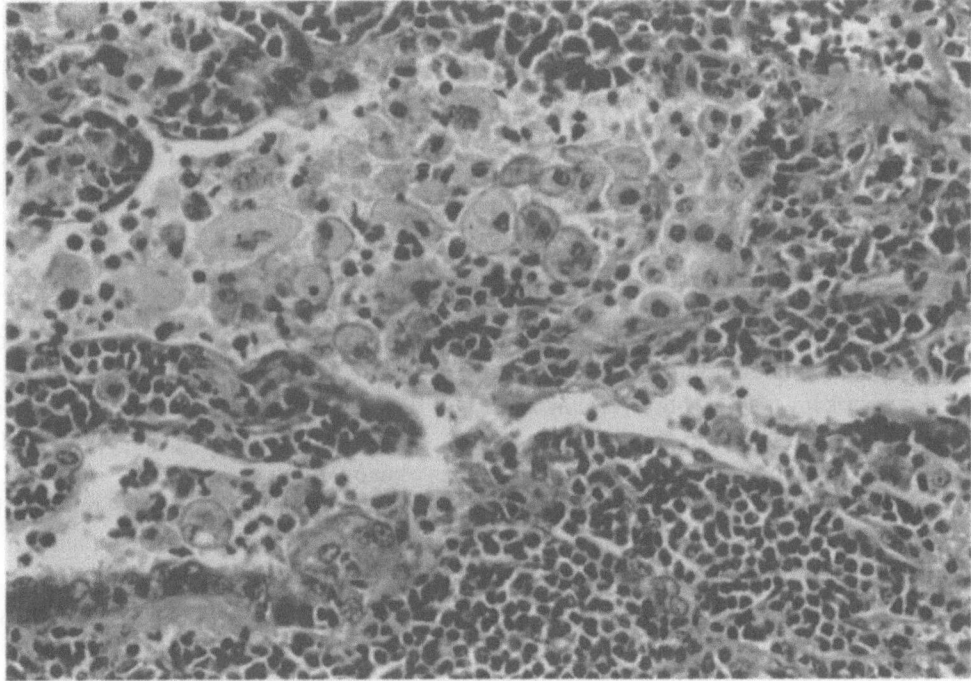

**Fig. 9.17.** Shows the edge of another focus of lymphocytes; part of a bronchiole in continuity with a short stretch of 'bronchiolised' alveolar lining; and many macrophages of varying size and content, some notably foamy. H & E, × 328

## General Commentary

Apart from the uncertainties always attending cytological aberrancies in situ of epithelium at any site, whether of squamous, transitional or intermediate character, borderline problems within the respiratory tract largely concern the distinction between granulomatous and neoplastic lesions, and, clinically rather than morphologically, the marginal predictability of the bronchial adenoma. Lesions will be considered in broadly anatomical sequence though some, such as papillomatosis, may involve the respiratory tract not only in the nasal cavity but as far distal as the larynx and sometimes further.

### NOSE AND NASOPHARYNX

### Lethal Midline Granuloma

The term lethal midline granuloma is descriptive, not aetiologically definitive, and to that extent inadequate. The inadequacy would be the greater if a more accurate classification or subdivision were to carry with it therapeutic implications: Kassel and his colleagues (1969) claim that this may be so. These authors subdivide the entity into (a) midline malignant reticulosis, (b) Wegener's granulomatosis and (c) malignant lymphoma of one of the accepted morphological types (though, as is obvious, 'accepted' in the context of ML is a highly relative term), and have suggested that the midline reticulosis is more likely to respond to chemotherapy than the orthodox MLs, while Wegener's granulomatosis may respond to ". . . corticosteroids and probably to immunosuppressive agents".

A fourth entity may be concerned, namely, 'lymphomatoid granulomatosis', which, as Lee and co-workers (1976) observe, may be closely related in particular to the Wegener lesion. Points of distinction are the relative monotypism of the MLs, a notable polytypism amongst the cells of the midline reticulosis and a commonly prominent arteritic element in Wegener's granulomatosis. In describing their four examples of lymphomatoid granulomatosis, Lee and his colleagues stress both the marked polytypism of the infiltrate and the necrotising destruction of both arteries and veins: in one of their cases, the inadequacy of a needle biopsy had led to a wrong diagnosis of ML.

The lesion in Wegener's granulomatosis need not always suggest a malignant process. In one local case, the histology of the destructive and relentlessly progressive lesion in the nasopharynx, had throughout much more strongly suggested a tuberculous process (hence its non-inclusion in the local series). Necropsy, however, with its demonstration of widespread arteritis, established the diagnosis conclusively.

Of their 'midline malignant reticulosis', Kassel and colleagues draw the analogy with mycosis fungoides that the 'reticulosis' may remain for long confined to one type of tissue before eventual dissemination and death.

### Juvenile Angiofibroma

Most reported series of this lesion show an 80% or greater incidence in male subjects. The lesion is highly vascular and notoriously prone to recurrence and destruction of bone though no accurate assessment of aggressiveness can be deduced from the histology (the appearances could reasonably be described as those of exuberant erectile tissue). The destruction of bone must surely be due to more than simple pressure since equally bulky oedematous nasal polyps rarely behave in this way. A warning of the dangers of treatment of the lesion by radiotherapy, because of complications, is given by Fu and Perzin (1974). These same authors have contributed a valuable series of nine other papers on nonepithelial neoplasms of the nasal cavity, culminating in one on malignant lymphomas (Fu and Perzin, 1979).

### Papillomas and Carcinomas

Although papillomas and carcinomas may appear at any level in the respiratory tract, two forms of overgrowth deserve particular mention, the papilloma of nasal cavity and the state of papillomatosis.

The papillomas, sometimes subdivided descriptively into inverted, fungiform and cylindrical cell forms (Hyams, 1971), are characterised by marked epithelial hyperplasia, often in a festooned pattern, and a notable tendency to recurrence, almost certainly due to the difficulties of total removal. Cellular atypia comprises the borderline element but, in the opinion of Lasser and his colleagues (1976), a mild or moderate degree of atypia gives no dependable guidance to future behaviour: in their own words, "We believe it is not possible to predict accurately from the histological appearance which tumor will become malignant".

A measure of the statistical risk of carcinoma may be gained from the just-cited report of Hyams wherein, of 315 cases of nasal and paranasal papillomas, 20 were associated with carcinoma. In the opinion of Osborn (1970), whose series in the upper respiratory tract comprised 168 transitional cell papillomas and seven transitional cell carcinomas, "Whether the true incidence of malignant change is nearer to 2% or 5% is clearly a matter of histologic interpretation . . ." In cases of frank carcinoma, lesions of dominantly squamous differentiation are more aggressive than those still recognisably of transitional character: the anaplastic are the most aggressive.

The further point was made (and illustrated) by Osborn that the presence of papillomatous epithelium amid bone is not necessarily prognostically ominous but may be pseudo-invasion rather than invasion proper. Even so, to make the distinction in prospect rather than in retrospect cannot be easy.

*Papillomatosis*

Papillomatosis (sometimes 'multiple papillomatosis'), an uncommon lesion, may occur in the larynx and/or more distally and at any age but is seen most frequently and characteristically in the larynx in infants and children under 10 years of age, least frequently distal to the larynx, and in adults. Its recognition, typically in a child, is always accompanied by the hope that recurrence will stop at, or shortly after, puberty. This is usual but not invariable: in a formerly local case, the patient, after some 50 endoscopies, was still producing papillomas when last seen some years ago at age 22. Histologically, minor degrees of cellular atypia may be disregarded but changes sufficiently marked to raise doubts about carcinoma in situ are a mandatory indication for continued follow-up and, possibly, further biopsies (Altmann et al., 1955). According to Al-Saleem and his associates (1968), carcinoma occurs with great rarity in youth and then almost exclusively in patients treated at some time by radiotherapy: this form of treatment should therefore never be used.

## LARYNX

*Carcinoma In Situ*

For obvious reasons, the assessment and treatment of lesions in the larynx that may or may not be carcinoma in situ have implications much graver than in the case of comparable lesions in, say, the cervix uteri: potentially curative limited procedures such as mucosal stripping do not carry the near certainty of cure that cone biopsy can offer with the cervix. The difficulties for the histologist have been well displayed by the findings of Auerbach and his colleagues (1970). These workers examined post mortem the larynxes of 942 subjects dead of some cause other than carcinoma of the larynx, and showed a close association between epithelial aberrancy and cigarette smoking (as reported by them earlier in the case also of both bronchial and oesophageal epithelium). Of the 942 patients, 88 were in the category 'never smoked regularly'. Not only did the authors find a frank carcinoma in situ in some 16% of the subjects (but in none of the 88 or the 116 in the further category of 'ex-cigarette smokers'), but also cells with atypical nuclei somewhere within the larynx in 84% of the 942. With a frequency of epithelial atypia as high as this in a population effectively healthy so far as concerned the larynx, the histologist should be wary of over-diagnosis with biopsies from patients whose larynx is not healthy or at least has demanded biopsy.

In a single case report by Busuttil and his colleagues (1974), a patient, on laryngeal biopsy, was described as having many unusually aberrant giant cells within an already highly dysplastic epithelium. The possibility was considered of their having been induced by a herpes virus: the patient was, however, a moderately heavy cigarette smoker.

It would be useful to know how frequently, if at all, dysplastic changes such as these would regress on cessation of smoking. If, as seems likely, similar changes in bronchial epithelium can regress in at least their earlier stages, we should probably use a higher rather than a lower threshold for the diagnosis of carcinoma in situ in the larynx in the hope that the point of no return had not yet been reached.

An informative follow-up report on 81 patients with carcinoma in situ of the larynx has been given by Elman and his associates (1979): of 69 treated by external radiotherapy, 75% were still free of recurrence at ten years: among 12 treated by local surgery, essentially because the disease was more extensive, there were five recurrences. The interval to recurrence ranged between seven and 107 months.

The ability of folate deficiency to induce dysplastic change in epithelium was mentioned in connection with Case 9.1. The phenomenon was described many years ago as occurring not only in epithelia of the digestive tract but also in the respiratory tract (Graham and Rheault, 1954) in the cervix uteri during pregnancy (Blackledge and Goodall, 1973) and in the puerperium (van Niekerk, 1966): it may be at the least a cause for concern and sometimes for over-diagnosis. I recall an invitation to examine a preparation of sputum that contained abnormal cells. The cells were so enormous and bizarre as to seem beyond the capacity of even malignant neoplasia to produce. Folate deficiency was suggested as a likelier explanation, and this was found to be so (the clinical data requested after the diagnosis of folate deficiency was suggested revealed that the patient was pregnant). By then, however, a diagnosis of bronchial carcinoma had been issued. The revised diagnosis was fortunately available in time to prevent the further procedures that would otherwise certainly have followed.

### Granular-Cell Myoblastoma

Three examples of this lesion in the larynx have been described by Piquet and his colleagues (1969). The constituent tissue presents as little intrinsic threat here as it does elsewhere but some risk lies naturally in the possibility that a biopsy may be more superficial than in the case of, for example, the tongue, and show only the aberrant pseudo-epitheliomatous downgrowth. It would therefore be wise, where aberrant epithelium is not certainly epitheliomatous but perhaps only pseudo-epitheliomatous, to note whether the biopsy has been deep enough to include any underlying granular cell tissue that might have been present.

### Other Lesions

The *lymphocytic pseudo-tumour* (pseudo-lymphoma) has been reported in the larynx (Al-Saleem et al., 1970) and poses the same problems as it does when elsewhere of distinction from lymphocytic lymphosarcoma. In the case cited, radiotherapy had been used with rapid regression of the lesion, and the patient was well 7 years later. A usefully comprehensive account of benign and malignant *supporting tissue neoplasms* of the larynx including, for example, fibrosarcoma, lipoma, chondroma and even osteosarcoma, has been given by Batsakis and Fox (1970). In this article the pathologist will find helpful notes on prognosis, and the surgeon on both this and treatment. The *pseudo-sarcoma* of Lane (1957) and of other authors occurs in the larynx and has been mentioned already.

### Prognostic Assessment of Carcinoma

The significance of histologically demonstrable 'host response' to carcinoma in the larynx and hypopharynx has been analysed by Bennett and his co-workers (1971). Such factors as sinus histiocytosis and germ centre hyperplasia in nodes were found to be of limited value only, as also was the degree of lymphocytic or plasma cell infiltration of the neoplasm itself. Throughout, the factor most closely correlated with behaviour, in terms of both nodal spread and 5-year survival, was degree of histological differentiation, from 69% 5-year survival (and 25% incidence of nodal metastasis) to 26% survival (and 72% nodal metastasis) with Grade I and Grade IV respectively.

These observations are supplementary to others offered earlier by McGavran and his colleagues (1961) who paid particular attention to histological minutiae apart from degree of differentiation that might be prognostically helpful. In their own words, "The presence of cartilage invasion, thyrocricoid membrane penetration, pre-epiglottic space invasion, cervical soft tissue extension, or vessel invasion is not associated with a significantly higher rate of cervical metastases than when these findings are absent". They added that invasion of nerve sheaths was a better, and ominous, guide but one rarely available until after the larynx had been removed.

### BRONCHUS AND LUNG

Problems of two main kinds are likely, and they are of a different order. One is simply that of correctly identifying the type of an uncommon neoplasm (and of these there is no lack in the lung). The other is the more significant in practice since it is more frequent and of more immediate import, namely, that of deciding whether in a biopsy a mass of smallish round or oval cells are leucocytes, perhaps distorted and to some extent squashed, or the cells of an undifferentiated oat cell carcinoma. The problem is compounded by the fact that neoplastic cells are undoubtedly less robust and resilient than normal cells, and more prone to squashing than, in particular, healthy lymphocytes. The only safeguard is a resolve never to diagnose oat cell carcinoma on the evidence of other than perfectly preserved cells. Squashed cells will often be recognised on later evidence to have been indeed malignant (and in some biopsies will smoothly merge with undoubted carcinoma) but the risk of error with even mildly traumatised cells is too great to warrant a diagnosis even of 'suspicious' (there already is suspicion, otherwise the biopsy would not have been performed).

The foregoing is a matter of general relevance. Some individual lesions merit a further brief mention.

## Bronchial Adenoma: Oncocytoma

The behaviour of bronchial adenomas and carcinomas, and their relation to the APUD system, Kultschitzky cell and carcinoid tumour, is generally familiar. In a series of 24 patients with bronchial adenomas reported by Tolis and others (1972), 18 were of carcinoid type, four cylindromatous and two mucoepidermoid: of the 24 patients, four had died of the lesion or as a complication of treatment. The assessment of prognosis given by these workers is that some 10%–15% of the carcinoid type of lesion will metastasise to regional nodes but that, even so, over 90% of the patients are likely to recover fully after resection. Regional nodal metastasis per se is therefore not unduly ominous. However, this conclusion applies only to microscopic metastasis: grossly obvious metastasis is much more serious. The cylindromatous lesion had proved rather more aggressive, and the mucoepidermoid form rather less aggressive, than the carcinoid. A generally more serious outcome was reported by Turnbull and his associates (1972) from their experience with 61 cases (44 carcinoid, 12 mucoepidermoid, 5 adenoid cystic, or cylindromatous). Of patients with the carcinoid and adenoid cystic forms, only 59% and 60% respectively had survived for 5 years: all with the mucoepidermoid form had died during this period.

The histology of the lesion in an individual case of any of the three types usually offers little help in assessing prognosis. Correspondingly, the pathologist can do little more than identify the nature of the mass, and from this convey to the surgeon an indication of the statistical risk of spread. Not all adenomas are histologically monotypic. An example has been reported by Akhtar and his colleagues (1974) that showed a large variety of cell types including clear cells, ciliated cells, mucous elements and 'oncocytes'.

The microscopic appearance of the so-called *oncocytoma* is by definition distinctive even if the term is no more than descriptive. The histogenesis of the lesion, including its being possibly a carcinoid or an adenoma or sometimes one and sometimes the other, has been considered by Santos-Briz and his associates (1977) who conclude that "The cell of origin . . . is unknown". However, since these authors themselves mention the occurrence of oncocytes in the collecting ducts of bronchial glands, such cells seem a very plausible candidate. At the same time, the facts in local Case 9.5 raises another and doubtless rare possibility, namely, solitary metastasis from a cryptic carcinoma elsewhere, in this instance a neoplasm of the adrenal (if the pulmonary lesion in this patient was really a metastasis, the adrenal mass was indeed a carcinoma: if not, the adrenal lesion was a rather polymorphic adenoma, the patient having by coincidence developed also a pulmonary oncocytoma). A comment by Santos-Briz and his colleagues has particular relevance in this context, "In some areas tumor tissue resembled hepatic or adrenal cortex as in previously reported cases".

Any other comparable case occurring now could be profitably investigated and possibly diagnosed on ultramicroscopic evidence as had been done by Santos-Briz and, earlier, by Black (1969) and Fechner and Bentinck (1973).

## Benign Clear Cell (Sugar) Tumour

This neoplasm is mentioned, not because it is common, for indeed it is rare, but because the lesion it so closely resembles is common, or at any rate relatively common, namely, metastatic carcinoma of kidney. The clear cell tumour of lung was first described by Liebow and Castleman (1971). It is benign, more usually silent than symptomatic, and of still uncertain histogenesis though, as mentioned by Sale and Kulander (1976), the Kultschitzky cell, smooth muscle, and pericyte have been suggested as possible ancestors. In their account of the lesion, Liebow and Castleman mention, as a point of distinction from metastatic carcinoma of kidney, the absence of haemorrhage. However, as in the case described by Sale and Kulander, this need not be so: their own example was notably haemorrhagic.

Certain diagnosis rests on ultramicroscopy which will reveal a pattern of membrane-bound glycogen-filled vesicles that is quite distinctive (and known to occur otherwise only in the hepatocytes of Pompé's disease). The investigative implications for a patient whose benign clear cell tumour is wrongly diagnosed as metastatic renal carcinoma need no emphasis.

### The 'Tumourlet'

The multifocal pattern of a tumourlet is well recognised (see Figs. 9.8, 9.9, 9.10). That many such lesions are carcinoid tumours originating in the Kultschitzky cells of a bronchus or bronchiole seems certain, and for these the terms 'bronchial carcinoid, tumorlet type' (Churg and Warnock, 1976) or 'carcinoid tumorlet' (Ranchod, 1977) are appropriate. Whether all are of carcinoid character is less certain. Hitherto, as described for example by Spencer (1968), two varieties have been widely recognised, the carcinoid and the metaplastic/hyperplastic arising in a background of fibrosis and bronchiectasis. Of the 20 examples examined by Churg and Warnock, one-third were in scarred lungs, two-thirds in lungs with little or no scarring. Nevertheless, cells in 14 of the 15 cases tested were argyrophilic. Possibly, then, even the tumourlets seeming to arise purely by metaplasia or focal hyperplasia have their origin in Kultschitzky cells and are also carcinoids. Since, as noted by Spencer, the lesion has been produced experimentally in rabbits, further experiments might, pace species differences, clarify the matter.

In the opinion of Bonikos and his colleagues

(1976), the tumourlet, bronchial carcinoid and oat cell carcinoma may all have as their cell of origin ". . . the bronchial counterpart of the intestinal argentaffin cell". In view of the fickleness of silver staining, especially in necropsy tissue (the cells in Case 9.4 showed neither argentaffinity nor argyrophilia), accurate identification of the cells in an individual lesion is likely to depend increasingly on ultramicroscopy in a search for neurosecretory granules.

Tumourlets are most likely to be found at necropsy or incidentally after resection, and are thus of more academic than clinical significance. The few examples of the carcinoid variety reported to have metastasised have extended no further than regional nodes and have not been associated with the classical carcinoid syndrome.

### Granulomatous Lesions

Certain forms of granulomatous lesion may be difficult to distinguish from malignant neoplasms, in particular, the more xanthomatous forms from metastatic carcinoma of kidney: those with a prominently plasma cell population from myeloma: and others where monocytic cells predominate from a malignant lymphoma.

Four examples of the *xanthomatous form* were described by Titus and his colleagues (1962), with an account of earlier reports by others, of which one mass was virtually identical macroscopically with metastatic renal carcinoma. Microscopically, however, despite the occasional stromal cell in mitosis, the appearances in lesions of this kind are characteristically those of a lipo- or xantho-granuloma rather than a neoplasm: for the whole group, the term 'plasma cell granuloma' rather than 'inflammatory pseudotumour' is preferred by Bahadori and Liebow (1973). The question arises whether the xanthogranulomatous lesion is yet another form or expression of the histiocytoma: to the extent that the lesion is regarded by Bahadori and Liebow, and on ultramicroscopic evidence also by Kuzela (1975), as distinct from the sclerosing angioma of lung, this seems unlikely. All observers appear to agree that the lesion, whether predominantly xanthomatous or plasma-celled, is essentially inflammatory and wholly benign: no causative pathogen, however, has yet been identified.

A further lesion, the *'lymphomatoid granulomatosis'* of Liebow and his colleagues (1972) was mentioned earlier as one that may simulate a ML, as the name clearly suggests, and also occasionally precede a ML (as was the case in 13% of the 40 examples described by Liebow). In the words of these authors, the disease is seen typically in ". . . a young person, especially a man with a febrile pulmonary disease manifested radiographically by bilateral shadows resembling metastases in the peripheral and lower portions of the lungs . . .", and an appropriate scheme of investigation, largely immunological, is suggested for these circumstances.

The conditions most requiring to be distinguished from lymphomatoid granulomatosis are ML and Wegener's granulomatosis. Though predominantly a lesion of lung, the process was found by Liebow and his colleagues to involve not infrequently also the skin and kidneys (each of these sites in 45% of their patients), central nervous system (20%) and peripheral nerves (neuritis in almost 20%): the involvement of skin, they remarked, might draw attention to a pulmonary lesion as yet silent. A recent updating and expansion of the original Liebow series by the same group of workers (Katzenstein et al., 1979) gives valuable diagnostic and prognostic information. Of 148 traced patients, more than one-half (94 or 63.5%) had died of the disease, while 12% of the patients had developed a malignant lymphoma at some time during their course. The authors conclude that lymphomatoid granulomatosis is an entity separate from both Wegener's granulomatosis and ML but one with some features of each.

### Lymphomatous and Lymphomatoid Lesions

Lymphomatoid granulomatosis straddles the boundary between ML and granulomatous lesions but the form of ML most likely to figure in these circumstances is the histiocytic. The lymphocytic variety raises the same problems in the lung vis-à-vis pseudo-lymphoma as it does elsewhere, especially in the digestive tract as earlier noted, but its occurrence particularly in the lung has been described by Saltzstein (1963) in an analysis of 102 examples. Features found helpful by this observer as suggesting inflammation rather than neoplasia were the infiltrating cells' being of mixed types (though with mature lymphocytes predominating): the presence of true germ centres (in general the most depend-

able criterion): and noninvolvement of adjacent lymph nodes. The size, direction and mode of infiltration by the cells was of no help. However, as Saltzstein says, "A histological distinction between a benign and malignant lesion will not be possible in some instances", a conclusion well exemplified by the experience of McNamara and his colleagues (1969) with two of their three reported cases. In their Case 2, the lesion showed poorly differentiated lymphocytes and no germ centres, and an adjacent node was involved, yet, after incomplete excision and no further specific treatment, the patient was well 10 years later. In their Case 3, the lymphocytes were mature, occasional germ centres were present and there was no nodal involvement, yet the patient died just over 5 years later with generalised 'reticulum cell sarcoma'.

With the borderline case there is little more the pathologist can do than diagnose 'lymphoma or pseudo-lymphoma' and discuss the matter with the clinician: ancillary evidence might emerge. To label the lesion 'lymphoblastoma', as suggested by Scharkoff (1969) would seem to point too firmly towards the side of malignancy.

### Solitary Metastases, Their Implications

Occasions are few when a pulmonary malignant metastasis can be resected with realistic hope of cure, and actual cures are fewer still. Individual examples of success have been recorded over the years but a recent instructive account of the procedure has been given by Vidne and his colleagues (1976) in the case of 17 patients with, among them, metastasis from ten different types of neoplasm including carcinomas of breast and large gut, melanocarcinoma, fibrosarcoma and others. Four of the patients died within 30 months of resection but the remaining 13 were alive at 12–129 months later. The attempt at cure is thus well justified: however, the criteria used in the selection of patients are clearly crucial.

The indications for attempted excision, whether by pneumonectomy, lobectomy or wedge resection, are given by Vidne and his colleagues. They include a reasonable assurance not only that the pulmonary lesion is solitary and removable in toto but that the primary lesion also has been removed in toto, and that there are no metastases elsewhere. This last requirement may be the hardest to satisfy: as techniques improve for the detection of silent metastases, the number of patients initially considered suitable for resection may be reduced. At the same time, when all such investigations are negative, the likelihood of cure will be so much the greater.

## Conclusions

1) The descriptively termed *lethal midline granuloma* may be separable into 'midline malignant reticulosis': Wegener's granulomatosis: a malignant lymphoma.

2) The histology of nasal papillomas is an uncertain guide to prognosis.

3) Epithelial dysplasia with cellular aberrancy is common in the larynges of cigarette smokers: over-diagnosis of CIS is therefore a risk.

4) The prognosis in carcinoma of the larynx is closely correlated with degree of histological differentiation.

5) Of bronchial adenomas, the mucoepidermoid form may be more aggressive than the carcinoid and adenoid cystic forms.

6) Only ultramicroscopy can certainly distinguish between metastatic carcinoma of kidney and the rare, benign, clear-cell ('sugar') tumour of lung.

7) Granulomatous lesions of lung may simulate carcinoma, myeloma and malignant lymphoma. 'Lymphomatoid granulomatosis' has a high mortality.

8) With careful selection of patients, resection of metastases by partial or total pneumonectomy may significantly lengthen survival.

## References

Akhtar M, Young I, Reyes F (1974) Bronchial adenoma with polymorphous features. Cancer 33: 1572–1576

Al-Saleem T, Peale AR, Norris CM (1968) Multiple papillomatosis of the lower respiratory tract. Clinical and pathologic study of eleven cases. Cancer 22: 1173–1184

Al-Saleem TI, Peale AR, Robbins R, Norris CM (1970) Lymphocytic pseudotumor (pseudolymphoma) of the larynx. Report of a rare case and review of the literature. Laryngoscope 80: 133–136

Altmann F, Basek M, Stout AP (1955) Papillomas of the larynx with intraepithelial anaplastic changes. Arch Otolaryngol 62: 478–485

Auerbach O, Hammond EC, Garfinkel L (1970) Histologic changes in the larynx in relation to smoking habits. Cancer 25: 92–104

Bahadori M, Liebow AA (1973) Plasma cell granulomas of the lung. Cancer 31: 191–208

Batsakis JG, Fox JE (1970) Supporting tissue neoplasms of the larynx. Surg Gynecol Obstet 131: 989–997

Bennett SH, Futrell JW, Roth JA, Hoye RC, Ketcham AS (1971) Prognostic significance of histologic host response in cancer of the larynx or hypopharynx. Cancer 28: 1255–1265

Black WC (1969) Pulmonary oncocytoma. Cancer 23: 1347–1357

Blackledge GD, Goodall HB (1973) Changes in cervico-vaginal epithelium in gestational megaloblastic anaemia. Aust NZJ Obstet 13: 241–245

Bonikos DS, Archibald R, Bensch KG (1976) On the origin of the so-called tumorlets of the lung. Hum Pathol 7: 461–469

Busuttil A, Sandison AT, Bratten NT (1974) Polyploidal giant cells in a laryngeal biopsy. Lancet II: 469

Churg A, Warnock ML (1976) Pulmonary tumorlet. A form of peripheral carcinoid. Cancer 37: 1469–1477

Elman AJ, Goodman M, Wang CC, Pilch B, Busse J (1979) In situ carcinoma of the vocal cords. Cancer 43: 2422–2428

Fechner RE, Bentinck BR (1973) Ultrastructure of bronchial oncocytoma. Cancer 31: 1451–1457

Fu Y-S, Perzin KH (1974) Non-epithelial tumors of the nasal cavity, paranasal sinuses, and nasopharynx: A clinicopathologic study. I. General features and vascular tumors. Cancer 33: 1275–1288

Fu Y-S, Perzin KH (1979). Non-epithelial tumors of the nasal cavity, paranasal sinuses and nasopharynx. A clinicopathologic study. X. Malignant lymphomas. Cancer 43: 611–621

Graham RM, Rheault MH (1954) Characteristic cellular changes in epithelial cells in pernicious anemia. J Lab Clin Med 43: 235–245

Hyams VJ (1971) Papillomas of the nasal cavity and paranasal sinuses. A clinicopathological study of 315 cases. Ann Otol 80: 192–206

Kassel SH, Echevarria RA, Guzzo FP (1969) Midline malignant reticulosis (so called lethal midline granuloma). Cancer 23: 920–935

Katzenstein A-LA, Carrington CB, Liebow AA (1979) Lymphomatoid granulomatosis. A clinicopathologic study of 152 cases. Cancer 43: 360–373

Kuzela DC (1975) Ultrastructural study of a post-inflammatory "tumor" of the lung. Cancer 36: 149–156

Lane N (1957) Pseudosarcoma (polypoid sarcoma-like masses) associated with squamous-cell carcinoma of the mouth, fauces, and larynx: Report of ten cases. Cancer 10: 19–41

Lasser A, Rothfeld PR, Shapiro RS (1976) Epithelial papilloma and squamous cell carcinoma of the nasal cavity and paranasal sinuses. A clinicopathological study. Cancer 38: 2503–2510

Lee SC, Roth LM, Brashear RE (1976) Lymphomatoid granulomatosis. A clinicopathologic study of four cases. Cancer 38: 846–853

Liebow AA, Castleman B (1971) Benign clear cell ("sugar") tumors of the lung. Yale J Biol Med 43: 213–222

Liebow AA, Carrington CRB, Friedman PJ (1972) Lymphomatoid granulomatosis. Hum Pathol 3: 457–558

McGavran MH, Bauer WC, Ogura JH (1961) The incidence of cervical lymph node metastases from epidermoid carcinoma of the larynx and their relationship to certain characteristics of the primary tumor. A study based on the clinical and pathological findings for 96 patients treated by primary en bloc laryngectomy and radical neck dissection. Cancer 14: 55–66

McNamara JJ, Kingsley WB, Paulson DL, Dandade PB, Race GJ, Urschel HC (1969) Primary lymphosarcoma of the lung. Ann Surg 169: 133–140

Niekerk WA van (1966) Cervical cytological abnormalities caused by folic acid deficiency. Acta Cytol (Baltimore) 10: 67–73

Osborn DA (1970) Nature and behavior of transitional tumors in the upper respiratory tract. Cancer 25: 50–60

Piquet JJ, Blondy G, Leduc M, Decroix G (1969) Les tumeurs d'Abrikossoff du larynx. Ann Otol Laryngol (Paris) 86: 79–85

Ranchod M (1977) The histogenesis and development of pulmonary tumorlets. Cancer 39: 1135–1145

Sale GE, Kulander BG (1976) Benign clear cell tumor of lung with necrosis. Cancer 37: 2355–2358

Saltzstein SL (1963) Pulmonary malignant lymphomas and pseudolymphomas: Classification, therapy, and prognosis. Cancer 16: 928–955

Santos-Briz A, Terrón J, Sastre R, Romero L, Valle A (1977) Oncocytoma of the lung. Cancer 40: 1330–1336

Scharkoff T (1969) Zum Begriff "Lymphoblastom der Lunge". Zentralbl Chir 94: 287–296

Spencer H (1968) Pathology of the Lung, 2nd edn. Pergamon Press, London

Titus JL, Harrison EG, Clagett OT, Anderson MW, Knaff LJ (1962) Xanthomatous and inflammatory pseudotumors of the lung. Cancer 15: 522–538

Tolis GA, Fry WA, Head L, Shields TW (1972) Bronchial adenomas. Surg Gynecol Obstet 134: 605–610

Turnbull AD, Huvos AG, Goodner JT, Beattie EJ (1972) The malignant potential of bronchial adenoma. Ann Thorac Surg 14: 453–464

Vidne BA, Richter S, Levy MJ (1976) Surgical treatment of solitary pulmonary metastasis. Cancer 38: 2561–2563

# 10  Lesions of the Female Genital Tract

Borderline lesions are fully represented in the female genital tract. Mostly they form relatively well-recognised groups: the vulvar skin dystrophies; dysplasia, and in situ and microinvasive carcinoma of the cervix; the overgrowths of the endometrium and myometrium; the commoner neoplasms of ovary; and aberrancies of trophoblast.

## Local Series

Every lesion mentioned above is to some extent a borderline problem, and a full list of all that were seen will not be given. The analysis of local cases on this occasion will comprise: (a) an account of ten individual cases which appear to be usefully instructive or illustrative of a particular problem; (b) a comparison of figures over the 25 years for the total number of patients diagnosed as having cancer of various kinds, and the total number of patients thus diagnosed who died. A comparison of this type could give at least a general indication whether a significant degree of histological over-diagnosis had been practised. A brief commentary on the bipartite analysis will follow.

### CASE DATA

#### Case 10.1

Age, 54 years: vulvar irritation 'for many years'. The lesion was regarded as 'leukoplakia'. Vulvectomy was performed but details cannot be traced. The patient reappeared 15 years later, again with the same complaint and now with bilateral warty outgrowths on the labia and enlarged inguinal nodes. Carcinoma was diagnosed clini-

cally, and vulvectomy repeated with removal of the palpable nodes.

The epidermis was hyperkeratotic and irregularly hyperplastic with appreciable downgrowth in many areas but was reported as insufficiently aberrant to warrant diagnosis as carcinoma. The many lymph nodes examined were inflamed but contained no carcinoma.

Panel review of these sections when the patient was seen yet again 6 years later (v.i.) found some opinions in favour of 'early carcinoma' but most against (the after-history had not been disclosed).

The patient suffered recurrent pruritus and was re-examined 6 years later. The labial margins were again markedly nodular, there was an almost pedunculated mass posteriorly and the perivulval 'leukoplakia' was by now also extensively perianal. Tissue from the further vulvectomy specimen showed epidermal atrophy in some areas, marked hypertrophy with downgrowth in others (Figs. 10.1, 10.2) but again the combination of pattern and cell detail was considered insufficient evidence to justify diagnosis as carcinoma.

The patient died from an unrelated cause 4 years later, then aged 79. From the time of first treatment the disease had lasted 25 years. A diagnosis of carcinoma might have been made at the time of the second vulvectomy, 10 years before death. The later history shows that, if so, the diagnosis would have been an over-diagnosis. In the event, throughout, the diagnoses had been *appropriate*.

#### Case 10.2

Age, 49 years: with irregular menorrhagia (premenopausal).

The curetted material was scanty but showed

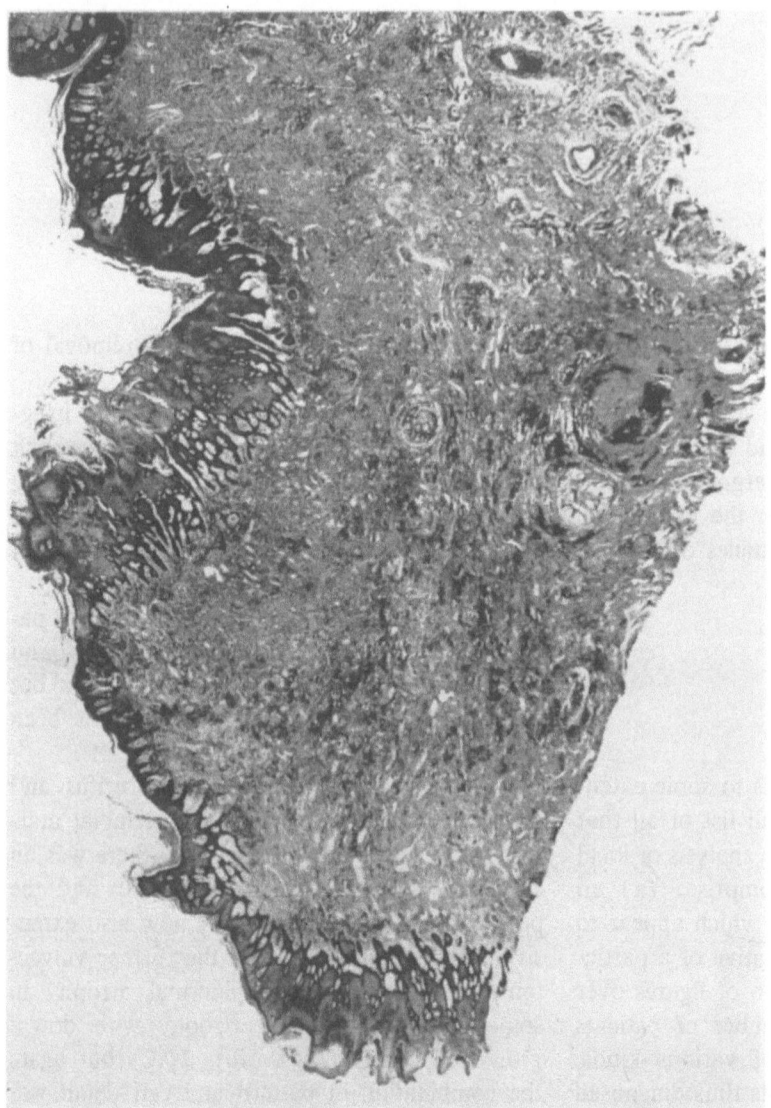

**Fig. 10.1.** The irregularity of the epidermis is evident as is a prominent degree of chronic inflammatory cell infiltration of the subjacent stroma. H & E, × 9

foci of 'back to back' glands of irregular outline and hyperchromatic, occasionally mitotically active, epithelium. The disturbance was reported as 'atypical hyperplasia'.

No further treatment was given, and the patient reappeared 3 years later still complaining of 'heavy irregular periods'. Curettage now showed unequivocal 'adenocarcinoma', confirmed in the excised uterus as involving an area of 3 × 2 cm on one wall and only minimally encroaching on the myometrium. She died 4 years later from an unrelated cause.

It is a matter of opinion whether the original designation as atypical hyperplasia was an appropriate diagnosis or an under-diagnosis. The material, as stated, was scanty. The suspicion must be that had it been ten times as great, adenocarcinoma would have been diagnosed; a further biopsy should perhaps have been sought. To this extent, the report may have been an *under-diagnosis*.

## Case 10.3

Age, 57 years: vaginal bleeding 17 years after the menopause. Curettage produced a 'fundal polyp', reported microscopically as a 'mildly hyperplastic cystic polyp'. Hysterectomy followed within 6 weeks.

The general state of the endometrium was as shown in Fig. 10.3: most of the glands were cystic and atrophic, others that were smaller had

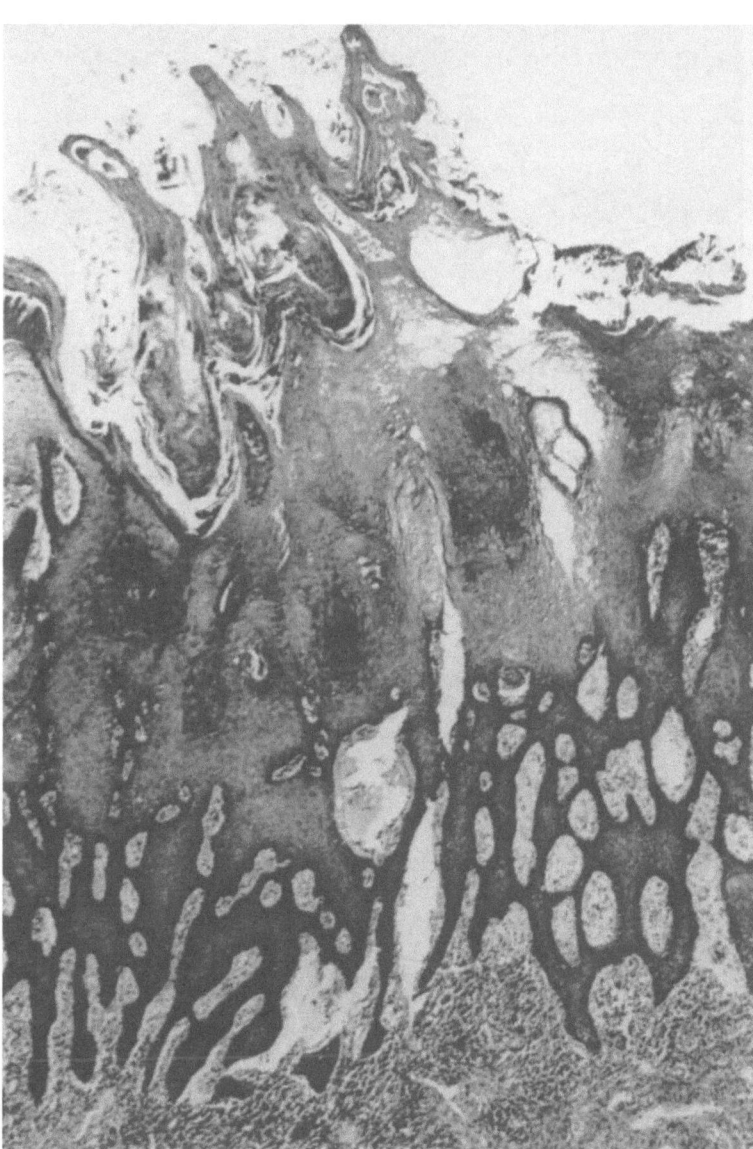

**Fig. 10.2.** Little can be gained from attempts to demonstrate a basement membrane in areas such as this. Irregular acanthosis of this degree was common. Subepidermal vesiculation, of which an area is seen in the upper part of the field, was extensive in some areas. H & E, × 45

a thicker epithelium with occasional cells in mitosis, but interest centered mainly on the circumscribed focus of paler glandular tissue at the lower right-hand corner of this figure.

Gland elements of all three types are seen in Fig. 10.4: atrophic-cystic in the centre; smaller, darker and hyperplastic to left; adenomatous or adenomatoid to right. In more detail (Fig. 10.5), the epithelium of the close-packed acinar tissue is multilayered and occasionally in mitosis though not unduly polymorphic. It was eventually agreed that the lesion be reported not as carcinoma but as an expression of 'atypical hyperplasia'.

The threat to the patient seemed minimal, and she remains well 10 years later. It is open to debate whether diagnosis of the lesion as *not* carcinoma has unfairly diminished local statistics for the incidence and cure of carcinoma corporis uteri by one unit. The clinical outcome, at any rate, suggests that the diagnosis was *appropriate*.

### Case 10.4

Age, 27 years: infertility and hypomenorrhoea. Curettage was performed.

The endometrial pattern was that shown in Fig. 10.6; that is, the classically borderline pattern of highly differentiated adenocarcinoma or (the phrase used at the time) 'adenoma malignum'.

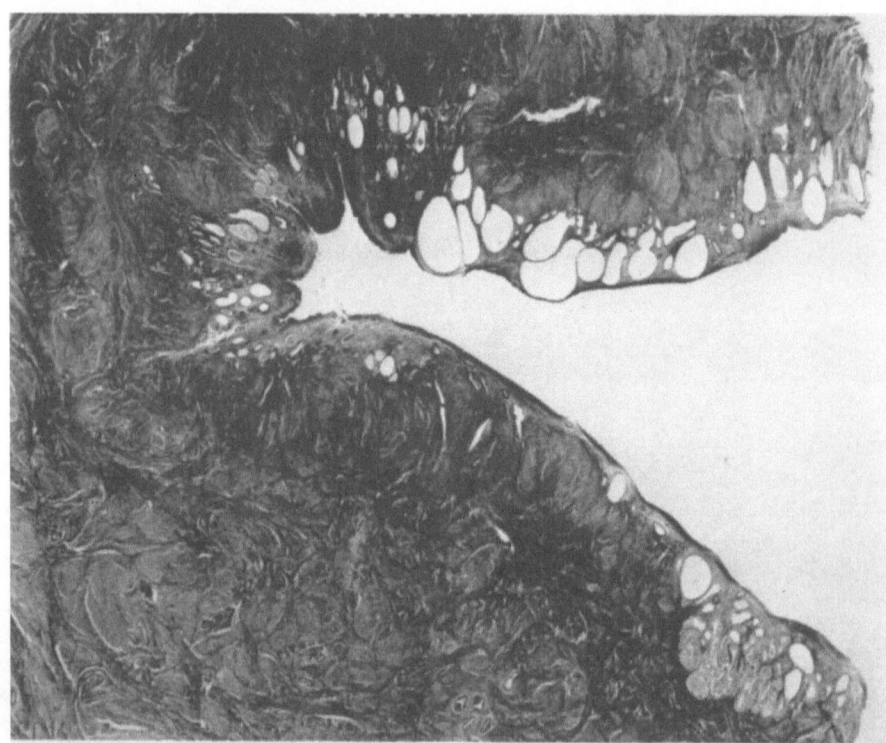

**Fig. 10.3.** The endometrium shows, from above right, atrophic cystic change, mildly hyperplastic smaller glands, almost total atrophy, then, at lower right, a circumscribed focus of paler tissue. H & E, × 9

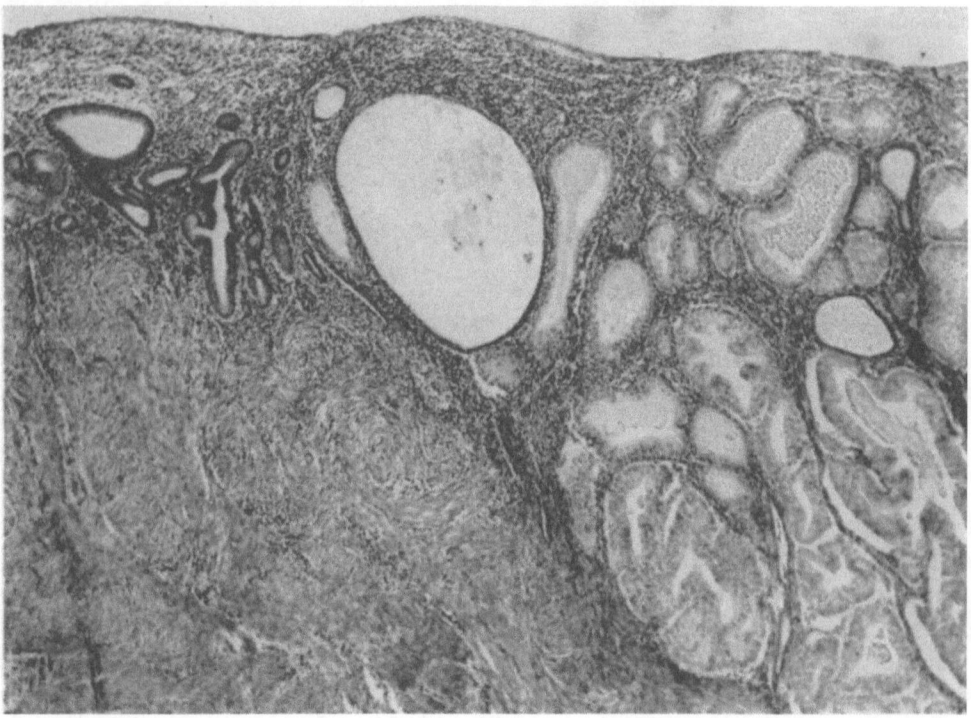

**Fig. 10.4.** Shows, in turn, relatively small glands with a thick epithelium, a cystic gland with atrophic epithelium, and the edge of the focus of paler multiacinar tissue. H & E, × 62

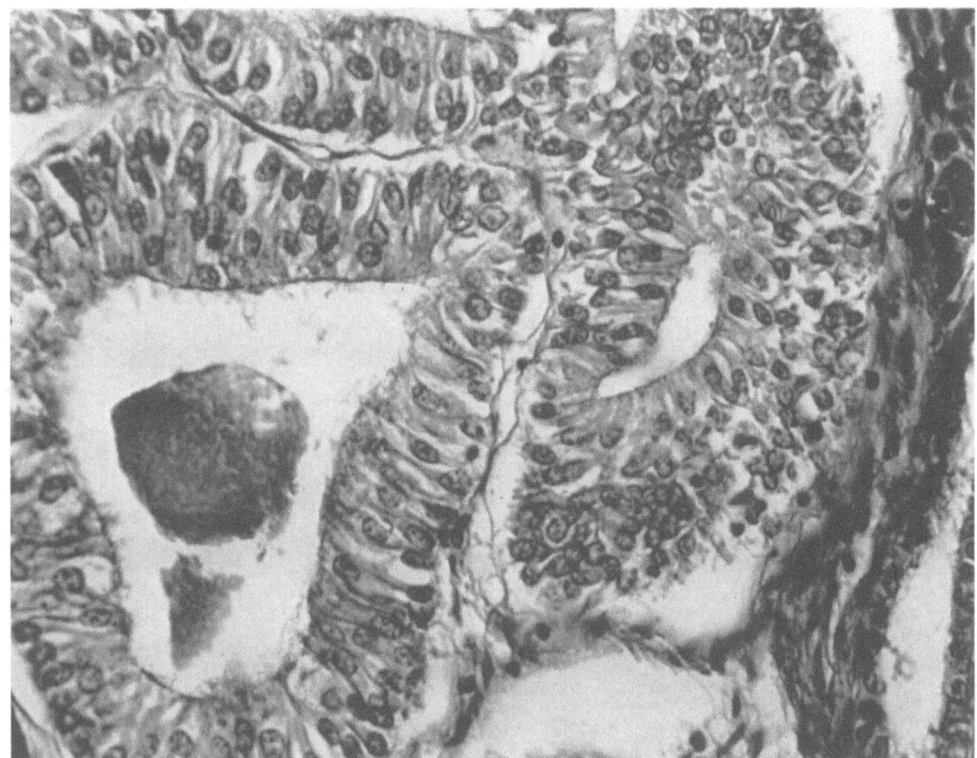

**Fig. 10.5.** The glands have a multilayered type of epithelium showing occasional mitotic divisions. H & E, × 493

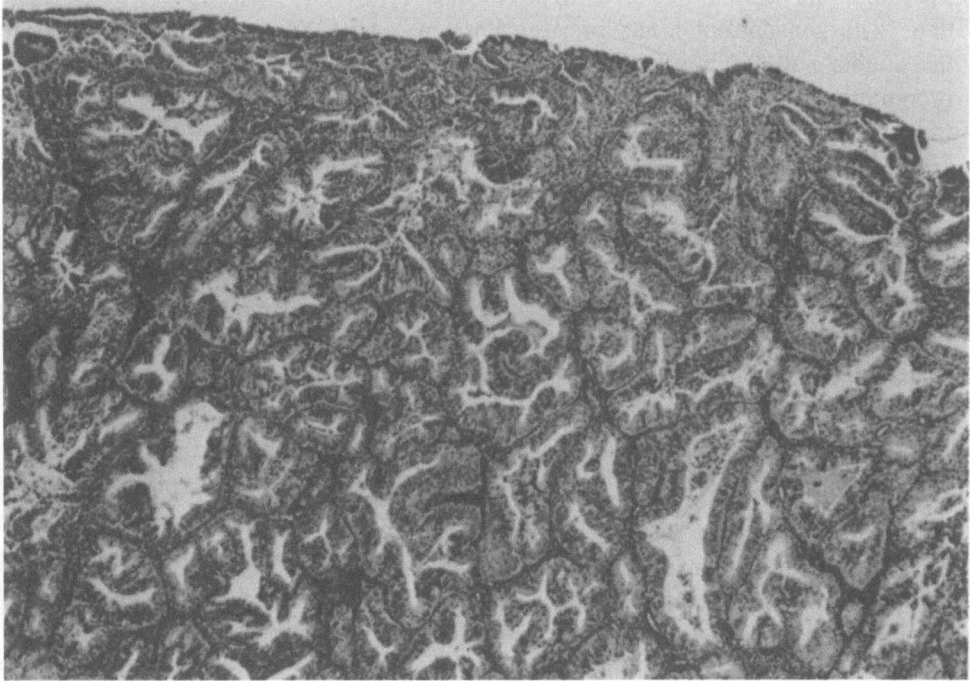

**Fig. 10.6.** The closely packed and rather irregular glands with overcellular epithelium were diagnosed as indicating well-differentiated glandular carcinoma, or, in older terminology, 'adenoma malignum'. H & E, × 53

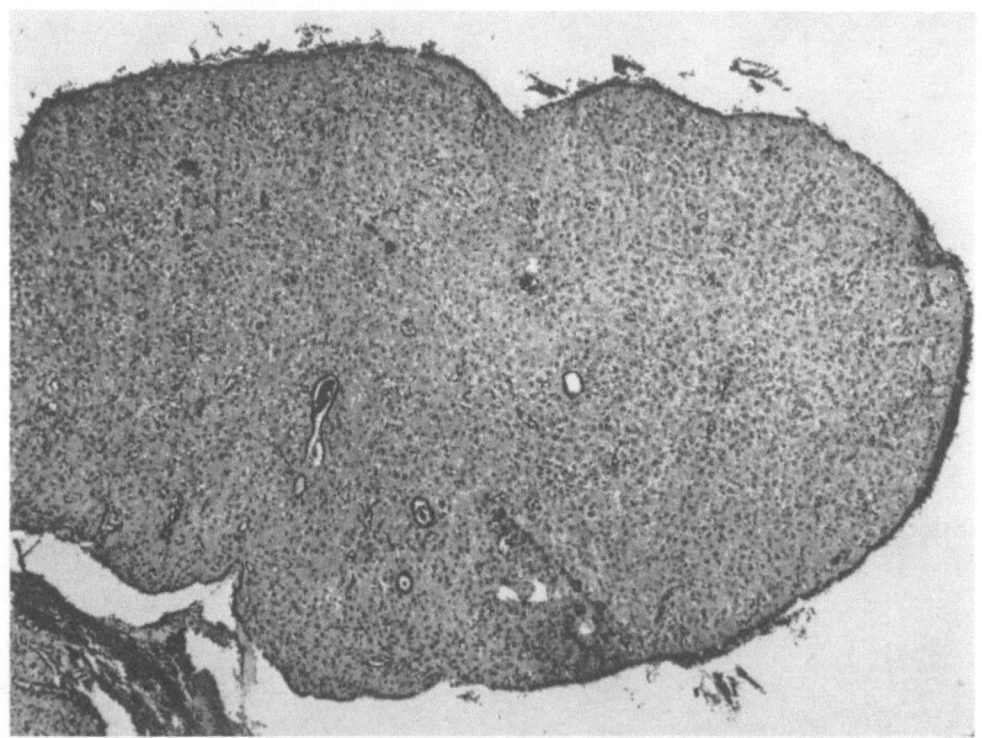

**Fig. 10.7.** Endometrium from the same patient after 2 months' treatment with progestogen preparations. H & E, × 53

The patient was anxious to become pregnant. Therefore, the decision was taken to use medication (with gonadotrophin and progestogens) in the double hope of averting hysterectomy and promoting fertility. Within weeks the endometrial pattern had changed to that shown in Fig. 10.7, the familiar dissociated conjunction of small glands and deciduoid stroma.

After 6 months, the patient had not conceived. Medication was stopped and, again within weeks, the endometrium had reverted to the 'adenoma malignum' pattern. For the next 4 years the cycle was repeated: medication with remission, nonmedication with regression, and all the time the patient was hoping to become pregnant. She was unsuccessful, and, after the 4 years, in the words of the case notes, patient and physician decided to 'call it a day'. Hysterectomy was performed, and the patient has remained well for the past 9 years. The often curious behaviour of endometrial adenocarcinoma, or what by all ordinary morphological criteria appears to be adenocarcinoma, in youth is mentioned later. In this instance the original diagnosis may reasonably be regarded as *appropriate*.

*Case 10.5*

Age, 27 years: found at caesarean section to have five fibroids up to 7 cm in diameter. Apart from foci of mucinous change, all had a typically whorled cut surface: they appeared to be well circumscribed.

A block was taken from each fibroid. Sections showed the pattern of quite highly cellular 'myoma'; all were reported as benign.

The patient appeared 8½ years later with abdominal pain and menorrhagia. Laparotomy showed a friable inoperable mass largely filling the pelvis and already involving the walls of bladder and rectum. She died 5 months later. The lesion was a spindle cell 'sarcoma'.

Some time later the sections of the original myoma were examined 'blind' by a group of pathologists; none would have diagnosed sarcoma, essentially because the cells were generally uniform and only occasionally in mitosis (fewer than 1 per 20 hpf in the most highly cellular areas). Despite the clinical outcome, the original diagnosis had to that extent been *appropriate*.

## Case 10.6

Age, 51 years: menorrhagia and abdominal swelling for 4 months. The excised uterus contained a well-circumscribed fibroid mass, almost spherical, 20 × 18 cm, widely degenerate and cystic, mottled brownish-red and yellow.

Representative sections showed variable vascularity and necrosis with appreciable nuclear polymorphism but no mitotic activity. The tissue was reported as not malignant: a degenerating 'myoma'.

The patient was seen again 6 months later. She had had a constant dull ache in the RIF since the hysterectomy and brisk vaginal bleeding for 2 days; a mass was palpable in the RIF. Biopsy was taken from 'vaginal vault granulations'.

Microscopy showed highly cellular, mitotically active tissue, virtually a malignant tissue culture, obviously a 'sarcoma'. Despite a full course of irradiation the lesion rapidly spread until the patient's death 9 months later.

One-half of the original 'fibroid' had been mounted as a museum specimen of degenerate myoma. When the obvious sarcoma was diagnosed, the specimen was demounted and serially sliced. No area appeared more suggestively sarcomatous than any other, or more suggestive than any of tissue originally sectioned. A further 30 blocks were taken but none of the sections showed tissue significantly different from that originally examined and reported as benign.

As in Case 10.5, despite the clinical outcome the original diagnosis had at least been technically *appropriate*.

## Case 10.7

Age, 16 years: increasing abdominal swelling; removal of left ovarian mass, 15 × 12 × 8 cm.

The mass was mucinous and finely locular (Fig. 10.8). Microscopically the epithelium in all the areas sectioned was uniform, minimally mitotic and typically that of a benign mucinous 'cystadenoma'.

Swelling recurred after 1 year and a further operation produced an even larger cyst, 22 × 18 × 12 cm, this time from the right ovary. There were small cystic nodules, 1 cm or less, on the pelvic peritoneum, and an area of indurated deep puckering at the rectosigmoid junction.

Histologically, the ovarian mass was again a simple mucinous cystadenoma: the peritoneal nodules and the rectosigmoid lesion (Fig. 10.9) were foci of 'adenocarcinoma'. Further blocks from the ovarian mass, and re-examination of the sections from the contralateral lesion earlier reported, revealed no areas even suggestive of carcinoma.

The problem was a variant of that, not unfamiliar, wherein one tries to decide whether, in a patient with carcinoma in both recto/sigmoid and ovary, the gut or the ovary is the source. In this instance, however, both ovarian tumours seemed wholly benign. On balance, it seemed (and still seems) likelier that one or other ovary had contained an area of carcinoma, undetected, that spread to the pelvis and colon, than that the lesion in colon was a coincidentally separate growth.

The patient was seen again 13 months later, when a nodule of carcinoma was excised from the laparotomy scar, and she died within the next 18 months.

## Case 10.8

Age, 25 years: lower abdominal pain and swelling. Laparotomy showed, mainly in the lower abdomen, peritoneal hyperaemia and thickening, much exudate and many fibrinous adhesions in company with apparently neoplastic nodules on bladder, colon and omentum, and replacement of the left ovary by a rough papillary mass, 10 × 6 × 5 cm.

The left ovarian mass was a 'papillary cystadenocarcinoma' (as was a 10-mm nodule later found in the slightly enlarged right ovary). The nodules elsewhere also contained similar tissue though most of their bulk was due to oedematous granulation tissue and exudate heavily infiltrated by leucocytes.

In view of the briskness of the inflammatory reaction, irradiation and intraperitoneal instillation of drugs were withheld; that is, no further specific treatment was given.

The patient remains fully fit 8 years later.

The borderline element here was not primarily histological, for the diagnosis was not in doubt, but secondarily it was so to the extent that all such lesions have about them an aura of unpredictability, and this was emphasised in the report. Such an outcome is always the hope in these circumstances but it rarely happens: the patient

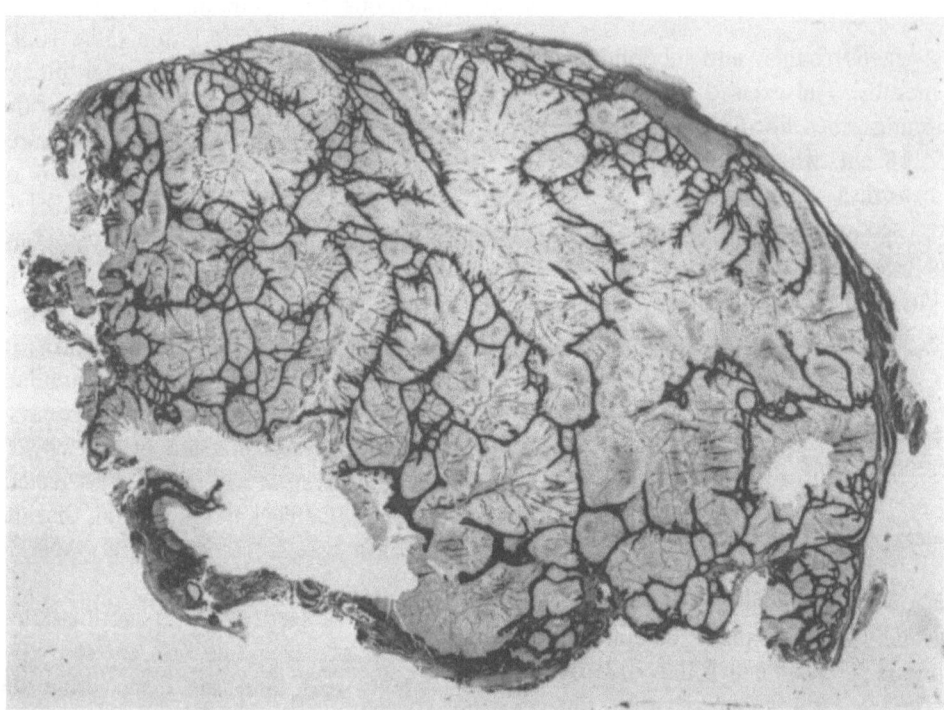

**Fig. 10.8.** Part of the multilocular mucoid tumour. Its epithelium was uniform and largely lacking in mitotic activity in all the areas examined. H & E, × 5

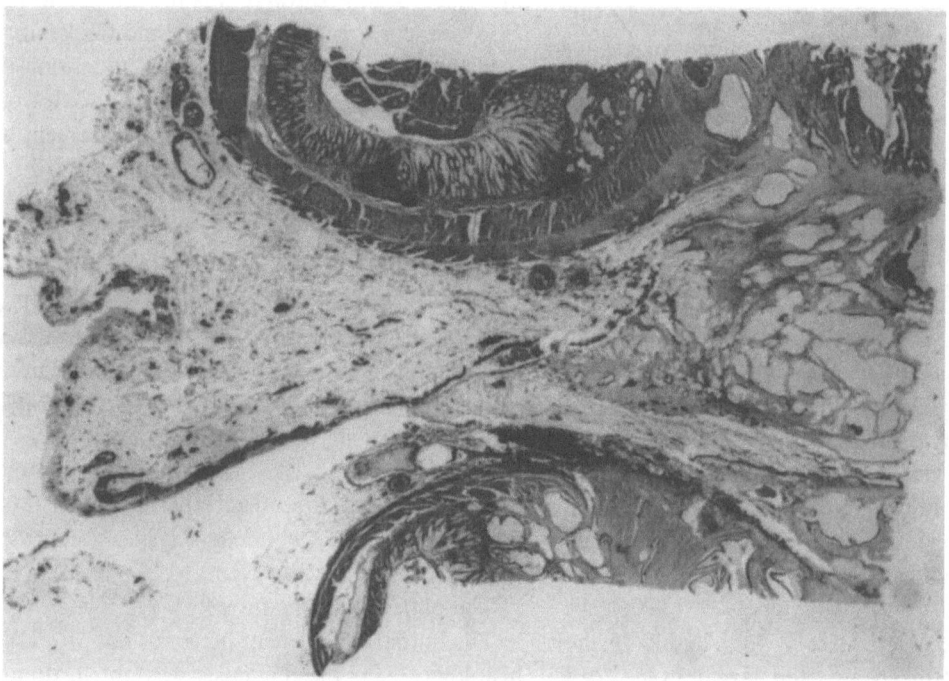

**Fig. 10.9.** Shows the outer part of an area of deep constriction in the wall of the colon. The inner half (*right*) of the space between the upper and lower stretches of muscularis propria is largely occupied by irregular glanduliform acini; at higher magnification their epithelium was malignant. Similar acini can be seen to be penetrating the outer layers of the muscularis propria. H & E, × 5

**Table 10.1.** Gynaecological cancer, 1948–1972 (local Region).

| Disease | Patients registered | Patients dead | Ratio diagnoses/deaths |
|---|---|---|---|
| Carcinoma, vulva/vagina | 205 | 180 | 1.13 : 1 |
| Carcinoma, cervix uteri | 1188 | 615 | 1.93 : 1 |
| Carcinoma, corpus uteri | 722 | 350 | 2.06 : 1 |
| Sarcoma, uterus | 65 | 48 | 1.35 : 1 |
| Carcinoma, ovary | 615 | 452 | 1.36 : 1 |

was fortunate in the intrinsic nature of the neoplasm she had. The significance of the inflammatory intensity remains a matter of speculation. Appropriateness of diagnosis is hardly at issue here.

### Case 10.9

Age, 31 years: irregular vaginal bleeding since normal delivery 5 months earlier: curettage produced tissue of unusual microscopic appearance.

The character of the tissue is shown in Figs. 10.10a and b. Little was lying free; most was present as a cellular infiltrate amid muscle. It was regarded as probably trophoblastic and therefore possibly choriocarcinomatous. The pattern was unfamiliar to the many pathologists, here and elsewhere, who saw it, but the possibility of its being an exaggerated form of benign chorionic invasion was mentioned. Mainly for this reason, no radical treatment was used.

The patient remained reasonably well after the curettage but irregular bleeding started again and a further curettage was performed 11 months after the first: tissue of the same type was still present. However, a comprehensive investigation 5 months later showed no abnormality in further curettings, chest X-ray or HCG assay. The patient became pregnant shortly thereafter and had a normal delivery 14 months after the first curettage.

There seems a strong possibility, later considered, that abnormal tissue of this kind represents the lower range of a continuum that stretches from benign chorionic invasion at one end to frank choriocarcinoma at the other. Although no firm diagnosis was given, the possibility put forward, and the consequently conservative treatment, was ultimately shown by events, fortuitously perhaps, to have been *appropriate*.

### Case 10.10

Age, 47 years: known carcinoma of cervix. Within 3 months of initial treatment by irradiation there was a large mass between uterus and bladder, also large external iliac lymph nodes of which four were received, the two largest each 15 × 10 mm.

The two smaller nodes were essentially normal. The two larger consisted largely of fat but one contained many well-formed glandular structures as shown in Fig. 10.11. In more detail (Fig. 10.12) they were lined by a single layer of uniform epithelium. Only their presence per se within a node raised the question of neoplastic metastasis, for their intrinsic appearance was wholly benign. Further, the lesion in cervix was typically epidermoid, and there were no foci of epidermoid carcinoma in any of the four nodes.

Despite the absence of unequivocally endometrial-type stroma around the glandular structures, this seemed certainly to be an example of 'pelvic nodal endometriosis' as described by Javert (1949). Appropriateness or otherwise of diagnosis is again hardly at issue here: correctness or incorrectness is, and with little doubt the diagnosis of endometriosis was correct.

### COMMENTARY ON LOCAL SERIES

Table 10.1 shows the numbers of patients diagnosed and registered as having cancer of different types, and the numbers notified to the local Registry as having died of these cancers during the same period[1]. For technical reasons (mainly because the Region is served by one department of radiotherapy) the figures refer to all patients originally diagnosed with the Region

---

[1] I am most grateful to Professor James Walker, University Department of Obstetrics and Gynaecology, Dundee, for permission to reproduce these figures.

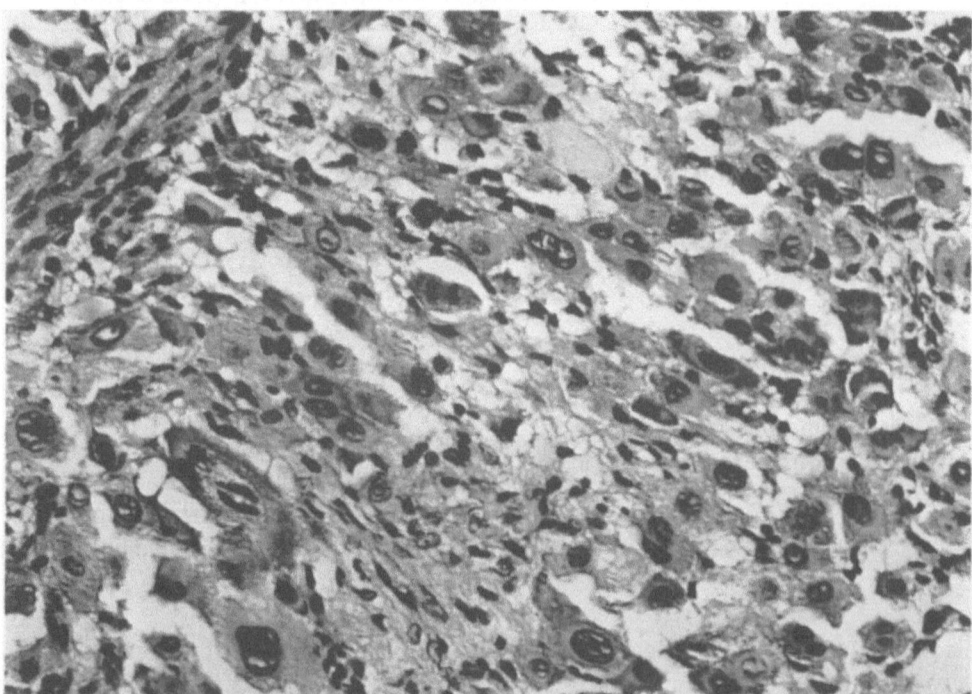

**Fig. 10.10a.** Large and appreciably aberrant cells, occasionally in mitosis, have largely replaced myometrium of which a band runs across the top left-hand corner of the field. H & E, × 320

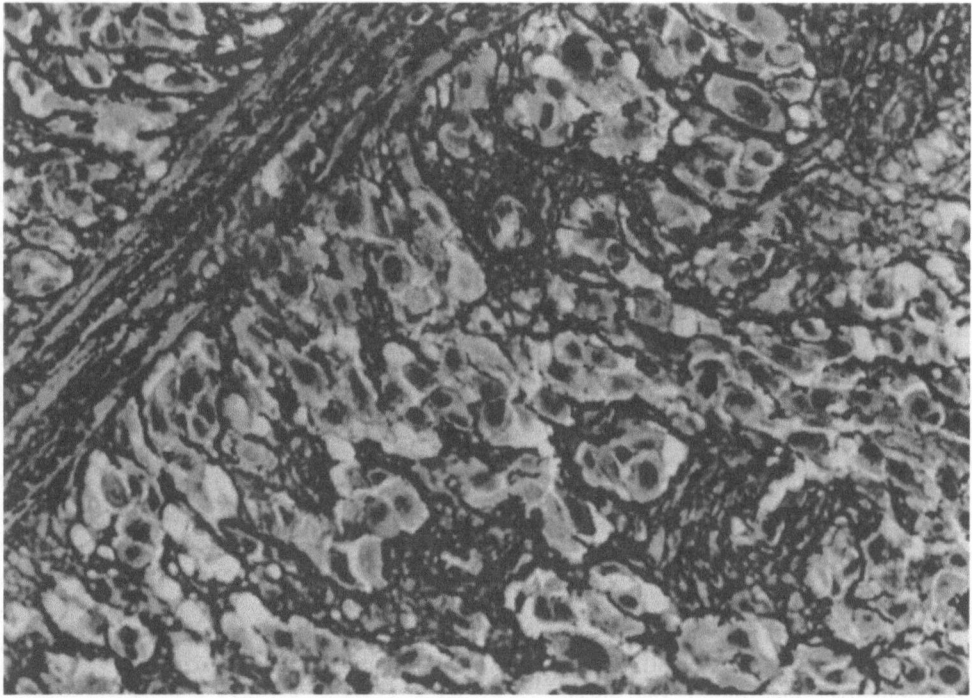

**Fig. 10.10b.** Reticulin staining of a deeper section from the same area shows the lack of an individually pericellular pattern, and the enclosure of clusters of cells indicative rather of an epithelial overgrowth. A pericellular pattern is seen, as expected, around the cells of the myometrial band (*top left*). H & E, × 320

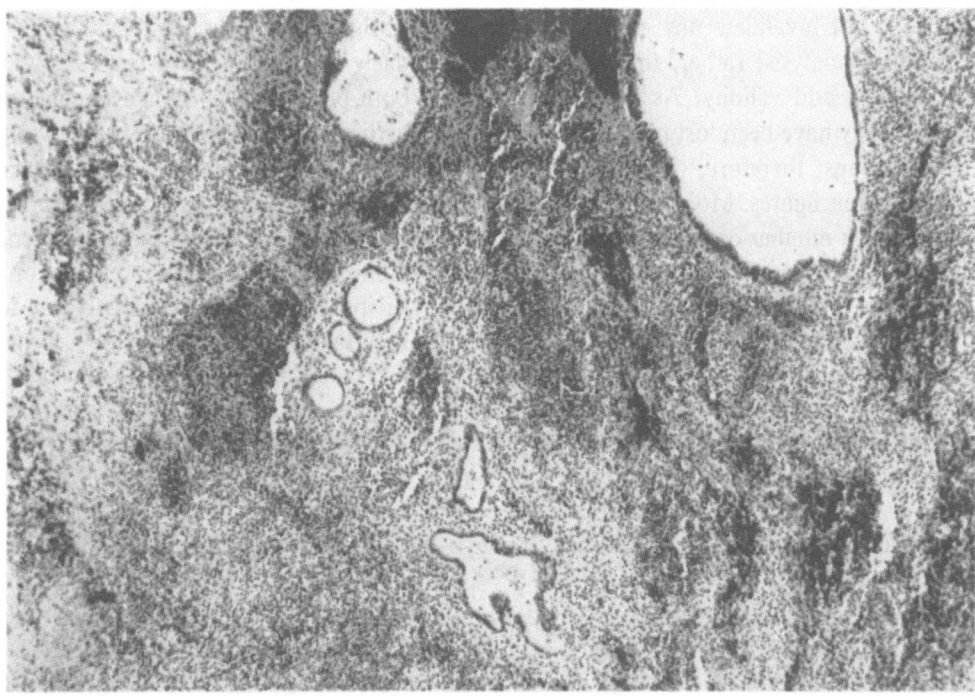

**Fig. 10.11.** Glandular structures are present within the substance of a lymph node. It was difficult to be sure whether any of the immediately surrounding cellular tissue was of an endometrial stromal character. H & E, × 62

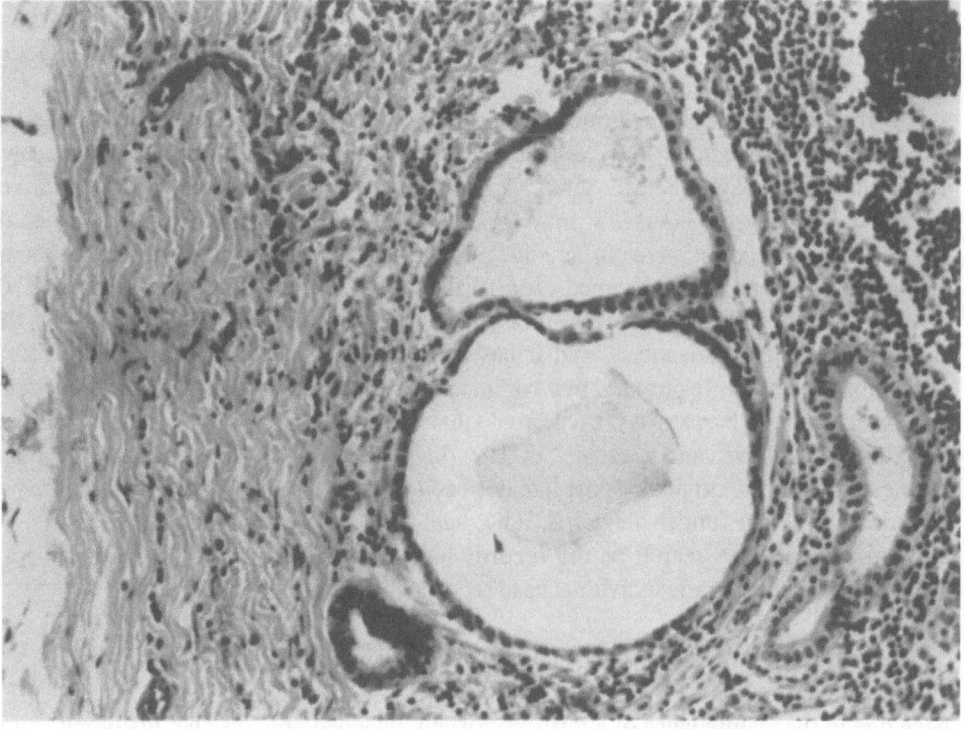

**Fig. 10.12.** The glandular structures had a lining of uniform epithelium throughout. They lie here immediately beneath the capsule of the node. H & E, × 238

(three hospitals), not within one hospital, but this need not invalidate any conclusions drawn from their analysis; rather, the larger numbers will tend to add validity. As many as 10% of patients may have been lost to follow-up in some of the groups; therefore, the figures for deaths are minimum figures. More important, however, an unknown number of patients, though figuring in the 'patients dead' column, died *having had* the disease (and possibly been cured), not *of* the disease. This certainly applies to the group 'carcinoma vulva/vagina' where the average age at diagnosis in a random sample of 50 cases was 69 years: many probably died simply of old age.

The figures for carcinoma of cervix do not include cases diagnosed as carcinoma in situ. All but six of the sarcomas of uterus were leiomyosarcomas.

No attempt will be made to analyse in detail the diagnostic validity and outcome of individual cases within each of the five groups in Table 10.1. Concern is rather with any general trend the figures may illustrate; and one reasonable conclusion seems possible. With figures for 'deaths/diagnoses' such as 187 out of 213 for carcinoma of vulva/vagina, and 50 out of 67 for sarcoma of the uterus, over-diagnosis has probably not been a prevalent habit. Further, in comparison with similar figures to be found in the literature, the same conclusion very possibly holds also for the other cancers.

It is true, of course, as mentioned earlier, that whereas an over-diagnosis may never be recognised, an under-diagnosis will tend always to emerge as such in due course. It may therefore be that some reports were originally underdiagnosed but were later redeemed on a further biopsy. This possibility is important in any analysis of the quality of diagnosis, and it has been given close attention. It prompts two comments: (a) where a first biopsy has been inadequate and unrepresentative, and a second or later biopsy conclusive, the original report has not been regarded as a true under-diagnosis, (b) such under-diagnoses as a search of the records has yielded are included in the individual case reports above.

The relatively low rate of over-diagnosis suggested by the figures in Table 10.1 may have been due to the maintenance of a fairly consistent diagnostic threshold over the years, and to the fact that the threshold has been higher rather than lower. Thus, the allowance for pseudo-epitheliomatous hyperplasia in the vulva, dubiously significant 'invasion' in the cervix, and both polymorphism and frequency of mitosis in myomas has been generous, while borderline overgrowths of the ovary have been demoted more often than promoted. Pathologists cannot sail so close to the wind unless cooperation of clinical colleagues, and supervision by them of their patients, are equally close; and that has fortunately been so here.

The significance of the so-called back-to-back pattern of endometrial glands has long been, and seems likely to remain, debatable. The pattern is one of the criteria by which 'atypical hyperplasia' is diagnosed, and this state is most commonly seen in patients around or shortly after the menopause. In these circumstances, hysterectomy is likely to follow, and the opportunity to study the natural history of the disorder disappears with the uterus. However, (see later) the discovery of the pattern during reproductive life is no indication for precipitate action: at the least it must prompt an enquiry about the possibility of a recent pregnancy or the ingestion of hormonal substances, for both these states may produce notably irregular endometrial patterns.

A borderline problem of which an example was met too recently to be included in the present series merits mention. The so-called adenomatoid tumour, best known as a lesion of uterine tube (or epididymis), may rarely occur in the myometrium, and, with irregular acinar elements, a content of mucin, and occasional mitoses, may closely resemble a metastatic adenocarcinoma. On purely histological grounds distinction between the two lesions may be difficult. In the case in question, a full search for a gastrointestinal carcinoma was negative and the patient remains well 3 years later. These facts leave little doubt that the lesion was indeed an adenomatoid tumour, and simultaneously serve to emphasise its high capacity for mimicry.

## General Commentary

### Vulva

Depending on the histology, and on the individual pathologist, a dystrophic lesion of vulvar and neighbouring skin may be given one of many names such as kraurosis, leukoplakia, lichen sclerosus et atrophicus, and examples may or may not include stretches of epithelium that are hyperplastic or doubtfully or certainly carcinoma. The extent to which this kind of lesion is precancerous is difficult to estimate: in series cited by Kaufman and his colleagues (1974) figures range from less than 1% to 25%. The reason for such variation can only be a lack of clear definition of the lesion by both clinician and histopathologist, and poorly based correlation between the findings of each.

The point was made earlier in connection with the skin as a whole that what matters in practice vis-à-vis cancer is the state of the epidermis, and on this is based the simple classification of dystrophic lesions of the vulva, by Kaufman and colleagues, into histologically hypertrophic, atrophic, and mixed forms. A substantially similar scheme has been formally proposed by a Committee (1976), and with it goes a recommendation that all such terms as kraurosis, leukoplakic vulvitis and the like be abandoned. The welcome simplification may have been stimulated in part by the results of modern treatment, for, in the opinion of Kaufman and his colleagues, "The presence of a vulvar dystrophy, when adequately treated, does not significantly predispose the patient to the development of vulvar carcinoma". The pathologist will remember that, with lesions he judges malignant, his opinion on adequacy of excision, depth of invasion and likelihood of metastasis will largely determine the type of later vulvectomy.

Paget's disease of the skin elsewhere than in nipple was also mentioned earlier as usually curable by excision. It may not always be so in the vulva. In a case described by Hart and Millman (1977) the lesion progressed over 10 years to invasive carcinoma with nodal metastasis.

Basal cell carcinoma behaves in the vulva as it does elsewhere. One of the rarely metastasising examples at this site has been described by Sworn and his colleagues (1979).

## CERVIX UTERI

Few lesions have generated as large a literature in the past 20 years as carcinoma of the cervix. Yet, despite the volumes of work and internationally recommended criteria for the defining of dysplasia, carcinoma in situ (CIS) and 'mi-

croinvasion', it is doubtful if much greater diagnostic uniformity prevails now than 20 years ago (widely varying diagnostic levels were still evident in the survey by Brudenell and his colleagues in 1973, and by Ringsted and his many coworkers in 1978). The reason is clear: the histoclinical correlation cannot be calculated. Dysplasia may not always progress to CIS, and CIS may not always progress to the frankly invasive form that all would accept as having significant lethal potential. Herein lies the nub of the debate on the significance of CIS and the value of population screening for its detection. As clearly exemplified in a short communication by Green (1979), the debate is even yet far from conclusion.

### Carcinoma In Situ

Slight diagnostic variation this way or that with the early epithelial lesions, from mild dysplasia to microinvasive carcinoma is fortunately a matter of epidemiological rather than main therapeutic importance but greater consistency, if attainable, should be sought. The microscopic staging of the lesions is so wholly subjective that any element open to objective assessment is welcome. One such is the mitotic frequency, and, within that, the individually aberrant mitotic figure. The mitotic frequency in lesions ranging from slight dysplasia to CIS in terms of the WHO recommendations (Poulsen et al., 1975) was found by Chi and his colleagues (1977) to increase in parallel with increasing epithelial disturbance: the increase was evident even if only the upper third of the epithelium was assessed. An objective scheme of grading could perhaps, therefore, be based on mitotic frequency in only the upper third.

The aberrant mitotic figure in its various forms (*see* Kirkland et al., 1967) is objectively demonstrable: therefore, it is a countable unit and as such a valuable unit, yet little or no use has been made of it. All are agreed on its constant, if variably frequent, presence in CIS: could it be used perhaps as the complete discriminator between CIS and the dysplasias, for much greater objectivity would be gained if it were? In the Panel Report by Govan and colleagues (1969), "bizarre mitoses" are admissible in *severe* dysplasia. In the WHO classification mentioned above, but in *mild* dysplasia, "Mitoses . . . occasionally are abnormal" even if, with normal mitoses, ". . . confined to the lower third of the epithelium". At present therefore, objective though it be, the aberrant mitosis despite its potential as an index would seem to be valueless, not only as a pointer to the threshold between dysplasia and carcinoma but even to the degree of dysplasia (uniformity could be achieved by the adoption of an arbitrary standard, say, $x$ normal, or one aberrant, mitosis per $y$ hpf in the upper third of the epithelium: but that is for international groups to consider; continued subjective assessment may be preferred). My own practice is to regard mitosis in the upper third, and more than an occasional aberrant form at any level, as an index of carcinoma. Rather unexpectedly, in his review of these lesions of the cervix, Christopherson (1977), though referring to normal mitotic figures, makes no mention of aberrant forms. The same article includes a warning of, and illustrates, a 'pseudo-invasive epithelial implant' that resulted from a punch biopsy.

*Microinvasive Carcinoma*

The definition of microinvasion is as much of a borderline problem as dysplasia or CIS. With 'breaching of the basement membrane' worthless, microinvasion is now often accepted as penetration of the carcinoma to a depth of no more than a specific number of millimetres beneath the pre-existing basal layer, as, for example, 5 mm in the series of Ng and Reagan (1969) and Christopherson and his colleagues (1976), 3 mm in the series of Seski and colleagues (1977) and 1 mm in that of Averette and others (1976). A depth of 5 mm is generous; few ingrowths as deep with squamous epithelium of similar pattern elsewhere would not be diagnosed as frankly invasive. It may be that the wish to conserve function, and the demonstrably high cure rates over the years, has led to a raising of the diagnostic threshold. Even so, pathologists well know that an ingrowth of 2 mm may be morphologically more sinister than one of 5 mm: observance of rigid criteria may ensure uniformity but is likely to leave the pathologist uneasy. Their own experience and survey of others' results have led Averette and colleagues to conclude that a 5-mm limit carries a significantly higher risk of nodal metastasis than the 1-mm limit they themselves use.

The apparent presence of neoplastic cells within vessels, here as elsewhere, is commonly held as prognostically ominous. Its significance and implications for therapy have been fully examined by Roche and Norris (1975). These authors stress the difficulty of knowing when a space is really a vessel ('capillary-like space' is the term they prefer) and conclude that ". . . neither invasion of what have been considered to be lymphatics nor a confluent pattern of stromal invasion should be a criterion for excluding either the diagnosis of microinvasion or treatment by simple hysterectomy". A substantially similar conclusion was reached by Christopherson and his colleagues in the survey just cited.

However, an analysis by Duncan (1978) of data in seven published series of patients with microinvasive carcinoma has shown that, of the combined total of 554, 47 had been reported as showing 'vascular channel involvement', and that, of these 47, 8 (17%) had developed nodal or other metastases. The matter remains debatable and calls for stricter histological scrutiny. The same problem, the reader will recall, applies in the case of borderline lesions of thyroid. 'Invasion of vessels' may be more often apparent than real, and even when real the correlation with viable metastasis is far from 100%.

A usefully critical analysis of the lesion in 265 patients by Sedlis and his associates (1979) clearly displays the problems of 'microinvasion': for example, in 50% of the cases, the original diagnosis was rejected on review, in most instances (99 patients) simply because microinvasion was considered not to be present. A particular merit of the analysis is that the authors lay down objective criteria for the pathologist and then associate the criteria with recommended forms of treatment. Thus, depth of invasion of 2 mm or more, extent of lateral spread of 4 mm or more, and presence of cells in capillary-like spaces are indications for radical hysterectomy or radiotherapy: lesser measurements, and absence of cells in CL spaces, are indications for simple hysterectomy. (These authors have shared the experience of others that "The 'break' through the basement membrane has not been found to be a particularly useful sign of invasion.")

Some other problems of borderline character in the cervix are diagnostically and prognostically relevant. The verrucous carcinoma, already mentioned, occurs here and causes the same problems of histoclinical discrepancy as elsewhere. An example has been described by Jennings and Barclay (1972). Pregnancy is reported to have no worsening effect on cervical carcinoma (Creasman et al., 1970; Fogh, 1972). The so-called Arias-Stella pattern of the endometrial glandular epithelium in pregnancy may appear also in glands in the cervix, and, with its nuclear polymorphism, might be mistaken for carcinoma (see later).

A borderline problem with therapeutic rather than 'benign or malignant?' implications is exemplified by cases where a cervical biopsy shows glandular carcinoma. Much may depend on the decision whether the lesion is an adenocarcinoma of the endocervix or the endometrium, for the treatment will be as for carcinoma of the cervix in the one, and carcinoma of the corpus in the other. The treatment of these lesions differs: and microscopic distinction between the two is not often simple. Use of the histochemical approach described by Moore and his colleagues (1959) will sometimes help to settle the issue. More recent histochemical techniques involving the use of lectins (Nicolson, 1974; Katsuyama and Spicer, 1978) are proving useful in distinguishing different types of mucin-secreting cells in at least physiological circumstances, and may be found applicable to the cervical lesions in question. Whether, however, their application to the mucins of neoplastic cells will prove equally dependable remains to be seen. The evident difference in CEA content between the two lesions, demonstrable in tissue sections by immunoperoxidase-staining as described by Wahlström and associates (1979), offers a further possible means of distinction.

## ENDOMETRIUM, THE GLANDULAR COMPONENT

### Atypical Hyperplasia

The glandular, and, in more detail, epithelial patterns that comprise atypical or adenomatoid hyperplasia are familiar; equally so are the prognostic problems they cause, succinctly expressed by TeLinde and his colleagues (1953) in the title of their paper, "What are the earliest endometrial changes to justify a diagnosis of endometrial cancer?"

Professional pathologists and others with a strong pathological interest have been trying for nearly a century, since the days of Cullen (1900), to define and identify these 'earliest endometrial changes', and none has succeeded; the borderline zone is little less broad than in 1900. The outcome could hardly be other than failure for the elementary reason that 'carcinoma' is not a particular kind of histological pattern but a disease. Histologically, apart from underlining the significance of the aberrant mitotic figure, attempts to describe and depict particular patterns of glandular and epithelial detail seem no more likely in the future to narrow the zone than they have in the past. The best we can do is to seek the closest degree of histoclinical correlation possible, and accept our limitations. Between the histologically normal at one end, and manifest carcinoma at the other, there is a rising gradient of morphological aberrancy. The gradient is smooth, and somewhere on it each pathologist will have his own step or threshold at which the diagnosis of carcinoma is thought proper. Below the threshold he is likely to use the term 'atypical hyperplasia' or an equivalent; however, if he does, he should be prepared to explain the implications to the clinician, for they are not instantly known to all.

The implication to be conveyed is that the lesion, unlike the almost innocuous cystic hyperplasias (innocuous, that is, qua precancerous condition; it is reckoned by Welch and Scully [1977] to be a cancer precursor in less than 0.4% of cases), represents a significant threat of subsequent carcinoma unless removed by either curettage or hysterectomy. To judge from experience with some cases on file in the Dundee University Department of Pathology, curettage can be curative for at least up to 20 years: hysterectomy, of course, should abolish the risk altogether. However, 'just to make sure', the endometrium of the excised uterus should be examined with total thoroughness, in 12 blocks or more if necessary. Should an area of undoubted carcinoma then be found, decision on further procedure will be the responsibility of the clinician, though he, in turn, may well seek help from the pathologist in trying to answer the question, How malignant is carcinoma of the endometrium?; for it is on the answer to this that the form of these further procedures will depend. The scope and implications of that question will be considered in the next section.

Meantime, for those patients on whom hysterectomy is not performed, what is the prognosis? As mentioned above, some patients at least have no further trouble after the initial curettage, and, in so far as 20 years is an acceptable measure of cure, are cured. In other patients the lesion may progress morphologically to a stage and degree that merits the diagnosis 'carcinoma'. The evidence for this demonstrable fact is mostly retrospective; that is, it is derived from the examination of curettings obtained, perhaps many years earlier, from patients now, on recurettage, found to have what is deemed to be carcinoma. Thus assessed, the risk to a patient with atypical hyperplasia of developing carcinoma was calculated by Campbell and Barter (1961), who divided the hyperplasia in 128 patients into three grades of increasing aberrancy, to be from 15% to 45%. By a slightly different but still retrospective analysis, Beutler and his colleagues (1963) found that of 3000 patients with carcinoma of the endometrium, 54 had had earlier atypical hyperplasia. However, none of these 54 patients and none of the 128 of Campbell and Barter was reported as having died of the carcinoma. Also, an attempt by Welch and Scully (1977) to calculate the risk led these observers to conclude that, for various reasons, of which earlier radiotherapy was one, they knew of ". . . no way to calculate from the data in the literature the magnitude of the risk . . ." In all, it appears that the threat to life represented by atypical hyperplasia is extremely small; the lesion diagnosed in these circumstances as carcinoma would seem mostly to be the 'histologist's cancer', the morphological aberrancy, rather than cancer, the life-threatening disease. That this is likely, gains added support from the further statement by Welch and Scully (who continue to use the term carcinoma in situ) that if 'carcinoma in situ' is extensive ". . . a diagnosis of invasive carcinoma is made with the realization that invasion of the stroma is often impossible to distinguish from proliferation and crowding of non-invasive atypical glands".

Nevertheless, it seems sound practice, on general pathological grounds and *pace* whatever other clinical considerations there may be, to regard atypical hyperplasia as an indication for hysterectomy, at least in the peri- and postmenopausal patient; with the patient who was initially treated by curettage alone, any further bleeding would be a virtually mandatory indication.

## Adenocarcinoma

Diagnostic uncertainty with the more aberrant hyperplasias implies a corresponding uncertainty with the less aberrant carcinomas, for one is the reciprocal of the other, yet the problem is rarely mentioned, at least in relation to the carcinomas. It is remarkable how many series of cases of endometrial carcinoma are published, and conclusions drawn, with no mention of the degree of confidence with which the diagnoses have been made; that is, with no mention of borderline lesions of which the pathologist had said, in effect, 'for practical purposes, carcinoma' rather than carcinoma outright. The omission is surprising in view of the bearing the decision has on figures of, for example, incidence, staging and cure. There are exceptions, of course, such as the series of Javert and Renning (1963), where cases of 'adenoma malignum'[2] are separately listed; that of Christopherson and his associates (1971), where ". . . cases of carcinoma in situ of the endometrium have been excluded from the histologically proved groups"; and that of Joelsson and colleagues (1973) where a 'Grade 0' was excluded as having morphological features ". . . suggestive but not proof of carcinoma" (they were designated 'adenocarcinoma in situ' nevertheless); but their scarcity emphasises the shortcomings elsewhere.

For manifest adenocarcinoma, many schemes of prognostic assessment have been proposed and with few exceptions depth of penetration of the myometrium has been the most reliable predictor. Apart from the important possible exception of certain circumstances in young women (*see* later), cases are few where a curette diagnosis of adenocarcinoma is not followed by hysterectomy. Therefore, with hysterectomy and the opportunity to see and directly measure in the uterus the extent and depth of penetration, the pathologist will have the best predictor literally in his hands: such histological factors as degree of differentiation, nuclear aberrancy and mitotic activity, are then of lesser significance. These

---

[2] The term 'adenoma malignum' is rarely seen now, and yet, in its paradoxical way, it expressed the problem very well. The equivalent term, 'carcinoma in situ' is also disappearing, and rightly, for in this context it is and always has been quite inappropriate: many a manifest carcinoma of the endometrium is equally manifestly still totally within the confines of the endometrium.

histological features would have the greater significance only if they were shown to be negatively correlated with depth of myometrial invasion; that is, if minimally aberrant carcinoma were often maximally invasive, and vice versa, and this seems not to be so.

There are schemes, such as those of Roman and his colleagues (1967) and of Cheon (1969), where various histological features have been allocated numerical values and prognostic 'scores' calculated, but only rarely has the attempt been made to assess the significance, or correlation with myometrial penetration, of any one of the features independently. One such is that of Austin and MacMahon (1969) in which the lesser degrees of nuclear atypia were associated with involvement of (a) the endometrium only, (b) superficial myometrium, and (c) deep myometrium in 81%, 72% and 52% of cases respectively. In other words, the more atypical the cells, the greater the invasiveness. Rather exceptionally (and, in view of some comments above, rather perversely!) these authors found depth of myometrial penetration less prognostically useful than nuclear grading. More in line with the majority view, Lewis (1971) reported that over 50% of patients with a carcinoma penetrating to within 2 mm of the serosa died, while, for four degrees of penetration from 'endometrium only' to 'within 2 mm of the serosa', the incidence of lymphatic nodal metastasis was nil, 2.1%, 12.5% and 41%. Detailed assessment of the histology is likely to add little greater precision.

Retrospective reviews of the histology of endometrial lesions diagnosed as carcinoma are much fewer than of, for example, lesions of lymph nodes. One such was that of Kempson and Pokorny (1968) where the diagnosis of carcinoma in 7 of 22 cases was changed to one of hyperplasia. Another was that of Keller and colleagues (1974) where, of 208 cases originally diagnosed as carcinoma, 48 were excluded since, ". . . histologic review failed to reveal definitive evidence of carcinoma". As the authors laconically say of these cases, "Their inclusion in the series would have improved the survival". It is unlikely that over-diagnosis of some 20% to 30% as found in these series is common but a tendency in this direction seems to exist. Quite the same considerations apply when borderline

tissue aberrancy is confined to endometrial polyps (Salm, 1972).

In view of the approach sometimes made to pathologists for their opinion, and because of the intrusion of borderline morphology, it seems appropriate to include a note on the effect on the endometrium and the risk of carcinoma in patients treated with oestrogens for whatever season, for example, postmenopausally or for gonadal dysgenesis, breast cancer or contraceptive purposes. According to Scully (1977), the risk of the development of carcinoma still cannot be accurately assessed, partly for epidemiological reasons, partly because it has probably been ". . . exaggerated to an unknown extent by the inclusion of cases of reversible atypical hyperplasia". A more recent survey of 451 oestrogen-users and 888 control nonusers by Antunes and his many colleagues (1979) assesses the risk for 'users' as compared with 'nonusers' as sixfold overall but ranging between 2.2-fold and 15-fold depending on dosage and duration of use. At the time of these authors' report, histological sections had been examined by the reviewing group from only 55 patients. The long-term outlook, in effect, the extent to which, again, the carcinomas in this series are morphological cancers rather than truly lethal cancers in potential, has yet to be determined.

### Adenocarcinoma in Youth

There may be doubt still whether the Stein-Leventhal syndrome really is a syndrome but there is ample evidence that, of women under 40 years of age diagnosed as having endometrial carcinoma, many have sclerocystic ovaries with or without such well-known associated conditions as severe menstrual disturbance, sterility, obesity, hypertension and diabetes mellitus. One of the earlier series, describing 46 such patients, was that of Sommers and his associates (1949); others have been analysed by Kempson and Pokorny (1968) and Peterson (1968). In the comparable series of Chamlian and Taylor (1970), endometrial hyperplasia in 14 of their patients progressed to become carcinoma over a period of from 1 to 14 years after initial diagnosis. Progression to carcinoma, when it occurs, is characteristically slow; furthermore, the carcinoma may even, apparently, regress completely after wedge resection of the ovaries or appropriate medication.

Apparent regression, as in one of the patients described by Fechner and Kaufman (1974), and even a later successful pregnancy (O'Neill, 1970), naturally raises questions about the validity and dependability of diagnosis and prognosis. These authors state the problem clearly, thus, "On purely morphological grounds, there appears to be no way to differentiate the endometrial adenocarcinoma which subsequently will have its malignancy reflected by myometrial invasion from the lesion which will not reappear after wedge resection of the ovaries". Further, from a study of their own cases and many described in the literature, Fechner and Kaufman report that ". . . not a single case of well-differentiated adenocarcinoma of the endometrium in a patient with Stein-Leventhal (syndrome) has been proved to metastasize, locally recur, or cause death . . ."; and substantially the same may hold for young women who do not have the Stein-Leventhal syndrome (Kempson and Pokorny, 1968).

The true biological status qua carcinoma of lesions of this kind is clearly debatable but the important implication in practice is that there is no need for precipitate hysterectomy: delay carries little risk, and conservative measures may cure. For the pathologist, the circumstances form a borderline problem of a particularly subtle sort: he cannot solve it but at least he must know it.

### Adenosquamous Carcinoma

The significance of epidermoid change in adenocarcinoma of the endometrium has been debated for decades. Recent reports have revealed a wider difference of opinion than has held hitherto.

For lesions in which both squamous epithelium and glandular epithelium are histologically malignant, the term 'adenosquamous carcinoma' (less suitably, 'mixed carcinoma') is now generally used. For those in which the squamous epithelium is histologically benign, i.e. a simple squamous metaplasia, the term 'adenoacanthoma' is still used by some workers, for example Salazar and associates (1977), but not by others, for example Haqqani and Fox (1976) who include neoplasms of this type in their group of adenocarcinoma. In the opinion of Salazar and his colleagues, the presence in an adenocarcinoma (AC) of squamous elements, whether histologi-

cally benign or malignant, is of no prognostic significance: "Adenocarcinomas of the endometrium with and without squamous elements should be regarded and approached as any pure AC". In the opinion of Haqqani and Fox, on the other hand, "The prognosis for patients with an endometrial adenosquamous carcinoma is very much worse than for women with a pure adenocarcinoma . . .".

The reason for such different findings in the US and the UK, which seem to be real, is uncertain and a matter of much interest but not relevant in the present context. The implication for the pathologist, at least in the UK, is that he will need to decide whether squamous elements in an adenocarcinoma of the endometrium are histologically malignant or not, and for this purpose Haqqani and Fox have given some guidance. In their experience, the main differences between simple metaplastic squamous epithelium and malignant squamous epithelium were:

*Metaplastic epithelium*
Intraglandular
In continuity with glandular epithelium
Does not infiltrate stroma

*Malignant epithelium*
Extraglandular
Not in continuity with glandular epithelium
Does infiltrate stroma

In addition, and as expected, there is in the malignant epithelium a variable degree of cellular polymorphism and mitotic activity, also requiring assessment; the problem is in miniature essentially the same as that of, for example, the solar keratosis of skin. Therefore, his total assessment of degree, type and extent of epidermoid change in an endometrial adenocarcinoma will determine on which side of the borderline between adenocarcinoma (or adenoacanthoma) and adenosquamous carcinoma the pathologist's diagnosis will lie; and the prognostic implications (again, at least in the United Kingdom) seem likely to be significantly different. The relation of the various types of lesion to penetration of the myometrium was not considered by Haqqani and Fox, and was for various reasons difficult to assess in the series of Salazar and his associates: in such a debatable area, further data on the invasiveness of the adenosquamous lesion are much needed.

## Clear Cell Carcinoma

The clear cell variant of adenocarcinoma occurs in the endometrium as well as elsewhere in the female genital tract; it is most familiar perhaps in the ovary but appears also in the cervix and vagina. Its histogenesis has long been debatable (a useful survey is given by Eastwood, 1978) but is not relevant here. An important matter is its resemblance to (metastatic) carcinoma of the kidney. The cells in both lesions commonly contain glycogen (Silverberg and De Giorgi, 1973; Kurman and Scully, 1976), though Eastwood found the amounts in the endometrial lesion to be variable, and separation of the two by ordinary means may be difficult. Ultramicroscopy, however, is reported as showing diagnostically different features (Silverberg and De Giorgi, 1973; Roth, 1974; Ohkawa et al., 1977). For those lacking ultramicroscopic resources, a useful point of differentiation is that the (almost certainly) Müllerian lesion quite frequently shows an admixture of typical or orthodox adenocarcinoma: areas of darker cells, it is true, frequently appear in the renal carcinoma but rarely do they closely resemble a typical adenocarcinoma of the endometrium.

A possibly misleading feature of the clear cell carcinoma is that it sometimes shows nuclear enlargement and polymorphism of the glandular epithelium closely resembling that of the Arias-Stella appearance of 'pregnancy' glands. The reciprocal danger also exists: the nuclear polymorphism of 'pregnancy' glands has itself been mistaken for carcinoma; further, the same polymorphic pattern may appear also in the glands of the endocervix, and be equally misleading there (Arias-Stella, 1959).

As with an orthodox endometrial adenocarcinoma, depth of myometrial penetration is the best guide to prognosis; patients with penetration deeper than 5 mm are much likelier to die than those with shallower lesions. Mitotic incidence, on the other hand, and rather unexpectedly, was found by Kurman and Scully (1976) to be of little value. These authors report a 5-year survival rate of 55.3%, that is, much lower than for the standard endometrial adenocarcinomas.

The clear cell carcinoma has become increasingly familiar as the neoplasm associated with the intake of diethylstilboestrol during pregnancy and consequent transplacental carcinogenesis (Herbst et al., 1974; Poskanzer and Herbst, 1977): to this extent at least its incidence has increased.

## ENDOMETRIUM, THE STROMAL COMPONENT, AND MYOMETRIUM

Overgrowths of endometrial stromal and myometrial origin are considered together in view of their close histogenetic relationship: they are the source of abundant debate.

Impressive accounts of the various lesions concerned, including the mixed mesodermal sarcoma and the carcinosarcoma, are given in the series of articles by Norris and his various colleagues on mesenchymal tumours of the uterus (Norris and Taylor, 1966, 1966a; Norris et al., 1966; Taylor and Norris, 1966; Norris and Parmley, 1975; Kurman and Norris, 1976) and the reader is referred to these for details. The present account will deal only with aspects of mainly borderline diagnostic importance, and with aspects of histogenesis for only so far as seems relevant.

The mainly debatable matters, for practical purposes, appear to be two:

1) Distinction of leiomyomas that are (a) hypercellular or bizarre, (b) 'epithelioid', from leiomyosarcomas.

2) The significance of hypercellular tissue resembling (a) endometrial stroma, (b) leiomyoma, that lies within the uterine wall and its vessels.

## Leiomyoma or Leiomyosarcoma?

In an early study, Kimbrough (1934) believed the best discriminator between benign and malignant leiomyomas to be the mitotic frequency. In general, this still holds. Lesions in 63 patients, all originally diagnosed as leiomyosarcoma (LMS) were reviewed by Taylor and Norris (1966) and reclassified on the basis of mitotic incidence (less than 10 or more than 10 mitotic figures per 10 hpf) as 24 cellular leiomyomas and 39 LMSs. Of the 24 patients, 21 were well (three were 'lost'); of the 39, 29 had died and 2 were still alive with recurrent or metastatic growth. Essentially similar results have been reported by Kempson and Bari (1970), Christopherson and colleagues (1972), and Hart and Billman (1978).

Discrepancies in the counting of mitoses in the same slides by different pathologists have been reported by Silverberg (1976), and some variation is not unexpected, but results such as those in the series just cited must be respected. To some extent the choice of a threshold is arbitrary but the mitotic index most generally agreed is (above or below) an average in the most highly cellular areas of 5 mitotic figures per 10 hpf (though still sometimes mentioned, it is difficult to believe that an experienced pathologist really has difficulty with pyknotic nuclei, squashed polymorphonuclears and the like: a mitotic figure is acceptable as a mitotic figure only if usable as illustration in a textbook).

Nuclear polymorphism is a less reliable predictor. It is true, as Novak and Woodruff (1974) remark, that ". . . although mitosis, regular or irregular, is the basic criterion for malignancy, nuclear pleomorphism is the rule in the most anaplastic lesions". Nevertheless, unlike mitotic activity, polymorphism lacks a comparably independent correlation with later metastasis and has been found quite unreliable as a criterion (see, for example, Taylor and Norris, 1966, and Christopherson and his colleagues, 1972).

These last authors have designated some leiomyomas that were ". . . so pleomorphic and cellular as to make one seriously consider sarcoma", as 'bizarre leiomyoma'; in their opinion, ". . . but for the lack of mitoses they were histologically malignant neoplasms". Such lesions formed part of a series of 81 tumours of smooth muscle, all originally diagnosed as sarcoma. Review on the basis of mitotic incidence yielded:

32 leiomyosarcoma  (24 known deaths)
31 cellular leiomyoma  (no known attributable deaths)
17 bizarre leiomyoma  (no known attributable deaths)

The combined evidence of this series and the others just cited leaves no doubt that the hypercellular myomas of the uterus are markedly prone to over-diagnosis: the wrongly diagnosed may be as many as the rightly diagnosed. It is no surprise that reported cure rates have ranged from 0% to 65% (Christopherson et al., 1972).

A further variant of the uterine myoma was described by Kurman and Norris (1976) as a 'leiomyoblastoma' (epithelioid or clear cell leiomyoma and plexiform tumourlet are synonyms).

The neoplasm shows a mixture of clear cells and eosinophilic cells of varying mitotic activity. Factors prognostically good are a predominance of clear cells, extensive hyalinisation and a circumscribed outline: factors prognostically bad are extensive necrosis and, though of reportedly lesser significance, mitotic activity. The authors recommend, nevertheless, that lesions showing less than, and more than, 5 mitoses per 10 hpf be termed epithelioid leiomyoma and epithelioid leiomyosarcoma respectively. Both clear cells and eosinophilic cells may contain glycogen. Cells of signet-ring contour may also be present but, of diagnostic significance, mucin staining of those in the series of Kurman and Norris was negative.

### Endometrial Pseudo-sarcoma

Suggestively sarcomatous patterns have been reported both in myomas (Fechner, 1968) and in the endometrium (Cruz-Aquino et al., 1967) in association with, and probably as a consequence of, progestogen therapy. The endometrial lesion, named pseudo-sarcoma by Cruz-Aquino and co-workers, is the more important in the sense that over-diagnosis of a lesion as endometrial sarcoma has more serious implications than over-diagnosis of a myoma as malignant. The dissociated pattern of underdeveloped glands and deciduoid stroma, so characteristic of progestogen influence, is partly maintained in the pseudo-sarcoma and would help to avoid error: glands in the just-cited cases had an atrophic appearance.

### Pseudo-sarcoma Botryoides

During pregnancy, but sometimes not during pregnancy, simple polyps of the cervix and elsewhere in the genital tract may become not only large and oedematous but aberrant enough microscopically to be misdiagnosed as sarcoma botryoides or mixed mesodermal tumour: and the mistake has been made. Two examples of the lesion during pregnancy were described by Elliott and his colleagues (1967), one in the cervix, the other in the hymen. Twenty-four examples occurring in the vagina were described by Norris and Taylor (1966b) who had seen also, in pregnant patients, three in the cervix and one in the labium majus. A feature that might particularly mislead the histologist is the presence, on occasion, of aberrant mitotic figures: these are mentioned in an especially helpful passage by Norris and Taylor that emphasises how broadly mimetic the lesion may be, thus, "Abnormal mitotic forms were found only in the 5 polyps having the most numerous atypical cells. These stromal cells resembled the atypical fibroblasts seen in giant cell cystitis, radiation dermatitis and in some examples of nodular (pseudosarcomatous) fasciitis and atypical fibroxanthomas of the skin. No atypical cells were found in the infants' polyps".

The only safeguard against misdiagnosis is awareness that the lesion exists. At the same time it seems proper to mention a possible source of under-diagnosis. One form of mixed mesodermal sarcoma, separately identified by Clement and Scully (1974) as *Müllerian adenosarcoma* (though in this instance only in the uterus and almost exclusively in the elderly), may be of insidiously benign appearance: indeed, in the words of these authors, the lesion is ". . . characterized by a mixture of malignant stromal and benign epithelial elements" to the point where the benign lesion described by Norris and Taylor may be very closely simulated. This variant of mixed mesodermal sarcoma or adenosarcoma appears to be much less aggressively malignant than the more familiar forms. A helpful recent account of the lesion has been given by Fox and his colleagues (1979).

*Stromatous, Stromatoid and Allied Overgrowths*

Lesions of many types make up this group, from the blatant sarcoma of endometrial stroma to the paradoxical 'benign metastasising myoma': and within it are borderline problems of different kinds. It is here, I believe, that histogenesis has relevance.

The uterus starts as a solid mass of mesenchyme that soon becomes canalised. The tissue immediately round the lumen becomes endometrium, with glandular and stromal component, and the rest becomes myometrium. The preamble may be platitudinous but its implication is that cells at any point in the uterus may at any time express the latent capacity they have to differentiate into glands, stroma, and muscle. Further, it seems reasonable to believe that this capacity may be expressed totally or partially, that any lesions arising will therefore be well

differentiated or poorly differentiated, and that any of the types of tissue, like any other tissue, may become neoplastic, whether benign or malignant.

On these assumptions, neoplastic tissue of stromal appearance is not inappropriate in the myometrium, even when quite unconnected with the endometrium (equally, not all foci of adenomyosis need necessarily have arrived in the myometrium by 'invading'). Neoplasms may be stromatous, stromatoid or myomatous, and may or may not include areas of glandular differentiation. Some examples of this tissue ectopia behave in a curious way, though this has no necessary association with their histogenesis. The less aggressive lesions, whether morphologically like muscle or like endometrial stroma, have a notable tendency to grow along channels, some of them certainly veins, others presumably lymphatics or smoothly expanded tissue spaces; and the reason for this is unknown. In some cases the invasive tissue may have grown from the medial coat of a vein, in others from a myoma (Norris and Parmley, 1975). Similar uncertainty surrounds the so-called 'benign metastasising myoma' (see below).

In their analysis of '53 endometrial stromal tumors', Norris and Taylor (1966) divided the 53 into 18 that were well circumscribed ('stromal nodules') and 35 that were infiltrating, subdivided on the basis of mitotic incidence (above or below 10 mitoses per 10 hpf) into stromal sarcoma (20 cases) and 'endolymphatic stromal myosis' (15 cases). Forms intermediate between the two infiltrating ones were few, and this has been my own experience. The quite sharply separable stromal sarcoma is typically a highly aggressive, mitotically active neoplasm, rarely difficult to diagnose. In the seven examples described by Yoonessi and Hart (1977), all seven patients died. Where diagnostic difficulty has arisen, the reason has been almost always not a histological but a nosological confusion with the much less aggressive lesions that microscopically so closely resemble the normal endometrial stroma, namely, the lesions known for a time as stromatous endometriosis (always quite inappropriate), then by a variety of names including stromatoid mural sarcoma (Park, 1949) and stromatosis, and most recently as the endolymphatic stromal myosis of Norris and Taylor. The term 'stromatoid mural sarcoma' (SMS) still seems appropriate; the tissue closely resembles endometrial stroma; it occurs predominantly within the wall of the uterus and need not involve the endometrium; it is always potentially recurrent and may metastasise. Little of this information is conveyed by either 'myosis' or 'stromatosis'.

*Stromatoid Mural Sarcoma.* Small islands of stromatoid cells are not uncommon in the myometrium (one is illustrated by Norris and Taylor, 1966), and may presumably be the source of a stromatoid sarcoma. The difficulty for the pathologist is to know when an overgrowth of tissue of this kind is neoplastic, and, if it is, how aggressive. For practical purposes it may be assumed that by the time an overgrowth has enforced hysterectomy it is neoplastic; that is, it is a sarcoma, albeit a sarcoma of low-grade malignancy. All are prone to local recurrence, mainly because, as the surgeon may see, cords of the typically whitish elastic tissue often extend far into the broad ligament. The pathologist may base his prognostic advice on degree of mitotic activity and margination: however, visible extension beyond the uterus obviously takes precedence, no matter how bland the histology.

*Intravenous Leiomyomatosis.* Uterine veins may be occupied also by muscular tissue, the intravenous leiomyomatosis (IL) of Norris and Parmley (1975). The lesion seems wholly analogous to the SMS with intraluminal extension: in SMS the occupant tissue has differentiated along stromal lines, in IL along muscular lines, to produce any of the many patterns of a leiomyoma. The lesion is intrinsically harmless but, as with the SMS, recurrence will follow if remnants are left in the pelvis, as happened in two of the cases of Norris and Parmley. The lesion has obvious relevance to the controversial 'benign metastasising myoma'.

*Benign Metastasising Myoma.* Metastasis from an apparently benign intrauterine myoma is a rare biological curio, mentioned here only as the logical extension of the entry into veins of stromatoid tissues as SMS, and muscular tissue as IL. Doubts have rightly been raised about the validity of some of the cases decribed but if tissue from a benign myoma can be implanted

and grow in a surgical scar, as Norris and Parmley record, there seems no adequate reason why similar tissue in uterine vessels should not sometimes escape to implant itself in either lymph nodes or lungs as described by Abell and Littler (1975) and Pocock and colleagues (1976) respectively. The experience of Horstmann and his colleagues (1977) with a patient who was found in early pregnancy to have what seemed to be multiple pulmonary fibroleiomyomatous hamartomas that later underwent total spontaneous regression led the authors to conclude that such lesions, as in the case of others described by earlier observers ". . . cannot be distinguished from benign metastasizing leiomyoma by either clinical, roentgenographic, or pathologic criteria and that all represent pulmonary metastases from a primary uterine neoplasm".

## Ovary

### Carcinoma

The long familiar difficulty surrounding the epithelial neoplasms of the ovary was formally acknowledged by inclusion in the relevant WHO classification (Serov et al., 1973) of a category of 'borderline' overgrowths characterised by most of the morphological criteria of malignancy while lacking ". . . obvious invasion of the stroma". Problems in the way of assessing 'invasion' have been sufficiently stressed already. They are no less with ovarian neoplasms than elsewhere, and, indeed, are greater in the ovary than in the case of, say, the cervix uteri where at least there is relatively well-defined layer of surface epithelium for comparison. In the opinion of Scully (1970), in relation particularly to the mucinous neoplasms, degree of papillarity and nuclear aberrancy are the main features of value in judging prognosis; assessment of invasion appeared too subjective to be reliable.

An attempt to gain greater objectivity by the use of 'discriminant functional analysis' of eight histological features in mucinous tumours was made by Blanco and his colleagues (1977). Their rather elaborate statistical calculations showed that discrimination could be made between benign and malignant lesions almost as well by analysis of three of the variables (nuclear aberrancy, degree of cellularity, and mitotic frequency) as of all eight; and the general conclusion was that ". . . by combining these factors . . . a fairly satisfactory prognosis can be made in the majority of cases". The analysis was a good attempt to gain greater prognostic precision from histology and may prove a useful prototype even if the results were probably less discriminant than the authors had hoped.

The formal acceptance of lesions as 'borderline' has revealed, and so in the future may lessen, the amount of over-diagnosis there has been in the past. A series of 688 mucinous tumours analysed in retrospect by Hart and Norris (1973) was found to include 136 in which the diagnosis originally made or considered was cystadenocarcinoma. Review brought a redistribution as 39 carcinomas, 97 borderline lesions; that is, the 'incidence' of carcinoma had been almost halved. In the days when therapy had only surgery, and sometimes irradiation, to offer, over-diagnosis had minor implication. Now, with potent cytotoxic agents available, the implications are more serious. Prognostically useful data were given by Dyson and her colleagues (1971) from their experience with lesions in 319 patients. Mitotic incidence was the best predictor: of patients with tumours showing on average less than one mitotic figure per one hpf, 96% were survivors at 5 years, whereas of those showing more than two figures per hpf only 7% survived. Nuclear atypicality was found to be "not a good guide"; areas of squamous epithelium (adenoacanthoma) did not worsen the prognosis.

Further helpful information has been provided by Scully (1970); for malignant and 'borderline' serous neoplasms, for example, the ten-year survival rates were 13% and 70% respectively. In practice, therefore, the pathologist can rely on the general principle that, with serous and mucinous neoplasms that are histologically aberrant but not blatantly malignant, the probability of survival is likely to be over 70%, and that, substantially in parallel, the less the nuclear aberrancy, the nearer the figure will be to 100%.

The papillary neoplasms of the ovary are those that most bring to mind the apparently spontaneous regression of cancer, seen in the complete resolution of a 'peritoneum full of secondaries' after removal of the primary mass. That the phenomenon exists is undoubted (Taylor, 1959): whether it truly is 'regression of cancer' is debatable and dependent on one's definition of cancer. The matter is not so much one of borderline structure, for the blandest of lesions may spread, as of borderline behaviour. Two views may be held on the relation between peritoneal spread and the primary mass: either removal of the mass removes the source of some metabolite, akin perhaps to the carcinogenic 'mitotic control protein' of Burch (1976), essential for survival of the metastases; or the cells of the metastases have a limited life, and removal of the primary tumour removes the source of successors. Whatever the explanation, the cells' behaviour is at least semicancerous. In practice, the occurrence is too rare to be allowed weight in prognosis: should spread have occurred, there can be only hope of regression (as happened in Case 10.8).

Survival rates at 5 years for other forms of epithelial overgrowth have also been given by Scully. For endometrioid carcinoma the figures are 55% when occurring alone, and 44% when, as not infrequently happens, there is coexistent carcinoma in the uterus. For the closely related clear cell carcinoma (already mentioned in relation to the endometrium) the figure is 37%.

Of ancillary factors with a bearing on prognosis, the significance of rupture of a cystic neoplasm with intraperitoneal spillage of the contents remains debatable. Rupture with spillage did not adversely affect the prognosis in the series of Hart and Norris (1973). In the series of Purola and Nieminen (1968), of 158 cases (all of which, however, were typical cystadenocarcinomas), puncture and suction of the contents had no adverse effects but rupture with spillage was associated with a reduction in 5-year survival of some 30% (the theoretical possibility remains that the tumours most prone to peritoneal implantation are also those most prone to rupture).

### Brenner Tumour

The Brenner tumour may be malignant, though only rarely: most are innocuous but a histologically intermediate form has been described by Roth and Sternberg (1971) as the 'proliferating Brenner tumor'. Structurally it resembles a low-grade papillary carcinoma of the urinary bladder and requires analogous assessment. None of the three examples reported by these authors had recurred at the time of reporting.

*Lipid Cell Tumour*

Lipid cell tumours are regarded by Taylor and Norris (1967) as a separable entity, likely to prove benign if less than 8 cm in diameter and if containing Reinke crystalloids. Extra-ovarian extension need not make the tumour uncurable but tumours ". . . exhibiting sufficient cytologic atypism to be considered histologically malignant probably will prove clinically malignant as well".

*Luteoma of Pregnancy*

A lesion that may mislead is the so-called luteoma of pregnancy (Sternberg and Barclay, 1966; Norris and Taylor, 1967). It may mislead mainly on account of its high cellularity and mitotic activity; not only may mitoses number up to one per 2 hpf, they may be aberrant (Sternberg and Barclay illustrate an unequivocal triaster). Available evidence suggests that the tumour regresses after the pregnancy. Removal is therefore probably unnecessary, at least if the mass is discovered incidentally as may happen at caesarean section, but it may be that only a frozen section will save the ovary; for this reason the pathologist must be aware of the potentially misleading histology. Neoplasms apart, the structure most likely to be simulated by the luteoma is the corpus luteum of pregnancy with its festooned outline and fibrous centre (recent local experience with a Krukenberg tumour during early pregnancy emphasised how substantial the difficulty of distinction from a luteoma can be). It should be recalled that simple ovarian neoplasms may undergo a rapid increase in size during pregnancy (Beischer et al., 1971) and also require assessment by, probably, frozen section.

Next in frequency after the epithelial neoplasms, and in line with overall incidence, problems of prognosis will arise with teratomas and, intrinsically more difficult to assess, granulosa-theca cell tumours.

*Teratoma*

The status of the cystic teratoma (dermoid cyst) is relatively straightforward. Almost 300 examples of malignant change therein have been reported (Climie and Health, 1968): 93% had developed carcinoma, and 90% of these were epidermoid; 7% developed sarcomas. Prognosis varied from good to grave, depending directly on the capsule's being intact or invaded. The occurrence and behaviour of sarcomas arising in teratomas has been given by Azoury and Woodruff (1971) in company with an account of ovarian sarcomas of both pure mesenchymal and paramesonephric types.

In one sense the status of the solid teratoma is also straightforward: the inclusion of "extra-embryonic tissue of yolk-sac origin" (Beilby and Parkinson, 1975) implies a virtual 100% mortality. Tissue of this kind includes apart from choriocarcinoma, any tissue with the relatively wide range of patterns that characterise the endodermal-sinus or yolk-sac tumour of the ovary. The important distinction is made by Beilby and Parkinson between embryonic-type tissue and the type of tissue implied by the widely used term 'embryonal carcinoma'. The tissue most easily recognised in a teratoma, whether cystic or solid, as morphologically identical with its counterpart in a normal embryo is neural tissue, characterised by its neural tubules and rosette formations. Such tissue may show impressive mitotic activity, hence the danger of its being diagnosed as malignant, but the activity is no more than would be appropriate in the embryo; it is in this sense truly embryonic and intrinsically benign. The possibility of confusion with 'embryonal carcinoma' exists, and is the reason for criticism of the term by Beilby and Parkinson. At the same time, even if the term should be rightly condemned, there is room for some other to describe the commonly present sheets of obviously malignant tissue that so closely resembles, but morphologically is not quite, choriocarcinoma: 'undifferentiated carcinoma' seems appropriate.

The clear separation of solid teratomas into those with and those without extraembryonic elements is, for prognostic purposes, an appreciable advance over schemes of grading suggested hitherto. Tissue of yolk-sac type may be a component of a teratoma at any site (Brown, 1976) and also form a pure yolk-sac tumour at the same sites even if no other tissue indicative of a teratoma can be found; at whatever site, the prognosis is uniformly bad. The possibilities of treatment of the lesion by chemotherapy (Wider et al., 1969) and its monitoring by alpha-fetoprotein (Wilkinson et al., 1973; Teilum et al., 1974) are relatively recent developments.

### Granulosa-theca Cell Tumour

The problem posed by the granulosa-theca cell tumours differs from that seen in the epithelial tumours. With the epithelial tumours the border-line zone between 'benign' and 'malignant' may be wide but histologically at least there are certainly benign neoplasms and certainly malignant neoplasms; there is a useful degree of correlation between structure and behaviour. With the granulosa-theca cell group there has seemed, until recently, almost no useful degree of correlation between structure and behaviour, hence the general reluctance to use the term granulosa cell carcinoma (the theca cell element is rarely a source of difficulty). However, recent observations by Fox and his colleagues (1975) on 92 patients with the granulosa cell lesion indicate that much of the uncertainty in the past has been due largely to too short follow-up of the patients.

Whereas Norris and Taylor (1968), from a series of 203 patients, reported a survival rate at 10 years with both pure granulosa cell and granulosa-theca cell tumours of 93%, Fox and his colleagues report that ". . . if no patient died from any other disease, approximately half of the women with this neoplasm would die, as a result of the tumour, within 20 years". In addition, these authors have identified seven features, some fixed, some variable, that are prognostically bad, namely, age over 40 years at diagnosis; abdominal symptoms; palpable mass; solid large tumour; bilaterality; extraovarian spread, and numerous mitotic figures. Of these, the pathologist can directly assess only the mitotic incidence, but even by itself this has no little predictive value. In the series of Fox and colleagues, for example, percentage survivals at 2 years and 20 years with nil mitoses were 96 and 75, whereas with 10 mitoses per 10 hpf the figures were 65 and 32. If, to these statistical probabilities, there is added the clinically based information just mentioned, prognosis can be given with some accuracy. Biologically, the term granulosa cell carcinoma is more appropriate than the non-committal granulosa cell tumour but whichever term is used the histological report should include some estimate of the likelihood of spread and metastasis.

The occurrence of the tumour in children and its relation to precocious puberty have been reviewed by Zangeneh and Kelley (1968) with no suggestion that the neoplasm behaves in any significantly different way in childhood. Two series of cases that they cite had a combined mortality of 12.5%.

Ovarian neoplasms in children (Editorial, 1971) present problems of clinical and therapeutic significance much more than histological.

An indication of spreading attempts to find a sharper separator of borderline neoplasms than the microscope is an account of the use of plasma ribonuclease as a possible index. Investigations by Sheid and his associates (1977) showed no difference in levels between controls and patients with benign ovarian tumours but increased levels in 21 of 22 patients with ovarian carcinoma of different types (most in clinical stages III and IV), and a return to normal values in all cases where ". . . postsurgical examinations indicated complete removal of malignant tissue".

### TROPHOBLAST

Trophoblast is a notorious source of borderline patterns in tissue. However, the clinical worries they cause have by now been largely abolished, though little credit for this goes to the pathologist. Histology has been replaced as assessor by the techniques of applied immunoendocrinology. So successful nowadays is care of the patient with a hydatidiform mole or a choriocarcinoma that an escapist report, 'Potentially malignant trophoblast: HCG supervision recommended', would almost suffice.

Be that as it may, most pathologists would still wish to identify the main areas where trophoblast is troublesome, namely: (a) when cytologically normal, and in company with normal villi, but apparently hyperplastic, (b) as unduly prominent benign chorionic invasion, (c) in any hydatidiform mole and (d) when aberrant in the absence of villi.

Hyperplasia may be simulated when a section has traversed the length of a cytotrophoblastic cell column; that is, the solid column of cells that extends from the tip of a villus, across the maternal blood lake, to the decidua. Whether hypercellularity otherwise is a true hyperplasia or the upper end of a normal distribution of cellular growth cannot be told: if cytologically normal, and in company with structurally normal villi, it appears to be clinically insignificant.

'Benign chorionic invasion'[3] is the proper term to apply to the harmless incursion of trophoblastic cells into the decidua. Some of the large cells may be altered decidual cells but most are chorionic. The process, however, may at times be excessive and far from harmless: there are degrees of incursion. The decidua may sometimes be almost completely replaced by large and polymorphic trophoblastic cells though with little remaining sign of decidual damage, and no haemorrhage. An example of this stage was illustrated in an earlier publication (Park, 1971, Fig. 4): the tissue on that occasion was obtained by curettage 7 days after an abortion.

A more exaggerated form of the phenomenon was seen in local Case 10.9, already described: the patient, to recall, had a successful pregnancy thereafter. The severest form is associated with the invasion and destruction of myometrium, and formation of an obvious mass in the uterus: it was exemplified by two personal cases described also in an earlier report and termed 'atypical choriocarcinoma' (Park, 1975). In each case hysterectomy was curative though, in one of the patients, only after a severe and prolonged illness (accompanied, inter alia, by a nephrotic syndrome). A series of 12 such cases was later described by Kurman and his colleagues (1976) as 'trophoblastic pseudo-tumor'.

With these lesions, the range of semineoplastic and neoplastic trophoblastic behaviour is complete, from the physiological benign chorionic invasion, through the atypical choriocarcinoma or 'trophoblastic pseudo-tumor' and the locally aggressive 'invasive hydatidiform mole', to the rapidly metastasising choriocarcinoma. Only at the lower end of the range is useful histoclinical correlation possible. Beyond that, as already indicated, the prognostic problems of borderline trophoblast, including that covering any hydatidiform mole and aberrant free-lying (non-villous) tissue, cannot be solved by the micro-

scope but with confidence by immunodiagnostic procedures alone.

None of the many attempts to establish or uncover a dependably prognostic correlation between degree of trophoblastic hyperplasia in a hydatidiform mole and its later behaviour has proved sound. All patients who have had a hydatidiform mole are at risk of subsequent choriocarcinoma but the risk may be minimised, if not almost abolished, by regular HCG assay. The scheme now operating in the United Kingdom (Editorial, 1972) provides facilities for the supervision of all such patients in the country. Death from postmolar choriocarcinoma is already of almost historical interest only.

ENDOMETRIOSIS

Foci of endometriosis may appear at many sites and represent some risk of misdiagnosis as glandular carcinoma. Simple frequency of distribution makes the risk greatest with deposits on the caecum and appendix, pelvic colon and rectum (see earlier), and in pelvic or external inguinal lymph nodes of which local Case 10.10 was an instance. A full account of the pathogenesis and possible distribution of endometriotic lesions was given by Javert (1949).

## Conclusions

1) Whatever the type of vulvar cutaneous dystrophy, prognosis depends on the histology of the epidermis.

2) The frequency of mitotic figures, normal and abnormal, in the upper third of the ectocervical epithelium is a possible objective basis for the definition of carcinoma in situ.

3) Microinvasion is widely defined as penetration of the carcinoma to a depth of up to 5 mm beneath the basal layer: 1 mm may be safer.

4) Apparent invasion of vessels in association with a microinvasive carcinoma of cervix has uncertain prognostic significance.

5) For therapeutic reasons, every attempt should be made to distinguish between the adenocarcinomas of cervix and corpus.

6) Atypical hyperplasia of the endometrium, even if untreated, represents a risk of potentially lethal adenocarcinoma of probably less than 5%.

---

[3] Though quite inappropriate, the alternative term 'syncytial endometritis' refuses to die; it appears in the WHO classification (Poulsen et al., 1975) and in the paper by Kurman and colleagues (1976) but at least is parenthesised in both cases. Most of the cells are not syncytial, and the process is not an inflammation.

Usually, however, its diagnosis is followed by hysterectomy: the natural history is thus hard to assess.

7) Cure rates for adenocarcinoma corporis are high: over-diagnosis may contribute to this.

8) Endometrial patterns in young women, especially those with sclerocystic ovaries, may be morphologically identical with adenocarcinoma, yet regress.

9) Adenosquamous carcinoma corporis has a geographically variable prognosis.

10) Clear cell carcinoma in both endometrium and endocervix may be misdiagnosed as the Arias-Stella pattern of pregnancy, and vice versa.

11) Uterine leiomyomas may show great nuclear atypia and are, hence, markedly prone to over-diagnosis. An arbitrary but reasonably dependable borderline is 5 mitoses per 10 hpf.

12) Pseudo-sarcomatous patterns may be induced in the endometrial stroma by progestogen therapy and in polyps by pregnancy.

13) The stromatoid mural sarcoma (stromatosis; endolymphatic myosis) must be distinguished from the sarcoma of endometrial stroma: the stromatoid lesion is much less aggressive but prone to pelvic recurrence.

14) A threshold of 10 mitoses per 10 hpf is a reasonably dependable separator of borderline adenocarcinomas of ovary.

15) The 'pregnancy luteoma' of ovary is wholly benign, and would probably regress spontaneously, but may show misleading mitotic activity.

16) The inclusion in a solid teratoma of ovary of tissue of extra-embryonic type is prognostically bad. Tissue of this kind must not be confused with ('normally' developing) neural tissue of ortho-embryonic type.

17) Half of the patients with a granulosa cell tumour may die therefrom within 20 years of resection.

18) Immunodiagnostic techniques have replaced histological techniques as guides to prognosis in patients with borderline lesions of trophoblast.

19) All patients who have had a hydatidiform mole should be under supervision, with HCG assay, for 2 years thereafter.

20) Endometriosis may be misdiagnosed as glandular carcinoma especially on the colon/rectum and in pelvis-related lymph nodes.

# References

Abell MR, Littler ER (1975) Benign metastasizing uterine leiomyoma. Multiple lymph nodal metastases. Cancer 36: 2206–2213

Antunes CMF, Stolley PD, Rosenshein NB, Davies JL, Tonascia JA, Brown C, Burnett L, Rutledge A, Pokempner M, Garcia R (1979) Endometrial cancer and estrogen use. Report of a large case-control study. N Engl J Med 300: 9–13

Arias-Stella J (1959) A topographic study of uterine epithelial atypia associated with chorionic tissue: Demonstration of alteration in the endocervix. Cancer 12: 782–790

Austin JH, MacMahon B (1969) Indication of prognosis in carcinoma of the corpus uteri. Surg Gynecol Obstet 128: 1247–1252

Averette HE, Nelson JH, Ng ABP, Hoskins WJ, Boyce JG, Ford JH (1976) Diagnosis and management of microinvasive (stage Ia) carcinoma of the uterine cervix. Cancer 38: 414–425

Azoury RS, Woodruff JD (1971) Primary ovarian sarcomas. Report of 43 cases from the Emil Novak Ovarian Tumor Registry. Obstet Gynecol 37: 920–941

Beilby JOW, Parkinson C (1975) Features of prognostic significance in solid ovarian teratoma. Cancer 36: 2147–2154

Beischer NA, Buttery BW, Fortune DW, Macafee CAJ (1971) Growth and malignancy of ovarian tumours in pregnancy. Aust NZJ Obstet Gynaecol 11: 208–220

Beutler HK, Dockerty MB, Randall LM (1963) Precancerous lesions of the endometrium. Am J Obstet Gynecol 86: 433–443

Blanco AA, Gibbs ACC, Langley FA (1977) Histological discrimination of malignancy in mucinous ovarian tumours. Histopathol 1: 431–443

Brown NJ (1976) Teratomas and yolk-sac tumours. J Clin Pathol 29: 1021–1025

Brudenell M, Cox BS, Taylor CW (1973) The management of dysplasia, carcinoma in situ and microcarcinoma of the cervix. J Obstet Gynaecol Br 80: 673–679

Burch PRJ (1976) The biology of cancer: A new approach. MTP Press, Lancaster

Campbell PE, Barter RA (1961) The significance of atypical endometrial hyperplasia. J Obstet Gynaecol Br 68: 668–672

Chamlian DL, Taylor HB (1970) Endometrial hyperplasia in young women. Obstet Gynecol 36: 659–666

Cheon H-K (1969) Prognosis of endometrial carcinoma. Obstet Gynecol 34: 680–684

Chi CH, Rubio CA, Lagerlöf B (1977) The frequency and distribution of mitotic figures in dysplasia and carcinoma in situ. Cancer 39: 1218–1223

Christopherson WM (1977) Dysplasia, carcinoma in situ, and microinvasive carcinoma of the uterine cervix. Hum Pathol 8: 489–501

Christopherson WM, Mendez WM, Parker JE, Lundin FE, Ahuja EM (1971) Carcinoma of the endometrium: A study of changing rates over a 15-year period. Cancer 27: 1005–1008

Christopherson WM, Williamson EO, Gray LA (1972) Leiomyosarcoma of the uterus. Cancer 29: 1512–1517

Christopherson WM, Gray LA, Parker JE (1976) Microinvasive carcinoma of the uterine cervix. A long-term followup study of eighty cases. Cancer 38: 629–632

Clement PB, Scully RE (1974) Müllerian adenosarcoma of the uterus. A clinicopathologic analysis of ten cases of a distinctive type of Müllerian mixed tumor. Cancer 34: 1138–1149

Climie ARW, Heath LP (1968) Malignant degeneration of benign cystic teratomas of the ovary. Review of the literature and report of a chondrosarcoma and carcinoid tumor. Cancer 22: 824–832

Commitee on Terminology (1976) New nomenclature for vulvar disease. Obstet Gynecol 47: 122–124

Creasman WT, Rutledge FN, Fletcher GH (1970) Carcinoma of the cervix associated with pregnancy. Obstet Gynecol 36: 495–501

Cruz-Aquino M, Shenker L, Blaustein A (1967) Pseudosarcoma of the endometrium. Obstet Gynecol 29: 93–96

Cullen TS (1900) Cancer of the uterus: Its pathology, symptomatology, diagnosis and treatment; also the pathology of diseases of the endometrium. Appleton, New York

Duncan ID (1978) Microinvasive squamous carcinoma of cervix in the Tayside Region of Scotland 1960–1973. Communication to Third World Congress on Cervical Pathology and Colposcopy, Orlando, California

Dyson JL, Beilby JOW, Steele SJ (1971) Factors influencing survival in carcinoma of the ovary. Br J Cancer 25: 237–249

Eastwood J (1978) Mesonephroid (clear cell) carcinoma of the ovary and endometrium. A comparative prospective clinico-pathological study and review of literature. Cancer 41: 1911–1928

Editorial (1971) Ovarian tumours in infants and children. Br Med J 4: 762–763

Editorial (1972) New follow-up of hydatidiform mole. Br Med J 4: 685–686

Elliott GB, Reynolds HA, Fidler HK (1967) Pseudosarcoma botryoides of cervix and vagina in pregnancy. J Obstet Gynaecol Br 74: 728–733

Fechner RE (1968) Atypical leiomyomas and synthetic progestin therapy. Am J Clin Pathol 49: 697–703

Fechner RE, Kaufman RH (1974) Endometrial adenocarcinoma in Stein-Leventhal syndrome. Cancer 34: 444–452

Fogh I (1972) Cancer colli uteri and pregnancy. Cancer 29: 114–116

Fox H, Agrawal K, Langley FA (1975) A clinicopathologic study of 92 cases of granulosa cell tumor of the ovary with special reference to the factors influencing prognosis. Cancer 35: 231–241

Fox H, Harilal KR, Youell A (1979) Müllerian adenosarcoma of the uterine body: A report of nine cases. Histopathol 3: 167–180

Govan ADT, Haines RM, Taylor CW, Woodcock AS (1969) The histology and cytology of changes in the epithelium of the cervix uteri. J Clin Pathol 22: 383–395

Green GH (1979) Screening and cervical cancer. Lancet I: 40

Haqqani MT, Fox H (1976) Adenosquamous carcinoma of the endometrium. J Clin Pathol 29: 959–966

Hart WR, Billman JK (1978) A reassessment of uterine neoplasms originally diagnosed as leiomyosarcomas. Cancer 41: 1902–1910

Hart WR, Millman JB (1977) Progression of intraepithelial Paget's disease of the vulva to invasive carcinoma. Cancer 40: 2333–2337

Hart WR, Norris HJ (1973) Borderline and malignant mucinous tumors of the ovary: Histologic criteria and clinical behavior. Cancer 31: 1031–1045

Herbst AL, Robboy SJ, Scully RE, Poskanzer DC (1974) Clear-cell adenocarcinoma of the vagina and cervix in girls: Analysis of 170 registry cases. Am J Obstet Gynecol 119: 713–724

Horstmann JP, Pietra GG, Harman JA, Cole NG, Grinspan S (1977) Spontaneous regression of pulmonary leiomyomas during pregnancy. Cancer 39: 314–321

Javert CT (1949) Pathogenesis of endometriosis based on endometrial homeoplasia, direct extension, exfoliation and implantation, lymphatic and hematogenous metastasis (including five case reports of endometrial tissue in pelvic lymph nodes). Cancer 2: 399–410

Javert CT, Renning EL (1963) Endometrial cancer. Survey of 610 cases treated at Woman's Hospital (1919–1960). Cancer 16: 1057–1064

Jennings RH, Barclay DL (1972) Verrucous carcinoma of the cervix. Cancer 30: 430–434

Joelsson I, Sandri A, Kottmeier HL (1973) Carcinoma of the uterine corpus. A retrospective survey of individualized therapy. Acta Radiol [Suppl] (Stockh) 334

Katsuyama T, Spicer SS (1978) Histochemical differentiation of complex carbohydrates with variants of the concanavalin A-horseradish peroxidase method. J Histochem Cytochem 26: 233–250

Kaufman RH, Gardner HL, Brown D, Beyth Y (1974) Vulvar dystrophies: An evaluation. Am J Obstet Gynecol 120: 363–367

Keller D, Kempson RL, Levine G, McLennan C (1974) Management of the patient with early endometrial carcinoma. Cancer 33: 1108–1116

Kempson RL, Bari W (1970) Uterine sarcomas. Classification, diagnosis, and prognosis. Hum Pathol 1: 331–349

Kempson RL, Pokorny GE (1968) Adenocarcinoma of the endometrium in women aged forty and younger. Cancer 21: 650–662

Kimbrough RA (1934) Sarcoma of uterus: Factors influencing results of treatment. Am J Obstet Gynecol 28: 12–17

Kirkland JA, Stanley MA, Cellier KM (1967) Comparative study of histologic and chromosomal abnormalities in cervical neoplasia. Cancer 20: 1934–1952

Kurman RJ, Norris HJ (1976) Mesenchymal tumors of the uterus. VI. Epithelioid smooth muscle tumors including leiomyoblastoma and clear-cell leiomyoma. A clinical and pathologic analysis of 26 cases. Cancer 37: 1853–1865

Kurman RJ, Scully RE (1976) Clear cell carcinoma of the endometrium. An analysis of 21 cases. Cancer 37: 872–882

Kurman RJ, Scully RE, Norris HJ (1976) Trophoblastic pseudotumor of the uterus. An exaggerated form of 'syncytial endometritis' simulating a malignant tumor. Cancer 38: 1214–1226

Lewis BV (1971) Nodal spread in relation to penetration and differentiation. Proc R Soc Med 64: 406–407

Moore RB, Reagan JW, Schoenberg MD (1959) The mucins of the normal and cancerous uterine mucosa. Cancer 12: 215–221

Ng ABP, Reagan JW (1969) Microinvasive carcinoma of the uterine cervix. Am J Clin Pathol 52: 511–529

Nicolson GL (1974) The interactions of lectins with animal cell surfaces. Int Rev Cytol 39: 89–190

Norris HJ, Parmley T (1975) Mesenchymal tumors of the uterus, V, intravenous leiomyomatosis. A clinical and pathologic study of 14 cases. Cancer 36: 2164–2178

Norris HJ, Taylor HB (1966) Mesenchymal tumors of the uterus. I. A clinical and pathological study of 53 endometrial stromal tumors. Cancer 19: 755–766

Norris HJ, Taylor HB (1966a) Mesenchymal tumors of the uterus. III. A clinical and pathologic study of 31 carcinosarcomas. Cancer 19: 1459–1465

Norris HJ, Taylor HB (1966b) Polyps of the vagina. A benign lesion resembling sarcoma botryoides. Cancer 19: 227–232

Norris HJ, Taylor HB (1967) Nodular theca-lutein hyperplasia of pregnancy (so-called 'pregnancy luteoma'). A clinical and pathologic study of 15 cases. Am J Clin Pathol 47: 557–566

Norris HJ, Taylor HB (1968) Prognosis of granulosa-theca tumors of the ovary. Cancer 21: 255–263

Norris HJ, Roth E, Taylor HB (1966) Mesenchymal tumors of the uterus. II. A clinical and pathologic study of 31 mixed mesodermal tumors. Obstet Gynecol 28: 57–63

Novak ER, Woodruff JD (1974) In: Novak ER (ed) Gynecologic and obstetric pathology, 7th edn. Saunders, London

Ohkawa K, Amasaki H, Terashima Y, Aizawa S, Ishikawa E (1977) Clear cell carcinoma of the ovary. Light and electron microscopic studies. Cancer 40: 3019–3029

O'Neill RT (1970) Pregnancy following hormonal therapy for adenocarcinoma of the endometrium. Am J Obstet Gynecol 108: 318–321

Park WW (1949) The nature of stromatous endometriosis. J Obstet Gynaecol Br 56: 759–776

Park WW (1971) Choriocarcinoma. A study of its pathology. Heinemann, London

Park WW (1975) Possible functions of nonvillous trophoblast. Eur J Obstet Gynecol Repro Biol 5: 35–46

Peterson EP (1968) Endometrial carcinoma in young women: A clinical profile. Obstet Gynecol 31: 702–707

Pocock E, Craig JR, Bullock WK (1976) Metastatic uterine leiomyomata. A case report. Cancer 38: 2096–2100

Poskanzer DC, Herbst AL (1977) Epidemiology of vaginal adenosis and adenocarcinoma associated with exposure to stilbestrol in utero. Cancer 39: 1892–1895

Poulsen HE, Taylor CW, Sobin LH (1975) Histological typing of female genital tract tumours. International histological classification of tumours, 13. WHO, Geneva

Purola F, Nieminen U (1968) Does rupture of cystic carcinoma during operation influence the prognosis? Ann Chir Gynaecol 57: 615–617

Ringsted J, Amtrup F, Asklund C, Baunsgaard P and 11 others (1978) Reliability of histo-pathological diagnosis of squamous epithelial changes of the uterine cervix. Acta Pathol Microbiol Scand (A) 86: 273–278

Roche WD, Norris HJ (1975) Microinvasive carcinoma of the cervix. The significance of lymphatic invasion and confluent patterns of stromal growth. Cancer 36: 180–186

Roman TN, Beck RP, Latour JPA (1967) Correlation of histologic grading with 5 yr survival rate in endometrial carcinoma. Am J Obstet Gynecol 97: 117–119

Roth LM (1974) Clear-cell adenocarcinoma of the female genital tract. A light and electron microscopic study. Cancer 33: 990–1001

Roth LM, Sternberg WH (1971) Proliferating Brenner tumors. Cancer 27: 687–693

Salazar OM, Papp EW de, Bonifiglio TA, Feldstein ML, Rubin P, Rudolph JH (1977) Adenosquamous carcinoma of the endometrium. An entity with an inherent poor prognosis? Cancer 40: 119–130

Salm R (1972) The incidence and significance of early carcinomas in endometrial polyps. J Pathol 108: 47–53

Scully RE (1970) Recent progress in ovarian cancer. Hum Pathol 1: 73–98

Scully RE (1977) Estrogens and endometrial carcinoma. Hum Pathol 8: 481–483

Sedlis A, Sall S, Tsukada Y, Park R, Mangan C, Shingleton H, Blessing JA (1979) Microinvasive carcinoma of the uterine cervix: A clinical-pathologic study. Am J Obstet Gynecol 133: 64–74

Serov SF, Scully RE, Sobin LH (1973) Histological typing of ovarian tumours. International histological classification of tumours, 9. WHO, Geneva

Seski JC, Abell MR, Morley GW (1977) Microinvasive squamous carcinoma of the cervix. Definition, histologic analysis, late results of treatment. Obstet Gynecol 50: 410–414

Sheid B, Lu T, Pedrinan L, Nelson JH (1977) Plasma ribonuclease. A marker for the detection of ovarian cancer. Cancer 39: 2204–2208

Silverberg SG (1976) Reproducibility of the mitosis count in the histologic diagnosis of smooth muscle tumors of the uterus. Hum Pathol 7: 451–454

Silverberg SG, Giorgi LS de (1973) Clear cell carcinoma of the endometrium. Clinical, pathologic, and ultrastructural findings. Cancer 31: 1127–1140

Sommers SC, Hertig AT, Bengloff H (1949) Genesis of endometrial carcinoma. II. Cases 19 to 35 years old. Cancer 2: 957–963

Sternberg WH, Barclay DL (1966) Luteoma of pregnancy. Am J Obstet Gynecol 95: 165–181

Sworn MJ, Hammond GT, Buchanan R (1979) Metastatic basal cell carcinoma of the vulva. Case report. Br J Obstet Gynaecol 86: 332–334

Taylor HB, Norris HJ (1966) Mesenchymal tumors of the uterus. IV. Diagnosis and prognosis of leiomyosarcomas. Arch Pathol 82: 40–44

Taylor HB, Norris HJ (1967) Lipid cell tumors of the ovary. Cancer 20: 1953–1962

Taylor HC (1959) Studies in the clinical and biological evolution of adenocarcinoma of the ovary. J Obstet Gynaecol Br 66: 827–842

Teilum G, Albrechtsen R, Norgaard-Pedersen B (1974) Immunoflourescent localization of alpha-fetoprotein synthesis in endodermal sinus tumor (yolk sac tumor). Acta Pathol Microbiol Scand [A] 82: 586–588

TeLinde RW, Jones HW, Galvin GA (1953) What are the earliest endometrial changes to justify a diagnosis of endometrial cancer? Am J Obstet Gynecol 66: 953–969

Wahlström T, Lindgren J, Korhonen M, Seppälä M (1979) Distinction between endocervical and endometrial adenocarcinoma with immunoperoxidase staining of carcinoembryonic antigen in routine histological tissue specimens. Lancet II: 1159–1160

Welch WR, Scully RE (1977) Precancerous lesions of the endometrium. Hum Pathol 8: 503–512

Wider JA, Marshall JR, Bardin CW, Lipsett MB, Ross GT (1969) Sustained remissions after chemotherapy for primary ovarian cancers containing choriocarcinoma. N Engl J Med 280: 1439–1442

Wilkinson EJ, Friedrich EG, Hosty TA (1973) Alphafetoprotein and endodermal sinus tumor of the ovary. Am J Obstet Gynecol 116: 711–714

Yoonessi M, Hart WR (1977) Endometrial stromal sarcomas. Cancer 40: 898–906

Zangeneh F, Kelley VC (1968) Granulosa-theca-cell tumor of the ovary in children. Am J Dis Child 115: 494–508

# 11 Some Miscellaneous Lesions

Each of the lesions in the local series comprising the background to this chapter had caused prognostic uncertainty either because the diagnosis was uncertain or because the lesion, though correctly identified at the time, had been shown by later events to have belied earlier apprehensions. In one of the cases the diagnosis was unequivocal (carcinoma of kidney) but the behaviour of the lesion examplified well the occasionally unpredictable character of the neoplasm. Some other borderline or possibly misleading lesions were recalled by these cases.

## CASE DATA

### Case 11.1

M (3 months). Failure to thrive. Admitted to hospital gravely ill with pyrexia, vomiting and sweating (sweating had been profuse from birth). X-ray showed a mediastinal mass. The mass, not adherent to lung, was enucleated.

The lesion was a highly cellular polymorphic neoplasm containing many foci of finely granular calcific deposit (Figs. 11.1, 11.2). Such stroma as was visible was finely fibrillar. The initial diagnosis of 'a sarcomatous growth' was later amplified to one of neuroblastoma. No rosette-like formations were present.

The patient remains well 28 years later (the profuse sweating had ceased from the time of operation). Remnants of the neoplasm, if any, still in situ after the enucleation had presumably either regressed or undergone maturation. These details bring up to date an earlier full account of the case (Alexander, 1951).

### Case 11.2

F (32 years) with backache, root pain and sensory loss related to D 10. The tissue removed was an oval extramedullary mass, 20 × 15 mm; it had been adherent to the dura.

The pattern was typically that of a meningioma of relatively high cellularity (Fig. 11.3). The degree of mitotic activity was over 6 per hpf in some areas: part of one such area is seen in Fig. 11.4. Adequacy of clearance was in doubt, and recurrence was mentioned in the report as quite likely to appear.

No further treatment was given. The patient recovered well and remains fully fit 12 years later. This case served to raise appreciably the threshold for optimism in later predictions about the likely behaviour of hypercellular meningiomas.

### Case 11.3

M (62 years) with 30-year history of personality disturbance. Recent history suggested presence of intracranial mass. Craniotomy revealed a unilateral haematoma replacing much of one frontal lobe. Parts of the wall of the haematoma were removed.

The cortical substance was coarsely granular and degenerative and included many nuclei of appreciably variable size and configuration (Fig. 11.5). Not all such cells were necessarily degenerate or dead to the extent that some were still engaged in mitotic activity (Fig. 11.6). The final decision, however, was that the process was one of degeneration and limited reaction rather than neoplasia.

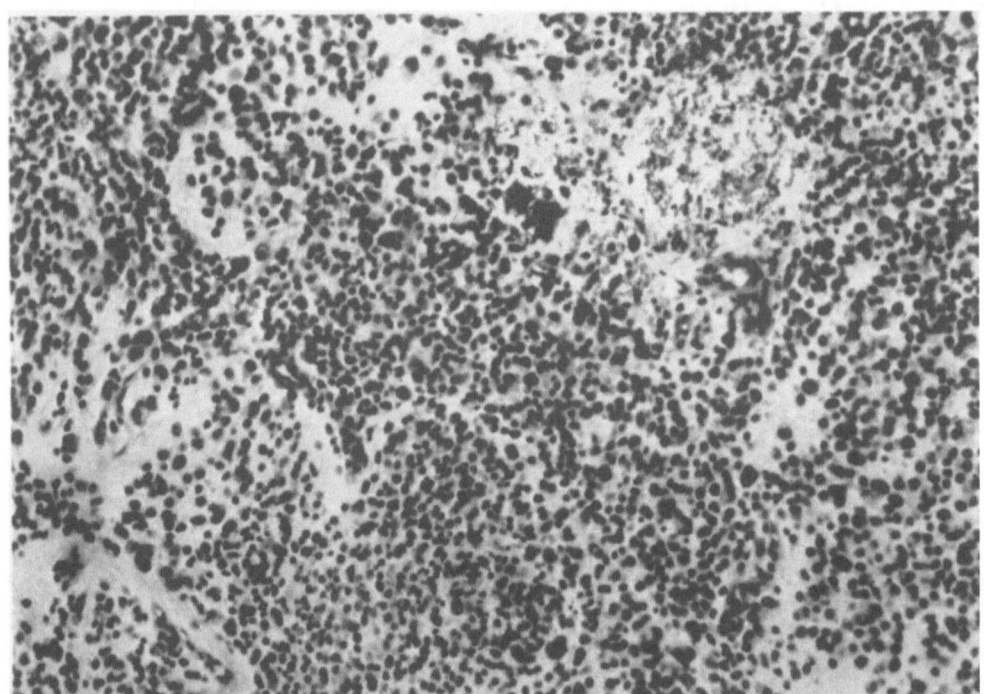

**Fig. 11.1.** At even this magnification, the polymorphism of the highly cellular tissue is evident. The finely granular focus at upper right represents calcific deposit of which there were many similar clusters. H & E, × 123

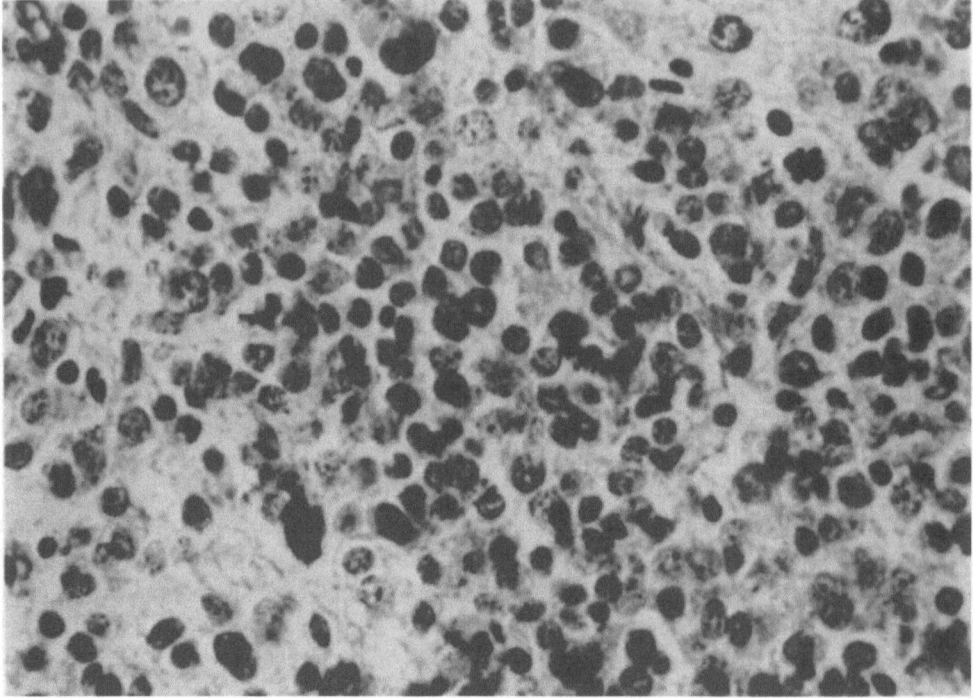

**Fig. 11.2.** The polymorphism is even more evident. The three mitoses in the field (*upper right-hand corner*; an obvious disaster *below upper edge towards left*; the pyknotic mass midway *between centre and lower left corner*) are a fair representation of the mitotic frequency. H & E, × 484

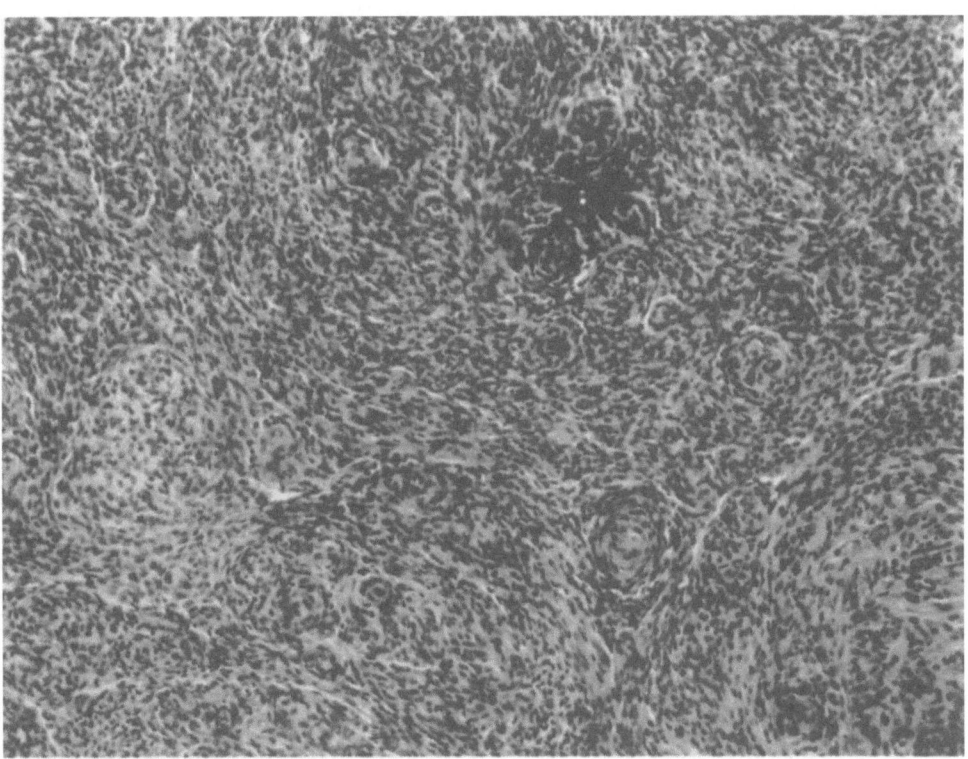

**Fig. 11.3.** Shows the broadly whorled pattern and high cellularity of the meningioma. H & E, × 140

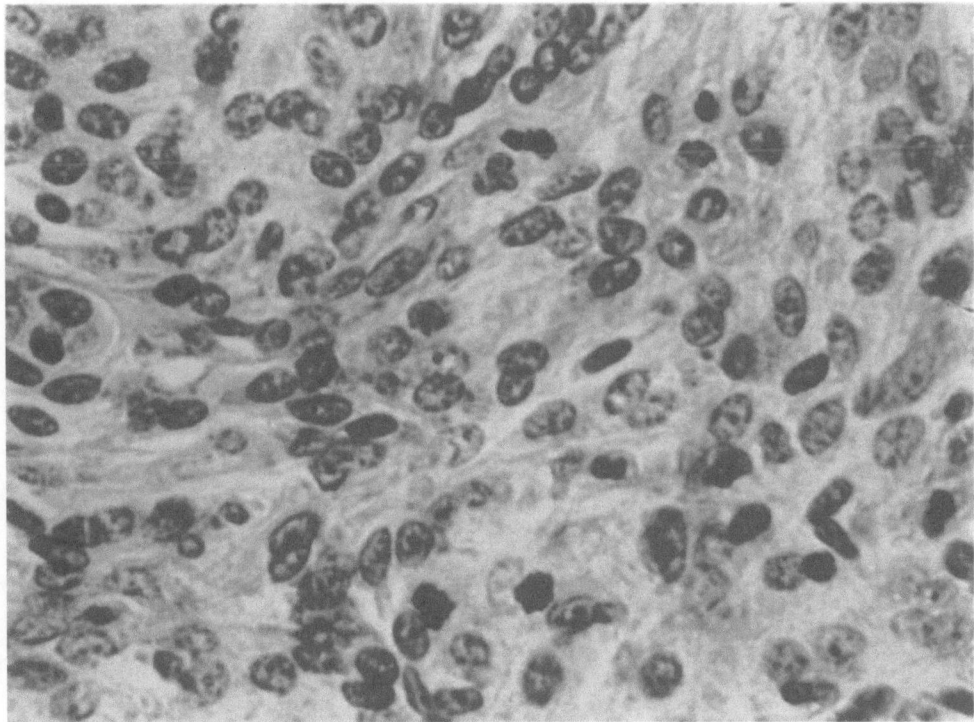

**Fig. 11.4.** In highly cellular areas such as this, mitotic figures, of which three are present in this field, were numerous. H & E, × 985

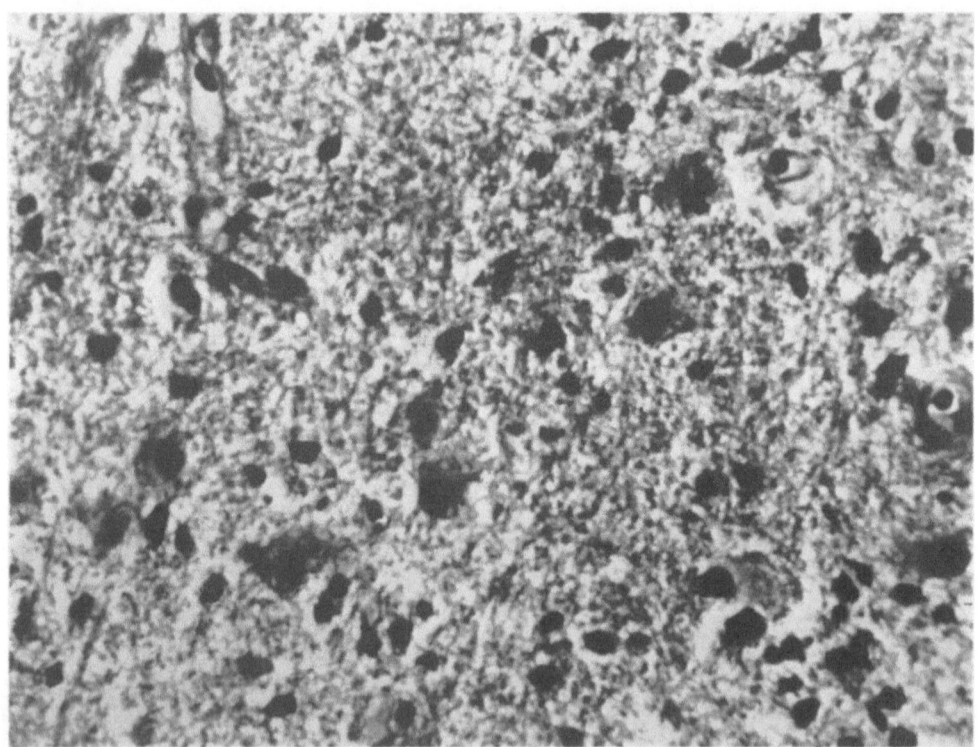

**Fig. 11.5.** Nuclear enlargement and polymorphism in cells around the edge of a haematoma. H & E, × 493

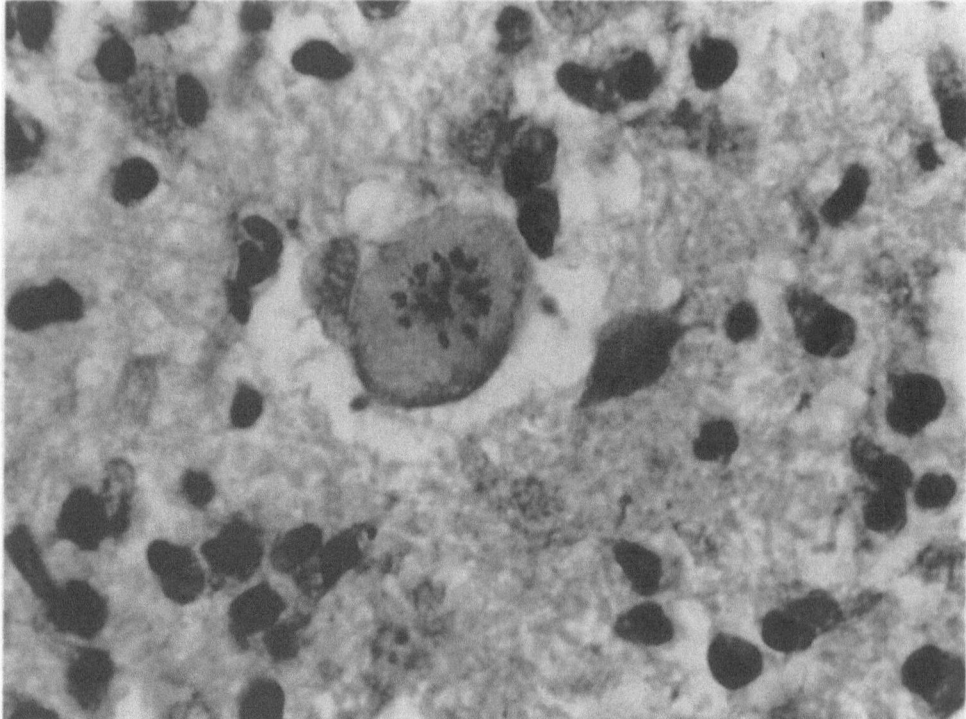

**Fig. 11.6.** Scattered cells in similar areas were in mitosis. They were presumably neuroglial. H & E, × 985

The patient recovered well from the operation but psychiatric disability persisted until his death 2 years later from bronchopneumonia generated by a bronchial carcinoma as revealed by necropsy. The brain showed only gliosis and vascular proliferation around the site of the earlier haematoma. There was no indication at necropsy of metastatic involvement of the brain, nor any suggestion on review of the original sections that metastasis had been the basis of the haematoma (the aetiology of the haematoma was never discovered: in view of the 30-year history, any direct relation to the psychiatric state seems quite improbable).

Mitotic activity and nuclear polymorphism in scattered cells, presumably astrocytic or microglial, did not on this occasion indicate neoplasia, primary or secondary.

## Case 11.4

M (51 years) with signs and symptoms of CNS disturbance. Fragmented material was received from an area of softening in the occipital region.

As in Case 11.3, the tissue had a generally degenerate appearance but in this instance finely rather than coarsely granular. Nuclei were again enlarged but mostly vesicular rather than pyknotic (Fig. 11.7). The similarity was continued by the presence of scattered large cells in mitosis, usually in areas where, for whatever reason, other nuclei were pyknotic (Fig. 11.8). The impression of degeneration rather than neoplasia prevailed, and the equivalent opinion was reported.

Further investigations preceded a further craniotomy with production of a 5-cm block of tissue containing an obvious vascular malformation with partial thrombosis and associated softening. The patient remains well 5 years later.

This specimen was received shortly after that of the preceding case and reinforced the belief that nuclear enlargement, polymorphism and occasional mitotic activity amongst presumably glial cells are not per se an indication of neoplasia.

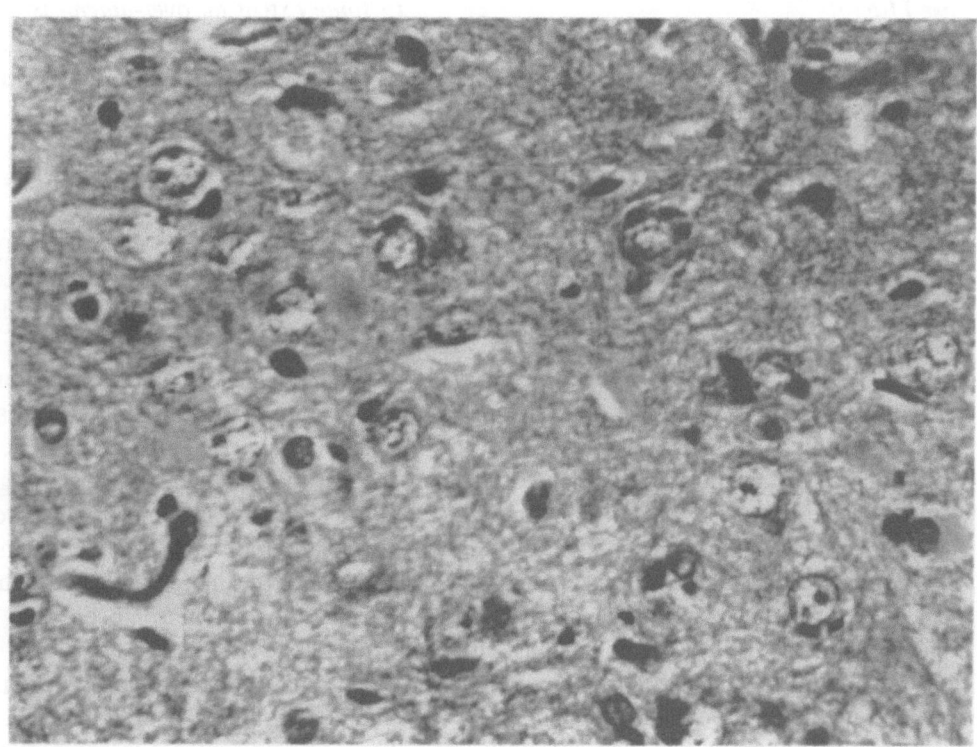

**Fig. 11.7.** A finely granular disorganised background containing cells with large vesicular nuclei. H & E, × 493

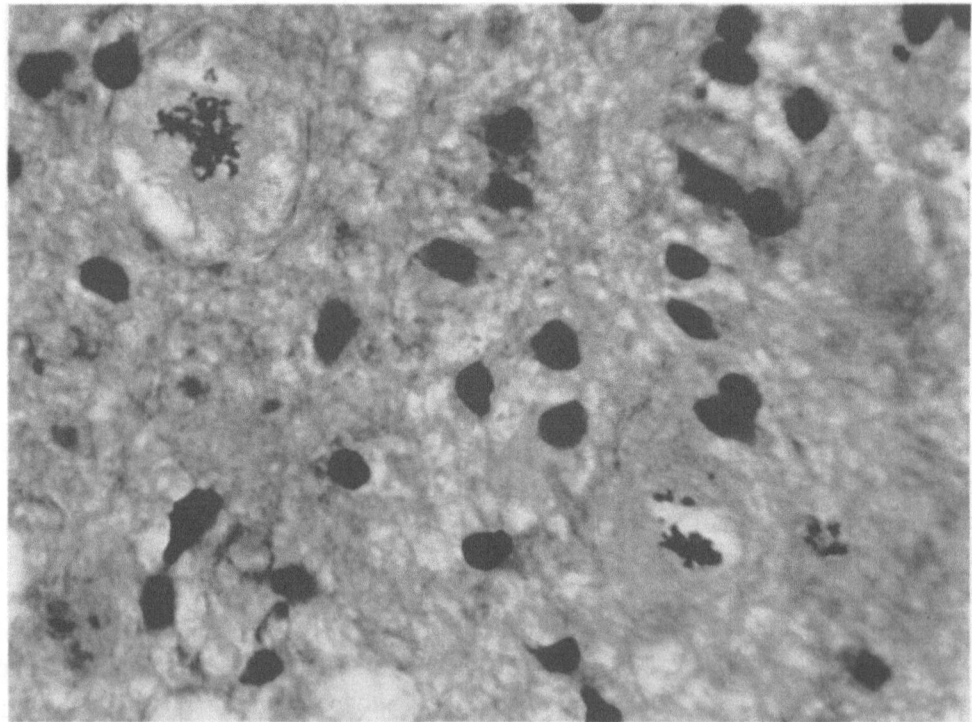

**Fig. 11.8.** Two of the nuclei are in mitosis, the larger possibly polyploid. H & E, × 985

*Case 11.5*

F (20 years) with a 5-mm yellowish nodule arising from the root of the iris and clearly visible through the cornea. It was removed by local iridectomy.

The pattern and composition of the nodule are shown in Figs, 11.9 to 11.12 inclusive. It had been described as a 'highly cellular and slightly pleomorphic mesoblastic tumour' and was diagnosed as a 'low-grade fibrosarcoma'. The eye was then removed.

There was no further trouble and the patient remains well 30 years later.

The degree of cellularity and pleomorphism were no greater than may be seen in many quite benign mesodermal tumours, and mitoses were very infrequent. The rather 'packeted' arrangement, most pronounced just beneath the deeply pigmented surface of the iris and emphasised by reticulin staining, is unusual for a myoma. However, despite the rather atypical reticulin pattern, this was the generally favoured diagnosis on review many years after the original events.

Designation of the lesion as sarcomatous was

to some extent an over-diagnosis in that probably little risk would have been entailed by waiting to observe the longer-term outcome of the iridectomy.

*Case 11.6*

F (48 years) with a 3-month history of increasing proptosis and downward displacement of the eye unaccompanied by pain or discoverable abnormality elsewhere. An oval 15 × 10 mm mass was excised from the wall of the orbital cavity.

Bisection showed a mottled cut surface, with small central cyst (Fig. 11.13). The pattern was 'mixed' to the extent of consisting of glanduliform structures in some areas, more solid sheets of vaguely epidermoid appearance in others (Fig. 11.14). In the more solid areas, the cells were considerably polymorphic and not infrequently in mitosis (Fig. 11.15).

The mass was diagnosed as an 'adenocarcinomatous mixed tumour of lachrymal gland'. There was no evidence in any part of the section to suggest that the nodule was once a lymph node, now wholly replaced by carcinoma.

The patient was further treated by radiotherapy, and the prognosis was considered to be not good.

The patient remains well 15 years later. Despite its cellularity and mitotic activity the lesion clearly had a low capacity for metastasis. Remnants, if any, had presumably been destroyed by the radiotherapy.

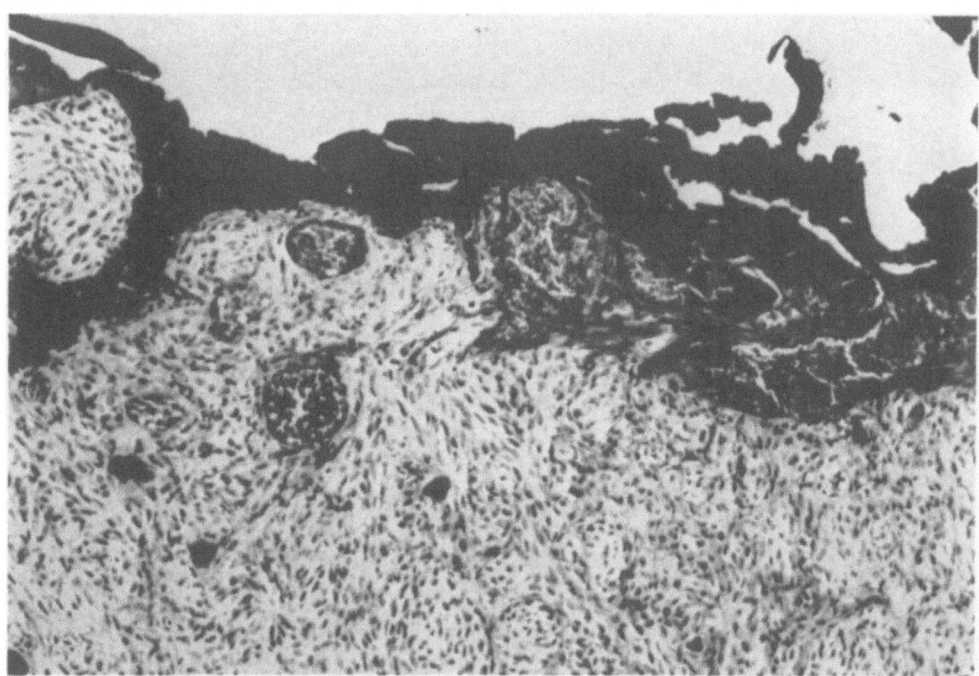

**Fig. 11.9.** Moderately highly cellular tissue extends downwards from immediately beneath the pigmented surface of the iris. H & E, × 123

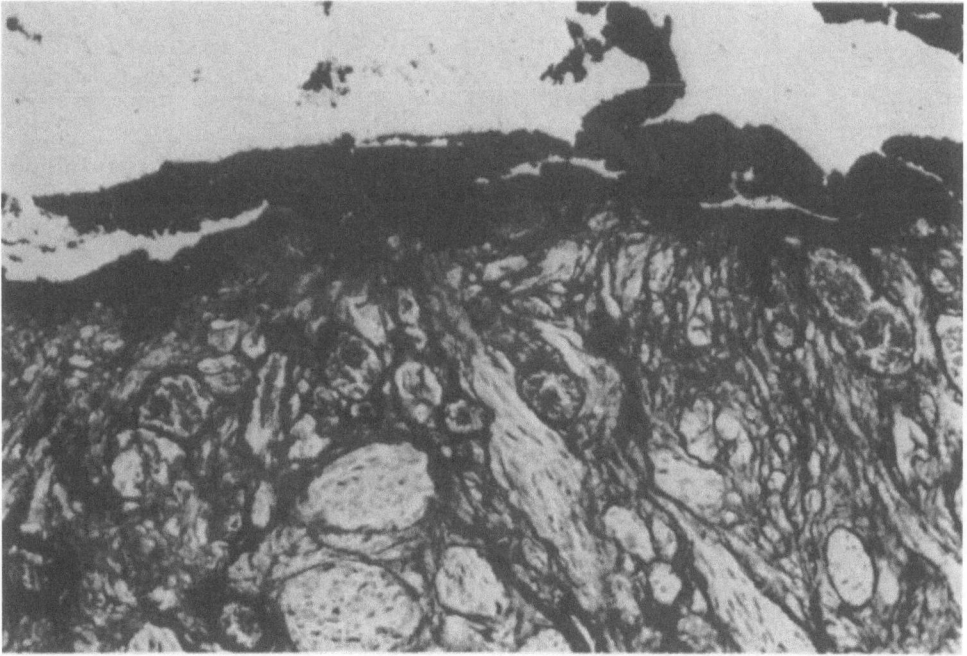

**Fig. 11.10.** A deeper section from the same block shows subdivision of the neoplastic tissue by a variably dense framework of reticulin fibres. Reticulin, × 123

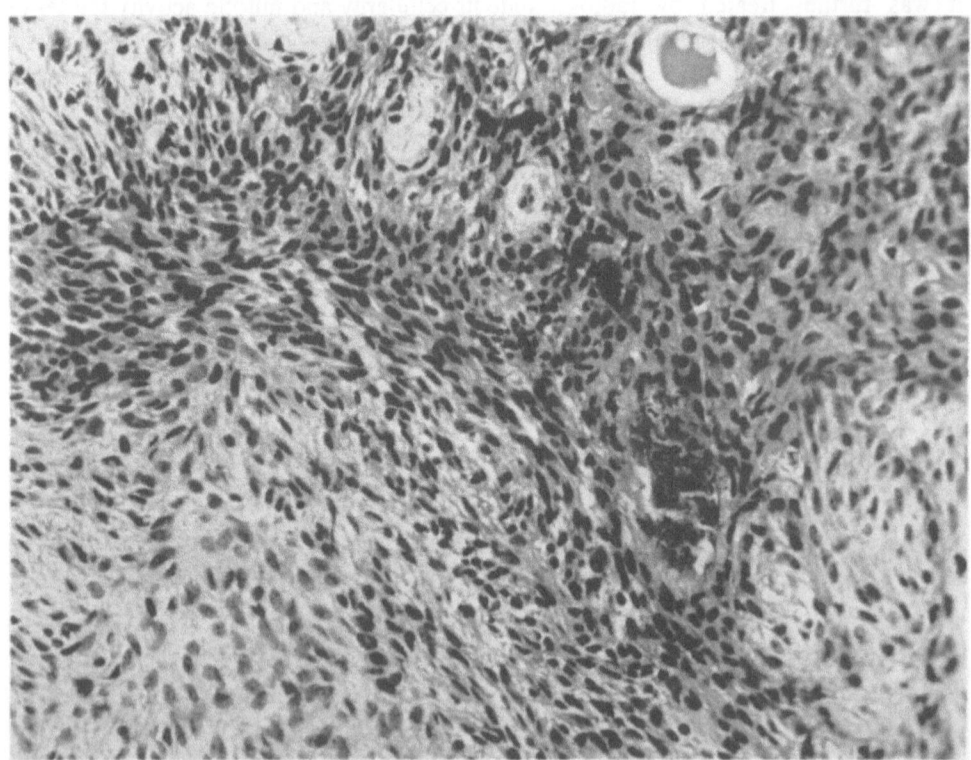

**Fig. 11.11.** The cells are not unduly polymorphic (and were only rarely in mitosis). The lumina along the upper edge are those of arterioles and venules. H & E, × 273

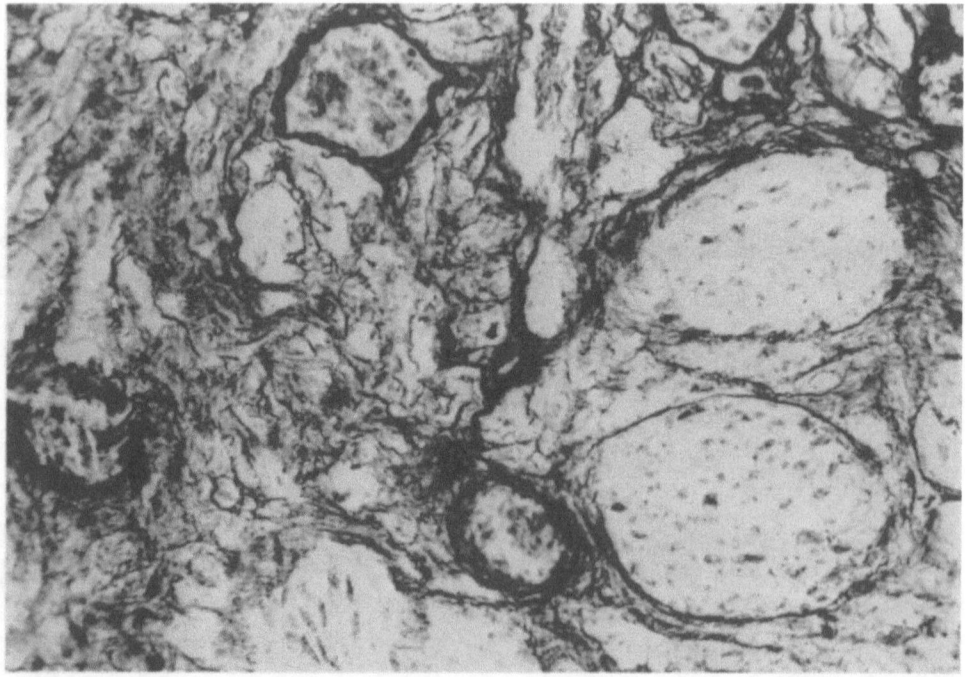

**Fig. 11.12.** An area, again from deeper in the same block, shows the reticulin framework thinning out towards the deeper part of the mass. In the deepest parts, representing 90% of the mass, it was wholly absent. Reticulin, × 273

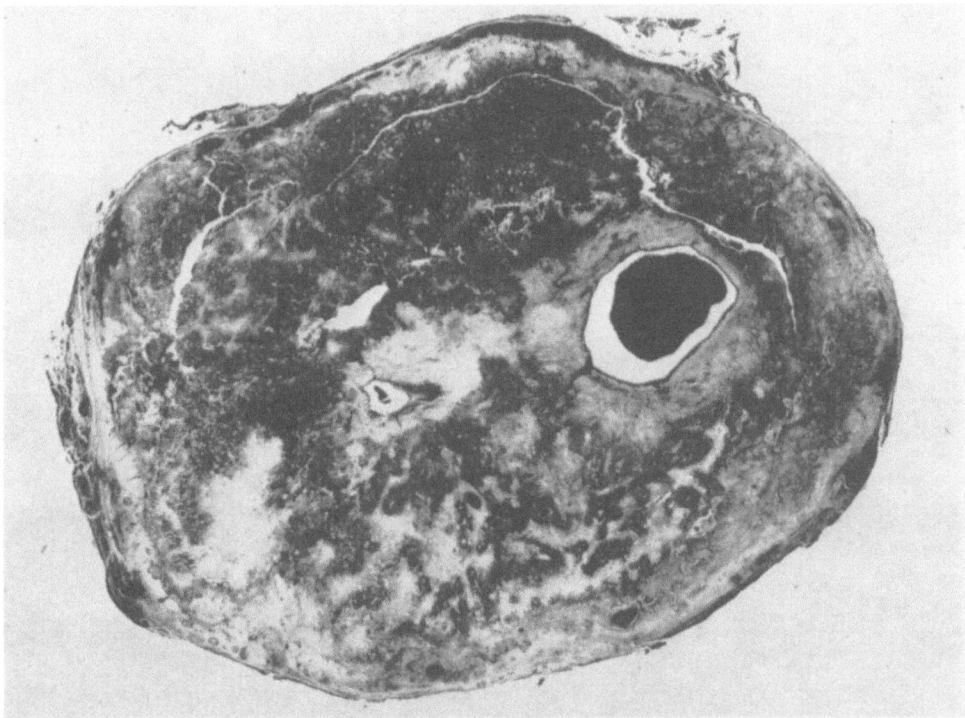

**Fig. 11.13.** The mass is well circumscribed. The cut surface is variably haemorrhagic, fibrous, and cystic. H & E, × 7

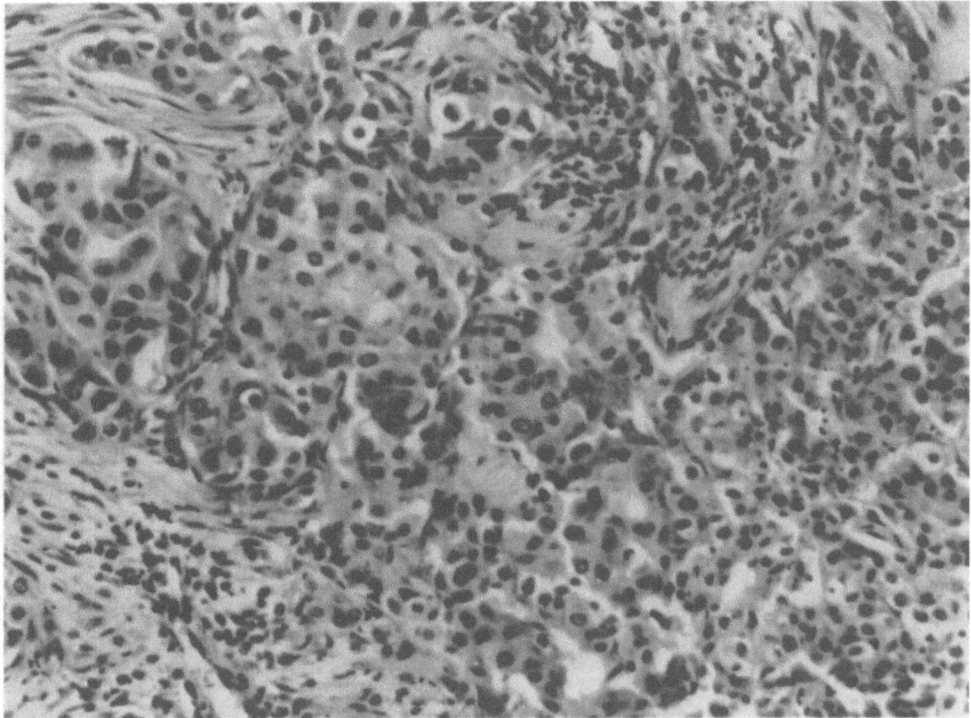

**Fig. 11.14.** One of the more glanduliform areas of the neoplasm. Elsewhere, cells of the same range of size formed a more epithelioid pattern. H & E, × 264

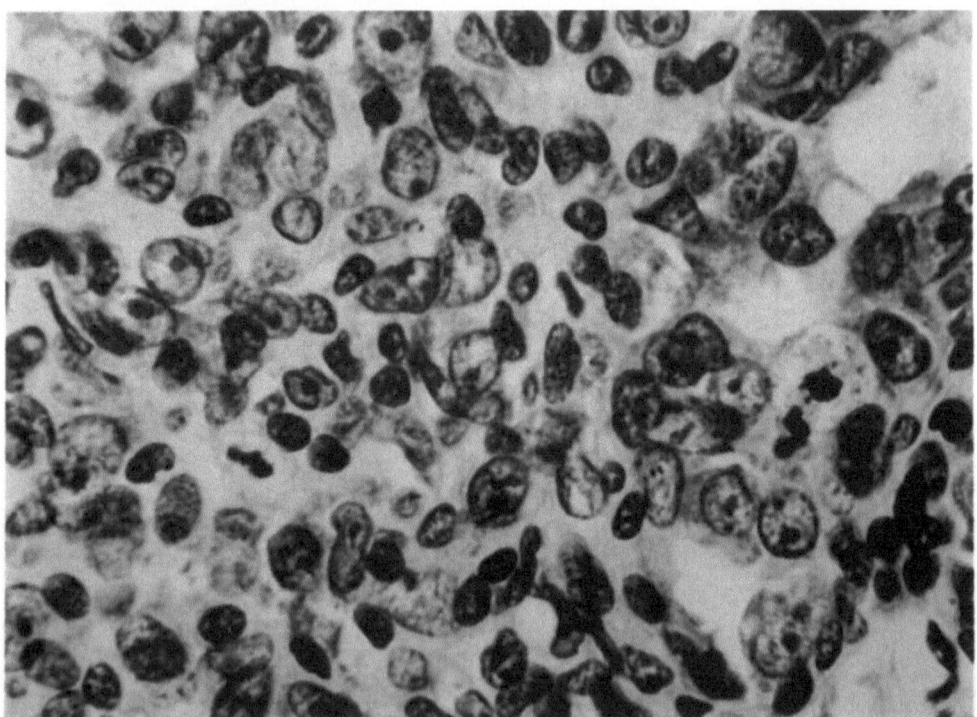

**Fig. 11.15.** Part of one of the more sheet-like areas where the cells showed considerable polymorphism and not infrequent mitoses (the diaster at *right* is obvious; a smaller figure lies in a corresponding position to *left of centre*). H & E, × 985

*Case 11.7*

F (62 years) with undue frequency of micturition. A 12-mm nodule was removed from the urethral meatus.

In some places, the investing epithelium was notably hyperplastic and extended quite deeply into the subjacent stroma: some such downgrowths were in continuity with underlying glands, which were themselves lined by hyperplastic epithelium, others were not so connected (Fig. 11.16). In detail, however, the cells of the hyperplastic epithelium were generally uniform throughout (Fig. 11.17).

The mass was diagnosed as 'a simple granulomatous urethral caruncle' but, because of the undue epithelial overgrowth, it was advised that the patient be seen again within a few months in case there should be any regrowth.

There were no sequelae, and the patient remained well until her unrelated death 11 years later.

*Case 11.8*

F (57 years) with pain in loin and haematuria: renal investigation was followed by nephrectomy. The kidney contained an oval mass, 10 × 8 cm, grossly indicative of primary carcinoma.

The lesion was clearly a carcinoma of kidney, atypical only in having many small foci of prominently papillary pattern.

Five years later a specimen was received as 'nodule from scar in flank' with minimal information about earlier events. With the earlier sections, the diagnosis was not in doubt but until their arrival the possibility had been considered of an adnexal carcinoma of skin of perhaps limited ability to metastasise (Figs. 11.18, 11.19).

The patient was still alive and well 8 years later, i.e. 13 years since the nephrectomy.

*Case 11.9*

M (81 years) with dark nodule in cleft between hallux and 1st toe, present for 'some years', but

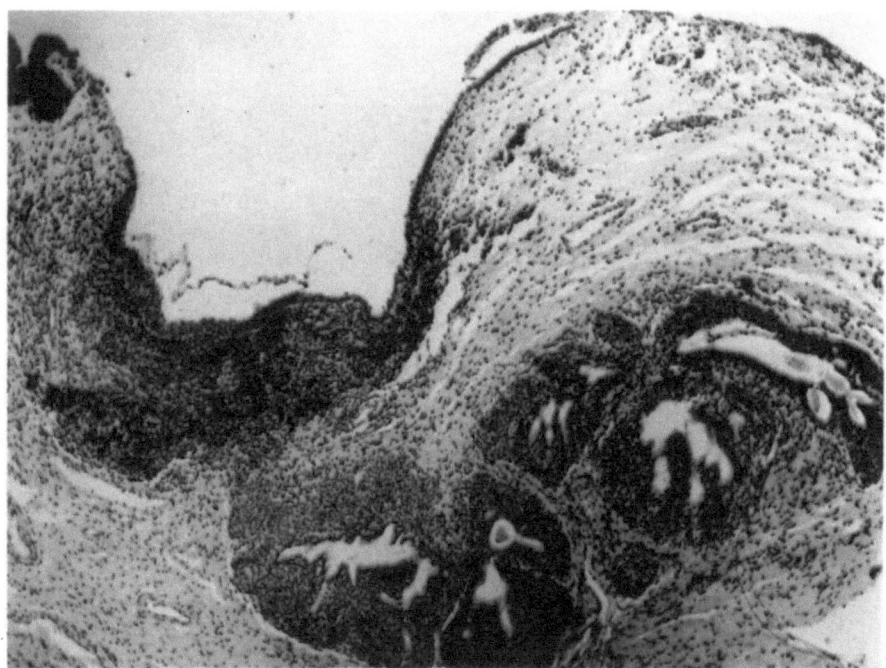

**Fig. 11.16.** The epithelial downgrowth to left of centre had probably developed in continuity with the overgrowth of the epithelium in the subjacent glands, though no such connection was demonstrated in sections deeper than this. Also, there were similar overgrowths of the surface epithelium in other areas totally devoid of underlying glands. H & E, × 56

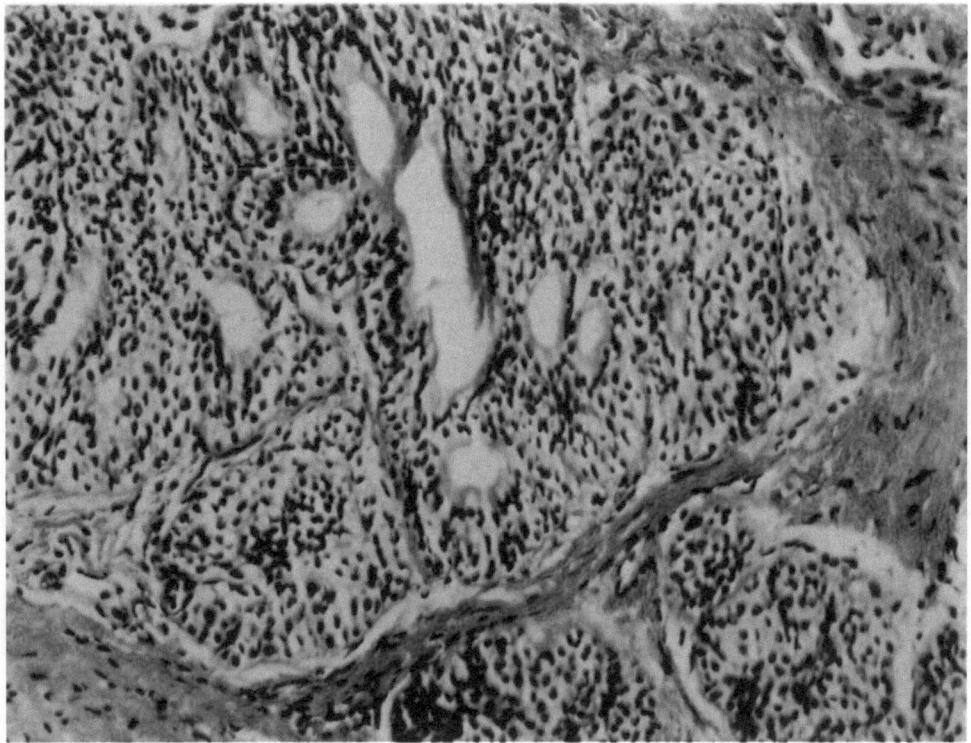

**Fig. 11.17.** Cytologically, the hyperplastic epithelium on the surface and, as here, around glands was generally uniform. H & E, × 246

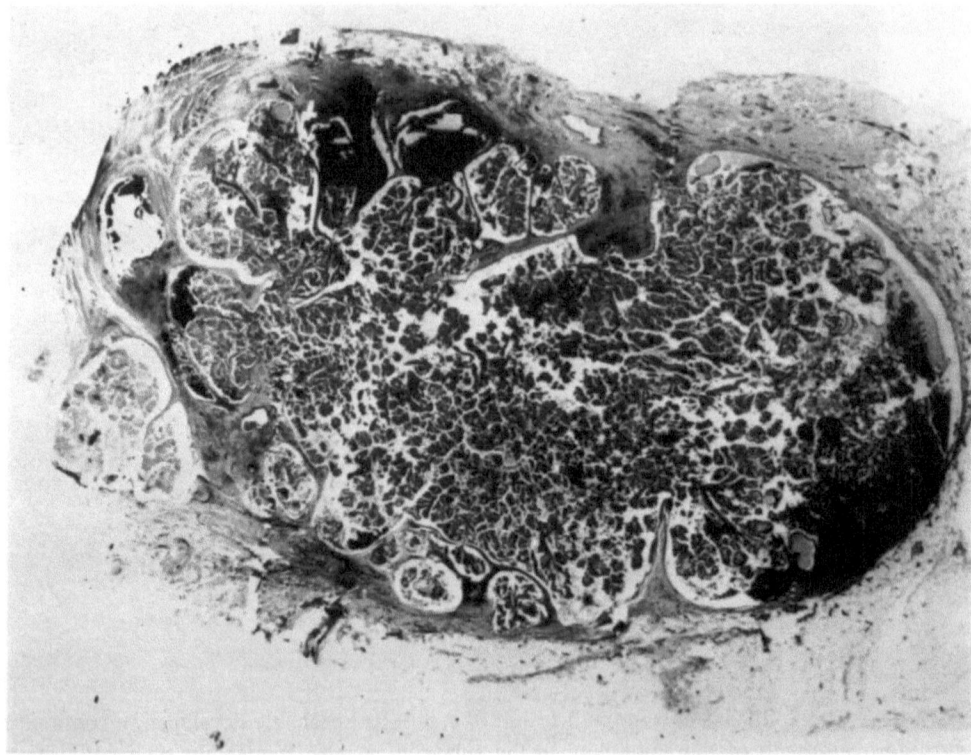

**Fig. 11.18.** The subcutaneous nodule. It was yellowish and haemorrhagic. H & E, × 9

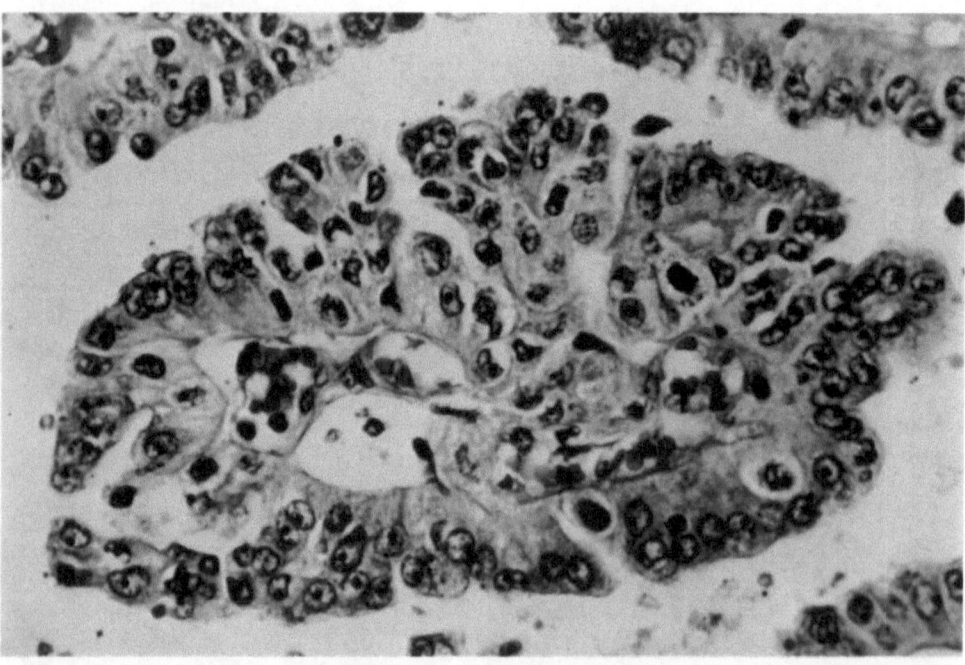

**Fig. 11.19.** The nodule was composed in essence of papillary structures of this kind. There are three mitotic figures in this single small frond, and this was reasonably representative of the degree of mitotic activity in general: in conjunction with this, the long survival is noteworthy. H & E, × 476

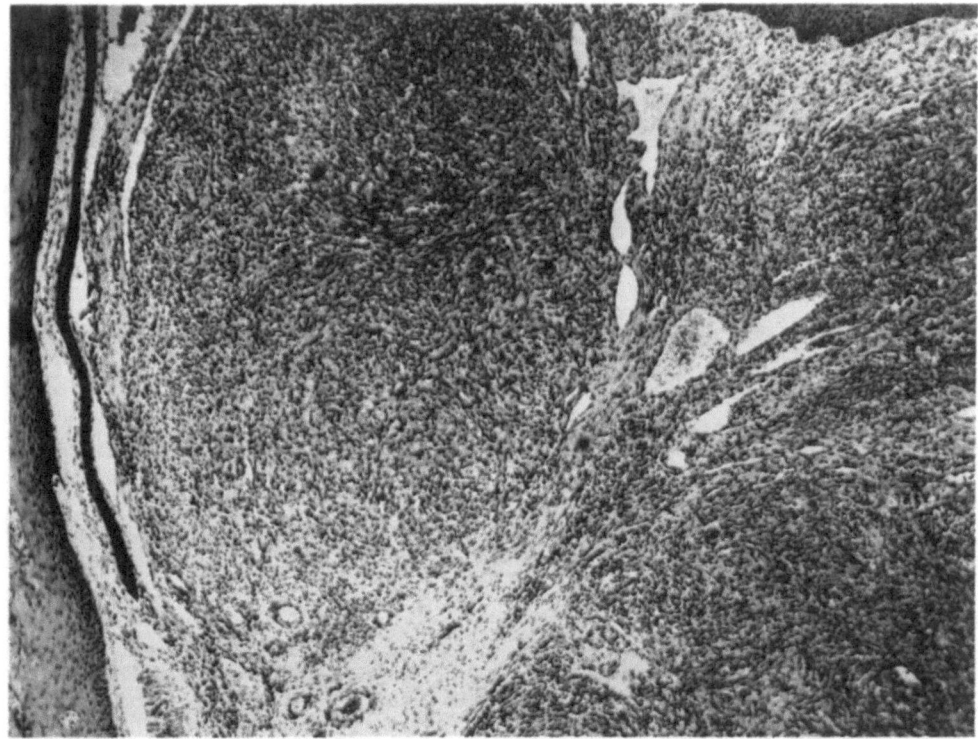

**Fig. 11.20.** The tissue is almost solidly cellular, and totally occupies the dermis. H & E, × 62

growing rapidly to 8 mm in diameter in past 3 months.

As shown in Fig. 11.20, the nodule was composed of highly cellular tissue extending throughout the dermis. In detail it was apparently vasoformative and sufficiently active mitotically to raise the question of angiosarcoma (Fig. 11.21). Reference was made in an earlier chapter to sections that were shown to a colleague from tropical Africa who had said that, if at home, he would probably have diagnosed them as Kaposi sarcoma: this was the case in question.

The mass was reported as an 'exuberant granuloma pyogenicum', and a warning given of possible recurrence, especially since completeness of excision was in doubt.

The area healed well and the patient was fully fit at last contact 4 years later. Lesions of the same kind occur in tropical countries and give rise to much differential diagnostic difficulty. A comparative study of granuloma pyogenicum and Kaposi's sarcoma has been made by Lee (1968) who believes that both lesions may develop in response to the same stimulus, nature as yet unknown: in granuloma pyogenicum the blood vascular endothelial cell is primarily in-

volved, in Kaposi's sarcoma a cell at some earlier stage of differentiation.

### Case 11.10

F (4½ years) with apparent 'swelling of glands' on right side of neck since attack of chicken pox 18 months earlier. The swelling appeared 'blue-ish'. A 15-mm nodule was removed and reported as 'haemangioma'.

Swelling reappeared and extended until, 18 months later, the upper edge lay behind the lobe of the ear. The material now removed comprised two masses of tissue, the larger 3 × 2 × 1 cm, with mottled red-purple and yellowish-white cut surface.

The reason for the variegated appearance of the cut surface is seen in Fig. 11.22: there is a mixture of variably distended or collapsed vascular spaces and foci of lymphoid tissue. The mixture is seen in more detail in Fig. 11.23. Some of the vascular channels had appreciably muscular walls, and many of these contained blood (Fig. 11.24): the thin-walled channels contained lymph.

The scattered lymphoid tissue was cytologi-

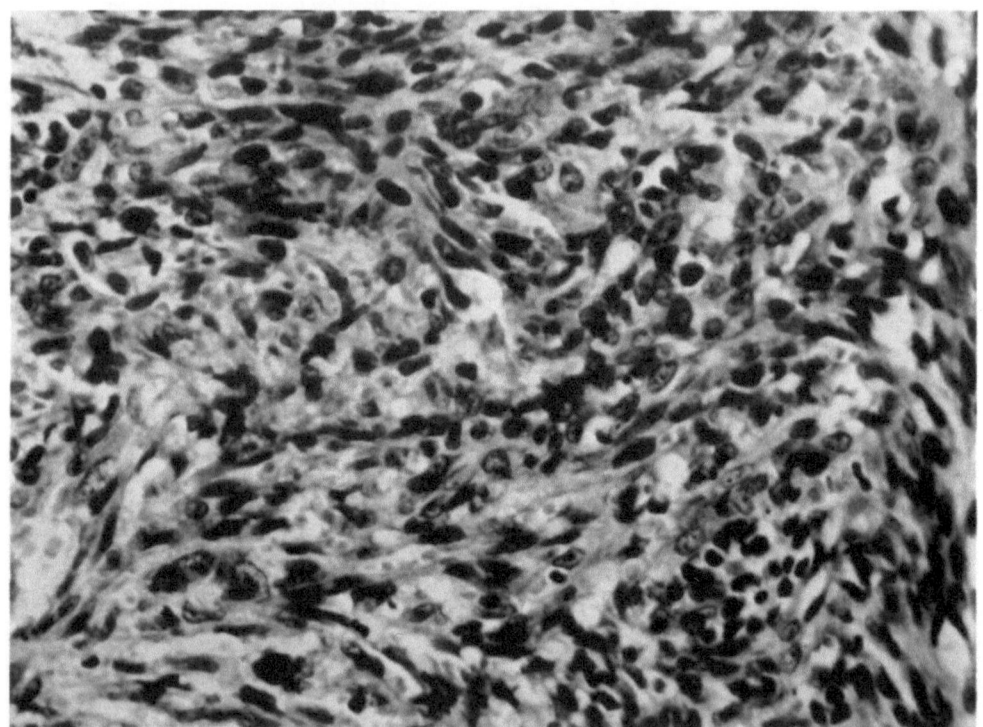

**Fig. 11.21.** The tissue was recognisably vasoformative in some places; mostly, as in this field, it formed continuous sheets of spindle cells. Three of the pyknotic masses in this field were cells in mitosis. H & E, × 493

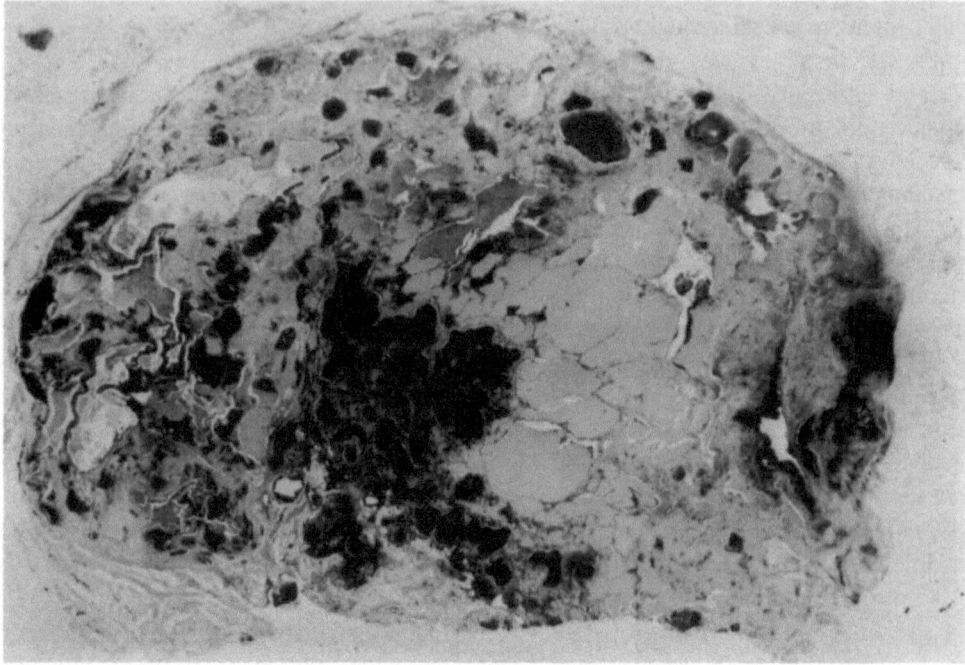

**Fig. 11.22.** The relatively large open channels towards right contained lymph: those in the left quarter of the field contained blood. The many dark foci just left of centre consisted of lymphoid tissue. The cut surface was correspondingly variegated. H & E, × 4

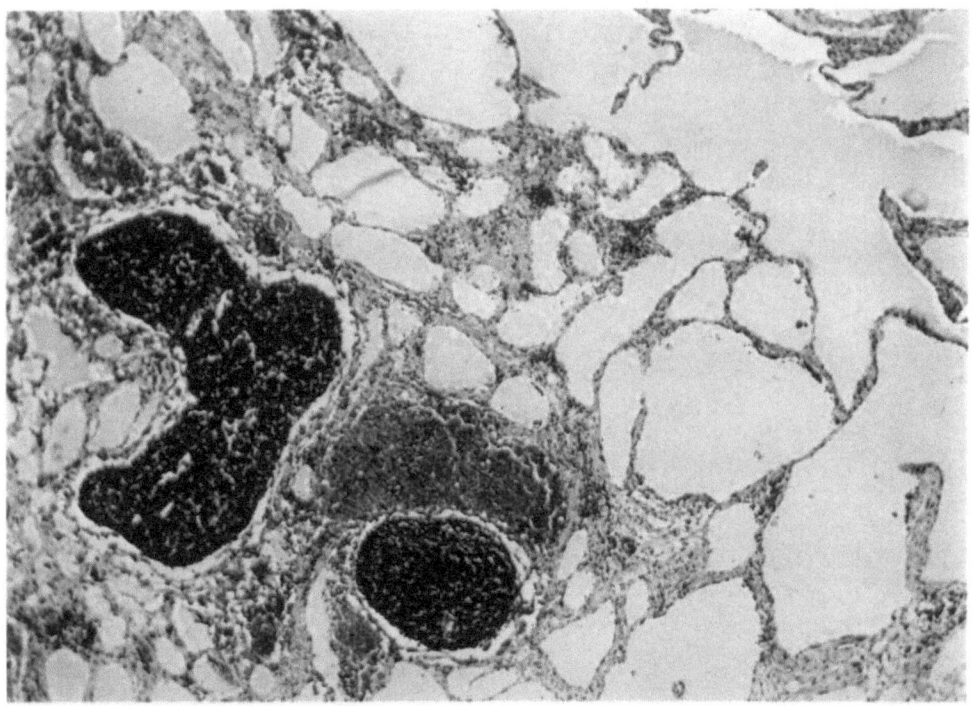

**Fig. 11.23.** Lymphangiomatous sinusoids and two foci of lymphoid tissue. The small area of moderately densely stained tissue above the lower lymphoid focus was an almost solid sheet of endothelial cells. H & E, × 60

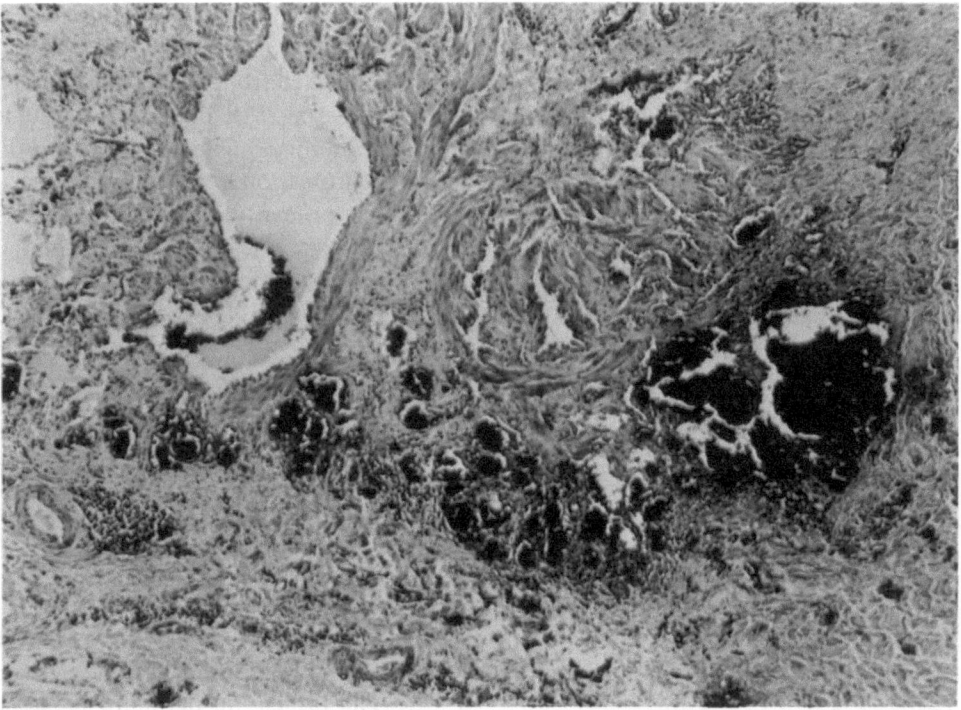

**Fig. 11.24.** An area of basically haemangiomatous character. The uppermost channels have notably muscular walls (and are mostly empty): the lowermost channels are smaller and have less muscular walls (and mostly contain blood). H & E, × 60

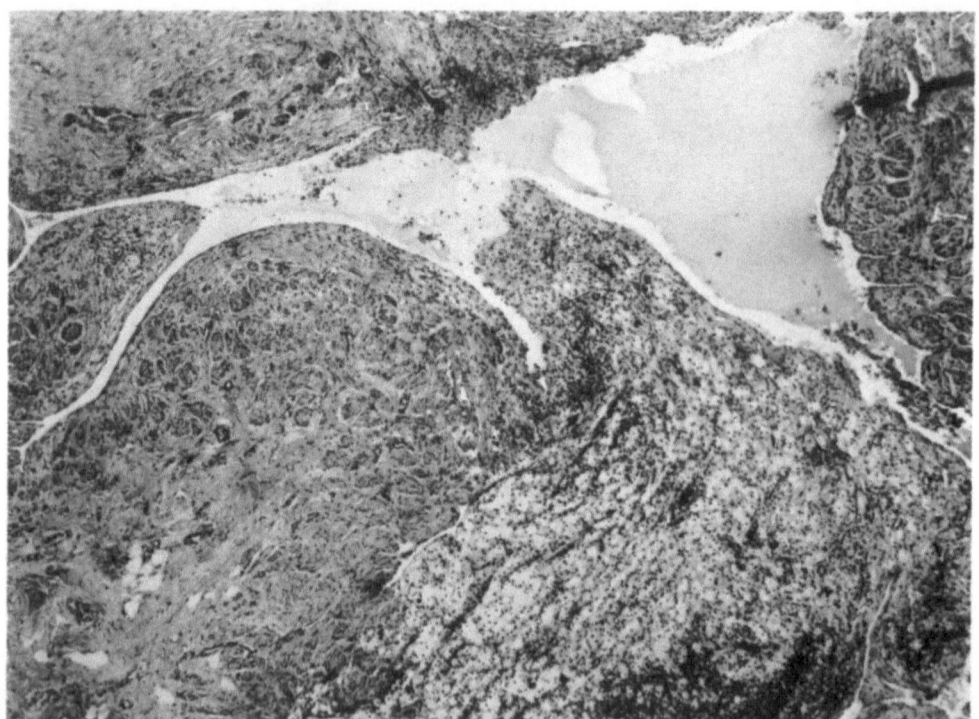

**Fig. 11.25.** Beside a lymphangiomatous sinusoid, endothelial cells are disposed either in small clusters (*lower left*) or as a finely fenestrated sheet (*lower right*). H & E, × 60

cally uniform and not a cause for concern. The stromal tissue, however, was condensed in places and highly cellular (Fig. 11.25), and scattered cells were in mitosis: it was believed to represent endothelial or angioendotheliomatous overgrowth. These features in conjunction with the clinical behaviour, namely, apparent recurrence to a greater size within 18 months, did cause concern but the lesion was believed to be essentially a lymph-haemangiomatous malformation, and benign; a form of 'hygroma'.

There was no recurrence and all has remained well for the 20 years thereafter to date. The generally held confidence that even exuberantly cellular and mitotically active endothelial tissue in infants and young children will regress was upheld.

## General Commentary

### NERVOUS SYSTEM

For reasons already mentioned, there is for this anatomical system no local series of cases com-

parable to those described in relation to other systems or organs. However, in particular, enough experience has been gained with material submitted from biopsies of intracranial lesions to reveal at least the nature of some of the main borderline problems. The lesions first mentioned, neuroblastoma and meningioma, are included not primarily because in the cases in question the diagnosis was greatly in doubt but as illustrating the difficulties sometimes of forecasting the outcome.

### Neuroblastoma

In Case 11.1, the neoplasm had been in the mediastinum, a location associated with an appreciably and unexpectedly better prognosis than any other. Of 27 children (2 weeks to 8 years) with mediastinal neuroblastoma reported by Filler and his colleagues (1972), 23 were alive at the time of reporting, 20 at more than 2 years, seven at more than 10 years since thoracotomy. The results are the more remarkable in that in 16 of the patients the lesion had already metastasised (including cervical nodes, 10; bone, 5): in the other 11 the tumour was confined to the mediastinum. Of the tumours, 8 were regarded as completely excised, 16 as incompletely excised, and 3 as inoperable. These results speak for themselves but some further points from this series may be cited as prognostically useful indicators. The lesions were subdivided histologically as 9 ganglioneuroblastoma (9 survivors); 15 neuroblastoma (13 survivors); 3 'primitive neuroblastoma' or sympathogonioma (1 survivor). Presence of lymphocytes amongst the neoplasms was of no prognostic significance. Only two patients showed an increased excretion of catecholamines (and for this the authors proffer an explanation). Four of the five patients with metastasis to bone died.

A significantly improved outlook for patients with mediastinal growths was found also by Mäkinen (1972) who suggested that a greater likelihood of early diagnosis, and thus of completeness of excision, might be a main contributory factor. Histologically, 'signs of maturation' such as vesicular nuclei, cytoplasmic processes and ganglion cells were found to be prognostically favourable as was degree of calcification (to recall, it was abundant in Case 11.1). Frequency of mitoses was of little predictive value. The series of Mäkinen comprised 54 patients: the 5-year survival rate was 24%. In a series of 133 patients described by Fortner and his co-workers (1968) the 5-year survival rate was 9.7%. Recurrence of a lesion later than 5 years after excision is evidently rare. One such case was reported by Richards and his colleagues (1976) where, after excision at age 3 months, a first recurrence at 10 years was followed by remission after therapy then further recurrence at the age of 19 and death within 12 months. The recurrence of neuroblastoma in the adult as reported by Mackay and associates (1976) was noted in an earlier chapter.

### Meningioma

There is fairly general agreement that the histoclinical correlation in the case of meningiomas is low. Not only is there no useful correlation between histological type and rate of recurrence (Wara et al., 1975), but highly cellular and mitotically active lesions, as in Case 11.2, may be rather unexpectedly cured, and lesions much less highly cellular and proliferative may, equally, unexpectedly recur and even metastasise. From their experience with 188 cases, all intracranial, Wara and colleagues found that lesions confidently believed at the time of first operation to be totally resectable were indeed so and were cured in almost 100% of cases: of cases where removal was thought probably incomplete, 74% recurred when radiotherapy was not used postoperatively but only 22% recurred when it was used.

A case of unusually long delayed recurrence of a spinal meningioma was reported by Svien and Wood (1957): re-excision was performed 23 years after the original excision, and the patient was well 4 years later. These authors commented on the much lower rate of recurrence of meningiomas in the spine than when in the skull: the explanation, they believed, was almost certainly simply a matter of easier access and therefore greater likelihood of total excision.

The structural variability of the meningioma is great: it has been briefly and well summarised by Kepes (1971), in a passage concerned particularly with histologically diagnostic problems and entitled "The Many Faces of Meningioma". Among lesions that may be simulated by one or more of the many faces are carcinomas. Some carcinomas, such as those of ovary and thyroid, mimic meningioma in containing psammoma bodies or calcospherites: some meningiomas mimic carcinoma in becoming in part mucinous. In general, the cells of a meningioma tend to have less clearly defined borders than those of a carcinoma, and they may even form something of a syncytium. With the occasional meningioma that contains melanin, distinction from a primary meningeal or even a metastatic melanocarcinoma may be impossible: much will depend on the amount of tissue available.

We are not concerned here with the problem, 'Obviously malignant but of what type?', and therefore not with the problem set by the tissue that might be, say, an amelanotic melanocarcinoma. However, in view of the therapeutic implications, two carcinomas frequently metastatic to the brain deserve mention nevertheless, carcinoma of kidney and choriocarcinoma. A metastatic carcinoma of kidney may closely resemble a haemangioblastoma, and the vascular lesion may be treatable (standard fixation for up to 24 h at any rate is unlikely in a carcinoma of kidney to reduce the glycogen to below a reasonably diagnostic level). The choriocarcinoma is highly important, not so much because its syncytial clusters can produce a puzzling haemorrhagic giant-celled lesion but:

a) Because it may cause intracranial haemorrhage, and do so by means of so few cells that their discovery in the wall of a lacerated blood-filled cavity is a lottery; the haemorrhage then may be well regarded as 'idiopathic';

b) Because choriocarcinoma, even of this severity, may still be curable.

It cannot be emphasised too often that any unusual or atypical or unduly puzzling disease, and certainly any intracranial haemorrhage, in a woman of reproductive age must be regarded as due to choriocarcinoma until proved otherwise (and that should not be difficult to arrange).

### Meningioma or Astrocytoma or Schwannoma?

Consideration of the two questions with which we are mainly concerned, namely, 'Whether malignant' and 'How malignant', requires that further attention be paid to the meningioma. A commoner problem in my own limited experience of neuropathological practice than any set by carcinomas has been that of distinguishing, for certain, between three neoplasms, namely, the meningioma, in particular the fibroblastic; astrocytoma, in particular the piloid; and the Schwannoma. There are some points that may be helpful towards making the distinction. The fibroblastic meningioma is likely to produce reticulin in a way the astrocytoma is not; also, astrocytes will usually be clearly demonstrable by gold sublimate staining (Cajal). These aids, however, will not be available for rapid opinion on a frozen section. Meningiomas, like some myomas, may mimic the palisading of a Schwannoma. However, the whorls in a meningioma typically surround a central capillary vessel; this is rarely so in a Schwannoma.

The element in a Schwannoma most likely to mimic and be wrongly interpreted as astrocytoma is the loose textured and somewhat microcystic Antoni B pattern with its stellate and often rather polymorphic cells. Reticulin staining should again help but again the problem on frozen sectioning remains. If the pathologist in these circumstances finds distinction between the three spindle-celled overgrowths impossible, his only course is to say so: there are few if any forms of treatment likely to be influenced by his decision that cannot wait the 48 h necessary for

paraffin sections, further staining procedures and the much better based opinion that will follow.

A staining reaction frequently found useful by my colleagues and me is the demonstration of alkaline phosphatase in the cells of many meningiomas as described by O'Connor and Laws (1963) and earlier observers. Many intracranial neoplasms were examined with this technique by these workers, and only in meningiomas were significantly positive results obtained. Many neoplasms showed positive staining of the walls of vessels but only in meningiomas were the neoplastic cells themselves found to stain. It is proper to note, however, that not all the meningiomas examined by O'Connor and Laws gave the reaction; in nine examples, five stained strongly, one was at 'trace' level, three were negative.

### Glioma or Gliosis?

The various diagnostic problems just examined have their prognostic implications but the implications are not all equally weighty. The decision that matters most is whether a lesion is a glioma or carcinoma, on the one hand, a benign spindle-celled neoplasm or only reparative or reactive gliosis, on the other. The difficulties of distinguishing an astroctyoma from the intrinsically benign meningioma and Schwannoma have just been considered. There remains that of trying to distinguish gliosis from glioma, in particular from the diffuse paucicellular fibrillary astrocytoma. In general, as described by Rubinstein (1972), reactive gliosis is characterised by a diffuse hyperplasia of cells that remain uniform and free of nuclear hyperchromatism, and show no mitotic activity: in his own words, "The discovery of mitotic figures in astrocytes is with one specific exception virtually diagnostic of neoplasia" (the exception is progressive multifocal leucodystrophy). The position seems to be that the zone of doubt between certain astrocytoma at one end and certainly reactive gliosis at the other is wider than in possibly any other comparable context: the counterpart fibroblast rarely causes a zone of doubt as wide as this.

An illustrative series of five photomicrographs taken successively along such a progression from virtually normal white matter to highly cellular glioblastoma multiforme is shown by Kepes (1971) with the accompanying comment, of one of the intermediate fields, that "The second section shows greater cellularity which could be due either to a neoplasm or to reactive gliosis around some other type of lesion". When even expert neuropathologists have this difficulty, the general pathologist need not feel unduly inadequate if at times he cannot give the neurosurgeon the certain answer he would like.

Cases 11.3 and 11.4 were included as instances where mitotic figures, even if scanty, were seen in biopsy tissue in circumstances where all the substantial retrospective evidence suggested a reactive process, not a neoplasm. The just cited statement of Rubinstein is the only comment I have found specifically concerned with mitotic activity in neuroglia: with the distinction between reactive gliosis and a neoplasm so important, mitotic figures either present or not present, and their frequency calculable, the matter seems worthy of further study.

### Chemodectoma

The chemodectoma is a classic example of a lesion whose future behaviour cannot be predicted with any assurance from the histology. This handicap has long been recognised, at least since the occasion when, on the evidence of intravascular extension, malignancy was diagnosed in an example described by Stout (1935) yet the patient was nevertheless well 16 years later. The same dissociation seemingly applies wherever the lesions occur, whether, for example, in the carotid body (Pryse-Davies et al., 1964: Whimster and Masson, 1970); glomus jugulare (Saldana et al., 1973); glomus intravagale (Murphy et al., 1970); or organ of Zuckerkandl (Brantigan and Katase, 1969). In sum, as Whimster and Masson say, microscopy is of value diagnostically but not prognostically.

The interesting opinion is offered by Saldana and his colleagues, from their studies of the lesion in a population living at high altitudes, that the chemodectoma may basically represent a state of hyperplasia, an undue response to a hypoxic stimulus, rather than neoplasia.

### Solitary Intracranial Metastases, Their Implications

As in the lung, so also the excision of apparently solitary metastases from the brain is sometimes successful. In a series of 51 cases analysed by Raskind and his colleagues (1971), 6 patients died within 2 weeks of craniotomy but 15 survived for at least 1 year (and 11 were still alive at the time of reporting).

An incidental but none the less interesting discovery during the survey was that 12 other patients suspected of having an intracranial metastasis had lesions of other kinds, namely, meningioma (4), glioma (3), chondroma (1) and haematoma (4, one in association with an angioma). There must be some possibility that, in the absence of such a survey, a growing intracranial mass in a patient in these circumstances would be regarded as metastatic and thus inoperable.

## THE EYE AND ORBIT

### Leiomyoma of Iris

The lesion of iris described in Case 11.5 was almost certainly a myoma. Iridectomy has proved curative for some such lesions, as reported for example by Moulton and Moulton (1948), Fleming (1948) and de Buen and associates (1971), and might well have been adequate treatment in the local example. Enucleation has been required in some cases either because of the size of the mass at the time of diagnosis or because local excision has been followed by regrowth. No examples of metastasis appear to have been recorded.

Earlier debate on histogenesis, whether the lesion is indeed a myoma rather than a neurilemmoma or even spindle cell melanocytic mass has been largely resolved by the ultramicroscopic studies of Meyer and his colleagues (1968) and Jakobiec and co-workers (1977). The features are those of smooth muscle cells.

A focal overgrowth that figures prominently in the differential diagnosis of myoma, whether of iris or ciliary body, is the curious 'pseudo-adenomatous hyperplasia' of the pigmentary epithelium of these structures in aged eyes. The true nature of the lesion seems still unsettled. In one account, Bérard and his colleagues (1969) used the designation 'benign papillary tumour' and mentioned the earlier use by others of adenoma, pseudo-adenoma, endothelioma and papillomatous hyperplasia. The term used by Hogan and Zimmerman (1962) is 'benign epithelioma (adenoma)' but so also, in another passage, 'pseudo-adenomatous hyperplasia' is used: their fig. 366 shows clearly the very substantial degree of cellular overgrowth that comprises both the substance of the nodules and their histologically borderline character.

### Borderline Orbital Growths

The term 'pseudo-tumour', already criticised on semantic grounds earlier in the text, is widely applied to lesions of the orbit. Its application here is especially unfortunate, for the term inevitably carries with it an aura of neoplasia, and orbital swellings due to neoplasia are far outnumbered by those due to inflammation. The term really has no place in the vocabulary of the pathologist.

However, in so far as it has pathological implications, the term concerns essentially the same problem as that met earlier in other areas, in particular in the lung and gut, namely, that of having to distinguish between, on the one hand, a malignant lymphoma or plasmacytoma, and, on the other, reactive lymphoid hyperplasia or a nonspecific plasma cell granuloma. Such non-neoplastic lesions as lipogranuloma, xanthogranuloma, myositis and vasculitis, all of which may cause swelling of the orbit, present their own histological problems but before he grapples with these the pathologist will have already decided that the morphological patterns lie on the non-neoplastic side of the borderline.

Case 11.6 was recollected as providing an occasion when consideration had to be given to the concept of 'pseudo-tumour' in clinical circumstances. The tumour itself, of lachrymal gland, was an illustrative example of probably the commonest neoplasm of the gland, the 'mixed' adenocarcinoma, where the diagnostic and prognostic difficulties are essentially the same as those inherent in similarly 'mixed' carcinomas at any site.

### URINARY TRACT

Some inflammatory lesions and forms of maldevelopmental overgrowth have at times been wrongly diagnosed as malignant, and the smooth biological and structural mergence of adenomas and carcinomas presents the same problems in the kidney as elsewhere, as, for example, in the liver.

### Xanthogranulomatous Pyelonephritis

The prevalence in this lesion of foam cells, especially in compact clusters, and the general destruction and distortion of architecture may lead to the erroneous diagnosis of carcinoma, as had happened in one of the four cases reported by Rios-Dalenz and Peacock (1966). These authors offered the advice that ". . . the absence of tubular formation, mitoses and nuclear polymorphism, the presence of abundant inflammatory infiltrate and the poor vascularity of the lesion (are) useful characteristics for distinguishing this benign condition from the hypernephroma". Liposarcoma may also require to be certainly excluded in some instances.

The points are made by Bennington and Beckwith (1975) that the xanthogranulomatous reaction may be essentially the same as that comprising 'malakoplakia', and, of more clinical significance, that either of these states may develop at any level in the urinary tract. The sites at which their borderline pseudo-carcinomatous patterns may appear obviously correspond.

### Hamartomas

Two forms of hamartoma represent a significant risk of over-diagnosis as malignant, as being either a Wilms' tumour or some form of sarcoma. Treatment is likely to be nephrectomy in any event, but diagnosis of a lesion as malignant may well be followed by radiotherapy and/or chemotherapy, and this has sometimes proved lethal.

In a series of 20 cases of the *leiomyomatous hamartoma* reported by Bogdan and his colleagues (1973), 17 had been initially diagnosed as either Wilms' tumour or sarcoma, and four of the infants had died in consequence of further therapy; the same had occurred in the case of the patient described by Kay and his associates (1966). A useful point of distinction from the Wilms' tumour is that, in the hamartoma, the epithelial component of the kidney is intrinsically normal throughout. A possibly misleading feature is that the usually prominent element of spindle-shaped smooth muscle cells may show much mitotic activity, up to four figures per hpf (Bogdan et al.); however, they show no significant pleomorphism, and there is typically neither haemorrhage nor necrosis. The lesion may contain occasional cysts and islands of cartilage, while its thin-walled sinusoids help to distinguish it from the other potentially misleading hamartoma, the angiomyolipoma, where vessels are notably thick-walled.

The *angiomyolipoma* was well described in a series of 32 examples by Farrow and his co-workers (1968). Here again, spindled smooth muscle cells are prominent, and in the experience of these authors may show ". . . scattered mitotic figures, hyperchromatism and moderate polymorphism. . . ." The presence of rather polymorphic giant cells amongst the also constantly prominent adipose tissue may add further to the impression of malignant neoplasia. In Farrow's series, three of the patients were children; in the others the lesion was frequently multifocal and had caused massive destruction of the kidney. The main danger to the patient is, again, the irradiation that may follow over-diagnosis of malignancy. The curious association of the lesion with tuberous sclerosis was fully exemplified in the series just cited.

An informative survey of malignant tumours of the kidney in childhood has been published by Young and Williams (1969), while a national study of the histology and behaviour of Wilms' tumour in the USA is currently in progress (Beckwith and Palmer, 1978).

### Renal Adenoma vs Carcinoma

The outlook for a patient with renal carcinoma is poor; reported 10-year survival rates are usually of the order of 20%–30% (Rafla, 1970; Skinner et al., 1971). Some patients, however, are able to resist the lesion for a long time, as, for example, in Case 11.9 where the patient was still alive 8 years after excision of a nodule of carcinoma recurrent in the scar 5 years after nephrectomy, and in the case of the patient reported by Takáts and Csapó (1966) where death occurred 37 years after the lesion had been diagnosed (and regarded at the time as inoperable).

The occasional success of resection for a solitary metastasis in the lung (Vidne et al., 1976) has been mentioned already. Somewhat comparable in its rarity is the regression of metastases after nephrectomy: two such cases were reported by Garfield and Kennedy (1972) who noted that only 27 other examples had been recorded at that time.

Debate on means of distinguishing between tubular adenomas and carcinomas was largely resolved by Bennington (1973). Until this time, the distinction was generally made arbitrarily: nodules up to 3 cm in diameter were accepted as adenomas, above 3 cm they were carcinomas (the general acceptance of size as the arbiter was tacit admission of the shortcomings of histology). A diagram produced by Bennington showed that, while some neoplasms smaller than 3 cm in diameter did metastasise, and some larger than 10 cm did not, there was, in general, a direct linear correlation between size and likelihood of metastasis, from less than 5% for masses less than 15 mm in diameter to some 85% for masses of 10 cm in diameter or more. There is thus a valuable scheme by which the pathologist may give to the surgeon a mathematically expressed likelihood of metastasis; and the probability may be refined further. Observers in most series have found the prognosis to be not surprisingly worsened by extracapsular extension of the neoplasm or by spread to regional nodes, and to be more unfavourable in patients over 60 years of age than under.

One form of adenoma provides an exception to the above assessment, the adenoma of 'oncocytic' character. Fourteen examples of the entity were described by Klein and Valensi (1976): all were larger than 3 cm in diameter (one was 13 cm in diameter) yet none had either recurred or metastasised.

### Carcinoma of Prostate

Carcinoma of the prostate is an important disease in that, as a population ages, so does the incidence of the carcinoma. However, accuracy in the calculation of figures of incidence and therefore curability may be blunted here, as with some other neoplasms, by a failure to make clear a distinction between 'cancer', the disease, and 'cancer', a histological pattern.

On the evidence of many surveys, cancer, in this instance carcinoma, has been said to be present in the prostates of up to 46% of men over age 50 years (Franks, 1954), or virtually one man in two of that age. Yet, as calculated by Fergusson (1970) from data for the UK, the number of men over 50 years who die from carcinoma of the prostate is of the order of 1 in 1700. This huge discrepancy has its origin in confused definition. When, as clinical histopathologists, we diagnose cancer, we imply a disease which, if untreated (and all too often even if treated), will significantly shorten the life of the patient; and our responsibility is, for purposes of prediction and therapy, to establish the appropriate histoclinical correlation as closely as we can. That is, we are regarding and diagnosing cancer as a life-shortening disease, and implying exactly that by our histological report. Therefore, we cannot in logic simultaneously use the term 'cancer' to refer to a condition present in half of the population at risk and also to a condition which will kill no more than one in 1700 of the same population. 'Cancer' (or carcinoma) is being used in the first sense to mean, not a life-shortening disease but a particular kind of histological pattern. With a virtually zero histoclinical correlation, the only explanation for the use of the term must be (or must have been) a belief that no form of growth other than that of malignant neoplasia could produce the tissue pattern or patterns in question. With acceptance of that premise, the *folie circulaire* is inevitable: any patient whose tissue shows the pattern has carcinoma of the prostate.

The histological patterns are well known, in particular the 'invasion' or occupation of possibly vascular lumina especially around nerves but also elsewhere by clusters of epithelial cells, and, to a lesser extent, foci of extreme or borderline microfollicular hyperplasia. Even if the lumina were certainly those of vessels, whether for blood or lymph, the near-zero correlation with metastasis would still make usage of the term 'carcinoma' quite inappropriate. However, as McNeal (1969) has noted in keeping with more modern observations, (a) perineural spaces are almost certainly not vessels, and (b) the prostate probably contains no lymphatics. Therefore, the strongest reason for believing the pattern to represent carcinoma has gone, and indeed (though still rather surprisingly supported by Mostofi and Price [1973] as ". . . the most reliable pathologic evidence for diagnosis of carcinoma of the prostate") the phenomenon is not even mentioned in some recent analyses of series of cases (see, for example, Epstein and Fatti, 1976; Kern, 1978).

There is need, nevertheless, for a term for lesions of this kind, for their academic interest is real. The terms incidental, occult and latent

carcinoma have been used, also prostatic microcarcinoma or PMC (Battaglia et al., 1979) and with some resulting confusion. However, the part to be criticised is not the adjective but the noun; it is 'carcinoma' that is difficult to justify. 'Pseudo-carcinoma' might suffice but some term at any rate less definitive than 'carcinoma' does seem desirable, otherwise statistics for the incidence and results of treatment of carcinoma proper of the prostate will continue to be hedged about by vagueness and doubt.

Many pathologists, from their experience, would probably agree with McNeal's belief that few carcinomas of prostate metastasise from a volume of less than 1 cm$^3$. Were foci of, say, 1 mm$^3$ a frequent source of metastasis, prostates originally reported as benign would be an embarrassingly frequent source of spread. In practice this is rare, almost certainly because the carcinomas that do metastasise are always large enough to be evident on 5-mm or even 10-mm gross sectioning and so be taken for microscopy. Matters, however, are different with the multiple fragments of tissue obtained at transurethral resection: the likelihood that even a 10-mm carcinoma will be 'missed' in these circumstances is high and, within reasonably practicable limits of sampling, difficult to minimise.

Given, then, a microscopically unequivocal carcinoma of prostate, it is proper to ask whether the pathologist can give to the clinician any guidance on likely behaviour. In general, in parallel with circumstances relating to the adenoma/carcinoma of kidney, it would be reasonable to regard a carcinoma of prostate as having a likelihood of metastasis of some 10% at a diameter of 10 mm, and one of some 80% at a diameter of 30 mm. Probably, also, the smaller the carcinoma, the longer the interval until metastases appear: with a mass 30 mm in diameter at the time of diagnosis, metastasis might already be diagnosable. A detailed multifactorial analysis of morphological features led Epstein and Fatti (1976) to conclude that only two were usefully predictive, the sharpness and degree of preservation of epithelial cell borders, and the degree of lymphocytic infiltration: carcinomas with indistinct cell borders and no lymphocytic infiltration were associated with a five-year survival of only 14.5%. According to both Byar and Mostofi (1969) and Silber and McGavran (1971), the prognosis for patients with manifest carcinoma is no different at ages under 50 years than over. The ability of prostatic carcinoma to produce a 'malignant retroperitoneal fibrosis' (Piper, 1969) was mentioned earlier.

Features or lesions that may show a superficial resemblance to carcinoma but that should rarely cause difficulty are foci of squamous or transitional cell metaplasia; unusually deep-seated paraurethral glands or diverticula; and the polytypic infiltrate of a nonspecific granulomatous inflammation. A likelier source of diagnostic error, well illustrated by Mostofi and Price (1973), is the inclusion in a section of part of an involutionary seminal vesicle: the epithelial cells lining the lumina here may show prominent nuclear enlargement and polymorphism, and be quite bizarre.

A distinction has been drawn, and is now widely recognised, between carcinoma of the prostate proper and carcinoma of the periurethral prostatic ducts (PUPDC). The distinction has clinical significance since, as Melicow and Usan (1976) emphasise, it implies some differences in clinical management: for example, PUPDC, ". . . indistinguishable from tumors arising in the posterior urethra," is non-androgen-dependent. Further, an account of 58 patients with the lesion is given by Kopelson and his colleagues (1978) who describe, as compared with the acinar lesion, the greater tendency of PUPDC to metastasise to liver and lungs, and the likelier therapeutic success of 'aggressive' radiotherapy than radical surgery.

BLADDER

*Overgrowths of Vesical Epithelium*

The genesis and significance of Brunn's nests, cystitis glandularis and cystitis cystica remain uncertain. In the opinion of Koss (1975) none of these variants of 'urothelial' overgrowth should be regarded as neoplastic: at the same time, the comment is added that ". . . there is histologic evidence of occasional association of cystitis glandularis and cystica and related abnormalities with bladder cancer, usually adenocarcinoma, and less commonly with urothelial carcinoma" (the term 'urothelium' seems to have been generally accepted; etymologically,

however, it is even less defensible than endo- or mesothelium). The possibility of confusion of cystitis glandularis with a glandular carcinoma is considerable. An example of total bladder involvement by the process reported by Bell and Wendel (1968) had been initially diagnosed on biopsy as glandular carcinoma but was correctly identified by further opinion. The treatment required was total cystectomy nevertheless.

The behaviour and implications of the transitional cell papilloma are too familiar to require comment here. A variant, however, merits a mention.

*Inverted Papilloma*

The inverted papilloma, so named because of an apparent reversal of the usual outside-inside relation between epithelium and stroma, appears almost exclusively in the region of the trigone and, significantly unlike the orthodox transitional cell form, has little or no tendency to recur or invade. In describing 20 examples, DeMeester and his colleagues (1975) concluded that the lesion arises ". . . from the irritated bladder mucosa of proliferative cystitis" and requires to be distinguished from both cystitis glandularis and its variant, cystitis cystica, and from papillary transitional cell carcinoma. The microscopic architecture of the lesion is essentially the same as may occur in some papillomas of the nasal cavity where, as mentioned earlier, the 'inverted' form may again comprise a subgroup.

*Precancerous Changes*

". . . it is immediately obvious that the microscopic criteria for the diagnosis of cancer in its non-invasive phases are arbitrary ones and subject to very wide observer variation" (Pugh, 1973).

The problem how best to estimate the future behaviour of dysplastic tissue is intrinsically the same in the bladder as elsewhere but it is met here less often (compared, for example, with biopsies of skin, cervix uteri, or even, nowadays, stomach). Unstable vesical epithelium is most likely to be found in bladders already containing a known lesion, in particular a papilloma or carcinoma, and the frequency and extent of such associated instability is great. In 100 cases of transitional cell carcinoma of the bladder, biopsy specimens from the mucosa away from the carcinoma were reported by Schade and Swinney (1968) to show 'precancerous changes' in over 80% (46 cases with atypical epithelium, 40 with carcinoma in situ). Similar results have been reported in relation to involvement of the ureter (Sharma et al., 1970) ureter and urethra (Cooper et al., 1973) and prostate (Seemayer et al., 1975). In five of these last authors' seven cases of CIS of the bladder, there was CIS also in ureters, seminal vesicles and vasa deferentia. An account of the natural history (and means of diagnosis and treatment) of carcinoma in situ of the bladder was given by Melamed and his colleagues (1964) who found ". . . clear and direct evidence of the potential for progression from in situ to invasive carcinoma after intervals of 8 to 67 months".

Achieving the compromise in these circumstances between the total removal of all potentially cancerous tissue and minimum mutilation is obviously a matter of skilled clinical judgement, and realistic conservatism will generally and understandably prevail.

Even with a lesion generally acceptable as papillary carcinoma of the bladder, prognosis remains uncertain. An attempt to achieve greater accuracy was made by Tiltman (1977) by ultramicroscopic examination of the silver staining band or basement membrane demonstrable between the epithelium and the fibrovascular core. The author's conclusion was that ". . . contrary to expectations, the presence or absence of invasion could not be used as an indication of subsequent behaviour".

### Adenomatoid Tumour of Epididymis

The adenomatoid tumour was earlier mentioned in relation to the female genital tract: a local example within the myometrium had strongly suggested a metastatic mucin-secreting carcinoma. The epididymal lesion also may mislead. An instance was reported by Hansen and Jensen (1969) in which the presence of neoplastic tissue within the substance of the testis, in conjunction with nuclear polymorphism, had led to a diagnosis of infiltration by 'solid adenomatous carcinoma', and consequent orchidectomy. The tissue here had shown no mitotic activity; similarly, mitotic figures were extremely few in the local intrauterine example. Mitotic scarcity

should at least suggest the possibility of the adenomatoid tumour in the genital tract of either sex; local excision is likely to cure.

### Urethral Caruncle

The frequency with which a seeming caruncle of the female urethra may prove to be a carcinoma was shown in an analysis of 394 'tumours' at that site by Marshall and his colleagues (1960). Of the 394 masses, 356 were caruncles, 17 were carcinomas. In practice, the important point to recall is that the constituent epithelial cells may be not only hyperplastic or metaplastic or both, they may also show also a disturbing degree of polymorphism.

The extent to which the morphology may mislead is well illustrated in the comment by Fox and Langley (1973) on the possible outcome of presenting a section of such a caruncle to a colleague for opinion in ignorance of the clinical data, thus, ". . . quite confident microscopists, misled by the dark staining, multilayered, transitional epithelium, have been known to misdiagnose a caruncle as carcinoma in situ of the cervix". Even so, it is not easy to understand why a histological pattern estimated to indicate CIS in the epithelium of the cervix should cease to indicate CIS in the epithelium of a caruncle.

### VASCULATURE

Case 11.9, an exuberant granuloma pyogenicum, and Case 11.10, recognised on its recurrence as a form of (cervical) hygroma, both caused concern at the time of diagnosis. The hygroma, with its abundant accompaniment of lymphoid tissue, recurrent at age 6 years and much larger than the original lesion, continued to be a source of lurking worry for some years thereafter but cure seems to have been achieved (treatment was purely surgical). To the extent that 'granulation tissue sarcoma' seemed a significant possibility in Case 5.19, this case also could have been included as relevant to this section.

A lesion certainly relevant here is the so-called intravascular angiomatosis, which Salyer and Salyer (1975) believe has fair claim to be regarded as a *pseudo-angiosarcoma*. The abnormal histological pattern is seen typically in organising thrombi and consists of a mixture of freely anastomosing small channels lined by prominent and sometimes atypical endothelial cells, occasionally in the form of cellular papillary projections. These authors suggest that distinction from an angiosarcoma may be made on several grounds: (a) the endothelial overgrowth is confined wholly or predominantly within vascular lumina, (b) mitotic figures are rare or absent, and (c) there are no solidly cellular areas devoid of vascular differentiation, and no areas of necrosis. In the light of events in Case 5.19, however, highly proliferative endothelium probably can be allowed an appreciable degree of mitotic activity and yet be seen as innocuous; any aberrant forms, on the other hand, would still have their usual ominous significance.

Another lesion which may simulate and be wrongly diagnosed as angiosarcoma is the so-called *angiolymphoid hyperplasia with eosinophilia* as seen in the skin. An example was described, with histochemical and ultrastructural details, by Castro and Winkelmann (1974) who include also a general survey of data in 47 other examples published earlier by other observers under various names including atypical pyogenic granuloma and papular angioplasia. The lesion appears typically as cutaneous and subcutaneous nodules in the head and neck. The constant histological feature, and the feature that comprises the pseudo-sarcomatous element, is the exuberant overgrowth of atypical or bizarre histiocyte-like endothelial cells, giving in all the pattern of an abnormal vascular proliferation. Prominent infiltration by eosinophil polymorphonuclears, histiocytes and lymphocytes, perhaps to the point of lymphoid follicle formation, is usual but not invariable and thus not a sine qua non for the diagnosis. The lesion, which is possibly an unusual response to some inflammatory stimulus, may have some relation to the general group of histiocytomas and thus, in particular, to the sclerosing angioma and fibroxanthoma.

There is continued debate on the interrelationships between endothelial cells, pericytes and smooth muscle cells, on the extent to which they are separately identifiable, share a common ancestry more specific than a 'primitive mesenchymal cell', or are morphologically interchangeable. It is not surprising, therefore, that an equivalent uncertainty surrounds their neoplastic expressions. Only few observations that seem to be relevant to clinical diagnostic difficulties will be made here.

## Hygroma

Few diagnostic problems are created by the hygroma that consists purely of distended lymphatic channels but the difficulties of total surgical removal may be formidable, especially when the mediastinum and deep tissues of the neck are involved. In some instances, as described by Willis (1960) and well exemplified in Case 11.10, there may be a prominent element of either smooth muscular tissue in the walls of the channels, or lymphoid tissue or both. The fact that the tissue removed at first biopsy in Case 11.10 was diagnosed as haemangioma is wholly in keeping with the conclusion by Willis that ". . . haemangiomas and lymphangiomas may not be sharply separable . . . (and) . . . that lesions of mixed structure occur".

The muscular tissue may be so prominent as to dominate the pattern. The lesion then becomes a candidate for diagnosis as *lymphangiomyoma*. Overgrowths of this type occur particularly in the mediastinum and were described in some detail by Pachter and Lattes (1963) who illustrated clearly the difficulties of classification in making the comment, "Whether or not the lesions, which we have described as being lymphangiomyomas or lymphangiopericytomas, might better be called vascular leiomyomas or venous hemangiomas will depend on the amount of muscle present as well as the interpretation placed on the nature of the vascular lumina".

A more widespread expression of the disorder, involving the lungs and retroperitoneum as well as the mediastinum, was described by Joliat and his colleagues (1973), as 'lymphangiomyomatosis'. The disorder occurs almost exclusively in women and is commonly characterised by chylous effusions.

The 'giant lymphoid hamartoma' was mentioned earlier as a lesion in the main, probably, of lymphoid rather than vascular dysgenesis even if many names for it have stressed the angiomatous element, as, for example, the 'angiomatous' lymphoid hamartoma of Tung and McCormack (1967) and others similar that they cite. The absence of any element of ectasia in the vessels, however, suggests that the entity is significantly different from the lymphangiomyoma even if the whole group is basically hamarto-matous in origin.

### Haemangiopericytoma

The first comprehensive account of haemangio-pericytoma was published some 30 years ago by Stout (1949), yet acceptance of the lesion as an entity has been slow. Much of the reason for hesitation has, I believe, been due to the apparent dependence of diagnosis on reticulin-stained sections and their detailed interpretation. Silver staining is a fickle process, and, with technique of even the highest quality, not a procedure that often enables one to say more than that 'on the whole' this pattern or that pattern predominates. Decision on the enclosure or non-enclosure of individual cells by reticulin fibrils is particularly difficult, and on this the diagnosing of haemangio-pericytoma has hitherto largely depended. In addition, the quality of some published photo-micrographs claiming to show characteristic and diagnostic reticulin patterns has not always in-duced confidence in the reader.

The difficulties have been in part resolved by the use of ultramicroscopy, to the point where Kuhn and Rosai (1969) and Battifora (1973), for example, believe that the parent cell of the neoplasm probably is the pericyte. However, the matter is not wholly settled. Thus, Hahn and his colleagues (1973) have emphasised the varia-tion there has been in descriptions of the ultra-microscopic morphology of the pericyte, and themselves examine the possibility that it may be a form of cell transitional between a 'mesen-chymal cell' and a smooth muscle cell. The size of the differential diagnostic problem is seen in the list of lesions these authors mention: glomangioma, haemangioendothelial sarcoma, undifferentiated or metastatic carcinoma, vascu-lar leiomyoma, leiomyoblastoma, treated malig-nant melanoma and vascular portions of a fibrosarcoma. To these may now be added cerebral haemangioblastoma and some forms of angioblastic meningioma which Popoff and co-workers (1974) believe may, instead, be also haemangiopericytomas. The essentially histo-genetic problem of distinguishing between these three lesions is clearly and fairly analysed by Russell and Rubinstein (1977).

The first difficulty surrounding the lesion is to identify it correctly, and clearly this is not easy, even on ultramicroscopy. The second problem then is to determine the prognosis, and this also is not easy: indeed, according to Stout and Lattes (1967), it cannot be done. In the words of these authors, "It is unfortunate that there are no known reliable criteria that will dis-tinguish the malignant from the benign hem-angiopericytomas". A more recent attempt to forecast the outcome has been described by McMaster and his associates (1975) from their experience with 60 cases. By using standard criteria such as mitotic frequency and degree of cellular anaplasia these workers divided the le-sions into benign, borderline and malignant classes: the deaths from metastasis in each group numbered 1/12, 6/16 and 23/32 respectively.

### Kaposi's Sarcoma

It would be presumptuous to comment at length here on this predominantly tropical lesion. From a recent histopathological study of 159 cases, mainly in skin, and of 16 examples in lymph nodes, O'Connell (1977, 1977a) had even yet to conclude that "The cause of Kaposi's sarcoma and the cell of origin are still uncertain". Elec-tron microscopy, tissue culture, and enzyme histochemistry have not completely resolved the problem. The neoplasms mentioned by this worker as diagnostic rivals are leiomyoma, leio-myosarcoma, fibrosarcoma and haemangioendo-theliosarcoma. The feature most helpful in distinguishing the lesion from these other growths is the presence in many of the neoplastic cells of eosinophilic hyaline globules rather similar to Russell bodies and usually smaller than an erythrocyte, of uncertain nature but possibly 'lysosomal degenerative bodies'.

## Conclusions

1) Neuroblastomas arising within the medi-astinum are prognostically less unfavourable than those arising elsewhere: fewer also than else-where secrete catecholamines in detectable amount. Examples of unduly delayed recurrence and of the appearance of the lesion in adults have been reported.

2) Certain distinction between meningioma, astrocytoma, and Schwannoma may be virtually impossible on frozen section; thereafter, special staining procedures should help. The demonstration of alkaline phosphatase in the cells of many meningiomas may be particularly helpful.

3) Distinction between glioma and gliosis depends largely on the representativeness of biopsy. The problem is likely to be greatest with the fibrillary astrocytoma, and may be insoluble on frozen section.

4) In assessment of chemodectomas, microscopy is of diagnostic but of almost no prognostic value.

5) With lesions of the orbit, distinction between lymphomatous and lymphomatoid overgrowths is as intrinsically difficult as it is elsewhere.

6) Lesions of kidney simulating carcinoma include xanthogranuloma and the leiomyomatous and angiomyolipomatous hamartomas.

7) Carcinomas of kidney have a probability of metastasis of some 5% when less than 15-mm diameter and of some 85% when 10-cm diameter or more. The conventional designation of masses smaller than 15-mm diameter as 'adenomas' is arbitrary and of no diagnostic or prognostic value.

Masses consisting wholly of cells of oncocytic character, whatever their size, appear to have a minimal tendency to behave as carcinomas.

8) Bladders containing a carcinoma are likely to bear areas elsewhere showing precancerous change; such changes may be present also in ureters and prostate.

9) Examples are few but urethral caruncles can be carcinomas.

10) Lymphangiomatous overgrowths are mostly hamartomas and occur mostly in mediastinum and neck. The not infrequent accompaniment of much smooth muscle and lymphoid tissue may raise the question of leiomyoma or malignant lymphoma but metastatically malignant behaviour is most unlikely.

11) The haemangiopericytoma remains an entity difficult to diagnose with assurance, and, even when diagnosed, of unpredictable outcome.

12) The nature and genesis of Kaposi's sarcoma remain uncertain; both it and granuloma pyogenicum may represent different responses to the same stimulus.

# References

Alexander RC (1951) Mediastinal neuroblastoma in an infant. Br J Surg 38: 517–518

Battaglia S, Barbolini G, Botticelli AR (1979) Early (stage A) prostatic cancer. IV. Methodological criteria for histopathological diagnosis. Virchows Arch (Path Anat) 382: 245–259

Battifora H (1973) Hemangiopericytoma: Ultrastructural study of five cases. Cancer 31: 1418–1432

Beckwith JB, Palmer NF (1978) Histopathology and prognosis of Wilms' tumor. Results from the first national Wilms' tumor study. Cancer 41: 1937–1948

Bell TE, Wendel RG (1968) Cystitis glandularis: Benign or malignant? J Urol 100: 462–465

Bennington JL (1973) Cancer of the kidney—etiology, epidemiology and pathology. Cancer 32: 1017–1029

Bennington JL, Beckwith JB (1975) Atlas of tumor pathology, 2nd ser, fasc 12. Tumors of the kidney, renal pelvis, and ureter. Armed Forces Institute of Pathology, Washington, D.C.

Bérard M, Bérard PV, Payan H (1969) Tumeur papillaire bénigne de l'épithélium non pigmenté du corps ciliaire (épithélioma bénin de Fuchs). Ann Oculist (Paris) 202: 457–462

Bogdan R, Taylor DEM, Mostofi FK (1973) Leiomyomatous hamartoma of the kidney. A clinical and pathologic analysis of 20 cases from the Kidney Tumor Registry. Cancer 31: 462–467

Brantigan CO, Katase RY (1969) Clinical and pathologic features of paragangliomas of the organ of Zuckerkandl. Surgery 65: 898–905

Buen S de, Olivares ML, Charlin C (1971) Leiomyoma of the iris. Report of a case. Br J Ophthalmol 55: 353–456

Byar DP, Mostofi FK (1969) Cancer of the prostate in men less than 50 years old: An analysis of 51 cases. J Urol 102: 726–733

Castro C, Winkelmann RK (1974) Angiolymphoid hyperplasia with eosinophilia in the skin. Cancer 34: 1696–1705

Cooper PH, Waisman J, Johnston WH, Skinner DG (1973) Severe atypia of transitional epithelium and carcinoma of the urinary bladder. Cancer 31: 1055–1060

Epstein NA, Fatti LP (1976) Prostatic carcinoma. Some morphological features affecting prognosis. Cancer 37: 2455–2465

Farrow GM, Harrison EG, Utz DC, Jones DR (1968) Renal angiomyolipoma. A clinicopathologic study of 32 cases. Cancer 22: 564–570

Fergusson JD (1970) Cancer of the prostate. Br Med J 4: 475–478

Filler RM, Traggis DG, Jaffe N, Vawter GF (1972) Favorable outlook for children with mediastinal neuroblastoma. J Pediatr Surg 7: 136–143

Fleming N (1948) A case of pigmented leiomyoma of the iris. Br J Ophthalmol 32: 885–892

Fortner J, Nicastri A, Murphy ML (1968) Neuroblastoma: Natural history and results of treating 133 cases. Ann Surg 167: 132–142

Fox H, Langley FA (1973) Postgraduate obstetrical and gynaecological pathology. Pergamon Press, Oxford

Franks LM (1954) Latent carcinoma of the prostate. J Pathol Bacteriol 68: 603–616

Garfield DH, Kennedy BJ (1972) Regression of metastatic renal cell carcinoma following nephrectomy. Cancer 30: 190–196

Hahn MJ, Dawson R, Esterly JA, Joseph DJ (1973) Hemangiopericytoma. An ultrastructural study. Cancer 31: 255–261

Hansen MM, Jensen JS (1969) Adenomatoid tumours of the testis and epididymis. Scand J Urol Nephrol 3: 157–159

Hogan MJ, Zimmerman LE (1962) Ophthalmic Pathology. An atlas and textbook, 2nd edn. Saunders, London

Jakobiec FA, Font RL, Tso MOM, Zimmerman LE (1977) Mesectodermal leiomyoma of the ciliary body. A tumor of presumed neural crest origin. Cancer 39: 2102–2113

Joliat G, Stalder H, Kapanci Y (1973) Lymphangiomyomatosis: A clinico-anatomical entity. Cancer 31: 455–461

Kay S, Pratt CB, Salzberg AM (1966) Hamartoma (leiomyomatous type) of the kidney. Cancer 19: 1825–1832

Kepes JJ (1971) In: Minckler J (ed) Pathology of the nervous system, chap 164. Differential diagnostic problems of brain tumors. McGraw Hill, London

Kern WH (1978) Well differentiated adenocarcinoma of the prostate. Cancer 41: 2046–2054

Klein MJ, Valensi QJ (1976) Proximal tubular adenomas of kidney with so-called oncocytic features. A clinicopathologic study of 13 cases of a rarely reported neoplasm. Cancer 38: 906–914

Kopelson G, Harisiadis L, Romas NA, Veenema RJ, Tannenbaum M (1978) Periurethral prostatic duct carcinoma. Clinical features and treatment results. Cancer 42: 2894–2902

Koss LG (1975) Atlas of tumor pathology, 2nd ser, fasc 11. Tumors of the urinary bladder. Armed Forces Institute of Pathology, Washington, D.C.

Kuhn C, Rosai J (1969) Tumors arising from pericytes. Ultrastructure and organ culture of a case. Arch Pathol 88: 653–663

Lee FD (1968) A comparative study of Kaposi's sarcoma and granuloma pyogenicum in Uganda. J Clin Pathol 21: 119–128

Mackay B, Luna MA, Butler JJ (1976) Adult neuroblastoma. Electron microscopic observations in nine cases. Cancer 37: 1334–1351

McMaster MJ, Soule EH, Ivins JC (1975) Hemangiopericytoma. A clinicopathologic study and long-term followup of 60 patients. Cancer 36: 2232–2244

McNeal JE (1969) Origin and development of carcinoma in the prostate. Cancer 23: 24–34

Mäkinen J (1972) Microscopic patterns as a guide to prognosis of neuroblastoma in childhood. Cancer 29: 1637–1646

Marshall FC, Uson AC, Melicow MM (1960) Neoplasms and caruncles of the female urethra. Surg Gynecol Obstet 110: 723–733

Meester LJ de, Farrow GM, Utz DC (1975) Inverted papillomas of the urinary bladder. Cancer 36: 505–513

Melamed MR, Voutsa NG, Grabstald H (1964) Natural history and clinical behavior of in situ carcinoma of the human urinary bladder. Cancer 17: 1533–1545

Melicow MM, Uson AC (1976) A spectrum of malignant epithelial tumors of the prostate gland. J Urol 115: 696–700

Meyer SL, Fine BS, Font RL, Zimmerman LE (1968) Leiomyoma of the ciliary body. Electron microscopic verification. Am J Ophthalmol 66: 1061–1068

Mostofi FK, Price EB (1973) Atlas of tumor pathology, 2nd ser, fasc 8. Tumors of the male genital system. Armed Forces Institute of Pathology, Washington, D.C.

Moulton EC, Moulton EC (1948) Leiomyoma of the iris. Am J Ophthalmol 31: 214–217

Murphy TE, Huvos AG, Frazell EL (1970) Chemodectomas of the glomus intravagale: Vagal body tumors, nonchromaffin paragangliomas of the nodose ganglion of the vagus nerve. Ann Surg 172: 246–255

O'Connell KM (1977) Kaposi's sarcoma: Histopathological study of 159 cases from Malawi. J Clin Pathol 30: 687–695

O'Connell KM (1977a) Kaposi's sarcoma in lymph nodes: Histological study of lesions from 16 cases in Malawi. J Clin Pathol 30: 696–703

O'Connor JS, Laws ER (1963) Histochemical survey of brain tumor enzymes. Arch Neurol 9: 641–651

Pachter MR, Lattes R (1963) Mesenchymal tumors of the mediastinum. III. Tumors of lymph vascular origin. Cancer 16: 108–117

Piper JV (1969) Malignant retroperitoneal fibrosis presenting as a vascular emergency. Br J Clin Pract 23: 390–391

Popoff NA, Malinin TI, Rosomoff HL (1974) Fine structure of intracranial hemangiopericytoma and angiomatous meningioma. Cancer 34: 1187–1197

Pryse-Davies J, Dawson IMP, Westbury G (1964) Some morphologic, histochemical, and chemical observations on chemodectomas and the normal carotid body, including a study of the chromaffin reaction and possible ganglion cell elements. Cancer 17: 185–202

Pugh RCB (1973) The pathology of cancer of the bladder. An editorial overview. Cancer 32: 1267–1274

Rafla S (1970) Renal cell carcinoma. Natural history and results of treatment. Cancer 25: 26–40

Raskind R, Weiss SR, Manning JJ, Wermuth RE (1971) Survival after surgical excision of single metastatic brain tumors. Amer J Roentgenol 111: 323–328

Richards MJS, Joo P, Gilbert EF (1976) The rare problem of late recurrence in neuroblastoma. Cancer: 1847–1852

Rios-Dalenz JL, Peacock RC (1966) Xanthogranulomatous pyelonephritis. Cancer 19: 289–296

Rubinstein LJ (1972) Atlas of tumor pathology, 2nd ser, fasc 6. Tumors of the central nervous system. Armed Forces Institute of Pathology, Washington, D.C.

Russell DS, Rubinstein LJ (1977) Pathology of tumours of the nervous system, 4th edn. Edward Arnold, London

Saldana MJ, Salem LE, Travesan R (1973) High altitude hypoxia and chemodectomas. Hum Pathol 4: 251–263

Salyer WR, Salyer DC (1975) Intravascular angiomatosis: Development and distinction from angiosarcoma. Cancer 36: 995–1001

Schade ROK, Swinney J (1968) Pre-cancerous changes in bladder epithelium. Lancet II: 943–946

Seemayer TA, Knaack J, Thelmo WL, Wang N-S, Ahmed MN (1975) Further observations on carcinoma in situ of the urinary bladder: Silent but extensive intraprostatic involvement. Cancer 36: 514–520

Sharma TC, Melamed MR, Whitmore WF (1970) Carcinoma in-situ of the ureter in patients with bladder carcinoma treated by cystectomy. Cancer 26: 583–587

Silber I, McGavran MH (1971) Adenocarcinoma of the prostate in men less than 56 years old: A study of 65 cases. J Urol 105: 283–285

Skinner DG, Colvin RB, Vermillion CD, Pfister RC, Leadbetter WF (1971) Diagnosis and management of renal cell carcinoma. A clinical and pathologic study of 309 cases. Cancer 28: 1165–1177

Stout AP (1935) The malignant tumors of the peripheral nerves. Am J Cancer 25: 1–36

Stout AP (1949) Hemangiopericytoma. A study of twenty-five new cases. Cancer 2: 1027–1054

Stout AP, Lattes R (1967) Atlas of tumor pathology, 2nd ser, fasc 1. Tumors of the soft tissues. Armed Forces Institute of Pathology, Washington, D.C.

Svien HJ, Wood MW (1957) Recurrence of a meningioma of the spinal cord after 23 years. Proc Mayo Clin 32: 573–578

Takáts LJ, Csapó Z (1966) Death from renal carcinoma 37 years after its original recognition. Cancer 19: 1172–1176

Tiltman AJ (1977) The identification and significance of early stromal invasion in papillary carcinoma of the urinary bladder. J Pathol 122: 91–94

Tung KSK, McCormack LJ (1967) Angiomatous lymphoid hamartoma. Report of five cases with a review of the literature. Cancer 20: 525–536

Vidne BA, Richter S, Levy MJ (1976) Surgical treatment of solitary pulmonary metastasis. Cancer 38: 2561–2563

Wara WM, Sheline GE, Newman H, Townsend JJ, Boldrey EB (1975) Radiation therapy of meningiomas. Amer J Roentgenol 123: 453–458

Whimster WF, Masson AF (1970) Malignant carotid body tumor with extradural metastases. Cancer 26: 239–244

Willis R (1960) Pathology of tumours, 3rd edn. Butterworth, London

Young DG, Williams DI (1969) Malignant renal tumours in infancy and childhood. Br J Hosp Med 2: 740–741, 744–752

# 12 General Assessment

... it seems fair to state that baselines or criteria for malignancy are not always clearly defined nor are they identical in the minds of equally capable pathologists. (Angevine, 1965)

... when carefully studied, human cancer provides its own experimental models and perhaps, in the last analysis, the only valid models. (Black et al., 1971)

Choriocarcinoma can be diagnosed with virtual certainty by hormonal assay. Otherwise, the diagnosis of cancer still rests on histology: and, histological 'proof' notwithstanding, the technique still has severe limitations. In the preceding chapters an attempt has been made by analysis of a local series of cases and a parallel survey of similar data published by others to estimate the extent of the limitations and thus the level of diagnostic accuracy.

Table 12.1 indicates, for most of the local series, the number of cases shown by their later behaviour to have been significantly over-diagnosed or under-diagnosed, or appropriately or inappropriately diagnosed, and, for comparison only, the number of cases of cancer of equivalent types diagnosed without qualification during the same period. In the few instances where the diagnosis has been classed as inappropriate, the inappropriateness had not had a significant bearing on the treatment of the patient or therefore on the clinical outcome.

For reasons mentioned in the earlier text, (a) of neoplasms of skin, only melanocarcinoma has been included in Table 12.1, and (b) lesions of the respiratory and female genital tracts, and those equivalent to the cases comprising Chapter 11, have not been included.

The main conclusions to be drawn from the survey are:

1) *Breast*. Lesions of the breast are histo-logically no more debatable than many that occur in other organs but the psychologically complex background against which they are seen is unique. Excision of the rectum or loss of a limb may be more physically disabling but in terms of psychological disability they are of an altogether lower order.

Technically, the pathologist meets most problems with the irregular hyperplasia that is sclerosing adenosis; in distinguishing between intraduct epitheliosis and intraduct carcinoma; and with the still highly debatable lesion known variably as LCIS or lobular neoplasia. It seems likely from the local data that, at least in the short term, mastectomy was performed on histologically inadequate evidence on four occasions, in each case an instance of over-diagnosis of epitheliosis as intraduct carcinoma.

2) *Thyroid*. Microfollicular adenomas are prone to over-diagnosis as follicular carcinoma: such, almost certainly, were the six over-diagnoses in the series. However, as has been stressed, virtual certainty that diagnosis of a lesion of thyroid as malignant was an over-diagnosis is, in retrospect, 'all very well'. Diagnosis in prospect is altogether different. Lesions of identical appearance may or may not metastasise, and until some new technique of discrimination becomes available, this 'mistake' will remain unavoidable.

3) *Lymph Nodes*. As expected, lymph nodes have provided more diagnostic variations than any other tissue. Of 40 borderline lesions, the reports issued on almost one-third proved inaccurate, yielding six over-diagnoses and eight under-diagnoses (the possibility remains, however, that some of the patients whose lesions were apparently over-diagnosed as ML may yet suffer recurrence). The 40 cases amounted to approximately one-quarter of the total of 173

**Table 12.1.** Summary of diagnoses.[1]

| | Cancers diagnosed | Borderline lesions | Quality of diagnosis | | | | Ratio b/a |
|---|---|---|---|---|---|---|---|
| | | | O/D | U/D | Appr. | Inappr. | |
| Breast | 1149 | 21 | 5 | 1 | 15 | | 1:55 |
| Thyroid | 33 | 26 | 6 | 1 | 19 | | 1:1.3 |
| Malignant lymphoma (HD) | 58 | 22 | 1 | 7 | 14 | | 1.2.6 |
| Malignant lymphoma (non-HD) | 75 | 18 | 1 | 3 | 14 | | 1:4.1 |
| Soft tissue | 51 | 36 | 7 | 4 | 20 | 5 | 1:1.4 |
| Bone/cartilage | 43 | 15 | 2 | 1 | 12 | | 1:2.9 |
| Melanocarcinoma | 78 | 24 | 1 | 5 | 17 | 1 | 1:3.3 |
| Digestive tract | 2260 | 26 | 2 | 4 | 20 | | 1.87 |

[1] Shows, for the 27 years under analysis and for various sites:
(a) The number of cancers diagnosed without qualification;
(b) The number of significantly borderline cases;
(c) The 'quality' of diagnosis as shown by later events (O/D, over-diagnosis; U/D, under-diagnosis; Appr, appropriate diagnosis; Inappr, inappropriate diagnosis);
(d) The ratio (b):(a).

cases received during the years under review where the diagnosis of ML was either firmly made (133) or seriously considered (the 40 borderline).

4) *Soft Tissue.* The notoriously oncomimetic character of many lesions of the soft tissues is well known. In the local series, two malignant lesions of lower limb were initially under-diagnosed, and, despite further treatment (amputation in one) both patients died. One of the two lesions should have been diagnosed as sarcomatous at the outset, when amputation might have been life-saving. In the second case, the histology became diagnostically sarcomatous only simultaneously with its spread: even on re-examination, the original tissue pattern would have not justified amputation.

Of seven cases over-diagnosed, only one patient lost a (lower) limb: the limb had to be removed by reason of extensive local tissue destruction, not primarily because of the over-diagnosis of the lesion as synoviosarcoma. However, the same mistake with tissue around, say, the knee, might have led to an unnecessary amputation.

5) *Bone.* In the one lesion that was significantly under-diagnosed, as osteoclastoma instead of osteosarcoma, even re-examination of the original sections gave no grounds for preferring the graver diagnosis. The histology of the lesion changed over a period of 5 years to that of a

fibrosarcoma: the original biopsy may have been inadequately representative. Neither of the two over-diagnoses led to amputation.

Misdiagnosis of cases of myositis ossificans or the aneurysmal bone cyst as osteosarcoma appears to have been avoided, a fortunate circumstance that owes much to ready access to and helpful cooperation from the Scottish Bone Tumour Registry.

6) *Skin.* Abandonment of amputation as primary treatment for uncomplicated melanocarcinoma of a limb has rendered the question of over- and under-diagnosis mainly academic: it thus remains a matter for speculation whether any of the patients who did die would have been saved by amputation. Excision of lymph nodes in continuity has rarely been practised in this area, and a similar speculation applies.

Even commoner and more problematical than the melanocytic lesions, though of lesser therapeutic significance, was the ? premycotic eruption. Of the total of 114 borderline lesions of skin included in the series (37 squamous or adnexal, 24 melanocytic, 53 infiltrative), the premycotic group accounted for nearly one-half. It seems unlikely that a relatively high proportion such as this can be appreciably reduced unless the diagnostic threshold is raised to the level where MF itself is being diagnosed.

7) *Digestive System.* The figures for this system in Table 12.1 may mislead in so far as

they suggest that of all the 2260 whole specimens or biopsies only 26 caused diagnostic concern. It seems proper, again, to stress that pleomorphic salivary adenomas and, with one exception each, intestinal polyps and carcinoid tumours have not been included, nor have many instances where initial concern, later resolved, was caused only by inadequate biopsy.

Throughout the digestive system as a whole, over-diagnosis of rectal lesions with consequent excision still represents the main danger, though, as in the breast and for the same reasons, techniques of more limited excision are increasingly being tried. Reassessment of the four cases under-diagnosed and the two cases over-diagnosed in this anatomical system, and formally included in Table 12.1, indicates two potentially avoidable 'casualties': one, the patient who received a course of radiotherapy (without sequelae for 21 years so far) for a benign lymphoepithelial lesion of the palate; the other, the youth whose rectal lymphoid polyp was over-diagnosed as a lymphosarcoma and led to colostomy. In neither of the two patients whose lesion was initially under-diagnosed (carcinoma of alveolus and oesophagus respectively) and who died, had the under-diagnosis led to either delay in or inappropriate treatment. Both were treated as for a malignant lesion from the outset. It is doubtful whether significant delay is ever caused by an oesophageal biopsy's being inadequate; the nature of the symptoms will demand either repeated biopsy or open operation or both.

8) Of other lesions, doubt remains whether the removal of an eye on one occasion was mandatory.

As the figures for cases over-diagnosed and cases under-diagnosed have emerged in Table 12.1, the numbers for each are by coincidence almost exactly the same (25 and 26) though with a distinct tendency towards one side or the other in different situations, as, for example, with lesions of breast, thyroid and the soft tissues, towards over-diagnosis, and, with those of ML and melanocarcinoma, towards under-diagnosis. Apart from the under-diagnosis of MLs, these tendencies are approximately in line with those cited from various series in the earlier text.

The reports in many of the quoted series, where borderline lesions have been reassessed

years later, when the outcome is mostly known, makes quite clear the fact that on many occasions cancer is over-diagnosed. Table 12.2 brings together data from most of the series of diagnostic revisions cited earlier in the text. The extent of over-diagnosis revealed is clearly substantial (in all the series combined it amounts to 26%) and on first reading almost alarming. Admittedly, the series are to some extent selected. For example, the 14 'sarcomas' of soft tissue, found on review to be not sarcomas, were all atypical fibroxanthomas: and the atypical fibroxanthoma is not a common lesion. Further, most of the commoner cancers, such as the carcinomas of breast, bronchus, stomach and large intestine, do not figure in the table, simply because no comparable retrospective series of these lesions have been found: the commonest cancers probably are being diagnosed with fair consistency and reliability. To this combined extent, namely, the selective character of the entries in Table 12.2 and the probable reliability of diagnosis of the commoner cancers, the data in the table are less profoundly disturbing than at first reading. Nevertheless, they are disquieting. They suggest, first, that, viewing the disease 'cancer' overall, as many as 5% or 10% of patients diagnosed as having cancer do not have cancer, and that statistics for both the incidence of a cancer and its cure are thereby impaired; second, with the less common cancers, such as those comprising Table 12.2, widely varying cure rates are less a measure of the clinicians' therapeutic successes than of their pathologists' diagnostic thresholds. Relatively consistent cure rates, as with carcinoma of the breast (pace LCIS), bespeak relatively consistent diagnostic levels. A tendency towards over-diagnosis is for obvious reasons unavoidable and understandable; the best hope of keeping the tendency within reasonable limits is a constant sharpening of histological criteria.

It bears repetition that, with the exception of a few otherwise illustrative or educative examples, only lesions represented by significantly borderline histological reports are included in this series of nearly 400 cases. How many, if any, breasts, uteri, rectums or stomachs, for example, may have been removed unnecessarily on the basis of lesions that were histologically marginal or equivocal but were diagnosed without qualification as malignant is not known, but they cannot have been many. In general, it has been the practice over the years, where doubt has persisted even after joint discussion with colleagues, to say so in the histological report, and this fact should have ensured the inclusion of virtually all such in the present series.

Before giving a brief summarising account of the main causes of diagnostic uncertainty and difficulty it may be appropriate to include here two lists of lesions of constant and continuing relevance to the practice of histopathology:

1) Benign lesions wherein certain distinction between 'benign' and 'malignant' may at times be virtually impossible:

Follicular adenoma of thyroid

Infectious mononucleosis: toxoplasmosis: drug-induced reactions, in lymph nodes

Atypical fibroxanthoma

Early callus: aneurysmal bone cyst: myositis ossificans

Mucosal patterns in ulcerative colitis

Pseudo-lymphomas in, especially, the gastro-intestinal tract

Apparent adenocarcinoma corporis uteri in youth

Exuberant granulation tissue.

2) Lesions diagnosable with confidence wherein the histology per se allows at best only a very approximate prediction of the likelihood of metastasis:

Medullary carcinoma of thyroid

Malignant mesenchymoma

Synovial sarcoma

Osteoclastoma

Ewing's tumour

**Table 12.2.** Data from series cited in earlier chapters that included details of diagnostic revisions.

| | 'Malignant' on original diagnosis | 'Not malignant' on review | Series[1] | Page no. present text |
|---|---|---|---|---|
| Thyroid | 345 (carc.: malignant adenoma) | 82 | Saxén et al. (1969) | 41 |
| Lymph node | 600 (HD) | 192 | Symmers (1968a) | 68 |
| Soft tissue | 330 (fibrosarcoma) | 34 | Pritchard et al. (1974) | 143 |
| | 50 ('soft tissue sarcoma') | 32 | Dahl (1976)[2] | 143 |
| | 14 (rhabdo-, fibrosarcomas) | 14 | Enzinger and Dulcey (1967) | 210 |
| Bone and cartilage | 657 ('sarcoma, osteogenic series') | 32 | McKenna et al. (1966) | 143 |
| | 75 (osteoclastoma) | 18 | Larsson et al. (1975)[3] | 250 |
| Skin | 25 (spindle-cell carcinoma) | 21 | Hudson and Winkelmann (1972) | 204 |
| | 144 (MF) | 69 | Epstein et al. (1972) | 269 |
| | 247 (melanocarcinoma) | 56 | Truax et al. (1966) | 275 |
| | 20 (melanocarcinoma, prepubertal) | 13 | Saksela and Rintala (1968)[4] | 275 |
| Digestive tract | 134 (malignant mixed salivary) | 35 | Gerughty et al. (1969) | 357 |
| | 10 (ML) | 3 | Saltzstein (1969)[5] | 365 |
| Endometrium | 208 (adenocarcinoma) | 48 | Keller et al. (1974) | 407 |
| | 22 (adenocarcinoma) | 7 | Kempson and Pokorny (1968) | 407 |
| Myometrium | 63 (LMS) | 24 | Taylor and Norris (1966) | 409 |
| | 81 (LMS) | 48 | Christopherson et al. (1972) | 410 |
| Ovary | 136 (mucinous carcinoma) | 97 ('border-line') | Hart and Norris (1973) | 413 |
| Kidney | 17 (Wilms' tumour, sarcoma) | 0 | Bogdan et al. (1973) | 440 |

[1] Refer to relevant chapter for complete reference.

[2] Total series (57) included also 7 cases diagnosed prospectively.

[3] Series of 75 divided originally into 33 'malignant', 42 'benign': diagnoses on revision, all 18 benign and not osteoclastoma.

[4] Histology not available in 3 of original 20.

[5] Nominal figures (10, 3) to represent author's statement that ". . . between one-fourth and one-half have been found to be pseudolymphomas".

Carcinoid tumour (except in appendix)
Bronchial adenoma
Chemodectoma
Haemangiopericytoma

## Comment in Summary

Diagnostic inaccuracy of some degree is inevitable: it cannot be overcome by the finest pathologist. One source of uncertainty or imprecision is insuperable: it bears directly on the statement made at the outset that diagnosis is prognosis, and, for the most part, a standard prognosis based on standard experience. The behaviour of a cancer of any individual type may be far from 'standard'. Carcinoma of the breast is again the exemplar, and all are familiar with the unpredictability and frequently long dormancy of the individual lesion here. The crucial element is the inherent biological variability of any individual lesion governed by what Gordon-Taylor (1959), in his account of the behaviour of carcinoma of the breast, called "The incomputable factor in cancer prognosis".

The behaviour of cancer extends from the indolent rodent ulcer to the choriocarcinoma that may arise, spread, and kill within the span of a single pregnancy. Probably no individual type of cancer has a range of behaviour as wide as this but the existence of significant variation is clear. Necropsy experience, or the long trouble-free survival of a patient whose excised lesion was massive enough to have been a potential source of metastases for possibly years, leaves little doubt that some cancers at any rate behave as does the rodent ulcer even though we cannot yet identify them in advance. Three periampullary carcinomas of duodenum with no metastases at necropsy, and two massive carcinomas of caecum from patients who survived long after excision, come to mind as instances where the histological diagnosis was straightforward and in no way borderline; yet the 'standard' prognosis was not fulfilled in practice. Histology fails as a predictor here but at least it 'fails safe'.

To what extent individual types of cancer possess such a range of biological variability, and how wide it is, is difficult to estimate (though, as well described by Smithers [1969], we are learning more of the tendency of some cancers to mature and subside, and of the rare but well-documented phenomenon of apparently total spontaneous regression [Lewison, 1976]), but the implications vis-à-vis treatment are evident. A patient will be fortunate or unfortunate accordingly as he has a cancer that metastasises late in its life or early; as a corollary, it may be that the range of survival in a group of patients is a measure less of the results of treatment than of the biological variability of the cancer they had.

The foregoing comments concern the histologically manifest cancers, and they are not the main concern of this treatise. Nevertheless, even though manifest, their correct identification may have therapeutic significance, as for example in the case earlier cited where the form of treatment of an adenocarcinoma in the cervix of the uterus may vary depending on the decision whether it is of endocervical or corporeal origin. Further, with an apparently metastatic deposit, 'Hunt the primary' is not always a sterile academic pursuit; the lesion might itself be primary. More immediately relevant than the manifest cancers are the earliest cancers and the problems they cause.

A cancer may be too early to be detectable by current techniques: if the earliest change is a monocellular mutation, this is obviously so and likely long to remain so. The conceptual difficulties inherent in the term 'earliness' in relation to cancer, the difference between structural earliness and biological earliness, are now well realised (clear analyses were provided by Kreyberg [1953] and Crile [1956] in their accounts of lesions in breast and the spreading of cancer respectively); and it is with the earliest structural changes that we enter the diagnostically difficult borderline zone, its width differing from lesion to lesion and pathologist to pathologist.

In practice, the problems of diagnosis of structurally early cancer grow all the time as biopsy by endoscope spreads. The implications have been mentioned already in the context of gastric carcinoma but they are generally relevant. The earlier the lesion, the less the degree of diagnostic asssurance, to the point where important statistics may suffer. The apparent incidence of a cancer may rise, and with it the cure rate, but the corresponding death rate may fail to fall; the reliability of diagnosis is then increasingly suspect.

Readers with an epidemiological interest may recall the paradox, statistical and biological, inherent in data published by Nieburgs and his colleagues (1957) in an account of the screening of a population for in situ carcinoma of the cervix. In comparing (a) the figures published by these workers for the incidence and prevalence of the disorder with (b) figures for the known mortality from cervical cancer, an Editorial (1958) reviewer remarked that ". . . a statistical poser pops up", namely, that there were in the series, ". . . eight and a half times as many cancers in situ as can be accounted for by deaths from cancer of the cervix". That is, if all carcinomas in situ progressed to potentially lethal carcinoma, then, even allowing gynaecologists a much higher cure rate than they themselves would claim, the number of women dying from cancer of the cervix was much smaller than it should have been. It may be that if all cancers were as open to early biopsy as cancer of the cervix, we should be in the same dilemma with every tissue.

No new criteria by which 'malignancy' may be histologically diagnosed have been discovered. We are still dependent for the calculations of our histoclinical correlations on the aberrancy of cells and departure from the structural norm in terms of 'invasion'. Even the electron microscope (EM) has not fulfilled early expectations. Many years ago a hope was expressed by Melnick (1932), perplexed by a seemingly simple myoma of stomach that metastasised, that "It may be that the future will reveal finer cytological characteristics of (smooth muscle) tumor cells not yet known. Cytological studies of tumor cells are few. Perhaps morphology here ends and physiology begins". The 'finer cytological characteristics' now have been revealed, and their recognition by electron microscopy is undoubtedly helpful; however, the help is almost always only towards distinguishing one type of malignant neoplasm from another, not towards distinguishing a malignant neoplasm from a benign. In a wide survey of the contribution of ultramicroscopy to the study of neoplasms, Bonikos and his colleagues (1976) state that

> While these differences between benign and malignant neoplasms do exist, electron microscopy is of little practical value in separating benign from malignant tumors since obvious

cases are easily diagnosed by light microscopy and borderline malignant neoplasms do not have ultrastructural features which allow them to be categorically classified as benign or malignant.

This remark was made particularly apropos neoplasms of soft tissue but nothing in the survey suggests that it has other than general relevance. There seems to be one exception, and it may be unique, namely, the earlier noted benign clear cell tumour ('sugar' tumour) of lung which may be distinguished with virtual certainty by EM, and only by EM, from the metastatic carcinoma of kidney.

Little remains to be added in commentary on the standard histological criteria of malignancy to the short lists of 'conclusions' at the end of the preceding chapters. For all its limitations and shortcomings, relatively high in some lesions benign, relatively low in some others malignant, mitotic incidence remains a valuable index: its general dependability was still being endorsed in the recent writings of three experienced pathologists reported simultaneously in a series of Editorials (1976). The aberrant mitotic figure, the nearest we have to an absolute criterion, is rarely seen other than in company with an excessive number of seemingly normal mitoses but at times, as for example in a papillary overgrowth of bladder or rectum, it could serve to move the diagnosis from the borderline zone into that of frank malignancy.

The other standard criterion, stromal invasion, has also been assessed to some extent already. No more will be said of the 'basement membrane'. Early stromal invasion may be particularly difficult to assess. The muscularis mucosae in the gastrointestinal tract is a useful frontier but the problem with hamartomatous overgrowths, and with benign epithelial displacement in polyps of the colon and rectum, will be remembered. In structures that lack a muscularis mucosae yet have a subjacent muscular stroma, such as gall bladder, endometrium and uterine tube, reliance has to be placed largely on assessment of detailed cytology. At yet other sites the problem may be more difficult still. Epithelial tissue within the thyroid, pancreas and prostate has, as it were, a right to be almost anywhere within the capsule, while in the breast there is not even a capsule. Again much depends on cytology, but all know how uniform and well differentiated small acinar structures may be in some areas of an elsewhere undoubted carcinoma in these organs. In the case of the prostate, a permeation of muscle bundles to the point where individual fibres are being separated is possibly the only certain indication of 'invasion'.

The presence of neoplastic tissue in vessels has, I believe, been overmuch emphasised as a prognostic indicator. Vessels may at times be not truly vessels but only seemingly so: reports are many of the detection of malignant cells in a vein or the inferior vena cava of a patient in whom metastases did not develop; also, a manifest vein may be blocked distal to the section by thrombus. The phenomenon is a worrying finding, of course, but is too often regarded (and reported) as indicating a virtually 100% certainty of metastasis. However, for the above reasons, this it does not indicate. Therefore, if a pathologist's report includes a mention of the occurrence, and it is rarely omitted, he is under a firm obligation to make his implications clear.

Invasion of nerves can be diagnosed microscopically with more assurance than invasion of vessels, but when present as the only abnormality to suggest 'malignancy', as may apply to the disorderly pancreas or prostate, its clinical significance at any rate is marginal if not minimal. Its occurrence in company with benign overgrowths of the breast was mentioned earlier. The presence in lymph nodes of naevus cells, melanophages, endometriosis and thyroid tissue has also been mentioned as in all instances a significant and possibly misleading simulator of malignant 'invasion'. In the case of thyroid tissue, however, true metastasis is much commoner than simulated metastasis.

In practice, in borderline lesions, neither cytological aberrancy nor apparent invasion is likely often to be used in isolation as the arbiter: a varying degree of both will contribute with, depending on site, mitotic incidence as the final weight that determines to which side the balance falls. Further, the pathologist will remember that, at all times but most starkly in the borderline case, the opinion he gives is basically one of statistical probability. The more nearly in this gray area he can express his opinion in terms of percentage, the more accurately and usefully will his clinically colleague be able to add it to the balance he himself has to weigh in planning his approach to the problems of the patient; and that is the raison d'être of clinical histopathology.

The rather uneven accession of lesions over the years, in particular the relative infrequency of lesions of the lung and CNS, has precluded the foregoing account's being in any sense a textbook. It is offered rather as a general pathologist's small vade mecum. A much more informative survey could be provided by a series of articles written by pathologists individually specialist in their fields, and that may yet be achieved: such a compilation will be an editorial project for some successor sometime.

# References

Angevine DM (1965) Some impressions concerning tissue diagnoses. Arch Pathol 80: 1–2

Black MM, Freeman C, Mork T, Harvei S, Cutler SJ (1971) Prognostic significance of microscopic structure of gastric carcinomas and their regional lymph nodes. Cancer 27: 703–711

Bonikos DS, Bensch KG, Kempson RL (1976) The contribution of electron microscopy to the differential diagnosis of tumors. Beitr Pathol 158: 417–444

Crile G (1956) Factors influencing the spread of cancer. Surg Gynecol Obstet 103: 342–352

Editorial (1958) Commentary on Nieburgs et al. (1957) (q.v.). Obstet Gynecol Survey 13: 706–707

Editorials (1976) Mitosis counting, I, II, III. Hum Pathol 7: 481–484

Gordon-Taylor G (1959) The incomputable factor in cancer prognosis. Br Med J 1: 455–462

Kreyberg L (1953) The significance of "early diagnosis" in breast cancer: A study of some common usages of the term. Br J Cancer 7: 157–165

Lewison EF (1976) Conference on Spontaneous Regression of Cancer. Natl Cancer Inst Monogr 44

Melnick PJ (1932) Metastasizing leiomyoma of the stomach. Am J Cancer 16: 890–902

Nieburgs HE, Stergus I, Stephenson EM, Harbin BL (1957) Mass screening of the total female population of a county for cervical carcinoma. JAMA 164: 1546–1551

Smithers DW (1969) Maturation in human tumours. Lancet II: 949–952

# Index[1]

Actinic reticuloid, 272
Adenitis, mesenteric, *114*, 136
Adenoacanthoma
  endometrial carcinoma, 408
  ovarian carcinoma, 413
Adenocarcinoid tumor, appendix, 364
Adenoma, bronchial, 385, 455
  oncocytic, renal, 441
  salivary, 357
  thyroid, *43*, 57
Adenoma malignum, *393*, 406
Adenomatoid tumour, 402
  vs adenocarcinoma, 402
  epididymis, 444
  vs testicular carcinoma, 444
  uterine tube, 402
  uterus, 402
Adenomatosis, nipple ducts, *16*, 25
Adenomyosis, uterus, 411
Adenosarcoma, Müllerian, 411
Adnexal adenoma/carcinoma, skin, 265
Adrenal carcinoma (metastatic) vs pulmonary oncocytoma, *377–380*
Age of patient, influence on diagnosis, 9–10
  bone, lesions of, 244–245
  mammary carcinoma, 33
  melanocytic lesions, 319–320
  neuroblastoma, 244–245
Age of patient, influence on prognosis
  endometrial carcinoma, 407
  mammary carcinoma, 33
  melanocarcinoma, 319
  renal carcinoma, 441
Albright syndrome, 254
Alkaline phosphatase
  meningioma, diagnostic significance, 438
  osteosarcoma, prognostic significance, 249
Alphafetoprotein (AFP), ovarian neoplasms, 415
Anaemia, refractory, association

with giant lymphoid hamartoma, 134
Aneurysmal bone cyst, 248, 249, 250, **252–253**
  vs angiosarcoma, 253
  vs fibrosarcoma, 253
  vs osteosarcoma, 252, 454
Angioma and allied lesions, 444–446; *see also* Haemangioblastoma; Haemangioma; Haemangiopericytoma
  angiofibroma, juvenile (nasal), 382–383
  irradiation, implications, 382
  angiolipoma, 198
  angiolymphoid hyperplasia with eosinophilia, 445
  vs angiosarcoma, 445
  angioma
    sclerosing, 445
    vertebral column, 253
  angiomatosis, intravascular, 444
  angiomyolipoma, renal, 197, 441
  angioplasia, papular, 445
  angiosarcoma, 208–209
    vs aneurysmal bone cyst, 253
    vs angiolymphoid hyperplasia with eosinophilia, 444
    gall bladder, *326*
    vs pseudoangiosarcoma, 445
Anus, mucoid carcinoma, *347*
Aponeurotic fibroma, juvenile, 206
Appendix vermiformis, adenocarcinoid tumour, 364
APUD system, bronchus, 385
Argentaffin carcinoma, *see* Carcinoid tumour
Arias-Stella phenomenon
  cervix uteri, 405
  vs clear cell carcinoma, 409
Arthropod bite granuloma, 271, **272–273**
Ascites, serosal metaplasia, 367
Asteroid bodies, giant cells, 212
Astrocytes, 438
  mitoses in, *421, 425*
Astrocytoma

diagnostic difficulties, 438
  vs meningioma vs Schwannoma, 438
Atypical fibroxanthoma, 202, 203–205; *see also* Fibroxanthoma, atypical
Audit, histopathological, 10–12

Basal cell carcinoma (BCC), 262, **265–266**
  vs carcinoid tumour, 266
  histiocytoma, simulation in association, 153
  metastases from, 265–266, 403
  morphoeiform, vs atypical fibroxanthoma, 204
  pseudoepitheliomatous hyperplasia associated, 266
  vulva, 403
Basement membrane, significance, 6; *see also* Invasion
  carcinoma, breast, 37
  carcinoma, urinary bladder, 444
  cervix uteri, 404
Basosquamous carcinoma, 265
Benign chorionic invasion, *399*, 415–416
Benign lymphoepithelial lesion (salivary), *326*, 358
Benign lymphoid polyp (rectum), *105*, 365
Benign metastasising goitre, 58
Benign metastasising myoma (uterus), 411, **412**
Biliary duct lymph node, inflammatory reactions, 134
Biopsy technique; *see also* Frozen section
  bony lesions, imprint preparations, 243
  breast, 14
  carcinoid tumour, 365
  intracranial neoplasms, alkaline phosphatase, 438
  lymph node sectioning (axillary), 36
  pancreas, 366–367

---

[1] Page numbers in *italic* refer to cases in the various Local Series either individually or as an entry in the relevant Tables under 'Local Series of Cases' or 'Local Series of Cases, Summarised Data'. Page numbers in **boldface**, when in a series, refer to the main entry for the subject concerned. Most of the more misleading tissue patterns appear as entries with the prefix 'Pseudo-' or within the groups 'Diagnostic revision' or 'Mitosis'. The entries 'entity *x* vs entity *y*' are included primarily as aide-mémoires.

Bladder urinary, lesions, 443–444
  carcinoma, 443–444
    cystitis cystica, 443
      glandularis, 443
        vs glandular carcinoma, 443
    papilloma, inverted, 443
      transitional cell, 443
    precancerous changes, 443–444
Blood vessel, invasion, 457; *see also*
    Vascular invasion; Pseudo-
    invasion; Stromal invasion
Blood vessels, lesions, 444–446
Blue naevus, vs atypical fibro-
    xanthoma, 204
Bone; *see also* Bone and cartilage
    (self-defining lesions, e.g.
    Aneurysmal bone cyst,
    Exostosis, indexed
    individually)
  biopsy technique, imprint
    preparations, 243
  callus vs chondrosarcoma vs
    osteosarcoma *222*, 247–250
  cherubism, 254
  clinical data, significance,
    240–242
  disappearing bone disease, 226
  fibrous dysplasia, 253–255; *see
    also* Fibrous dysplasia
  infarction, relation to malignant
    fibrous histiocytoma, 255
  malignant fibrous histiocytoma,
    255
  malignant round cell tumour,
    differential diagnosis,
    244–245
  mesodermal hamartoma, 197
  radiotherapy, possible contra-
    indications, 254
Bone and cartilage, lesions
  callus vs osteosarcoma vs
    chondrosarcoma, 247–250
  chondroma vs chondrosarcoma,
    245–247
  diagnosis, clinical vs histological
    evidence, 242
  inflammatory patterns vs
    neoplastic patterns, 242–245
  malignant neoplasms, compara-
    tive mortality, 221
Bone and cartilage, local series of
    cases, 221–240
  results on review, 222
  summarised data, 222
Breast, local series of cases, 14–27
  results on review, 16
  summarised data, 15
Breast, lesions
  adenomatosis, nipple ducts, *16*,
    25
  carcinoma
    adenoid cystic, 32
    age of patient
      influence on diagnosis, 33
      influence on prognosis, 33
    basement membrane,
      significance, 37
    contralateral breast, 29, **37**
    cytology, 14
    'early' and 'late', 35, 455

elastosis, 36
epithelial-stromal junction
    (ESJ), 37
frozen section, 30
in situ, lobular (LCIS), 28–30
intraduct, *16*, 27, **30–32**
  cribriform pattern, 31
  late recurrence, 455
lymph nodes, involvement/
    assessment, 35–37
  mast cells, prognostic
    significance, 37
  occult metastasis, 36
  sectioning technique, 36
  sinus histiocytosis, 36
  vs malignant lymphoma, 38
  metastatic, vs histiocytoma,
    204
'minimal', 29
needle biopsy, 14
Paget's disease, 32
population screening, 37
pregnancy, influence, 33
prognosis, assessment,
    33–38
R-S cell, seeming presence in,
    125
size of neoplasm, influence on
    prognosis, 35
squamous cell, 33
'staging', influence on
    prognosis, 34–35
tylectomy, 13
cystosarcoma phyllodes, 33
dysplasia, 28
  neural invasion, innocuous, 36
  vascular invasion, innocuous,
    36
elastosis, 36
epithelial-stromal junction
    (ESJ), 37
epitheliosis, *16*, 31
fibroadenoma, *16*
fibrocystic disease (FCD), 28
lactational hyperplasia
    (adenosis), *16*
malignant lymphoma, vs
    carcinoma, 38
nipple duct adenomatosis, *16*
Paget's disease, 32
papillomatosis, *16*
pseudoinvasive patterns, 36, 37
pseudolymphoma, 38
sclerosing adenosis, *16*
stromal invasion, assessment, 37
Brenner tumour, 413
Bromoderma, pseudoepithelioma-
    tous hyperplasia, 263
Bronchus and lung, lesions of,
    384–388
adenoma, 385
  histoclinical correlation low,
    455
carcinoid tumour, 385
carcinoma, R-S cell, seeming
    presence in, 125
clear cell (sugar) tumour,
    385–386
granuloma, plasma cell, 386
  xanthomatous, 386

granulomatosis, lymphomatoid,
    386
hamartoma, fibroleiomyo-
    matous, 412
  lymphangiomyomatous, 445
metastases, resection, therapeutic
    value, 387–388
oncocytoma, *377–380*, 385
pseudotumour, inflammatory,
    386
'shock' lung, pseudosarcomatous
    pattern, 209
tumourlet, 386
Brucellosis vs malignant
    lymphoma, 137
Brunn's nest, 443


Calcification, focal
  neuroblastoma, prognostic value,
    *421*, 437
  salivary neoplasms, prognostic
    value, 357
Callus, misleading appearances,
    *222*, 247–250, 454
Cancer
  'early' and 'late', 35, 455
  qua systemic disorder, 6, 208
Carcinoembryonic antigen (CEA),
    10
  adenocarcinoma uteri, diagnostic
    value, 405
  granular cell myoblastoma, 210
Carcinogenesis, transplacental, 409
Carcinoid tumour, 363–365
  adenocarcinoid, appendix, 364
  vs basal cell carcinoma, 266
  biopsy requirements, 365
  bronchus, 385
  vs carcinoma simplex, 364
  diagnostic revision, 364
  histoclinical correlation low, 455
Carcinoma
  adenoid cystic
    breast, 32
    salivary tissue, 265
    skin, 265
  adenosquamous, endometrium,
    408
  adnexal, skin, 265
  anaplastic, vs atypical
    fibroxanthoma, 204
  argentaffin, *see* Carcinoid tumour
  basal cell, *see* Basal cell
    carcinoma
  basosquamous, 265
  clear cell
    female genital tract, 409
      vs Arias-Stella phenomenon,
        409
    lung, 385–386
  clinically cryptic, thyroid, 62
  combined (oesophagus), 360
  embryonal, 414
  endometrioid, 413
  'indolent mucoid' (stomach), 361
  metastatic
    vs histiocytoma, 204
    vs malignant fibrous
      histiocytoma (bone), 255

vs malignant lymphoma, *105*, 137
vs myeloma, 243–244
microinvasive (cervix uteri), 404
mucinous, vs meningioma, 437
mucoepidermoid, 358
mucoid (anus), *347*
salivary, 357–358
simplex, vs carcinoid tumour, 364
spindle-celled, 194
vs atypical fibroxanthoma, 204
diagnostic revision, 204
vs melanocarcinoma, 194
vs pseudosarcoma, 358–359
squamous cell, *see* Squamous cell carcinoma
undifferentiated, vs haemangiopericytoma, 446
verrucous
cervix uteri, 405
oesophagus, 360
oral cavity, 356
radiotherapy, implications, 264
skin, 264
Carcinoma in situ (CIS)
bladder, urinary, 444
breast, lobular (LCIS), 28–30
cervix uteri, 403–404
endometrium, 406
large intestine, 363
larynx, 383–384
oesophagus, 360
pancreatic duct, 367
seminal vesicle, 444
skin, 266
small intestine (I$^{131}$), 362
stomach, 360
ureter, 444
vas deferens, 444
Carcinosarcoma (endometrium), 409
Carotid body, chemodectoma, 439
Cartilage, *see* Chondro- entries
Caruncle, urethral, *430*, 444
Cases analysed, local series
bone and cartilage, 221–240
breast, 14–27
digestive tract, 325–356
female genital tract, 391–402
lymph nodes, 71–124
miscellaneous lesions, 423–436
respiratory tract, 371–380
skin
epithelial (non-melanocytic), 260–261
melanocytic, 275–311
mycosis fungoides and comparable conditions, 267–268
soft tissues, 144–194
thyroid, 42–57
total local series, 1–3, 452
Cat-scratch disease vs malignant lymphoma, 136
Cell(s); *see also* Epithelioid cell; Giant cell
eosinophil polymorphonuclear angiolymphoid hyperplasia, 445
Hodgkin's disease, 127

epithelioid
epithelioid sarcoma, 214
lymphomas and ? lymphomas, 130
fibroblast, atypical
atypical fibroxanthoma, 411
cystitis, giant cell, 411
nodular fasciitis, 411
radiation dermatitis, 411
Kultschitzky, 385, 386
mast cell (axillary nodes), prognostic significance, 37
melanocarcinoma, constituent types, 313
mycosis cell, 269–270
myofibroblast, 209
pericyte, 386, 445, **446**
Reed-Sternberg, 124–125; *see also* R-S cell
signet ring (epithelioid myoma), 410
smooth muscle, relation to pericyte, 446
T-cell, relation to mycosis fungoides, 271
Cellular blue naevus (CBN), *277*, 314
Cervix uteri, 403–405
Arias-Stella phenomenon, 405
carcinoma
adenocarcinoma, vs adenocarcinoma corporis, 405
clear cell, 409
in situ, 403–404
apparent vascular invasion, 404
'invasion', 403
microinvasive, 404
retroperitoneal fibrosis (idiopathic), simulated, 207
verrucous, 405
dysplasia, 403
folate deficiency, association, 384
pseudoinvasion, stromal, post-biopsy, 404
pseudosarcoma botryoides, 410
'Checkerboard' pattern (proliferative myositis), 210
Chemodectoma, 439
histoclinical correlation low, 455
Cherubism, 254
Childhood
angiofibroma (nasal), juvenile, 206
aponeurotic fibroma, juvenile, 206
fibroma, recurrent digital, 206
fibromatoses, 206
fibrosarcoma, 207–208
granulosa cell tumour, 415
'hand tumours', 207
Hodgkin's disease, 128
melanocytic tumours, 9, 316, 319–320
melanoma, juvenile, 316
neuroblastoma, *427*, 436
ovarian neoplasms, 415
pseudosarcoma botryoides, 410

salivary neoplasms, *326*, 358
synovial sarcoma, 214
Chloasma, progestogens and, 319
Chondroblastoma, 247
Chondroma, *222, 245*
fibromyxoid, 247
vs juvenile aponeurotic fibroma, 206
larynx, 384
periosteal, 246
site, prognostic significance, 246
Chondromatosis, synovial, 246
Chondromyxoid fibroma (CMF), *222*, 247
late recurrence, 247
Chondrosarcoma, 245
bimorphic, 246
vs callus, 247–250
fibrosarcoma, association, 246
fibrous dysplasia, 254
myxoid, extraskeletal, 213
osteoid tissue, significance, 249
vs osteosarcoma, 247–250
osteosarcoma, association, 246
Choriocarcinoma, 5, 415–416
'atypical', *399*, 416
intracranial metastasis, diagnostic difficulties, 437
mimetic capacity, 437
ovarian teratoma, 414
Chorion, benign chorionic invasion, *399*, 415–416
Chylous effusion, 445
Ciliary body, pseudoadenomatous hyperplasia, 439
Clinical data, significance, 8–10
bony lesions, 240–242
keratoacanthoma, 9, 262
mycosis fungoides, 269
Composite lymphoma, 129
Computer analysis
epidermal overgrowths, 262
Hodgkin's disease, 70
ovary, mucinous tumours, 412–413
pattern recognition, 5
Condyloma
acuminatum, 264
'giant', 264
Corpus luteum (pregnancy) vs luteoma, 414
Correlation, histoclinical
basis of diagnosis, 3
low level, lesions listed, 454–455
'Criteria of malignancy', 6–8, 456–457
Cyst
aneurysmal bone, 252–253; *see also* Aneurysmal bone cyst
dermoid (ovary), 414
unicameral bone, 254
Cystitis
cystica, 443
giant cell, atypical fibroblasts, 411
glandularis, 443
Cystosarcoma phyllodes, 33

Decision theory, 5
Denture hyperplasia, *327*, 357

Dermatitis (radiation), atypical fibroblasts, 411
Dermatofibroma, *147*
Dermatofibrosarcoma protuberans (DFSP), *147*, 202–203
    fibroxanthoma, relation, 206
Dermatopathic lymphadenopathy, vs ML, 132–133, 135
Dermoid cyst (ovary), 414
Desmoid tumour, *147*, 207
Desmosomes, synovial sarcoma, 213
Diagnosis, histopathological
    age of patient, influence, 9, 33, 244, 316, 319–320
    'blind' approach, 8
    false-positive, false-negative, 7
    rationale, 3–6
    statistics, influence on, 453, 455, *see also* Diagnostic revision
Diagnostic revision (*and see* Table 12.2)
    carcinoid tumour, 364
    carcinoma, spindle-celled (skin), 204
    endometrium, carcinoma, 407
    kidney, sarcoma, 197, 440
    leiomyosarcoma (myometrium), 410
    liposarcoma, 199
    malignant lymphoma, 67–69
    melanocytic lesions, 275
    mycosis fungoides, 269
    osteoclastoma, 250
    osteosarcoma, 249
    ovary, carcinoma, 413
    salivary neoplasms, 357
    sarcoma, epithelioid, 214
    soft tissues, lesions, 143, 214
    thyroid, carcinoma, 41, 57, 63
    thyroid, malignant lymphoma, 61
    Wilms' tumour, 440
Diethylstilboestrol (carcinogenesis), 409
Digestive tract; *see also* entries for various organs
    local series of cases, 325–356
        results on review, 325
        summarised data, 326
    carcinoid tumour, 363–365; *see also* Carcinoid tumour
    malignant lymphoma, 365–366
    plasma cell lesions, 366
    pseudolymphoma, 365–366
Disappearing bone disease (massive osteolysis), 226
Drug-induced reactions (lymph node) vs malignant lymphoma, 135, 454
Duodenum
    carcinoma, periampullary, 362
    hamartoma, *326*, 361
Dysplasia, epithelial
    bladder, urinary, 442
    breast, 28
    cervix uteri, 403
    epidermis, 262
    folate deficiency, production by, 384

jejunum, 362
larynx, 383
prostate, 444
ureter, 444
urethra, 444
vulva, *391*, 402–403
Dysplasia, fibrous (bone), 253–255; *see also* Fibrous dysplasia

'Early gastric cancer' (EGC), 360
Eccrine poroma, malignant, *308*, 311
Elastosis (mammary lesions), 36
Enchondroma, 246, 248
Endodermal sinus tumour, 414
Endolymphatic stromal myosis (uterus), 411
Endometriosis, 367, **416**
    lymph node, 137, *399*
    rectum, *326*, 367
Endometrium, glandular component, 405–409
    adenoacanthoma, 408
    'adenoma malignum', *393*, 406
    'back-to-back' glands, 402
    carcinoma
        adenocarcinoma, *393*, 405, **406–408**
            vs adenocarcinoma cervicis, 405
            vs Arias-Stella phenomenon, 409
            diagnostic revision, 407
            oestrogens, response to, 407
            progestogens, response to, *396*
            youth, occurrence in, 407–408, 454
        adenosquamous, 408
        clear cell, 409
    carcinosarcoma, 409
    hyperplasia, atypical, 402, **405–406**
    polyp, 407
Endometrium, stromal component, 409–412
    pseudosarcoma, 410
    sarcoma, 411
        mixed mesodermal, 409
        stromatoid mural, 411, **412**
    'stromal nodules', 411
    stromal overgrowths, 411–412
    stromatosis, 411
Eosinophil granuloma
    digestive system, 365
    skin, 272
Eosinophil polymorphonuclear cell; *see also* Eosinophil granuloma
    angiolymphoid hyperplasia, 445
    Hodgkin's disease, 127
Epidermis; *see also* Pseudo-epitheliomatous hyperplasia; Skin
    dysplasia, 262
    histiocytoma, changes associated, 153
    leukodystrophy ('leukoplakia'), 356
    overgrowths, computer-analysis, 262

pseudocarcinomatous pattern (podophyllin), 264
Epidermodysplasia verruciformis, 264
Epididymis, adenomatoid tumour, 444
Epithelial inclusions (lymph node), 36, 37
Epithelial-stromal junction (ESJ), breast, 37; *see also* Basement membrane
Epithelioid cell
    epithelioid sarcoma, 214
    lymphoma, ? lymphoma, 130
Epithelioid sarcoma, 214
    diagnostic revision, 214
    vs granuloma, 214
    vs nodular tenosynovitis, 214
Epithelioma adenoides cysticum, 265
Epitheliosis, mammary, *16*, 31
Epulis, melanotic, *287*
Ewing's tumour (sarcoma), 243–244
    extraskeletal, 185
    histoclinical correlation low, 454
Exostosis, solitary, *222*, 235
Extramammary Paget's disease (EMPD), 266
Eye and Orbit, 439–440
    ciliary body, pseudoadenomatous hyperplasia, 439–440
    iris, leiomyoma, *426*, 439
    melanocytic tumour, 439
    neurilemmoma, 439

Fasciitis, nodular (pseudosarcomatous), *147*, 200
    atypical fibroblasts, 411
    vs liposarcoma, 199, 200
Fat; *see also* Lipo- entries
    necrosis, vs liposarcoma, 199
    neoplasms, 198–200
Female genital tract, local series of cases, *391*–402; *see also* entries under various organs
Fibroblast
    atypical, in various lesions, 411
    'facultative', 201
Fibroblastic lesions, 144, *147*; *see also* other Fibro- entries
Fibrocystic disease (FCD), breast, 28
Fibroma
    chondromyxoid (CMF), *222*, 247
    juvenile, aponeurotic, 206
        vs chondroma, 206
    non-ossifying, *222*, *228*, 253–254
        vs malignant fibrous histiocytoma, 255
    ossifying, 253–254
        vs fibrous dysplasia, 254
    recurrent digital, *147*, 206
    qua histiocytoma, 169
Fibromatoses, juvenile, 206
Fibromatosis, plantar, *147*
Fibrosarcoma, *147*, 207–208
    vs aneurysmal bone cyst, 253

vs atypical fibroxanthoma, 203,
205
childhood, 207–208
chondrosarcoma, association, 246
vs desmoplastic melanocarcinoma, 313
vs fibrous dysplasia, 254
vs granulation tissue, 165
vs haemangiopericytoma, 446
larynx, 384
late recurrence, 208
malignant mesenchymoma, relation, 197
Paget's disease, association, 254
post-irradiation, 208
pulmonary metastases resected,
387
thyroid, 61
Fibrosis
lymph node, 129, 131, 134, 135
retroperitoneal, idiopathic
vs Hodgkin's disease, 207
vs metastatic carcinoma, 207
Fibrous cortical defect, 253–254
Fibrous dysplasia (bone), *222*, 251,
**253–255**
chondrosarcoma, association, 254
vs fibrosarcoma, 254
myxoma, association, 196
vs ossifying fibroma, 254
vs osteoclastoma, 254
osteosarcoma, association, 254
Fibrous histiocytoma, 201–206; *see
also* Histiocytoma/fibrous histiocytoma
malignant (MFH), bone, 250
Fibroxanthoma, atypical, 201, **203–
205**
atypical fibroblasts, 411
vs extraskeletal osteosarcoma,
212
vs fibrosarcoma, 205
vs liposarcoma, 204
vs malignant lymphoma, 204
vs pseudosarcoma, skin, 263
vs sarcomas, 454
Fibroxanthoma, malignant, 200,
205–206
R-S cell, seeming presence in,
*125*
vs giant cell tumour, extraskeletal, 212
vs myxofibrosarcoma, 206
Fibroxanthosarcoma, 205–206; *see
also* Fibroxanthoma, malignant
DFSP, relation to, 206
Folate deficiency, effects on epithelium, 384
Follicular lymphoma, 70, *105*
Formalin pigment, vs melanin, 319
Fracture, *see* Callus, 247–250
'Frog spawn' pattern (chondroblastoma), 247
Frozen section
breast, 30
intracranial lesions, 438
lymph node, 131
melanocytic lesions, 316–317
ovary, in pregnancy

luteoma, 414
neoplasms, 414
pancreas, 367
thyroid, 58
Fungal infections, pseudoepitheliomatous hyperplasia, 263

Gall bladder, angiosarcoma, *326*
Ganglioneuroblastoma, 437
Gastro-intestinal tract, malignant
neoplasms, comparative mortality, 144
Germinoblastoma, 70
Giant cell(s)
aneurysmal bone cyst, 253
asteroid bodies, 212
bony lesions, soft tissue, 211–213
fibroblastic lesions, 250–255
osteoclastomatous, nature, 252
proliferative myositis, 210
Giant cell reparative granuloma vs
osteoclastoma, 252
Giant cell tumour
bone, 251–252
soft tissue, 211–212
Giant condyloma, 264
Giant lymphoid hamartoma, **134**,
445
vs malignant lymphoma, 132–
133
Glioblastoma multiforme, tissue
patterns, 438
Glioma/gliosis, distinction, 438–
439
Glomangioma, vs haemangiopericytoma, 446
Glomus intravagale, jugulare
chemodectoma, 439
Glossitis mediana rhombica, 357
Glycogen
clear cell carcinoma, female
genital tract, 409
epithelioid leiomyoma (myometrium), 410
Ewing's tumour, 243
Pompé's disease, 386
renal carcinoma vs haemangioblastoma, 437
'sugar' tumour (lung), 385–386
Granular cell myoblastoma, *147*,
209–210
carcinoembryonic antigen, 210
larynx, 384
pseudoepitheliomatous hyperplasia, 263
Granular cell pseudotumour, disseminated, 209
Granulation tissue
myofibroblast, 209
sarcoma, 169, **208–209**
vs sarcoma, *165*, *167*, 454
Granuloma
arthropod bite, 271, **272–273**
biliary duct nodes, 134
eosinophil
digestive system, 365
skin, 272
giant cell reparative, 252
histiocytosis, oleogranulomatous,
134

Hodgkin's disease, 127
lipophagic, peritoneum, 367
midline, lethal, 382
oleogranuloma, 134
plasma cell
digestive tract, 366
pulmonary, 386
prostate, 443
pulmonary
plasma cell, 386
xanthomatous, 386
pyelonephritis, xanthogranulomatous, 440
pyogenicum, 209
atypical, 444
exuberant, *433*
vs Kaposi's sarcoma, 209
vs epithelioid sarcoma, 214
xanthomatous, pulmonary, 386
Granulomatosis
lymphomatoid, 137–138, 272,
382, 386
Wegener's, 382, 387
Granulosa-theca cell tumour, 415


Haemangioblastoma
vs haemangiopericytoma, 446
vs renal carcinoma, 437
Haemangioma, 445
Haemangiopericytoma, 446
vs angioblastic meningioma, 446
vs haemangioblastoma, 446
histoclinical correlation low, 455
Haematoma-sarcoma, 208–209
Haemorrhage, intracranial, choriocarcinoma, 438
Halo naevus, 193
Hamartoma
duodenal, *326*, 361
giant lymphoid, **134**, 445
vs malignant lymphoma, 132–
133
mesenchymoma qua, 197
mesodermal, various tissues, 197
pulmonary, fibroleiomyomatous,
412
renal
angiomyolipoma, 441
leiomyomatous, 440–441
Hand, tumours of, childhood, 207
Hand-Schüller-Christian disease, *99*
vs SHML, 134
Hashimoto's disease, 61, 62
Heart, myxoma, 196
Hemisomatectomy, 247
Heredity, in malignant lymphoma,
*81*, *123*, 128
Herpes zoster
Hodgkin's disease, behaviour,
128
nodes, vs malignant lymphoma,
*117*, 132–133, 135
Hibernoma, 198
Histiocyte, R-S cell, relation, 125
Histiocyte/reticulum cell overgrowth, lymph nodes, 130
Histiocytoma/fibrous histiocytoma,
benign and malignant, *147*,
201–206

Histiocytoma (*continued*)
angiolymphoid hyperplasia with eosinophilia, relation, 445
epidermal abnormality associated, 153
vs fibrous cortical defect, 254
vs metastatic carcinoma, 204
myxoid form, 195
vs neuronaevus, *277*
recurrent digital fibroma, relation, 169
sclerosing angioma, relation, 445
Histiocytosis
malignant, 137
oleogranulomatous, 134
sinus (SH), lymph node, 112, **134**
with massive lymphadenopathy (SHML), 112, 134
vs metastatic carcinoma, 205
X, 134
vs malignant lymphoma, 132–133
skin, 272
Histoclinical correlation
basis of diagnosis, 3
low level, lesions listed, 454–455
Histological 'proof', 3
Histology
'blind' assessment, 8–9
'para-normal', 7
Histometric analysis
Hodgkin's disease, 70
'leukoplakia', 262
Histopathological diagnosis, *see* Diagnosis, histopathological
Hodgkin's disease, 124–128; *see also* Malignant lymphoma
'atypical', 71
childhood, 128
classification, 70
diagnosis, computer-assisted, 5
diagnostic revision, 67–69
eosinophil polymorphonuclears, 127
focal involvement, lymph nodes, 127
granulomas, 127
hereditary factor, *81, 123*, 128
herpes zoster, 128
histometric analysis, 70
vs idiopathic retroperitoneal fibrosis, 207
immunology, 127–128
keratoacanthoma, 263
Lennert lymphoma, relation, 130
pregnancy, 128
prognosis, 126–127
Reed-Sternberg cell, 124–125; *see also* Reed-Sternberg cell
vascular invasion, 127
Hydantoin drugs, lymph nodes, 136
Hydatidiform mole, 5, **415–416**
Hygroma, *433*, 445–446
Hyperplasia
angiolymphoid, with eosinophilia, 445
atypical, endometrium, 402, **405**
atypical, pancreatic duct, 367
denture, *327*, 357

non-specific reactive lymph node, 131, 132–133
pseudoadenomatous, ciliary body, iris, 439
pseudoepitheliomatous, 263; *see also* Pseudoepitheliomatous hyperplasia
Hyperthyroidism, carcinoma of thyroid, 62

I$^{131}$, small intestine, effects, 362
Immunoblast, pleomorphic, relation to R-S cell, 125
Immunoblastic lymphadenopathy, 130, **135**
vs malignant lymphoma, 132–133
Immunology, Hodgkin's disease, 127
Imprint preparations
bony lesions, 243
lymph node, 71
Inclusions
eosinophil
Kaposi's sarcoma, 446
recurrent digital fibroma, *167*, 206
epithelial, lymph nodes, 137
Infarction
bone, relation to malignant fibrous histiocytoma, 255
lymph node, *109*
Infectious mononucleosis
vs malignant lymphoma, 136, 454
mitotic aberrancy, 7
R-S cell, seeming presence in, 125
Intestine, large, *see* Large intestine
Intracranial neoplasms, frozen section, 438
Invasion; *see also* Basement membrane; Pseudoinvasion; Pseudocarcinomatous pattern
cervix uteri (microinvasion), 403
lymph nodes, capsular transgression, 131
melancarcinoma, prognostic value, 312
stromal, 456–457
breast, dysplasias, 37
pancreas, 366, *456*
prostate, 456
thyroid, *43*, 456
tonsil, capsular permeation, *355*, 359
vascular, 457
angiomatosis, intravascular, 444
breast (dysplasias), 36
cervix uteri, carcinoma, 404
chemodectoma, 439
endo/myometrial overgrowths, 411–412
Hodgkin's disease, 127
prostate, carcinoma, 442
thyroid lesions, 58

Iris
hyperplasia, pseudoadenomatous, 439
leiomyoma, *426*, 439

Joints, *see* Synovial lesions, 213–214
Junctional naevus, 266, **314**
Juvenile
angiofibroma (nasal), 382–383
aponeurotic fibroma, 206
fibromatoses, 206–207
melanoma, 316

Kaposi's sarcoma, 200, **446**
eosinophil inclusions, 446
vs granuloma pyogenicum, 209, **433**
lymph nodes, vs malignant lymphoma, 135
Keratoacanthoma, 9, 262–263
histiocytoma, simulation in association, 153
Hodgkin's disease, behaviour in, 263
Keratosis
oral, 262
seborrhoeic, 260, 262
senilis, 262
Kidney
adenoma, 441
oncocytic, 441
angiomyolipoma, 441
carcinoma
vs adenoma, 441
vs clear cell carcinoma, 409
vs haemangioblastoma, 437
late recurrence, 441
vs malakoplakia, 440
vs 'sugar' tumour (lung), 386
vs xanthogranuloma (lung), 386
vs xanthogranulomatous pyelonephritis, 40
hamartoma
angiomyolipoma, 441
leiomyomatous, 440
vs Wilms' tumour, 440
pyelonephritis, xanthogranulomatous, 440
sarcomas, diagnostic revision, 197
Wilms' tumour, 440–441
Kiel classification (lymphomas), 70
Kraurosis vulvae, 403
Krukenberg tumour vs luteoma of pregnancy, 414
Kultschitzky cell, 385, 386

Lachrymal gland, carcinoma, *426*, 440
Large intestine, 362–363; *see also* Digestive tract; Rectum
carcinoma, pulmonary metastases resected, 387
in situ, 363
eosinophil granuloma, 365
polyp, 362–363
pseudomalignant patterns, 363

'transitional mucosa', 363
ulcerative colitis, carcinoma, 363
Larynx, 383–384
    carcinoma in situ, 383–384
    dysplasia, 383
    fibrosarcoma, 384
    granular cell myoblastoma, 384
    lipoma, 384
    pseudosarcoma, 384
    stromal neoplasms, 384
Lateral aberrant thyroid, 42, 59
Latency
    carcinoma
        breast, 455
        kidney, 430, 441
    chondromyxoid fibroma, 247
    fibrosarcoma, 208
    melanocarcinoma, 320
    meningioma, spinal, 437
    neuroblastoma, 437
Lectins, possible diagnostic value
    (adenocarcinoma uteri), 405
Leiomyoblastoma, 410
    vs haemangiopericytoma, 446
Leiomyoma, 409–410
    bizarre, 409–410
    epithelioid (clear cell), 410
    iris, 426, 439
    vs leiomyosarcoma, 409–410
    vascular, vs haemangiopericy-
        toma, 446
Leiomyomatosis, intravenous
    (uterus), 412
Leiomyosarcoma (LMS)
    diagnostic revision, 410
    epithelioid (stomach), 361
    vs leiomyoma, 409–410
    vs pseudosarcoma (skin), 263
Lennert lymphoma, 124, **130**
Lentigo maligna, 277, 314–316
Leukodystrophy, epithelial, 356
    progressive multifocal, astro-
        cytes, 438
'Leukoplakia', **261–262**
    oral cavity, 356–357
    vulva, 391, 403
Lichen planus, 262
    hypertrophicus, 260
    sclerosus et atrophicus, vulva,
        403
Lipid cell tumour, ovary, 414
Lipoma, 198
    angiolipoma, 198
    angiomyolipoma, 197, 441
    infiltrating, 198
    larynx, 384
Liposarcoma, 147, 199–200
    vs atypical fibroxanthoma, 204
    pyrexia, 199
    vs xanthogranulomatous
        pyelonephritis, 440
Liver, Pompé's disease, 386
Lobular carcinoma in situ (LCIS),
    breast, 28–30
Local series, total cases analysed
    451–453; see also Cases ana-
    lysed, local series
Lung, see Bronchus and lung
Lupus erythematosus, lymph nodes

vs malignant lymphoma, 69,
    132–133, 135
Luteoma, pregnancy, 414
Lymph node; see also Malignant
    lymphoma
    adenitis, mesenteric, 114, 136
    biopsy technique, 36, 71
    brucellosis, vs ML, 132–133, 137
    capsular transgression, 131
    carcinoma, metastatic, vs ML
        105, 137
        thyroid, vs ML, 61
    cat-scratch disease, vs ML, 132–
        133, 136
    data recording, 71
    dermatopathic lymphadenopathy,
        vs ML, 132–133, 135
    diagnostic revision, 67–69
    drug-induced reactions, vs ML,
        132–133, 135, 454
    endometriosis, 137, 399, 416
    enlargement, prognostic signifi-
        cance, 69
    epithelial inclusions, 36–37, 137
    epithelioid cells, 130
    fibrosis, 131
        biliary duct nodes, 134
        vascularised sinusoidal, 135
    focal involvement, Hodgkin's
        disease, 127
    frozen section, 131
    granuloma
        Hodgkin's disease, 127
        oleogranulomatous histiocyto-
            sis, 134
    herpes zoster, vs ML, 117, 132–
        133, 135
    histiocyte/reticulum cell over-
        growth, 130
    histiocytosis
        oleogranulomatous, 134
        X, vs ML, 132–133, 134
    hyperplasia, non-specific reac-
        tive, vs ML, 117, 131, 132–
        133
    immunoblastic lymphadeno-
        pathy, 130, 132–133, 135
    infarction, 109
    infectious mononucleosis, vs
        ML, 132–133, 136, 454
    Kaposi's sarcoma
    lupus erythematosus, 69, 132–
        133, 135
    lymphopathia venereum, vs ML,
        132–133, 136–137
    mast cell, prognostic signifi-
        cance (mammary carci-
        noma), 37
    melanin within, 318
    melanocarcinoma, metastatic, vs
        ML, 137
    naevus cells within, 137, 318
    necrosis, 131
    occult metastasis (mammary
        carcinoma), 36
    post-vaccinial reaction, vs ML,
        132–133, 135
    psammoma bodies, diagnostic
        significance (cervical), 59

pseudocarcinomatous pattern
    (glandular inclusions), 36
rheumatoid arthritis, vs ML,
    132–133, 134
sectioning/sampling technique,
    36
sinus histiocytosis (SH)
    biliary duct nodes, 134
    carcinoma
        breast, 36
        stomach, 361
    with massive lymphadenopa-
        thy (SHML), 134
    vs ML, 132–133, 134
syphilitic adenitis, vs ML, 132–
    133, 134
thyroid tissue content (cervical),
    43, 59
toxoplasmosis, vs ML, 132–133,
    136, 454
vascular proliferation, 131
'vascular transformation', 135
Lymph nodes, local series of cases,
    71–124; see also Hodgkin's
    disease; Malignant lymphoma;
    Pseudolymphoma
    results on review, 72
    summarised data, 74, 105
Lymphadenectomy, melanocarci-
    noma, 317–319
Lymphadenopathy
    dermatopathic, 135
    immunoblastic, 130, 135
Lymphangioma, 445
Lymphangiomyoma, 445
Lymphangiomyomatosis, 445
Lymphangiopericytoma, 446
Lymphatics, lesions of, 445–446
Lymphoepithelial lesion, benign,
    326, 358
Lymphoepithelioma, 326
Lymphoid hamartoma, angioma-
    tous, R-S cell, seeming pres-
    ence in, 125
Lymphoid hyperplasia, angiofol-
    licular, 134
Lymphoma
    benign (rectum), 105, 365
    malignant (ML), 67–130
        lesions simulating, 130–138
Lymphomatoid granulomatosis,
    **137–138**, 272, 382, 386–387
Lymphomatoid papulosis, 272
Lymphomatoid pityriasis liche-
    noides, 272
Lymphopathia venereum, vs ML,
    136–137
Lymphoplasia, cutaneous, 271

Malakoplakia, vs renal carcinoma,
    440
Malignant fibrous histiocytoma,
    201, 205
    bone, 250, **255**
        vs non-ossifying (non-osteo-
            genic) fibroma, 255
        vs osteoclastoma, 255
Malignant lymphoma (ML), 67–
    130; see also Hodgkin's dis-
    ease; Malignant lymphoma,

Malignant lymphoma (*continued*)
  lesions simulation; Pseudo-
    lymphoma
  bone, 243–244
  classification, 69, 70
  composite, 129
  diagnostic revision, 67–69
  digestive tract, 365–366
  follicular, 70
  heredity, *81, 123,* 128
  Hodgkin's disease, 124–128
  Lennert lymphoma, 124, 130
  lymphomatoid granulomatosis,
    relation, 386–387
  malignant fibrous histiocytoma
    (bone), association, 255
  Mikulicz disease, association,
    358
  mycosis fungoides, association,
    269
  nasal cavity, 382
  non-Hodgkin, 128–130
  'starry sky' appearance, 129
  stomach, 361
  thyroid, 61
    diagnostic revision, 61
    vs lymphoid hyperplasia, 42
Malignant lymphoma, lesions
  simulating, 130–138
  brucellosis, 137
  carcinoma
    breast, 38
    melanocarcinoma, 137
    metastatic, *112,* 137
    thyroid, 61
  cat-scratch disease, 136
  dermatopathic lymphadenopathy,
    135
  drug-induced lymphadenopathy,
    135, 454
  giant lymphoid hamartoma, 134
  herpes zoster, *117,* 132–133, 135
  histiocytosis X, 134
  hyperplasia, non-specific re-
    active, 131
  immunoblastic lymphadenopa-
    thy, 135
  infectious mononucleosis, 136,
    454
  Kaposi's sarcoma, 135
  lupus erythematosus, 69, 135
  lymphomatoid granulomatosis,
    137–138
  lymphopathia venereum, 137–
    138
  post-vaccinial lymphadenopathy,
    135
  rheumatoid arthritis, 134
  SHML, 134
  syphilitic adenitis, 134
  toxoplasmosis, 136, 454
Massive osteolysis ('disappearing
  bone disease'), 226
Mast cell (axillary nodes), prognostic significance, 37
Mediastinum
  giant lymphoid hamartoma, 134
  hygroma, 445
  lymphangiomyoma, 445
  neuroblastoma, *421,* 436

Melanin
  vs formalin pigment, 319
  in lymph node, 318
Melanocarcinoma, *277,* 274–320
  amelanotic, *277*
  childhood, 9, 316, 319–320
  classification, 311–312
  constituent cells, 313–314
  desmoplastic, 313
  diagnosis
    age of patient, influence, 316,
      319–320
    frozen section, 316–317
    revision, 275
  vs EMPD, 266
  vs haemangiopericytoma, 446
  latency, 320
  lentigo maligna, *277,* 314–316
  lymphadenectomy, 317–319
  vs malignant eccrine poroma,
    *277,* 308
  vs malignant lymphoma, 137
  meningeal, 437
  vs meningioma, 437
  metastatic, latency, 320
  pregnancy, interrelations, 319
  prognostic assessment, 312
  'pseudomelanoma', 317
  pulmonary metastases resected,
    387
  R-S cells, seeming presence in,
    125
  regression, 320
  'scoring', prognostic, 312
  spindle-celled
    vs atypical fibroxanthoma, 204
    vs carcinoma, spindle-celled,
      194
    vs fibrosarcoma, 313
    vs pseudosarcoma, skin, 263
  subungual, 318
  superficial spreading, 311, 317
  trauma, relation, 317
'Melanoma', term condemned, 274
Melanoma, juvenile, 9, 316
Melanonaevus; *see also* Naevus
  childhood, 9, 316, 319–320
  vs EMPD, 266
  lentigo maligna, relation, 315
  pregnancy, 319
Melanotic epulis, *287*
Meninges
  melanocarcinoma, 437
Meningioma, *421,* 437–438
  angioblastic, vs haemangioperi-
    cytoma, 446
  vs astrocytoma vs Schwannoma,
    438
  vs carcinoma
    melanocarcinoma, 437
    mucinous, 437
    thyroid, 437
  latency (spinal), 437
Mesenchymoma
  benign and malignant, *147,* 196–
    198
  feminising, 196
  malignant
    fibrosarcoma, relation, 197

  histoclinical correlation low,
    454
  vs myositis ossificans, 198
Mesenteric adenitis, vs ML, *114,*
  136
Metaphyseal fibrous defect, 253–
  254
Metaplasia
  peritoneum, 367
  prostate, 443
  squamous
    cystosarcoma phyllodes, 33
    endometrium, carcinoma, 409
    ovary, carcinoma, 413
Metastasis
  basal cell carcinoma, 265–266
  basosquamous carcinoma, 265
  benign metastasising goitre, 58
  benign metastasising myoma
    (uterus), 411, **412**
  resection, therapeutic value
    intracranial, 439
    pulmonary
      osteoclastoma, 252
      renal carcinoma, 441
      various neoplasms, 387–388
  squamous cell carcinoma, 264
Mikulicz disease, *326,* 358
Miscellaneous cases, local series,
  423–436
Mitosis, aberrant
  cervix uteri (CIS), role as dis-
    criminator, 403
  innocuous
    atypical fibroxanthoma, 204
    infectious mononucleosis
      (liver), 7
    luteoma of pregnancy, 414
    mesenteric adenitis, 136
    nodular tenosynovitis, 213
    pseudosarcoma botryoides,
      410
    reparative tissue, 6–7
  counting, 410
Mitotic control protein, 413
Mitotic incidence, prognostically
  equivocal
  atypical fibroxanthoma, 204
  basal cell carcinoma, 266
  clear cell carcinoma (endo-
    metrium), 409
  fibrosarcoma (childhood), 207
  liposarcoma, 199
  lymph nodes, abnormal, 123
  osteosarcoma, 249
  thyroid, lymphomatoid lesions,
    61
Mixed mesodermal tumour, 196,
  409
  Müllerian adenosarcoma variant,
    411
  vs pseudosarcoma botryoides,
    411
Molluscum contagiosum, 271
  sebaceum, 9; *see also* Kera-
    toacanthoma
Monomorphism, term examined,
  269
Mortality, comparative: malignant
  neoplasms

bone and cartilage, 221
  gastrointestinal system, 144, 221
  soft tissues, 144
Mucha-Habermann disease, 272
Müllerian adenosarcoma, 411
Muscle, skeletal; *see also* Leio-;
    Myo-; Rhabdo- entries
  mesodermal hamartoma, 197
  myositis ossificans, 210–211
  myxoma, intramuscular, 196
  proliferative myositis, 210
  pseudolymphomatous infiltrate,
    136
Mycosis cell, 269–270
Mycosis fungoides and comparable
    conditions, 267–273
  R-S cell, seeming presence in,
    125
Myeloma, *222*, 242–245
  extramedullary (EMP), 243
    vs SMB vs myelomatosis, 243
  vs inflammatory lesions, 242
  vs metastatic carcinoma, 243–
    244
  non-secretory, 243
  solitary, 239
    of bone (SMB), 243
Myelomatosis, R-S cell, seeming
    presence in, 125
Myoblastoma, granular cell, **209–**
  **210**, 384
Myofibroblast, 209
Myoma
  benign metastasising (uterus),
    411, **412**
  cutis, *147*
Myometrium
  adenocarcinoma corporis, in-
    vasion, 407
  adenomyosis, 411
  leiomyoblastoma, 410
  leiomyoma (bizarre; epithelioid;
    clear cell), 409
  leiomyomatosis, intravenous, 412
  leiomyosarcoma, *396, 397*, 409–
    410
  myoma, benign metastasising,
    411, **412**
  plexiform tumourlet, 410
Myositis, proliferative, *see* Pro-
    liferative myositis
Myositis ossificans, *147*, 210–211
  vs callus, 248
  vs malignant mesenchymoma,
    198
  vs osteosarcoma, 210, 454
Myxofibrosarcoma, vs malignant
    fibroxanthoma, 206
Myxoma, 195–196
  cardiac, 196
  fibrous dysplasia (bone), associa-
    tion, 196


Naevus
  blue, vs atypical fibroxanthoma,
    204
  cellular blue (CBN), *277*, 314
  compound, *277*
  'halo', 320

intradermal, *277*
junctional, *277*
  lentigo maligna, relation, 314
  vs Paget's disease, 266
Spitz, *277*, 314, **316**
Naevus cells in lymph nodes, 137,
  318
Nasal cavity
  granuloma, lethal midline, 382
  malignant lymphoma, 382
  papilloma, 382–383
  reticulosis, malignant midline,
    382
Necrosis
  focal, salivary neoplasms, prog-
    nostic value, 357
  lymph node, 131
Necrotising sialometaplasia, 357
Nerve, mesodermal hamartoma,
  197
Nervous system, lesions, 436–439
Neuroblastoma, 243–244, *421,*
  436–437
Neurofibroma, *147*
Neurofibrosarcoma, *147*
Nihilism, therapeutic, 3
Nipple
  adenomatosis, ducts, *16*
  Paget's disease, *32*, 266
Nodular tenosynovitis, *147*, 213
  vs epithelioid sarcoma, 214
Non-Hodgkin lymphoma, 128–130;
    *see also* Malignant lymphoma
Non-ossifying fibroma, 253–255


Oesophagus, lesions, 359–360
Oestrogens, endometrium, effects,
  407
Oleogranuloma (lymph node), 134
Omentum, serosal metaplasia, *326,*
  367
Oncocytic adenoma (kidney), 441
Oncocytoma, pulmonary, *377–380,*
  385
Oral cavity
  benign lymphoepithelial lesion,
    *326*, 358
  denture hyperplasia, 357
  glossitis mediana rhombica, 357
  keratosis, 262
  leukoplakia, 356
  palate, neoplasms, 358
  verrucous carcinoma, 356
Oral contraceptives, *see* Pro-
    gestogens
Orbit
  lachrymal gland, carcinoma, *426,*
    440
  pseudotumour, 440
Osseous tumour, soft tissue, pseu-
    domalignant, 211
Ossifying fibroma, *see* Fibroma,
    ossifying, 253–254
Osteoblastoma, 250
  osteoid osteoma, relation, 250
  pseudomalignant, 250
Osteoclastoma
  extraskeletal, 211

aneurysmal bone cyst, relation,
  212
malignant, soft tissue lesions re-
    sembling, 211
skeletal, *222*, 251–252
  diagnostic revision, 250
  vs fibrous dysplasia, 254
  vs giant cell reparative granu-
    loma, 252
  grading, 252
  histoclinical correlation low,
    454
  vs malignant fibrous histiocy-
    toma, 255
  vs non-ossifying fibroma, 252
  osteoid tissue, 252
  Paget's disease associated, 252
  pulmonary metastases re-
    sected, 252
Osteoid osteoma, 250
  giant (osteoblastoma), 250
Osteoid tissue
  in chondrosarcoma, significance,
    249
  in proliferative myositis, 210
Osteolysis, massive ('disappearing
    bone disease'), 226
Osteomyelitis, *222*, 242
  vs myeloma, 242
Osteosarcoma, *222*, 249–250
  alkaline phosphatase, prognostic
    significance, 249
  vs aneurysmal bone cyst, 248,
    249
  biopsy procedure, prognostic
    implications, 250
  vs callus, 247–250
  vs chondrosarcoma, 247–250
  chondrosarcoma, association,
    246
  diagnostic revision, 249
  extraskeletal, 211
    vs atypical fibroxanthoma, 212
    post-irradiation (thorotrast),
      212
  fibrous dysplasia, association,
    254
  grading, 249
  intraosseous, 249
  larynx, 384
  vs malignant fibrous histio-
    cytoma, 255
  regression, 250
Ovary, lesions, 412–415
  adenoacanthoma, 413
  Brenner tumour, 413
  carcinoma, *397*, 412–413
    clear cell, **409**, 413
    diagnostic revision, 413
    embryonal, 414
    endometrioid, 413
    metastatic, vs meningioma, 437
    mucinous, 413
    regression, *397*, 413
    spillage from, 413
  dermoid cyst, 414
    leakage from, 367
  endodermal sinus tumour, 414
  frozen section, tumours in preg-
    nancy, 414

Ovary, lesions (*continued*)
  granulosa-theca cell tumour, 415
  Krukenberg tumour vs luteoma
    of pregnancy, 414
  lipid cell tumour, 414
  luteoma, pregnancy, 414
  neoplasms
    childhood, 415
    plasma ribonuclease, 415
  sarcoma, 414
  terstoma, 414–415
  tumours, in pregnancy, 414
  yolk sac tumour, 414
Paget's disease
  bone
    fibrosarcoma, association, 254
    osteoclastoma, association, 252
  extramammary (EMPD)
    vulva, 403
    vs junctional naevus vs
      melanocarcinoma, 266
  nipple
    vs junctional naevus, 32, 266
Palate, neoplasms, 358
Pancreas
  biopsy problems, 366–367
  frozen section, 367
  duct hyperplasia, atypical (CIS),
    367
  peudocarcinomatous pattern,
    366
Papilloma
  inverted
    nasal cavity, 382
    urinary bladder, 443
  transitional cell, urinary bladder,
    443
Papillomatosis
  oesphagus, 360
  respiratory tract, 382–383
Papular angioplasia, 445
Papulosis, lymphomatoid, 272
Parapsoriasis, atrophic, 269
Pattern-recognition, computer-
    based, 5
Pautrier microabscess
  actinic reticuloid, 272
  mycosis fungoides, 267–271
Pericyte, 445, 446
Peritoneum
  lipophage granuloma, 367
  metaplasia, *326*, 367
  ovarian cyst rupture, reaction,
    413
Periurethral prostatic ducts, carci-
    noma (PUPDC), 443
Peutz-Jehgers syndrome, 363
Pharynx, neoplasms, 358
  pseudosarcoma, 358–359
'Pill', *see* Progestogens
Pityriasis lichenoides, vs ML, 272
Placenta, 415–416
  carcinogenesis, transplacental,
    409
  trophoblastic overgrowths, 415–
    416
Plantar fibromatosis, *147*
Plasma cell lesions, digestive tract,
    *105*, 366

plasmacytoma vs plasma cell
    granuloma, 366
  stomach, *105*
Plasmacytoma vs sinusoidal fibrosis
    (lymph node), 135; *see also*
    Myeloma
Podophyllin, pseudocarcinomatous
    pattern, 264
Poikiloderma atrophicans, 269
Polymorphism, term examined, 269
Polyp
  benign lymphoid (rectum),
    *105*, 365
  endometrium, 407
  gastric, 360
  large intestine, *326*, 362–363
Polytypia, term examined, 269
Pompé's disease, 386
Poroma, malignant eccrine, *308*,
    311
Pregnancy
  after endometrial carcinoma,
    408
  Arias-Stella phenomenon
    cervix uteri, 405
    vs clear cell carcinoma, 409
  corpus luteum vs luteoma, 414
  influence on prognosis
    carcinoma, breast, 33
    Hodgkin's disease, 128
    liposarcoma, 199
    melanocarcinoma, 319
  Krukenberg tumour vs luteoma,
    414
  lactational hyperplasia (adeno-
    sis), *16*
  luteoma, ovary, 414
  ovarian neoplasms
    enlargement, 414
    frozen section, 414
  pseudosarcoma botryoides, 410
  transplacental carcinogenesis,
    409
  trophoblastic overgrowths,
    415–416
Probability, significance in diag-
    nosis, 5, 9
Progestogens, effect/influence
  chloasma, 319
  endometrium, carcinoma, *396*,
    410
  melanonaevi, 319
  pseudosarcoma, endometrium,
    410
Prognosis, influence of age; *see
    also* Childhood; Pregnancy,
    influence on prognosis
  carcinoma
    breast, 33
    endometrium, 407
    kidney, 441
    melanocarcinoma, 319–320
Proliferative myositis, *147*, 210
  osteoid tissue in, 210
  R-S cell, seeming presence in,
    125
  vs Trichinella spiralis (tissue
    response), 145
'Proof', histological, 3

Prostate
  carcinoma, 441–443
    vs idiopathic retroperitoneal
      fibrosis, 207, 443
    vs involutionary seminal
      vesicle, 443
    lesions simulating, 443
    microcarcinoma (PMC), 441
  granuloma, 443
  metaplasia, 443
  periurethral ducts, carcinoma
    (PUPDC), 443
  pseudocarcinomatous pattern,
    442
Psammoma bodies
  carcinoma, thyroid, diagnostic
    significance, 59
  meningioma vs carcinoma, ovary
    (metastatic), 437
  vs carcinoma, thyroid (meta-
    static), 437
Pseudoadenomatous hyperplasia,
    ciliary body, 439–440
Pseudoangiosarcoma, 444
Pseudocancers, general, 4
Pseudocarcinomatous pattern; *see
    also* Pseudoepitheliomatous
    hyperplasia; Pseudoinvasion
  epidermis, podophyllin-induced,
    264
  lymph node, glandular inclu-
    sions, 36
  pancreas, 366
  polyp, intestinal, 363
  prostate, 456
Pseudoepitheliomatous hyperplasia,
    263
  arthropod bite, 272
  basal cell carcinoma, 266
  bromoderma, 263
  cutaneous lymphoid hyperplasia,
    271
  fungal infection, 263
  granular cell myoblastoma, 263
  oral cavity, 357
  vulva, 402
Pseudoinvasion; *see also* Invasion;
    Pseudocarcinomatous pattern
  neural, breast (dysplasias), 36
  stromal
    cervix uteri, post-biopsy, 404
    intestinal polyps, 363
    pancreas, 366
    prostate, 456
    thyroid, *43*, 456
  vascular
    breast (dysplasias), 36
    Spitz naevus, 316
    thyroid, 58
Pseudoleukaemia cutis, 271
Pseudolymphoma, 137, 454; *see
    also* Malignant lymphoma,
    lesions simulating
  breast, 38
  digestive tract, 365–366
  larynx, 384
  lung, *380*, 387
  muscle (infiltrate), 136
  skin (infiltrate), 271–273

Pseudomalignant osseous tumour, soft tissue, 211
Pseudomalignant osteoblastoma, 250
Pseudomelanoma, 317
Pseudosarcoma, 143, 193–196
    angiolymphoid hyperplasia with eosinophilia, 445
    angiomatosis, intravascular, 444
    atypical fibroxanthoma, **203–205**, 263
    botryoides, 410–411
    endometrium, 410
    fasciitis (nodular), 199, **200**
    larynx, 384
    lung ('shock' lung), 209
    myositis ossificans, 210
    pharynx, *326*, 358–359
    proliferative myositis, 210
    skin, 263
    upper digestive/respiratory tracts, 358–359
Pseudotumour, 4
    granular cell, disseminated, 209
    lung, inflammatory, 386
    orbit, 440
    trophoblastic, *399*, 416
Pyelonephritis, xanthogranulomatous vs renal carcinoma, 440
Pyogenic granuloma, *see* Granuloma pyogenicum
Pyrexia, in liposarcoma, 199

Radiation dermatitis, atypical fibroblasts, 411
Radiotherapy, possible contraindications
    bony lesions, 254
    desmoid tumour, 207
    fibrosarcoma, 208
    juvenile angiofibroma (nasal), 382
    papillomatosis, respiratory tract, 383
    thorotrast, 212
    verrucous carcinoma, 264
Rectum; *see also* Large intestine
    benign lymphoma (polyp), *105*, 365
    carcinoid tumour, 364
    endometriosis, *326*, 367
Reed-Sternberg cell, 124–125
    vs mycosis cell, 125, 270
    non-Hodgkin lesions, seeming presence in, 125
    vs plasma cell, 366
Regression
    carcinoid tumour, 365
    desmoid tumour (post-menopausal), 207
    endometrium, carcinoma, 407
    fibrosarcoma, childhood, 208
    lung, multiple hamartomas, 412
    lymphadenopathy, immunoblastic, 130
    melanocarcinoma, 320
    neuroblastoma, *421*, 436
    osteosarcoma, 250

ovary
    carcinoma, *397*, 413
    luteoma, 414
    renal carcinoma (metastases), 441
Reinke crystalloids, prognostic significance, 414
Reparative lesions, *145–147*, 208–209; *see also* Granulation tissue
Respiratory tract, local series of cases, 371–380; *see also* entries under various organs
    papillomatosis, 382–383
        irradiation, implications, 383
    'shock' lung, pseudosarcoma, 209
'Reticulum cell sarcoma', 69, 71
Retroperitoneum
    fibrosis, idiopathic
        vs Hodgkin's disease, 207
        vs metastatic carcinoma, 207, 443
    fibroxanthoma, 202
    liposarcoma, *147*, 199–200
    lymphangiomyomatosis, 445
Rhabdomyosarcoma, 198
    vs atypical fibroxanthoma, 204
    post-traumatic, 208
Rheumatoid arthritis (lymph nodes), vs ML, 132–133, 134
Ribonuclease, plasma (ovarian neoplasms), 415
Round-cell tumours (bone), assessment, 244–245
Rubeola, R-S cells, seeming presence in, 125
Rye classification, 70

Salivary neoplasms, 357–358
    adenoma, 357
    carcinoma, 357–358
        adenoid cystic, 265
        childhood, *326*, 358
        diagnostic revision, 357
        focal calcification, prognostic value, 357
        focal necrosis, prognostic value, 357
Salivary tissue; *see also* Salivary neoplasms
    benign lymphoepithelial lesion, *326*, 358
    necrotising sialometaplasia, 357
Sarcoid, Spiegler-Fendt, 271
Sarcoma; *see also* Angio-; Chondro-; Fibro- entries
    botryoides, 410
    epithelioid, 214
    Ewing's, 243–244
        extraskeletal, 185
    fibroxanthosarcoma, 205
    germinoblastic, 70
    granulation tissue, 169, 208–209
    haematoma-sarcoma, 208–209
    immunoblastic (with mycosis fungoides), 271
    Kaposi's, 446
    kidney, 197

lymphomatous, *see* Malignant lymphoma
leiomyosarcoma, 410
    epithelioid, 361
    mixed mesodermal, 196, 409
    ovarian, 414
    post-irradiation
        fibrosarcoma, 207–208, 254
        osteosarcoma, extraskeletal (thorotrast), 212
    spindle-celled, 313
    'staging' of, 214–215
    stomach (non-lymphomatous), *326*, 361
    stromatoid mural (uterus), 411, 412
    synovial, *147*, 213–214
    teratoma (ovarian), 414
Schwannoma vs meningioma vs astrocytoma, 438
Sclerema neonatorum, vs liposarcoma, 199
Seborrhoeic keratosis, histiocytoma-associated simulation, 153
Seminal vesicle
    carcinoma in situ, 444
    involutionary, vs prostatic carcinoma, 443
Serosal metaplasia, *326*, 367
Sézary syndrome, 271
'Shock' lung, pseudosarcomatous pattern, 209
Sialometaplasia, necrotising, 357
Sinus histiocytosis (SH), lymph nodes, *see* Lymph node, SH; Histiocytosis
Skin, lesions; *see also* Epidermis; Pseudoepitheliomatous hyperplasia (and self-defining lesions indexed individually)
    actinic reticuloid, 272
    adnexal neoplasms, 265
    carcinoma
        basal cell, 265; *see also* Basal cell carcinoma
        basosquamous, 265
        spindle cell, diagnostic revision, 204
        squamous cell, 259–262
            metastasis, 264
    eccrine poroma, malignant, *308*, 311
    eosinophil granuloma, 272
    epidermal abnormalities with histiocytoma, 153
    histiocytosis X, 272
    immunoblastic lymphadenopathy, 130
    lymphocytic infiltrations, 271–273
    lymphomatoid papulosis, 272
    lymphoplasia, 271
    mesodermal hamartoma, 197
    premycotic eruption, 269
    pseudoleukaemia, 271
    pseudolymphomatous infiltrate, 271–273
    pseudosarcoma, 263

Skin, local series of cases
  epidermis (non-melanocytic),
    260–261
    summarised data, 261
  mycosis fungoides and compara-
    ble conditions, 267–269
    summarised data, 268
  melanocarcinoma, 275–311
    results on review, 276
    summarised data, 277
Small intestine, 361–362; see also
  Digestive tract
  mucosal changes, I¹³¹, 362
Soft tissues, lesions (self-defining
    lesions indexed individually)
  bony neoplasms, 211–213
  diagnostic revision, 143
  malignant neoplasms, compara-
    tive mortality, 144
  osteosarcoma, 211
  pseudomalignant osseous tu-
    mour, 211
Soft tissues, local series of cases,
    144–194
  results on review, 146
  summarised data, 147
Solitary myeloma, bone (SMB),
    239
Spindle-celled carcinoma (skin),
    diagnostic revision, 204; see
    also Carcinoma, spindle-celled
Spitz naevus, 277, 314, 316
Squamous cell carcinoma, 259–262;
    see also Carcinoma, verrucous
  metastasis, 264
  pseudosarcoma (pharynx), asso-
    ciation, 358
'Stade éphélide', 314
'Starry sky' appearance, 129, 134
Statistics, histopathological diag-
    nosis, influence, 453, 455; see
    also Diagnostic revision
Stein-Leventhal syndrome, 408
Stomach, 360–361
  carcinoid tumour, 326, 364
  carcinoma, 360–361
    'early gastric cancer' (EGC),
      360
    indolent mucoid, 361
  leiomyosarcoma, epithelioid, 361
  malignant lymphoma, 361, 365
  plasmacytoma, 105
  polyp, 360
  sarcoma, non-lymphomatous,
    326, 361
  ulcer-cancer, 326, 361
Storiform pattern, 202, 205–206,
    255
Stromatoid mural sarcoma (SMS),
    411, 412
Struma lymphomatosa, 43, 61–62
'Sugar' tumour (lung), 385–386
Sympathogonioma, 437
Syncytial endometritis, 416
Synovial lesions, 144–145, 147,
    213–214
  chondromatosis, 246
  sarcoma, 147, 213–214

histoclinical correlation low,
    454
villonodular synovitis, 202
Syphilis, lymphadenitis, vs ML,
    132–133, 134
Systemic disturbance
  giant lymphoid hamartoma
    (various), 134
  pyrexia (liposarcoma), 199

T-cells, mycosis fungoides, 270
Technique, biopsy, see Biopsy
  technique; Frozen section
Tenosynovitis, nodular, 213
  vs epithelioid sarcoma, 214
Teratoma, ovary, 414
Testis, adenomatoid tumour vs
  carcinoma, 444
Theca cell tumour, 415
Thorotrast, extraskeletal osteo-
  sarcoma, complication, 212
Thrombus, pseudoangiosarcoma,
    444
Thymoma (lymphocytic), R-S cell,
  seeming presence in, 125
Thyroid, lesions
  adenoma, microfollicular, 43,
    57–59
    vs adenomatoid nodule, 57
    vs carcinoma, 57, 454
  carcinoma, 59–63
    chronic thyroiditis, relation, 62
    clinically cryptic, 62–63
    diagnostic revision, 41, 57, 63
    follicular, 41, 43, 63
      metastasis first expression,
        41
    hyperthyroidism, 62
    vs 'lateral aberrant thyroid',
      42, 59
    medullary, 60–61
      calcitonin, in diagnosis, 60
      histoclinical correlation low,
        454
      ultramicroscopy, in diag-
        nosis, 60
    metastatic, vs meningioma,
      437
    vs ML, 61
    multifocal, 60
    necrosy incidence, 62
    papillary, 43, 59–60
    psammoma bodies, signifi-
      cance, 59
  fibrosarcoma, 61
  frozen section, 58
  Hashimoto's disease, 61, 62
  hyperplasia vs carcinoma, 42,
    43, 60
  'lateral aberrant', 42, 45, 59
  lymphoid hyperplasia vs ML, 42
  lymphoreticular neoplasms,
    61–62
  malignant lymphoma, 61–62
    diagnostic revision, 61
  solitary nodule, 58
  stromal invasion, 43, 456
  struma lymphomatosa, 43, 61–62
  vascular invasion, 58

Thyroid, local series of cases,
    42–57
  results on review, 42
  summarised data, 43
Thyroid tissue, cervical nodes, 59
Thyroiditis, chronic, relation to
  carcinoma, 62
'Tissue culture' pattern, 200
Tissue patterns
  checkerboard (proliferative
    myositis), 210
  cribriform (breast), 31
  frog spawn (chondroblastoma),
    247
  starry sky (lymph node), 129,
    134
  storiform (DFSP), 202, 205–206
  tissue culture (fasciitis), 200
Tongue, glossitis mediana rhombica, 357
Tonsil, pseudolymphomatous
  permeation, 326, 359
Toxoplasmosis, vs ML, 132–133,
    136, 454
'Transitional mucosa', large in-
    testine, 363
Trichoepithelioma, 265
Trichinella spiralis, tissue response,
  vs proliferative myositis, 145
Trophoblast, 415–416
  benign chorionic invasion, 399,
    415–416
  hyperplasia, 5
  pseudotumour, 399, 416
Tube, uterine, adenomatoid tumour, 402
Tuberculosis, pulmonary, nodal
  reaction vs ML, 117
Tuberous sclerosis, angiomyolipoma (renal), association,
    197, 441
Tumourlet
  myometrium, 410
  pulmonary, 386

Ulcer, gastric, endoscopy, 360
Ulcer-cancer (peptic), 326, 360
Ulcerative colitis
  vs carcinoma, 454
  carcinoma in, 363
Ultramicroscopy
  chondrosarcoma, 246
  condyloma acuminatum, 264
  dermo-epidermal junction, 6
  diagnosis of cancer, relevance,
    456
  epithelial-stromal junction
    (ESJ), breast, 37
  lung, tumourlet, 386
  melanocytic lesions, 275
  thyroid, medullary carcinoma, 60
Unicameral bone cyst, 254
Ureter, carcinoma in situ, 444
Urethra, caruncle, 430, 444
Urinary tract, 440–444
Uterus, see Cervix uteri; Endometrium; Myometrium

Vagina
  carcinoma, clear cell, 409
  pseudosarcoma botryoides, 410
Vas deferens, carcinoma in situ,
  444
Vascular invasion, *see* Invasion,
  vascular
Vascular proliferation, lymph node,
  131
  transformation, lymph node, 135
Vasculature, lesions, *see* Angioma
  and allied lesions; Lymphatics
Vertebral column, angioma, 253
Vulva, 402–403

basal cell carcinoma, 403
dystrophy, *391*, 402
kraurosis, 403
'leukoplakia', *391*, 403
lichen sclerosus et atrophicus,
  403
Paget's disease, 403
pseudosarcoma botryoides, 410

Wegener's granulomatosis, 382,
  387
Wilms' tumour, 440, 441
  vs leiomyomatous hamartoma,
  440

Xanthogranuloma, vs liposarcoma,
  199, 440
Xanthoma, fibrous, 200, 201–206;
  *see also* Fibroxanthoma
juvenile, skin, 272

Yersinia enterocolitica, pseudotuberculosis, 137
Yolk sac tumour, 414

Zuckerkandl, organ of, chemodectoma, 439